American
Medical
Association

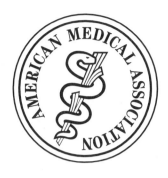

D1447739

Health Care Almanac

*Every person's guide to the thoughtful
and practical sides of medicine.*

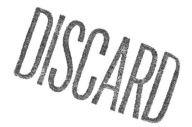

Cataloging Data

Health care almanac—2nd ed. / editor, Lorri A. Zipperer.
    p. cm.
    Includes bibliographical references and index.
    ISBN 0-89970-900-1

    1. Health Services—United States—encyclopedias. 2. Medicine—United
States—encyclopedias. 3. Societies, Medical—United States—encyclopedias. 4.
American Medical Association. I. Zipperer, Lorri A., 1959- II. American Medical
Association.
W 13 H4344 1998

ISBN: 0-89970-900-1

OP 311797

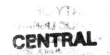

BP28:97-765:4M:12/97

Experience is by industry achieved
And perfected by the swift course of time.

William Shakespeare
Two Gentlemen of Verona
Act I, scene 3

Contents

American Medical Association

Preface

Physicians, practice managers, medical librarians, insurance companies, law firms, management consultants, and the public have long turned to the American Medical Association (AMA) for help in locating the information they need regarding medical care and health care. As a members' organization, the AMA makes a number of major efforts to compile and publish information in a useful form that will help physicians and their patients. *Health Care Almanac* is the result of one such effort.

This book will be of special interest, for example, to those trying to locate a support group for their particular disease, a specialty society or voluntary health group, convenient definitions of many medical occupations and health care delivery terms, or organizational background about the AMA and quick summaries of the AMA's major policies. A wealth of other information is included, some targeted to physicians on topics such as developing patient satisfaction surveys, licensure information and resources, and quality telemedicine.

Positive responses to the first edition of *The Health Care Almanac* convinced the AMA that it was crucial to update this book and offer a new edition. Organizations change their names or merge, phone numbers and addresses change, and new terms are coined frequently, but one constant remains: the AMA's commitment to provide high-quality, reliable information to the medical profession and to the public.

This revised edition places a strong emphasis on ethics, in keeping with the AMA's recent initiatives in this area. Information about the AMA's new Ethics Institute, background on terminal care and advanced directives, and a copy of the patient bill of rights are just a few of the highlights of this volume. No matter what your question about health or medicine, the AMA wishes you the very best in your research.

Percy Wootton, MD

Percy Wootton, MD
American Medical Association President
1998–1999

Introduction

Updating the *Health Care Almanac* (1995) offers an opportunity to build on a tradition of service begun by the AMA Library's phone reference and referral function, one that is now dispersed throughout the Association. The *Almanac's* philosophy is based on bringing an information professional's insight and support to bear in an effort to aid users who span the globe in their search for access to the medical community and its unique body of knowledge and process.

The changes to the first edition are healthy ones. This edition of the *Almanac* has taken on a broader resource vision than its predecessor to reflect the influx and influence of electronic communications and resources. Web sites are now included to provide information and easy access to the health care arena for both patient and practitioner. Glossaries have been added to some sections, including Managed Care, Tort Reform, and Medicare, adding value to the referral information that appeared in the earlier edition. An End of Life section and an expanded Safety section are two new additions. And we've retained such favorites as state association and government office lists, the National Library of Medicine's *Current Bibliographies in Medicine*, and *A Piece of My Mind* essays that illustrate and offer access to the ever-changing field of medicine.

The AMA section lends a uniqueness to our publication for those interested in organized medicine in general and the AMA in particular. The AMA celebrated its sesquicentennial in 1997, and a timeline of the evolution of the organization, as well as historical essays, illustrate some of what has been accomplished since the AMA's inception in 1847. The AMA section of the book then exhibits the Association's continuing evolution by describing the world's largest physician organization, presenting general organizational units, and defining various current activities at the AMA. Bibliographies of select AMA Council reports—including the Council on Ethical and Judicial Affairs, the Council on Scientific Affairs, and the Council on Medical Service—that cannot be found elsewhere enrich the clinical and socioeconomic references found in the *Almanac*. They truly illustrate the broad range of knowledge developed by the Association.

Acknowledging the range of subject matter in the *Almanac*, we also must note that this publication does not intend to be all-inclusive. We heeded certain considerations in an effort to make this an affordable tool for individuals, managed care organizations' administrative staffs, private practitioners, and those in allied health fields who have no convenient access to a medical library or a professional librarian. Comprehensiveness in the full sense of the word—there are no X,Y, or Z chapters—was not a goal. "See" and "See also" mentions and complete bibliographic references within the text were sacrificed to keep the book a reasonable length. We have provided instead an in-depth index and a list of sources to service cross-referencing needs. Also, we remind users of the abbreviated nature of the *Almanac;* a visit to a public, university, or medical library and to listed Web pages provides a richer base from which to conduct more extensive research. These limitations aside, the *Almanac* successfully puts the expertise of information professionals at the AMA in your hands at a reasonable cost.

With this edition of the *Health Care Almanac* we continue a tradition of assistance to people who need to know more. We strive to give patients a place to start when asking tough questions. We aim to empower physicians, administrators, and other professionals to find quick and easy answers to questions their professions present to them daily. We welcome the interest of anyone who seeks an entryway into the intriguing world of medicine.

How to Use the *Almanac*

There are three sections to the *Almanac*. The first, and largest, section is organized as a dictionary-style directory, arranged alphabetically by subject. This section includes the names of organizations that may be able to provide readers with information on specific subjects. The second section outlines the major administrative units of the American Medical Association and is there to guide professionals who need assistance from the AMA to the appropriate areas of the Association. The third section contains tools to help you navigate the *Almanac*: The source list and index guide you quickly to the information you need.

Directory chapters

These chapters include several types of entries, each with a unique purpose.

Listings

The listings are primarily addresses of professional organizations, associations, or government entities. They should be used as the starting point in a search for information. We have broadened the access points by including e-mail and Web addresses when possible, with the caveat that these addresses change very rapidly. Readers looking for information on Volunteerism should look in Chapter V and use those listings to call or write for help with their particular concerns. Generally speaking, these groups do not constitute their own headings. For instance, the National Committee for Quality Assurance (NCQA) is listed under "Quality," reflecting the organization's primary purpose, not in Chapter N under its name. The names of organizations are directly accessible through the index. Please keep in mind that the inclusion of any of the educational programs, therapies, or organizations as listings in the *Almanac* does not represent an endorsement of a product or group by the American Medical Association. We are merely recognizing each entity's particular place in the medical arena. Listings of AMA policies, also included periodically, are clearly labeled to distinguish them from other sorts of text materials.

Essays

A variety of essays are presented in the *Almanac*. These serve as initial information sources or as "food for thought" and, coupled with the listings, give readers an introduction to a subject. The original source materials referenced here are indicated by a three- or four-letter code at the end of each essay that refers the reader to the source list for the *Almanac*. The date of each source has been included to add value to the information.

Journal of the American Medical Association (JAMA) materials

The Journal is represented in several formats, and those included in the *Almanac* only suggest the range of topics covered therein. Consulting the *JAMA* index published with each volume of *JAMA* or monitoring the appropriate areas of the AMA Web page will lead interested readers to a wide variety of materials from this weekly publication. *JAMA* articles are provided for readers who would like to know more about a particular subject. They serve a "read more about it" purpose and offer a more detailed discussion of a topic than would

normally appear in the *Almanac*. Abstracts, when available, are attached to give a more complete picture of the article. These abstracts also appear in the lengthy bibliographies in the AMA section of the Diagnostic and Therapeutic Technology Assessment opinions and the reports of the AMA's Council on Scientific Affairs and the Council on Ethical and Judicial Affairs.

JAMA Theme Issues are single issues that concentrate on one subject. For example, *JAMA* regularly looks at clinical issues associated with smoking. A brief synopsis of what is covered accompanies the citation for the issue.

Poetry and Medicine and *A Piece of My Mind* entries both offer the reader depictions of medicine not usually presented in a reference book. We hope these pieces add depth to the subject entries they supplement.

American Medical News materials

Reports on current socioeconomic issues and business concerns in medicine are presented through a selection of articles from the AMA's weekly newspaper. Articles are fully cited and are either included in their entirety or as informative excerpts. Topics covered include Gulf War syndrome, medical marijuana, and management issues. Again, monitoring the AMA's Web page will lend access to the materials presented in this weekly publication.

US government materials

Too numerous to fully cite each time they appear, the bulk of the government information is Department of Labor definitions of health care–related professions, such as "nurses, registered," or "dietitians." These are designated by the symbol (DOT-1991). Other federal offices and special activities are also described through the use of a variety of government sources.

American Medical Association

Developed as a guide for professionals who need or want to be in contact with the AMA, this section outlines the areas physicians and other professionals would most likely need to gain access to. Not every AMA department, publication, or initiative is mentioned. Again, in the interest of space, this section best serves as a ready guide to units within the AMA, the general goals of the Association, and some specific AMA departments. Staff contacts were not included since roles, duties, and phone numbers can change quickly.

Display Copies

Over the years, many requests for certain items "in a framable format" have been received by the Association. We hope these designed pages are suitable.

Sources

The *Almanac's* reference materials are listed here in alphabetic order by code. Each entry includes the full title, publisher, date, authors, and format, if applicable. Ninety percent of the materials used in the *Almanac* are published by, and available for purchase through, the AMA or can be obtained from a public or medical library.

Index

"See" and "See also" references were too numerous to include in the first two sections of the *Almanac*. Therefore, the index is intended to serve cross-referencing needs. Association names are listed in full, although only popular acronyms are included (ie, HCFA, AHA). Clinically oriented materials, mostly included in the various bibliographies, are indexed under medical terminology, but medical terms generally are not included unless actually used in the text. For instance, there is no reference to "Neoplasms—see Cancer."

Acknowledgments

About the Editor

Lorri A. Zipperer received a Master of Arts degree in Library and Information Studies from Northern Illinois University in 1991. Experience in preparing online bibliographic research and doing phone reference work early in her career at the AMA contributed greatly to the content of this book. She has published in the professional literature and presented on the strengths an information professional can bring to an organization that are applicable beyond the library environment. Her current position as Information Project Manager of the National Patient Safety Foundation at the AMA allows for even further application of that philosophy. Ms Zipperer has received awards for her work on the *Almanac*, as well as in exploring the role of information in the corporate environment.

Acknowledgments

The *Almanac* is a prime example of how a team approach to publishing can work. This remains true throughout each version of the publication and greatly adds to its richness. The submissions of text and the production help given by numerous individuals made the project move smoothly. Many, from a variety of departments, gave of their time in the spirit of cooperation to make the book come into being.

Pat Dragisic, Consumer Books—Whose editorial skill and knowledge of the AMA helped pull the AMA sections together.

Fran Dyra, Marketing—Who advocated for the publication despite the editor's hectic schedule and helped keep the energy level high.

Jane Kenamore, Records and Archives Management —Who provided editorial, historical review of the publication.

J. D. Kinney and Julie Breo, Marketing—Whose creative ideas and support for the book helped us get noticed!

George Kruto—Who has been with us since the beginning and whose consistent indexing expertise adds tremendous value to the publication.

Jean Roberts, Product Line Development—Who stepped in for Tom Sharpe and offered patient support throughout the production and editorial process.

Tom Sharpe, Product Line Development at the AMA—Whose belief in the *Almanac* and support for its editor are still felt, even though he has left the Association.

JoAnne Zipperer—Whose effectiveness at research and diligent hours of address verification brought to life the cyberspace component of the book.

Todd Bake—who coordinated design and final production.

Certain AMA employees contributed their support, their expertise, and the resources of their departments to portions of the *Almanac*, adding greatly to this AMA-wide effort:

Sharon Ali, Publishing Operations, and Anne White Michalski, Marketing Information and Fulfillment, from the original team, who assisted in the proofing, initial verification, and overall research support.

Ashish Bajaj, Resident Physician Services

Corrie Benson and Kalaveeta Dean, Product Line Development

Larry Goldman, Mental Health

Rose Heald, Health Care Financing

Mary Ellen Johnston and Melanie Parenti, Database and New Media

Eileen Keane, Accreditation Council of Graduate Medical Education

Karla Kinderman and Carol O'Brien, Health Law

Kevin O'Neil and Nina Sandlin, *American Medical News*

Also acknowledged are the many authors and departments who produced materials that helped to augment the pages of this book and lent a watchful eye in helping with the myriad address changes that take place instantaneously once a book like this is completed.

Support and acknowledgment by the special library community and colleagues there, especially Rebecca Corliss, add credence to the value of this publication and of the librarian's role in the publishing process.

Finally, in transitioning from the Health Law Division to the National Patient Safety Foundation during the course of this project, Health Law's support for this publication and its editor was always present and is valued. My gratitude to my colleagues at the Foundation—Marty Hatlie, Jill Blim, Eleanor Vogt, Charlotte Miller, and Michelle Ewing—for their support and for sharing my time with this project over the last 8 months, and to Ross Vagnieres, again, for being there.

Lorri Zipperer

Editor

A

Abbreviated Injury Scale

Abbreviated Injury Scale
(Released every 5 years—Current revision 1990)
Association for Advancement of Automotive Medicine
2350 E Devon Ave, Ste 205
Des Plaines, IL 60018
847 390-8927   Fax 847 390-9962
E-mail: AAAMI@aol.com

Abbreviation of Specialties

Alphabetic Codes for *American Medical Directory:* AMA
Codes for Self-designation of Practice Specialties

A   Allergy
ADL   Adolescent Medicine (Pediatric)
ADM   Addiction Medicine
ADP   Addiction Psychiatry
AI   Allergy & Immunology
ALI   Allergy & Immunology/Clinical and Laboratory Immunology
AM   Aerospace Medicine
AMI   Adolescent Medicine (Internal Medicine)
AN   Anesthesiology
APM   Pain Management (Anesthesiology)
AS   Abdominal Surgery
ATP   Anatomic Pathology
BBK   Blood Banking/Transfusion Medicine
CBG   Clinical Biochemical Genetics
CCA   Critical Care Medicine (Anesthesiology)
CCG   Critical Cytogenetics
CCM   Critical Care Medicine (Internal Medicine)
CCP   Pediatric Critical Care Medicine
CCS   Surgical Critical Care (Surgery)
CD   Cardiovascular Disease
CDS   Cardiovascular Surgery
CG   Clinical Genetics
CHN   Child Neurology
CHP   Child and Adolescent Psychiatry
CLP   Clinical Pathology
CMG   Clinical Molecular Genetics
CN   Clinical Neurophysiology
CRS   Colon & Rectal Surgery
CTS   Cardiothoracic Surgery

D   Dermatology
DDL   Clinical and Laboratory Dermatological Immunology
DIA   Diabetes
DMP   Dermatopathology
DR   Diagnostic Radiology
EM   Emergency Medicine
END   Endocrinology, Diabetes and Metabolism
ESM   Sports Medicine (Emergency Medicine)
ETX   Medical Toxicology (Emergency Medicine)
FOP   Forensic Pathology
FP   Family Practice
FPG   Geriatric Medicine (Family Practice)
FPS   Facial Plastic Surgery
FSM   Sports Medicine (Family Practice)
GE   Gastroenterology
GO   Gynecological Oncology
GP   General Practice
GPM   General Preventive Medicine
GS   General Surgery
GYN   Gynecology
HEM   Hematology (Internal Medicine)
HEP   Hepatology
HMP   Hematology (Pathology)
HNS   Head & Neck Surgery
HO   Hematology/Oncology
HSO   Hand Surgery (Orthopedic Surgery)
HSP   Surgery of the Hand (Plastic Surgery)
HSS   Surgery of the Hand (Surgery)
ICE   Cardiac Electrophysiology
ID   Infectious Disease
IG   Immunology
ILI   Clinical and Laboratory Immunology (Internal Medicine)
IM   Internal Medicine
IMG   Geriatric Medicine (Internal Medicine)
ISM   Sports Medicine (Internal Medicine)
LM   Legal Medicine
MFM   Maternal & Fetal Medicine
MG   Medical Genetics

MDM   Medical Management
MM   Medical Microbiology
MPD   Internal Medicine/Pediatrics
MPH   Public Health and General Preventive Medicine
N   Neurology
NCC   Critical Care Medicine (Neurological Surgery)
NEP   Nephrology
NM   Nuclear Medicine
NP   Neuropathology
NPM   Neonatal-Perinatal Medicine
NR   Nuclear Radiology
NS   Neurological Surgery
NSP   Pediatric Surgery (Neurology)
NTR   Nutrition
OAR   Adult Reconstructive Orthopedics
OBG   Obstetrics & Gynecology
OBS   Obstetrics
OCC   Critical Care Medicine (Obstetrics & Gynecology)
OFA   Orthopedics, Foot and Ankle
OM   Occupational Medicine
OMO   Musculoskeletal Oncology
ON   Medical Oncology
OP   Pediatric Orthopedics
OPH   Ophthalmology
ORS   Orthopedic Surgery
OSM   Sports Medicine (Orthopedic Surgery)
OSS   Orthopedic Surgery of the Spine
OT   Otology
OTO   Otolaryngology
OTR   Orthopedic Trauma
P   Psychiatry
PA   Clinical Pharmacology
PCC   Pulmonary Critical Care Medicine
PCH   Chemical Pathology
PCP   Cytopathology
PD   Pediatrics
PDA   Pediatric Allergy
PDC   Pediatric Cardiology
PDE   Pediatric Endocrinology
PDI   Pediatric Infectious Disease
PDO   Pediatric Otolaryngology
PDP   Pediatric Pulmonology
PDR   Pediatric Radiology
PDS   Pediatric Surgery (Surgery)
PDT   Medical Toxicology (Pediatrics)
PE   Pediatric Emergency Medicine (Emergency Medicine)
PEM   Pediatric Emergency Medicine (Pediatrics)

PFP   Forensic Psychiatry
PG   Pediatric Gastroenterology
PH   Public Health and General Preventive Medicine
PHO   Pediatric Hematology/Oncology
PIP   Immunopathology
PLI   Clinical and Laboratory Immunology (Pediatrics)
PLM   Palliative Medicine
PM   Physical Medicine & Rehabilitation
PMD   Pain Medicine
PN   Pediatric Nephrology
PO   Pediatric Ophthalmology
PP   Pathology, Pediatric Pathology
PPR   Pediatric Rheumatology
PS   Plastic Surgery
PSM   Sports Medicine (Pediatrics)
PTH   Anatomic/Clinical Pathology
PTX   Medical Toxicology (Preventive Medicine)
PUD   Pulmonary Disease
PYA   Psychoanalysis
PYG   Geriatric Psychiatry
R   Radiology
REN   Reproductive Endocrinology
RHU   Rheumatology
RIP   Radioisotopic Pathology
RNR   Neuroradiology
RO   Radiation Oncology
RP   Radiological Physics
SCI   Spinal Cord Injury
SM   Sleep Medicine
SO   Surgical Oncology
SP   Selective Pathology
TRS   Trauma Surgery
TS   Thoracic Surgery
TTS   Transplant Surgery
U   Urology
UM   Underseas Medicine
UP   Pediatric Urology
VIR   Vascular and Interventional Radiology
VS   Vascular Surgery
(PCD–1997)

Contact local Medicare carriers for 2-digit codes for Medicare forms.

Abdominal Surgery

American Society of Abdominal Surgeons
675 Main St, Melrose, MA 02176
617 665-6102   Fax 617 665-4127

Abortion

RU-486 gets FDA nod, but obstacles to wide use linger

Diane M. Gianelli
AM News Oct 7, 1996 p68

Those who claim that RU-486 will dramatically increase the number of abortion providers and make the procedure a more private experience for women may be overstating the case, says one abortion provider group.

"While we support making RU-486 available, we don't believe that this is going to significantly increase the pool of physicians who perform abortions," said Ron Fitzsimmons, executive director of the National Coalition of Abortion Providers. But the announcement last month that the Food and Drug Administration had given conditional approval to the drug, which induces a non-surgical abortion, was hailed in a Washington Post editorial as a move that will "trigger enormous social change." The Post predicted the pill "will be available in almost every doctor's office." The National Abortion and Reproductive Rights Action League also has high hopes for RU-486, saying it will offer women "a private alternative to the violence and harassment at abortion clinics."

Expanded access questioned

But Fitzsimmons, whose group represents 220 abortion providers, predicts that with few exceptions, the pill will be dispensed by the clinics that are already performing surgical abortions. The political climate surrounding abortion and the ongoing harassment of providers make more provider-recruits unlikely, he said. Fitzsimmons added that physicians who prescribe RU-486 abortions in their private offices would be tracked down by anti-abortion activists and subjected to the same harassment that clinics now face.

But the biggest roadblock, Fitzsimmons said, may be practical considerations. The procedure requires at least three visits and can take up to five days, using more staff time than a surgical abortion, he said. It will thus be more expensive for clinics that offer the pill. The longer time frame poses another potential concern, Fitzsimmons added: the possibility of a woman changing her mind about the abortion in mid-treatment or failing to keep each of the appointments required by the regimen.

Some clinic-based providers also have safety concerns with the drug, Fitzsimmons added. "There are some clinics out there that think this is anti-woman. There are many more medical side effects" with RU-486 than with surgical abortions, he said, such as heavy bleeding. Fitzsimmons said many of his clinics are also are worried about liability related to the new method.

William A. Ledee, a spokesperson for Unimed, a professional liability insurance agency that insures many abortion doctors, added that physicians who do not already perform surgical abortions may have difficulty obtaining liability coverage for RU-486 abortions. Furthermore, Ledee said, it's unlikely that most doctors' policies will cover them for prescribing RU-486 for at least a year, even if they already do surgical abortions. The insurers need time to study the risks involved "so they can be in a position to determine what premiums to charge." Doctors considering prescribing RU-486 abortions would be prudent to alert their carriers ahead of time, Ledee advised.

Clinics less than enthusiastic

"There are so many permutations of this," said Fitzsimmons. "People make it sound as if you just drop a pill. It's much more complicated." In fact, he said, "if we did a poll right now, 90% of our clinics would say, 'We don't want this. It's a pain.' " But many will eventually start to offer it if their competition does, he predicted. And if testimony before the FDA's Reproductive Health Drugs advisory committee last summer is any indication, a number of clinics are already poised to begin. Participants in recent US trials reported high levels of satisfaction with the RU-486 regimen.

A spokesperson for Advances in Health Technology, the group created to market the drug, expects RU-486 will be on the market sometime next year.

The drug, also known as mifepristone, will initially be distributed only to physicians who already provide abortions. They will be trained in the use of the drug by the marketing company. During phase two, the drug will be distributed to doctors who do not currently do abortions.

Susan Allen, MD, who heads Advances in Health Technology, told the FDA advisory committee last summer that her group would require phase-two doctors to learn how to perform surgical abortions before they would be allowed to prescribe medical ones with RU-486.

But members of the FDA panel reacted negatively to that recommendation and asked why the physician prescribing RU-486 couldn't have a backup surgeon available if the patient failed to abort and needed a surgical abortion.

Dr. Allen appears to have heeded that advice. Through a spokesperson, she said that physicians who wish to prescribe mifepristone must have the skills to date a pregnancy, diagnose an ectopic pregnancy, and either have the skills to perform a surgical abortion or have access to emergency backup. The group has not yet defined "emergency backup," the spokesman said.

Induced termination of pregnancy before and after *Roe v Wade:* trends in the mortality and morbidity of women

Council on Scientific Affairs, American Medical Association
JAMA 1992 Dec 12, 268(22):3231-39

Abstract: The mortality and morbidity of women who terminated their pregnancy before the 1973 Supreme Court decision in Roe v Wade are compared with post-Roe v Wade mortality and morbidity. Mortality data before 1973 are from the National Center for Health Statistics; data from 1973 through 1985 are from the Centers for Disease Control and The Alan Guttmacher Institute. Trends in serious abortion-related complications between 1970 and 1990 are based on data from the Joint Program for the Study of Abortion and from the National Abortion Federation. Deaths from illegally induced abortion declined between 1940 and 1972 in part because of the introduction of antibiotics to manage sepsis and the widespread use of effective contraceptives.

A

Deaths from legal abortion declined fivefold between 1973 and 1985 (from 3.3 deaths to 0.4 death per 100,000 procedures), reflecting increased physician education and skills, improvements in medical technology, and, notably, the earlier termination of pregnancy. The risk of death from legal abortion is higher among minority women and women over the age of 35 years, and increases with gestational age. Legal-abortion mortality between 1979 and 1985 was 0.6 death per 100,000 procedures, more than 10 times lower than the 9.1 maternal deaths per 100,000 live births, between 1979 and 1986. Serious complications from legal abortion are rare. Most women who have a single abortion with vacuum aspiration experience few if any subsequent problems getting pregnant or having healthy children. Less is known about the effects of multiple abortions on future fecundity. Adverse emotional reactions to abortion are rare; most women experience relief and reduced depression and distress.

Public health policy implications of abortion

American College of Obstetricians and Gynecologists
409 12th St SW
Washington, DC 20024-2188
202 638-5577   Fax 202 484-8107

Abortion Clinics, Referral to

Planned Parenthood Federation of America
810 Seventh Ave
New York, NY 10019
212 541-7800   Fax 212 245-1845
Web address: http://www.igc.apc.org/ppfa

Academic Health

Association of Academic Health Centers
1400 16th St NW, Ste 720
Washington, DC 20036
202 265-9600   Fax 202 265-7514

Accent Reduction

American Speech-Language-Hearing Association
10801 Rockville Pike
Rockville, MD 20852
800 638-TALK—Referral to a speech pathologist
800 638-8255   301 897-5700
E-mail: irc@asha.org

Accounting

5 fast ways to manage cash

AM News Dec 6 1993 p43

Make it easy for patients to pay
Include a self-addressed, postage-paid envelope with the bill. You pay for the postage only if it's used.

If vendors give you 30 days to pay, get them the money on the 30th day.

That gives your money more time to generate interest or be available for emergencies.

Ask for discounts
Vendors may offer discounts for purchases or quick payments.

Bill more often
You may not want to bill every day, but don't do it every six weeks either. It's your money, go get it.

Deposit cash daily
No excuses. Get the money to the bank so it can work for you.

Follow your money: how tight are your controls?

Mike Mitka
AM News Dec 20, 1993 p17

Use this checklist to find out how your accounting practices stack up.
1. Are the following accounting records kept up to date and balanced monthly:
   a. Checkbook balance?
   b. Cash disbursement journal?
   c. Payroll cards?
   d. Accounts receivable control log?
2. Is a chart of accounts used?
3. Are all doctors' personal funds completely segregated from the business?
4. Are all employees required to take annual vacations?
5. Are all employees handling funds bonded?
6. Are "medical/dental" one-write systems used for cash receipts, payment activity, payroll and cash disbursement?
7. Are patient visit slips pre-numbered and controlled?
8. Are monthly statements sent to all patients?
9. Does someone other than the person receiving mail cash receipts produce and mail patient invoices?
10. Does someone other than the bookkeeper open the mail and list receipts before forwarding them to bookkeeper?
11. Is the listing of the receipts subsequently traced to the cash receipts journal?
12. Do you use pre-numbered receipts for over-the-counter cash payments?
13. Are checks immediately stamped "for deposit only" by the mail opener?
14. Do you verify the patients-per-day sheet against appointment schedule daily?
15. At the end of each day, are day sheets totaled and balanced, and a bank deposit completed?
16. Can this procedure be done without the staff person working overtime?
17. Are cash receipts deposited daily?
18. Is there a policy that patient account receivable cards can't be removed from the "business area" of the office by staff or doctors?
19. Are patient account receivable cards tied in monthly to a control and periodically purged of old uncollectible or nonactive accounts?
20. Are account adjustments and write-offs approved and initialed by a doctor and recorded on a memo ledger?
21. Is one person responsible for supply purchasing and inventory with a cross-trained backup?
22. Is a vendor/inventory file maintained identifying each inventory item, its suppliers, prices and reorder points?
23. Are prenumbered purchase orders and checks used?

24. Are supply orders verified against shipping documents?
25. Is supporting documentation (purchase order, invoice) reviewed by doctor before authorizing payment?
26. Are invoices canceled (stamped 'paid') when paid?
27. Are all disbursements made by check?
28. Is the doctor's signature required on all checks, including payroll checks?
29. Does the doctor sign checks only after they are completely filled out?
30. Are all voided checks retained, mutilated and accounted for?
31. Does the doctor review the bank reconciliation?
32. Is one person responsible for petty cash fund?
33. Is petty cash kept in a lockable cash box?
34. Are petty cash reconciliation and receipts reviewed by doctor before authorizing a replenishment check?

Accreditation

Definition and benefits of accreditation

Accreditation is a process of external peer review in which a private, nongovernment agency or association grants public recognition to an institution or specialized program of study that meets established qualifications and educational standards, as determined through initial and subsequent periodic evaluations. The process encourages educational institutions and programs to continuously evaluate and improve their processes and outcomes. Accreditation helps prospective students identify institutions with programs that meet standards established by and for the field(s) in which they are interested and assists those who wish to transfer from one institution to another. For institutions, accreditation protects against internal and external pressures to modify programs for reasons that are not educationally sound, involves faculty and staff in comprehensive program and institutional evaluation and planning, and stimulates self-improvement by providing national standards against which the institution can evaluate the program it sponsors.

Accreditation also benefits society by providing reasonable assurance of quality educational preparation for professional certification, registration, or licensure. It may be used, along with other considerations, as a basis for determining eligibility for some types of federal assistance and for identifying institutions and programs for the investment of public and private funds.(AHRP–1997)

Continuing medical education

Accreditation Council for Continuing Medical Education
515 N State St, Ste 7340
Chicago, IL 60610
312 464-2500   Fax 312 464-2586

Graduate medical education

Accreditation Council for Graduate Medical Education
515 N State St, Ste 2000
Chicago, IL 60610
312 464-4920

Hospitals, ambulatory surgical facilities, long-term nursing homes

Joint Commission on Accreditation of Healthcare Organizations
One Renaissance Blvd
Oakbrook Terrace, IL 60181
630 916-5600   Fax 630 792-5001
Web address: http://www.jcaho.org

Medical schools

AMA Department of Undergraduate Medical Education
515 N State St, Chicago, IL 60610
312 464-5000, ext 4691

Accreditation, Health Professions

Accreditation Council for Occupational Therapy Education
American Occupational Therapy Association
4270 Montgomery Ln, PO Box 31220
Bethesda, MD 20824-1220
301 652-2682   Fax 301 652-7711

American Art Therapy Association
1202 Allanson Rd
Mundelein, IL 60060
847 949-6064   Fax 847 566-4580

Commission on Accreditation of Allied Health Education Programs
35 E Wacker Dr, Ste 1970
Chicago, IL 60601-2208
312 553-9355   Fax 312 553-9616
E-mail: caahep@mcs.net

Commission on Accreditation/Approval for Dietetics Education
The American Dietetic Association
216 W Jackson Blvd
Chicago, IL 60606-6995
312 899-0040, ext 4872   Fax 312 899-4817
E-mail: bmitche@eatright.org

Commission on Dental Accreditation of the American Dental Association
211 E Chicago Ave
Chicago, IL 60611-2678
312 440-2718   Fax 312 440-2915
Web address: http://www.ada.org

Commission on Opticianry Accreditation
10111 Martin Luther King Jr Hwy, Ste 100
Bowie, MD 20720-4200
301 459-8075   Fax 301 577-3880

Council on Academic Accreditation in Audiology and Speech-Language Pathology
American Speech-Language-Hearing Association (ASHA)
10801 Rockville Pike, Rockville, MD 20852
301 897-5700   Fax 301 571-0457

Council on Accreditation of the National Recreation and Park Association
2775 S Quincy St, Ste 300
Arlington, VA 22206-2236
703 578-5570   Fax 703 671-6772

Council on Rehabilitation Education (CORE)
1835 Rohlwing Rd, Ste E
Rolling Meadows, IL 60008
847 394-1785   Fax 847 394-2108
E-mail: patters@polaris.net

Joint Review Committee on Educational Programs in
Nuclear Medicine Technology
350 South 400 East, Ste 200
Salt Lake City, UT 84111-2938
801 364-4310 Fax 801 364-9234
E-mail: jrcnmt@lgcy.com

Joint Review Committee on Education in
Radiologic Technology
20 N Wacker Dr, Ste 900
Chicago, IL 60606-2901
312 704-5300 Fax 312 704-5304
E-mail: jrcert@mail.idt.net

National Accrediting Agency for Clinical
Laboratory Sciences
8410 W Bryn Mawr Ave, Ste 670
Chicago, IL 60631-3415
773 714-8880 Fax 773 714-8886
E-mail: NAACLS@mcs.net
Web address: http://www.mcs.net/~naacls

Commission on Accreditation of Allied Health
Education Programs
35 E Wacker Dr, Ste 1920, Chicago, IL 60601-2208
312 553-9355 Fax 312 553-9616
Web address: http://www.caahep.org

Acne

Skincare Help Line
800 222-SKIN (800 222-7546)

Acoustic Neuroma

Acoustic Neuroma Association
PO Box 12402, Atlanta, GA 30355
404 237-8032 Fax 404 237-2704
Web address: http://neurosurgery.mgh.harvard.edu/ana

Acupuncture

Acupuncture has been part of Chinese medicine for
thousands of years. Its proponents state that the body's
vital energy (Ch'i or Qi) circulates through "meridians"
along the surface of the body. They also state that illness
and disease result from imbalances or interruptions of
Ch'i, which can be corrected by acupuncture. The treatment is applied to 'acupuncture points,' which are said to
be located along the meridians. The existence of meridians or acupuncture points has never been scientifically
validated.

Traditionally, acupuncture, as now practiced, involves the
insertion of stainless steel needles into various body areas.
Low-frequency current may be applied to the needles to
produce greater stimulation. Other procedures used
separately or together include:
• moxibustion (burning or floss or herbs applied to the
  skin);
• injection of sterile water, procaine, morphine, vitamins
  or homeopathic solutions through the inserted needles;
• placement of needles in the external ear
  (auriculotherapy); and
• acupressure (use of manual pressure).

Some practitioners espouse the traditional Chinese view
of health and disease and consider acupuncture and its
variations a valid approach to the full gamut of disease.

Others reject these trappings and claim that acupuncture
offers a simple way to achieve pain relief.

Acupuncture was introduced in the United States about
1825 but generated little interest until President Richard
M. Nixon's 1972 visit to China. Since then, it has been
promoted for the treatment of pain and a variety of other
problems.

All states permit acupuncture to be performed—some by
physicians alone, some by lay acupuncturists under medical supervision, and some by unsupervised laypersons. In
1990 the National Accreditation Commission for Schools
and Colleges of Acupuncture and Oriental Medicine was
recognized by the US Secretary of Education as an accreditation agency. This recognition is not based upon
the scientific validity of what is taught but upon other
criteria. Many insurance companies cover acupuncture
treatment if performed by a licensed physician, but Medicare and Medicaid generally do not. Acupuncture needles
are considered "investigational" devices by the FDA and
are not approved for the treatment of any disease.
(ALT-1993)

Acupuncturist: Administers specific therapeutic treatment of symptoms and disorders amenable to acupuncture procedures, as specifically indicated by supervising
physician: Reviews patient's medical history, physical
findings, and diagnosis made by physician to ascertain
symptoms or disorder to be treated. Selects needles of
various lengths, according to location of insertion. Inserts needles at locations of body known to be efficacious
to certain disorders, utilizing knowledge of acupuncture
points and their functions. Leaves needles in patient for
specific length of time, according to symptom or disorder
treated, and removes needles. Burns bark of mugwort
tree in small strainer to administer moxibustion treatment. Covers insertion area with cloth and rubs strainer
over cloth to impart heat and assist in relieving patient's
symptoms. (DOT-1991)

Resources

American Academy of Medical Acupuncturists
5820 Wilshire Blvd, Ste 500
Los Angeles, CA 90036
800 521-2262 213 937-5514 Fax 213 937-0959

National Commission for the Certification for
Acupuncture
1424 16th St NW, Ste 501
Washington, DC 20036
202 232-1404 Fax 202 462-6157

Addiction Medicine/ Addictionology

American Society of Addiction Medicine
4601 N Park Ave Arcade, Ste 101
Chevy Chase, MD 20815
301 656-3920 Fax 301 656-3815
E-mail: usamoffice@aol.com

Adolescent Health

Guidelines for Adolescent Preventive Services (GAPS)

GAPS is a set of recommendations that assist primary care providers to organize the content and periodicity of clinical preventive services for adolescents. The GAPS project has produced the only set of clinical preventive services recommendations for adolescents; it serves as a resource for health professionals and as a model for public-private ventures.

JAMA Theme Issue: Adolescent Health

JAMA 1993 Mar 17; 269(11)

This issue of the Journal focuses on topics in medicine that present unique concerns in regard to adolescent patients. Articles on confidentiality in the use of health services, sports participation, and low-birth-weight infants are presented.

Adolescence: Medical Education for Adolescent Health

Medical Education: Although specialty medical education in adolescent medicine is strong, many primary care physicians feel that they lack the necessary skills and information to manage the complex biopsychosocial problems of adolescents. Medical organizations should develop creative, new educational approaches for teaching the principles and techniques of adolescent health care to nonspecialists who see the majority of adolescents in office practices.

Greater involvement of medical students and residents in community field experiences would increase physician sensitivity to the broad nature of adolescent health problems. Valuable field experience could include working with schools, drug rehabilitation programs, correctional facilities, or volunteer groups that sponsor adolescent health programs, such as health hot lines and mentoring programs.

Education modules could be developed for entire office-based medical practices that include the medical, clerical, and nursing staff. The modules would sensitize all office staff to the needs and concerns of adolescents and develop their skills when dealing with adolescents. The goals of this approach would be increased utilization of medical services by adolescents, greater satisfaction with medical services, and increased compliance by adolescents.

Partnership and Advocacy: Because most adolescent health problems cut across medicine, education, juvenile justice, and social service, the development and dissemination of successful programs require interdisciplinary cooperation and coordination. Although much has been done on behalf of adolescents, many recent initiatives have had a limited impact because they were developed and implemented without the support and input of others working in the same area. Organized medicine must continue to develop partnerships with the many groups involved in adolescent health. More effective advocacy and use of resources results from a strong unified voice.

In 1988, the AMA established the AMA Adolescent Health Coalition, consisting of 31 organizations involved in adolescent health. The members of the coalition represent medical specialty societies, government agencies, private foundations, and membership organizations in the health and social service professions. The Coalition provides a vehicle for disseminating information about adolescent health and discussing major issues and initiatives in the area.

Many specialty and state medical societies have successfully advocated for comprehensive health education curricula and prevention programs in unintentional injury, adolescent drug use, unintended pregnancy, and other areas of adolescent health.

Better organization and coordination of resources is critically needed at the national, state, and local levels. The development of a coordinating council in the federal government to monitor funding and public policy related to adolescent health should be considered. In addition, organized medicine should also promote and participate in state- and community-level coordinating committees consisting of public and private groups involved in health, education, youth service, advocacy, and policy making.

Organized medicine will continue its role and expand its vigilance to ensure that adolescents receive the health education and health services they need to become healthy and productive adults. In the future, organized medicine is likely to become increasingly involved in issues related to (*a*) adolescents' access to health care services (eg, Medicaid coverage, services to underserved youth, availability of school-based health centers, drug testing of students, and confidentiality issues), (*b*) the coordination and integration of health, education, and social services for adolescents, and (*c*) preventive services for adolescents. (ADK-1990)

Adolescent Health Policy Compendium. 1994
American Medical Association; Chicago. Four volumes.
OP0189694

Code Blue: Uniting for Healthier Youth
A report by school boards across the US of recommendations to improve the health of adolescents, 52pp
Available from:
National Association of State Boards of Education
1012 Cameron St, Alexandria, VA 22314
703 684-4000

Resources

AMA Department of Adolescent Health
515 N State St, Chicago, IL 60610
312 464-5570

Society for Adolescent Medicine
1916 NW Cooper Oaks Circle
Blue Springs, MO 64014
816 795-8336   816 224-8010

Youth Suicide Prevention
11 Parkman Way, Needham, MA 20192-2863
617 738-0700   Fax 617 566-1423

Adoption

National Adoption Center
1500 Walnut St, Ste 701, Philadelphia, PA 19102
800 TO-ADOPT   215 735-9988   Fax 215 735-9410

Advance Directives

AMA Policy

Decisions to Forgo Life-Sustaining Treatment for
Incompetent Patients. (H-140.970) CEJA Rep. D, A-91

The AMA believes that:

(1) Advance directives (living wills and durable powers of
attorney for health care) are the best insurance for individuals that their interests will be promoted in the event
that they become incompetent. Generally, it is most
effective if the individual designates a proxy decisionmaker and discusses with the proxy his or her values
regarding decisions about life support.

(2) Without an advance directive that designates a proxy,
the patient's family should become the surrogate decision
maker. Family includes persons with whom the patient is
closely associated. In the case when there is no person
closely associated with the patient, but there are persons
who both care about the patient and have some relevant
knowledge of the patient, such relations should be involved in the decision-making process, and may be appropriate surrogates.

(3) It is the responsibility of physicians to provide all
relevant medical information and to explain to surrogate
decision makers that decisions should be based on substituted judgment (what the patient would have decided)
when there is evidence of patients' preferences and values. If there is not adequate evidence of preferences and
values, the decision should be based on the best interests
of the patient (what outcome would most likely promote
the patient's well-being).

(4) Institutional ethics committees should be established
for the purpose of facilitating sound decision making.
These ethics committees should be structured so that a
diversity of perspectives, including those from outside
medicine, are represented.

(5) The surrogate's decision should almost always be
accepted by the physician. However, there are four situations that may require either institutional or judicial
review and/or intervention in the decision-making process. These situations are when (*a*) there is no available
family willing to be the patient's surrogate decision
maker; (*b*) there is a dispute among family members and
there is no decision maker designated in an advance
directive; (*c*) a health care provider believes that the
family's decision is clearly not what the patient would
have decided if competent; and (*d*) a health care provider
believes that the decision is not a decision that could
reasonably be judged to be in the patient's best interests.
Decisions based on a conflict of interest generally would
not be in the patient's best interest. In these four cases,
the guidelines outlined in the report should be followed.
In particular, when there are disputes among family
members or between family and health care providers,
the use of ethics committees specifically designed to

facilitate sound decision making is recommended before
resorting to the courts.

(6) Judicial review for decisions about life-sustaining
treatment should be a last resort. It is strongly encouraged that when judicial review is necessary, in
nonemergency situations, the courts should determine
who is to make treatment decisions, including appointing
a guardian, rather than making treatment decisions.

(7) When a permanently unconscious patient was never
competent or had not left any evidence of previous preferences or values, since there is no objective way to ascertain what would be in the best interests of the patient,
the surrogate's decision should not be challenged as long
as the decision is based on the decision maker's true
concern for what would be best for the patient.

(8) In the case of seriously ill or handicapped newborns,
present and future interests of the infant must be considered. Due to the complexities involved in deciding about
life support for seriously ill newborns, physicians should
specifically discuss with parents the risks and uncertainties
involved. When possible, parents should be given time to
adjust to the shock of the situation and absorb the medical information presented to them before making decisions about life-sustaining treatment. In addition, counseling services and an opportunity to talk with couples
who have had to make similar decisions should be available to the parents.

(9) Due to the complexity of decisions for permanently
unconscious patients and newborns, an ethics committee
should be available, whenever possible, to facilitate the
surrogate's decision making.

(10) Hospitals and other health care facilities should
establish protocols regarding assessment of decision-
making capacity, informing patients about advance directives, identifying surrogate decision makers, the use of
advance directives, substituted judgment and best interests in decision making, and the procedures for challenging the decision of a surrogate. These protocols should
be in accordance with the CEJA preceding guidelines.

Resources

*Advance medical directives: a guide to living wills and
powers of attorney for health care.* Patient and physician
brochures are available from the AMA.

Choice in Dying—The National Council for the
Right to Die
200 Varick St, 10th Fl, New York, NY 10014-4810
800 989-WILL   212 366-5540   Fax 212 366-5337
E-mail: cid@choices.org

Medical Directive
c/o Harvard Medical School Health Letter
164 Longwood Ave, Boston, MA 02115
Medical Directive forms:
$5 for 2 forms with a self-addressed, stamped envelope

Advertisements—Television and Radio

Complaints and Inquiries:
Federal Trade Commission
Pennsylvania Ave at Sixth St NW
Washington, DC 20580
202 326-2222
E-mail: antitrust@ftc.gov
Web address: http://www.ftc.gov

Aerospace Medicine

Aerospace Medical Association
320 S Henry St, Alexandria, VA 22314
703 739-2240   Fax 703 739-9652

Board Certification in Aerospace Medicine:
American Board of Preventive Medicine
9950 W Lawrence Ave, Ste 106
Schiller Park, IL 60176
708 671-1750   Fax 708 671-1715

Aesculapius, Staff of

The AMA logo is the Staff of Aesculapius, not the caduceus (which is the winged staff of Hermes [Roman—Mercury] entwined with two serpents)

A Piece of My Mind

One snake or two?

Robert E. Rakel, MD
JAMA 1985 April 26; 253(16): 2369

The staff of Aesculapius has represented medicine since about 800 BC, and most authorities support its use as the symbol of medicine. The Encyclopedia Britannica agrees: "This staff is the only true symbol of medicine."

Why, then, is the caduceus, which had never been chosen to represent medicine until after 1800, so frequently being adopted as the symbol of medicine? And is the twin-serpent magic wand of Hermes (later the Roman Mercury), messenger of the gods and protector of merchants and thieves, an appropriate symbol for the medical profession?

The word caduceus is derived from a Greek root meaning "herald's wand." The Romans were said to have used caduceus as badge of neutrality among heralds seeking peaceful negotiations with the enemy.

Hart[1] notes that the beginning of the use of the caduceus as a medical symbol in the United States dates back to 1856, when it was selected by the US Marine Hospital Service to designate the noncombatant nature of the medical corps. The Surgeon General's crest of 1818, which was designed for this purpose and contained the single-snake staff of Aesculapius, was somehow ignored. This omission was compounded in 1871, when the caduceus became the symbol of the Public Health Service, and in 1902, when it was adopted by the US Army Medical Corps.

The popularity of the caduceus today is probably attributable to its being more aesthetically appealing than the staff of Aesculapius. The symmetry of the wings atop a staff and the double snakes is more balanced than the staff and single snake of Aesculapius.

Purists, however, fervently profess and staunchly defend the staff of Aesculapius, emphasizing that from its inception it has represented the ideals of medicine. It is not clear whether Aesculapius was a famous physicians who practiced in Thessaly, Greece, around 1200 BC and who subsequently was deified, or whether he was just a Greek god without human origin. In any event, more than 300 temples incorporating many therapeutic measures that remain popular today—such as diet, rest, drugs, and massage—were established in his honor throughout Greece and Rome.[2]

There is general agreement among scholars that the snake, whether it be one or two around a staff, is an appropriate symbol for the healing art. In addition to representing wisdom, learning, and fertility, it stands for longevity and restoration of health. The snake, after all, appears to regenerate by shedding its skin, thereby assuming a new life. The serpent also was considered a potent force against disease and was thought to protect children from epidemics if they touched its skin.

The debate begins over whether Aesculapius or Hermes is the most appropriate representative of medicine. The Greek lyric poet Pindar described Aesculapius in this way:

A gentle craftsman who drove pain away,
Soother of cruel pangs, a joy to men,
Bringing them golden health.[3]

Aesculapius provides medicine with a purely ethical and noncommercial image, in contrast to Hermes, the god of commerce, who is usually depicted with a full purse. The cunning and craftiness of Hermes also made him the protector of thieves and outlaws, an association medicine may well wish to avoid. In Homer's "Hymn to Hermes," Apollo says:

This among the Gods shall be your gift...
To be considered as the Lord of those who swindle,
housebreak, sheepsteal and shop-lift.
A schemer subtle beyond all belief....[4]

Hermes is not only associated with the marketplace and a fat purse, he is also a god of dreams, magic, and sleep. His image adorns graves, and he is said to conduct departed souls to Hades—a role physicians should rightfully shun. The number 4 was sacred to Mercury, so the Romans named the fourth day of the week "dies murcurii," or Wednesday, in his honor.[5] It is probably only a coincidence that this has become known as the physician's favorite "day off"—or perhaps this is Mercury's most legitimate tie to the medical profession.

Aesculapius, the god of medicine, was never represented as using the caduceus. Indeed, his staff first appears in history around 800 BC as a staff or rod around which a single snake is entwined.[5] Greek mythology explains this staff by describing how Aesculapius discovered a magical herb when he observed a snake rejuvenate a previously dead companion by placing the herb in its mouth.[6]

The caduceus, representing neutrality, noncombatant, and peace, will remain the symbol for military medicine. It will, no doubt, also continue to be embraced by others who prefer for aesthetic reasons its balance and symmetry.

A There is insufficient reason, however, for it to be the symbol for all of medicine. Those who respect the past and value the circumstances under which symbols are born will prefer the staff of Aesculapius, insisting that it more accurately reflects the ideals of the profession.

References

1. Hart GD: The earliest medical use of the caduceus. *Can Med Assoc J* 1972;107:1107-1110.

2. Schouten J: The Rod and Serpent of Asklepios. *New Yorker,* Elsevier North Holland Inc, 1967.

3. Hamilton E: *Mythology.* Boston, Little Brown & Co, 1942.

4. Ingpen R, Peck WE (eds): *The Complete Works of Percy Bysshe Shelley.* New York, Charles Scribner's Sons, 1928.

5. Stenn F: The symbol of medicine. *Q Bull Northwestern Univ Med Sch* 1958;32:74-87.

6. Bunn JT: Origin of the caduceus motif. *JAMA* 1967;202:163-167.

Aging

What every doctor needs to know about aging and health care spending

AM News: Member Matters May 23/30 1994 p22D

Many people believe aging of the US population is one of the major forces behind today's rapidly growing health care spending.

A number of often-cited facts seem to support this assertion. The elderly consume four times as much of medical care as people younger than 65. The 65 and older population will continue to grow at an increasing rate. Population increase for seniors ages 75 and older will grow more than 30 percent per year.

But data summarized by the AMA Center on Health Policy Research show that the aging population makes a relatively small contribution to growth in overall health care expenditures.

How much has the aging population stimulated health care spending during the last 50 years?
Researchers estimate that aging was responsible for only about 15 percent of the more than 400 percent increase in per capita health care expenditures between 1950 and 1987. They also say aging was unimportant when compared with other factors—especially the growth of medical technology.

How does this compare with more recent increases in personal health care spending?
From the mid-'80s to early '90s, contributions to health care costs by aging Americans was relatively small, with the largest annual increase in spending, 1.4 percent, for nursing homes.

Will the growing number of the elderly increase health care costs in the near future?
The US Congressional Budget Office finds the increasing elderly population will only modestly add to the growth of health care spending over the next decade.

The aging population will account for less than 1% of the expected 9.8 percent average annual growth in personal health care spending between 1992 and 2000. Economic projections indicate that the aging population will in-crease health care spending by an average of only 0.5 percent annually.

What causes the ever-increasing growth in health care spending?
The following three factors will have a major impact on health care spending in the next few years:
- Overall inflation will account for 50 percent of the cost increase.
- Medical-specific inflation and medical technology will each account for about 25 percent.
- Spending for long-term care will be more strongly affected by population aging than other health care categories including physician care, hospitalization and personal health care.

How do aging baby-boomers contribute to health care spending?
From 1985 to 1990, researchers found that baby boomers, defined as Americans born between 1947 and 1955, were responsible for only a small portion of increased health care spending.

After 2005, when the first baby boomers retire, their contributions to health care spending will increase significantly.

What are the political implications?
Targeting health care spending for the very old will not produce any substantial savings.

What will increase health care spending in the next 10 years?
Economists predict future growth in demand for medical care will be generated by technological progress—bringing new products to market that reduce the pain, discomfort and inconvenience of medical procedures.

JAMA Theme Issue: Aging

JAMA 1995 May 3; 273(17)

Articles in this issue include discussions on improving the quality of long-term care, risk factors for falls, incontinence and functional dependence, and Alzheimer's disease incidence.

Resources

Administration on Aging
330 Independence Ave SW, Rm 4640
Washington, DC 20201
202 619-0641
E-mail: esec@ban-gate.aoa.dhhs.gov
Web address: http://www.aoa.dhhs.gov

American Aging: Trends and Projections:
Federal Council on the Aging
330 Independence Ave SW, Rm 4342
Washington, DC 20201
202 619-2451

American Association for International Aging
1900 L St NW, Ste 510
Washington, DC 20036-5002
202 833-8893   Fax 202 833-8762

American Health Assistance Foundation
15825 Shady Grove Rd, Ste 140
Rockville, MD 20850
800 437-2423   301 948-3244   Fax 301 258-9454

Children of Aging Parents (CAPS)
Woodbourne Office Campus, Ste 302A
1609 Woodbourne Rd, Levittown, PA 19057-1511
800 227-7294   215 945-6900   Fax 215 945-8720

National Institute on Aging
National Institutes of Health
Department of Health and Human Services
9000 Rockville Pike, Bethesda, MD 20892
301 496-1752
Web address: http://www.nih.gov/nia

Aging, State Departments of

Alabama Commission on Aging
770 Washington Ave, Ste 470
Montgomery, AL 36130
334 242-5743   Fax 334 242-5594

Alaska Department of Administration
Senior Service Division
State Office Bldg, 7th Floor
PO Box 110209, Juneau, AK 99811-0209
907 465-3250   Fax 907 465-4716

Arizona Department of Economic Security
Aging and Community Service Division
PO Box 6123, Phoenix, AZ 85007
602 542-6572   602 542-5339

Arkansas Department of Human Services
Division of Aging and Adult Services
Donaghey Plaza S, PO Box 1437
Little Rock, AR 72203
501 682-8521   Fax 501 686-6836

California Health and Welfare Agency
Department of Aging
1600 K St, 4th Fl, Sacramento, CA 95814
916 322-5290   Fax 916 324-1903

Colorado Department of Social Services
Division of Aging and Adult Services
1575 Sherman St, 8th Fl, Denver, CO 80203
303 620-4147   Fax 303 866-4214

Connecticut Department of Social Services
Elderly Service Division
25 Sigourney St, Hartford, CT 06106
203 424-5274   Fax 203 424-4960

Delaware Department of Health and Social Services
Division of Aging, Delaware State Hospital
1901 N DuPont Hwy, New Castle, DE 19720
800 223-9074   302 577-4660   Fax 302 577-4510

District of Columbia Diversity and Special
Services Office Aging Office
441 4th St NW, Ste 900, Washington, DC 20001
202 724-5622   Fax 202 724-4979

Florida Department of Health and Rehabilitative Services
Office of Aging and Adult Services
1317 Winewood Blvd, Tallahassee, FL 32399-0700
904 488-8922   Fax 904 922-2993

Georgia Department of Human Resources
Aging Service Office
2 Peachtree St NW, Atlanta, GA 30303
404 984-2023   Fax 404 657-5255

Hawaii Office of the Governor Aging Office
Old Federal Building
335 Merchant St, Rm 241
Honolulu, HI 96813
808 586-0100   808 586-0185

Idaho Office on Aging
PO Box 83720, Boise, ID 83720-0007
208 334-3833   Fax 208 334-3033

Illinois Department of Aging
421·E Capitol Ave N0100
Springfield, IL 62702-1789
217 785-2870   Fax 217 785-4477

Indiana Family and Social Service Administration
Disability, Aging and Rehabilitation Service Division
402 W Washington St, Rm W341
Indianapolis, IN 46204
317 232-1147   Fax 317 233-4693

Iowa Department of Elder Affairs
236 Jewett Bldg, 914 Grand Ave
Des Moines, IA 50309
515 281-5188   Fax 515 281-4036

Kansas Department on Aging
915 SW Harrison, Rm 122-S, Topeka, KS 66612-1500
913 296-4986   Fax 913 296-0256

Kentucky Human Resources Cabinet
Department for Social Services
Aging Services Division
275 E Main St, Frankfort, KY 40621
502 564-6930   Fax 502 564-5002

Louisiana Governor's Office of Elderly Affairs
4550 N Blvd, 2nd Fl, Box 80374
Baton Rouge, LA 70898-3074
504 925-1700   Fax 504 925-1749

Maine Department of Human Services
Elderly and Adult Services Bureau
State House, Station 11, Augusta, ME 04333
207 624-5355   Fax 204 287-3005

Maryland Office on Aging
301 W Preston St, Rm 1004
Baltimore, MD 21201-2374
401 225-1100   Fax 410 333-7943

Massachusetts Department of Elder Affairs
1 Ashburton Pl, 5th Fl, Boston, MA 02108
617 727-7750   Fax 617 727-9368

Michigan Office of Services to the Aging
611 W Ottawa St, 3rd Fl, PO Box 30026
Lansing, MI 48909
517 373-8230   Fax 517 373-4092

Minnesota Department of Human Services
Aging and Adult Services Program Division
444 Lafayette Rd, St Paul, MN 55155
612 296-2770   Fax 612 297-1949

Mississippi Department of Human Services
Div of Aging & Adult Services
PO Box 352, Jackson, MS 39205-0352
601 359-4480   Fax 601 359-4477

Missouri Department of Social Services
Division of Aging
615 Howerton Ct, PO Box 1337
Jefferson City, MO 65109
314 751-8535   Fax 314 751-3203

Montana Office of the Governor
Aging Services Bureau
Capitol Station, PO Box 8005, Helena, MT 59604
406 444-5900   Fax 406 444-5956

Nebraska Department on Aging
301 Centennial Mall S, 5th Fl
PO Box 95044, Lincoln, NE 68509-5044
402 471-2306   Fax 402 471-4619

Nevada Department of Human Resources
Aging Service Division
505 E King Street, Rm 600
Carson City, NV 89710
702 687-4400   Fax 702 687-4733

New Hampshire Department of Health
and Human Service
Division of Elderly and Adult Services
115 Pleasant St, Annex Bldg 1
Concord, NH 03301-3843
603 271-4394   Fax 603 271-4643

New Jersey Department of Community Affairs
Division on Aging
101 S Broad St, CN 800, Trenton, NJ 08625-0800
609 292-4833   Fax 609 392-4339

New Mexico State Agency on Aging
La Villa Rivera Bldg
224 E Palace Ave, Santa Fe, NM 87501
505 827-7640   Fax 505 827-7649

New York State Office for the Aging
Agency Bldg 2, Empire State Plaza, Bldg 2, 5th Fl
Albany, NY 12223-0001
518 474-4425   Fax 518 474-0608

North Carolina Department of Human Services
Division of Aging
PO Box 29526, Raleigh, NC 27626-0526
919 733-3983   Fax 919 715-4645

North Dakota Department of Human Services
Division on Aging Services
S600 E Blvd Ave, State Capitol, Judicial Wing
Bismarck, ND 58505
701 328-2577   Fax 701 328-2359

Ohio Department of Aging
50 W Broad St, 9th Fl, Columbus, OH 43266-0501
614 466-7246   Fax 614 466-5741

Oklahoma Department of Human Services
Aging Services Division
Sequoyah Memorial Office Bldg
2400 N Lincoln Blvd, PO Box 25352
Oklahoma City, OK 73125
405 521-2327   Fax 405 521-6458

Oregon Department of Human Resources
Division of Senior and Disabled Services
500 Summer St NE, Salem, OR 97310-1015
503 945-5811   Fax 503 373-7832

Pennsylvania Department of Aging
MSSOB, 6th Fl, 400 Market St, Harrisburg, PA 17120
717 783-1550   Fax 717 772-3382

Puerto Rico Department of Social Services
Division of Geriatrics
PO Box 11398, Santurce, PR 00910
809 722-7400   Fax 809 721-6510

Rhode Island Department of Elderly Affairs
160 Pine St, Providence, RI 02903
401 277-2894   Fax 401 277-1490

South Carolina Department of Health
and Human Services
Office on Aging
PO Box 11369, Columbia, SC 29211
803 253-6177   Fax 803 253-4173

South Dakota Department of Social Services
Office of Program Management
Adult Services on Aging Department
Kneip Bldg, 700 Governors Dr
Pierre, SD 57501-2291
605 773-3656   Fax 605 773-4855

Tennessee Commission on Aging
500 Deaderic St, 9th Fl, Nashville, TN 37243-0860
615 741-2056   Fax 615 741-3309

Texas Department on Aging
PO Box 12786, Capitol Station, Austin, TX 78741
512 444-2727   Fax 512 440-5290

Utah Department of Human Services
Division of Aging and Adult Services
PO Box 45500, Salt Lake City, UT 84145-5500
801 538-3910   Fax 801 539-4016

Vermont Agency of Human Services
Office on Aging and Disability
State Complex, 103 S Main St
Waterbury, VT 05671-0204
802 241-2220   Fax 802 241-2979

Virginia Department of Health and Human Resources
Department on Aging
700 E Franklin St, 10th Fl
Richmond, VA 23219-2327
804 225-2271   Fax 804 371-8381

Washington Department of Social and Health Services
Bureau of Aging and Adult Services
PO Box 45040, Olympia, WA 98504-5010
360 586-3768   Fax 360 586-5874

West Virginia Department of Health and Human
Resources, Aging Commission
State Complex, 1900 Kanawha Blvd
Charleston, WV 25305
304 558-3317   Fax 304 558-0004

Wisconsin Department of Health and Social Services
Division of Community Services, Bureau on Aging
1 W Wilson St, PO Box 7850
Madison, WI 53707
608 266-3840   Fax 608 266-2579

Wyoming Department of Health
Aging Division
Hathaway Bldg, Rm 139, Cheyenne, WY 82002
307 777-7986   Fax 307 777-5340

AIDS

A Piece of My Mind

Joshua knew

Liana Roxanne Clark, MD
JAMA 1993 Dec 22/29; 270(24): 2902

Joshua knew before I did that it was time. I went to see him just as I had done numerous mornings before. He lay on his bed, still, except for the slow rise and fall of his chest. His sallow skin was lined with fine blue veins. I drew closer, avoiding the tangle of tubing and wires that sprouted from him like roots from a plant. His small hands rested delicately on his distended belly. He was a small boy, appearing much younger than his 5 years. He slept peacefully, his sandy-blonde, sleep-tousled hair decorating his pillow. His round cheeks were spattered with brown freckles. A clear oxygen mask covered an upturned nose and slightly agape mouth.

I nodded to his mother, who sat ever present at his bedside. As I leaned over to listen to his chest with my stethoscope, Joshua awakened. His teal blue eyes fixed on my face.

"I don't need this anymore," he said, and pulled off the oxygen mask. "I'm ready to die now."

I looked at his mother, trying to hide my shock. For three weeks I had struggled to make this child well enough to go home for what would inevitably be his last Christmas. Now, on December 17, Joshua was telling me that the fight was over. His mother reached to take his hand and I backed away from the bed. Joshua had drifted back into unconsciousness. I felt a lump forming in my throat, and I knew that tears would soon follow.

As I left the room, I struggled to regain control of my emotions. I had felt so helpless, standing by, watching Joshua die, bit by bit, unable to heal him. Looking through his hospital room window, I saw his mother speaking to him, pausing to kiss him softly on the forehead. She seemed so strong, while I felt as if I were being torn apart.

As I turned away, I saw Joshua's father walking toward the room. I leaned back heavily against the wall, as if seeking strength from the building itself. Covered with the faces of gaily colored smiling clowns, the wall was a stark contrast to my solemn expression. He approached me, searching my face for some sign of hope. Slowly, I managed to form the words, to tell him that Joshua was ready to die. He set his jaw grimly and went inside. I followed reluctantly.

Both parents now stood next to him. They murmured softly, telling him how much they loved him. I stood at a short distance, willing myself not to cry. I turned to watch the monitor, focusing intently on the tiny tracings. Gradually as I watched, the heartbeat became slower and slower, until it stopped. His parents held Joshua as they cried in their grief. Mechanically I moved forward, put the stethoscope in my ears, placed the diaphragm on Joshua's chest, and listened to the silence. He was gone.

I mumbled condolences to the parents and hurried from the room. Walking rapidly down the hall, looking neither right nor left, finally I reached the stairwell. After closing the door behind me, I sat heavily on the concrete steps. A soft wail emanated from some place deep within me. Warm tears began to flow down my cheeks as I wept quietly for Joshua. Soon, however, angry sobs racked my body as all the frustration and impotence overwhelmed me. After a while, I could cry no longer. So I sat, tracing patterns on the dusty stair, asking myself the unanswerable questions.

Why couldn't I have saved my little Joshua?

Why does AIDS have to win every time?

JAMA Theme Issue: AIDS

JAMA 1996 July 10; 276 (2)

AIDS has been a selected topic of JAMA (see also June 9, 1993, and August 10, 1994, issues) on several occasions over the past 12 years. This recent issue focuses on Zidovudine therapy, the recommendations of an international panel of experts regarding antiretroviral therapy for HIV infection, and prevalence data from 1984 to 1992.

Resources

AIDS Archive
Gerber Hart Library and Archive
3352 N Paulina, Chicago, IL 60657
773 883-3003

Business response to AIDS
An initiative by the Centers for Disease Control and Prevention to provide workplace awareness and eductional materials to companies that wish to increase their effectiveness in this area.

National AIDS Clearinghouse
800 458-5231

Clinical Trials Information
800 TRIALS-A (800 874-2572)
M-F 9 am-7 pm EST
Web address: http://www.actis.org

HIV early care: guidelines for physicians, 2nd edition
AMA Department of HIV/AIDS
515 N State St, Chicago, IL 60610
312 464-5563

AIDS—Education

American Alliance for Health, Physical Education, Recreation and Dance
1900 Association Dr, Reston, VA 22091
703 476-3400   Fax 703 476-9527
Web address: http://www.TAHPERD.sfasu.edu/aahperd/aahperd.html

Child Welfare League of America
440 1st St NW, Ste 310
Washington, DC 20001
202 638-2952   Fax 202 638-4004
(Publications and videos)

AIDS
155 Wilson Blvd, Ste 700, Rosslyn, VA 22209

Public Health Service
Office of Public Affairs, Rm 721-H
200 Independence Ave SW
Washington, DC 20201

Guidelines for HIV-infected children
American Academy of Pediatrics
141 Northwest Point Blvd, PO Box 927
Elk Grove Village, IL 60009-0927
800 228-5005   847 228-5005   Fax 847 228-5067
E-Mail: Kidsdocs@aap.org
Web address: http://aap.org

Living with AIDS
(Videotape regarding home health care for AIDS patients)
National Center for Homecare
Education and Research
350 Fifth Ave, New York, NY 10011
212 560-3300

National PTA
700 N Rush, Chicago, IL 60610
312 787-0977

AIDS
Surgeon General's pamphlet
PO Box 14252, Washington, DC 20044
For bulk orders: 800 458-5231

Teens and AIDS: Playing It Safe
American Council on Life Insurance
Dept 190, 1001 Pennsylvania Ave NW
Washington, DC 20004-2599
800 942-4242   202 624-2000   Fax 202 624-2319

Contact for free facts on AIDS:
American Red Cross/Public Health Service

AIDS—Education for Health Care Professionals

Prevention tips

AM News Oct 10, 1994 p18

Ask
Be willing to bring up and talk about sensitive issues.

Be open
Share information in a non-judgmental manner.

Take histories
Routinely complete thorough sex and drug histories.

Use cueing devices
Checklists and stickers on medical files are useful reminder tools.

Individualize and personalize
Refer to behaviors that apply to the patient and personalize your message.

Be specific
Giving general information about risk factors is often not enough to motivate behavior change. Target specific behaviors to be changed. Consider drafting a patient "contract."

Use continuing medical education
Special training programs can increase knowledge and improve counseling techniques. (Some states require such participation.) Contact your local, state, or specialty medical society, or call the Federal Health Resources and Services Administration at 301 443-6364.

Give test results in person
Even negative STD and HIV anti-body testing results should be given face to face, to allow an opportunity for behavioral counseling.

Take small steps
Focusing on incremental progress can be more effective than trying to make global changes.

Aids Education and Training Centers (ETCs)

AIDS Education and Training Centers (ETCs) are a national network of 17 centers designated for the education and training of health care providers to counsel, diagnose, and treat persons at risk of and infected with HIV. These centers also disseminate information about HIV resources, drug trials, and referrals. ETCs have a responsibility for designated geographic areas.

NY/Virgin Islands ETC
Serving New York and the Virgin Islands
212 305-3616   Fax 212 305-6832

Northwest AIDS ETC
Serving Washington, Alaska, Montana, Idaho, Oregon
206 720-4250   Fax 206 720-4218

Great Lakes to Tennessee Valley ETC
Serving Ohio, Michigan, Kentucky, Tennessee
313 962-2000   Fax 313 962-4444

Pacific AIDS ETC—Western Division
Serving Nevada, Arizona, Hawaii, California
209 252-2851   Fax 209 454-8012

Pacific AIDS ETC—Southern Division
Serving Riverside, San Bernardino, Los Angeles, Orange, Ventura, Santa Barbara counties
213 342-1846   Fax 213 342-2051

Emory AIDS Training Network
Serving Southern Alabama, Georgia, North Carolina, South Carolina
404 727-2929   Fax 404 727-4562

Delta Region AIDS ETC
Serving Arkansas, Louisiana, Mississippi
504 568-3855   Fax 504 568-7893

Mountain Plains Regional AIDS ETC
Serving North and South Dakota, Utah, Colorado, New Mexico, Nebraska, Kansas, Wyoming
303 355-1301   Fax 303 355-1448

Midwest AIDS Training and Education Center
Serving Iowa, Minnesota, Wisconsin, Illinois, Indiana, Missouri
312 996-1373   Fax 312 413-4184

Mid-Atlantic AIDS ETC
Serving W Virginia, Delaware, Virginia (excluding Arlington, Fairfax, Loudon, Prince William, Stafford counties), Maryland (excluding Montgomery, Prince Georges, Calvert, Charles, Frederick counties)
804 828-2447   Fax 804 828-1795

New England AIDS ETC
Serving Connecticut, Maine, Massachusetts, New Hampshire, Rhode Island, Vermont
617 566-2283   Fax 617 566-2994

AIDS ETC for TX and OK
Serving Texas and Oklahoma
713 500-9205   Fax 713 500-9198

Pennsylvania AIDS ETC
Serving Pennsylvania
412 624-1895   Fax 412 624-4767

New Jersey AIDS ETC
201 982-3690 Fax 201 982-7128

Florida AIDS ETC
305 672-2100 ext 3533 Fax 305 538-9301

Puerto Rico AIDS ETC
809 759-6528 Fax 809 764-2470

District of Columbia AIDS ETC
Serving metropolitan Washington, DC, area (including MD counties of Montgomery, Prince Georges, Calvert, Charles, Frederick, and VA counties of Arlington, Fairfax, Loudon, Prince William, Stafford)
202 865-6249 Fax 202 745-3731

AIDS—Hotlines—National

AZT Hotline
800 843-9388

San Francisco AIDS Foundation
PO Box 426182, San Francisco, CA 94142
415 487-3000 Fax 415 487-3009

Centers for Disease Control and Prevention
American Social Health Association
800 342-AIDS

Johns Hopkins AIDS Service
(Information on AIDS drug trials; describes trial eligibility requirements)
301 955-4345

National AIDS Information Clearinghouse
(operated by the Centers for Disease Control and Prevention)
Box 6003, Rockville, MD 20854-6003
800 458-5231

National AIDS Hotline
800 342-2437

Spanish
800 344-7432

Hearing Impaired (TTY-TDD line)
800 243-7889

National AIDS Testing
800 356-2437

National Association of People With AIDS
1413 K St NW, Washington, DC 20005
202 4898-0414 Fax 202 898-0435

National Gay Task Force/Gay Lesbian Crisis Line
800 221-7044

Physician Link, list of MDs with expertise in AIDS treatment and research
800 344-5500

Teen-staffed AIDS hotline
800 234-TEEN 5-9 pm EDT 2-6 pm PDT
Monday through Saturday

US Public Health Service Hotline
800 342-2437 (recorded message)
800 342-7514
(questions answered, information on NIH experimental AIDS treatment)

Statistics on AIDS
(tape recorded message set up by the Centers for Disease Control and Prevention)

National Statistics
404 330-3020

State and City Statistics
404 330-3022

Statistics by Transmission Categories
404 330-3021

AIDS—Hotlines—Statewide

Alabama
800 228-0469 (M-F 8 am-8 pm)

Alaska
800 478-2437 (M-F 9 am-6 pm)

Arizona
800 334-1540 (M-F 8 am-5 pm)

Arkansas
800 364-2437

California, Northern
800 367-2437

California, Southern
800 922-2437

Colorado
800 252-2437

Connecticut
Department of Health, AIDS Coordinator
Statewide Hotline 800 203-1234

Delaware
800 422-0429

DC, Washington
Metro DC AIDS Task Force 800 332-7432
Hotline 202 332-2437

Florida
Statewide Hotline 800 352-2437
Spanish
800 545-7437

Georgia
Statewide Hotline 800 551-2728
AIDS Atlanta 404 872-0600

Hawaii
800 321-1555

Idaho
800 677-2437

Illinois
800 243-2437
(will provide list of free and confidential testing sites)
Chicago
Howard Brown Clinic
945 W George, Chicago, IL 60657
312 871-5777 (fee for test)

Indiana
800 848-2437 (M-Sat, 10 am-8 pm)

Iowa
800 445-2437 (7 days/24 hours)

Kansas
800 232-0040 (M-F 9 am-9 pm)

Kentucky
800 840-2865 (M-F 8 am-8 pm)

Louisiana
800 992-4379 (M-F, 2 pm-10 pm S-S, 2 pm-8 pm)

Maine
800 851-2437 (M-F, 9 am-5 pm)

Maryland
Statewide Hotline 800 638-6252
Baltimore
Baltimore Health Education Resource Organization
800 553-3140
Spanish
301 949-0945

Massachusetts
Statewide Hotline 800 235-2331
Boston
Fenway Community Health Center
617 267-7573

Michigan
800 827-2437
Spanish
800 826-7437
(M-F 9 am-9 pm S-S 9 am-5 pm)

Minnesota
800 248-2437

Mississippi
800 826-2961 (24 hours)

Missouri
800 533-2437 (24 hours)

Montana
800 233-6668 (24 hours)

Nebraska
800 782-2437 (9 am-11 pm)

Nevada
800 842-2437

New Hampshire
800 752-2437 (M-F, 8:30 am-4:30 pm)

New Jersey
Statewide Hotline 800 624-2377

New Mexico
800 545-2437

New York State
800 872-2777 (M-F, 2 pm-8 pm; S-S, 10 am-6 pm)
Spanish
800 233-7432
800 541-2437 (Information Tapes)

North Carolina
800 733-7301 (M-F, 9 am-5 pm)

North Dakota
800 472-2180 (M-F, 8 am-5 pm)

Ohio
800 332-2437 (M-F, 9 am-11 pm; S-S, 9 am- 6 pm)

Oklahoma
800 535-2437 (24 hours)

Oregon
800 777-2437 (M-F, 10 am-9 pm; S-S, noon-6 pm)

Pennsylvania
800 662-6080 (M-F, 8 am-4:30 pm)

Puerto Rico
800 981-5721

Rhode Island
800-726-3010 (M-F, 9:30 am-8 pm)
Spanish
800 442-7432 (M-F, 4:30 pm-8 pm)

South Carolina
800 322-2437 (24 hours)

South Dakota
800 592-1861 (M-F, 8 am-5 pm)

Tennessee
800 525-2437 (M-F, 8 am- 4:30 pm)

Texas
800 299-2437 (M-F, 8 am-12 pm, 1 pm-5 pm)

Utah
800 366-2437 (24 hours)
Salt Lake City 801 487-2100 (24 hours)

Vermont
800 882-2437 (M-F, 8 am-4:30 pm)

Virginia
800 533-4138 (M-F, 8:30 am-5 pm)
Spanish
800 322-7432

Virgin Islands
809 773-2437

Washington
800 272-2437 (M-F, 8 am-5 pm)

West Virginia
800 642-8244 (M-F, 8:30 am-8 pm)

Wisconsin
800 334-2437

Milwaukee
414 273-2437 (M-F, 9 am-9 pm; S-S, 11 am-5 pm)

Wyoming
800 327-3577 (M-F, 8 am-5 pm)

Air Pollution

Air and Waste Management Association (AWMA)
1 Gateway Center, 3rd Fl, Pittsburgh, PA 15222
800 270-3444   412 232-3444   Fax 412 232-3450

Environmental Protection Agency
401 M St, SW, Washington, DC 20460
Public Information: 202 260-4700
Web address: http://www.epa.gov

Alcoholism

AMA Policy

Alcoholism as a Disability (H-30.995) CSA Rep. H, I-80;
Reaffirmed: CLRPD Rep B, I-90

(1) The AMA believes it is important for professional and layman alike to recognize that alcoholism is in and of itself a disabling and handicapped condition. (2) The AMA encourages the availability of appropriate services to persons suffering from multiple disabilities or multiple handicaps, including alcoholism. (3) The AMA endorses the position that printed and audiovisual materials pertaining to the subject of people suffering from both alcoholism and other disabilities include the terminology "alcoholic person with multiple disabilities or alcoholic

person with multiple disabilities or alcoholic person with multiple handicaps." Hopefully, this language clarification will reinforce the concept that alcoholism is in and of itself a disabling and handicapping condition.

AMA Policy

Alcohol Advertising and Depiction in the Public Media (H-30.984) BOT Rep. Q, A-86; Reaffirmed: Sunset Report, I-96

The AMA recommends (1) that additional well-designed research be conducted under impartial and independent auspices to provide more definitive evidence on whether, and in what manner, advertising contributes to alcohol abuse; (2) that producers and distributors of alcoholic beverages discontinue advertising directed toward youth, such as promotions on high school and college campuses; (3) that advertisers and broadcasters cooperate in eliminating television program content that depicts the irresponsible use of alcohol without showing its adverse consequences (examples of such use include driving after drinking, drinking while pregnant or drinking to enhance performance or win social acceptance); (4) that health education labels be used on all alcoholic beverage containers and in all alcoholic beverage advertising (with the messages focusing on the hazards of alcohol consumption by specific population groups especially at risk, such as pregnant women, as well as the dangers of irresponsible use to all sectors of the populace); and (5) that the alcohol beverage industry be encouraged to accurately label all product containers as to ingredients, preservatives and ethanol content (by percent, rather than by proof).

Resources

AL-ANON Family Group Headquarters
PO Box 862, Midtown Station
New York, NY 10018-0862
800 356-9996   212 302-7240   Fax 212 869-3757

Alcoholics Anonymous World Services
475 Riverside Dr, New York, NY 10163
212 870-3400   Fax 212 870-3003
Web address: http://www.alcoholics-anonymous.org

American Society on Addiction Medicine
4601 N Park Ave, Arcade Ste 101
Chevy Chase, MD 20815
301 656-3920   Fax 301 656-3815
E-mail: usamoffice@aol.com

Children of Alcoholics Foundation
PO Box 4185, Grand Central Station
New York, NY 10163-4185
800 359-COAF   212 754-0656   Fax 212 754-0664

National Clearinghouse for Alcohol and Drug Information
Good Executive Blvd, WILCO Bldg, Ste 402
Box 2345, Rockville, MD 20852
301 468-2600

National Council on Alcoholism
800 NCA-CALL (800 622-2255)

National Institute of Alcohol Abuse and Alcoholism
National Clearinghouse for Alcohol Information
9000 Rockville Pike, Bethesda, MD 20892
301 443-3860
Web address: http://www.niaaa.nih.gov

Drunk Driving
Mothers Against Drunk Driving
511 E John Carpenter Frwy, #700
Irving, TX 75062
800 GET-MADD   214 744-6233   Fax 214 869-2206

National Commission Against Drunk Driving
11900 L Street NW, Ste 705
Washington, DC 20036
202 452-6004 Fax 202 223-7012

National Safety Council
1121 Spring Lake Dr, Itasca, IL 60143-3201
630 285-1121   Fax 630 285-1315 (brochure available)
Web address: http://www.nsc.org

Allergy

JAMA Theme Issue: Allergic and immunologic diseases

1992; Nov 25, 268(20)

This *JAMA Primer on Allergic and Immunologic Diseases* represents a continuing effort to provide up-to-date information on applied immunology. Although the JAMA *Primer* traditionally has been directed toward medical students and copies are sent to all US medical students, previous editions have been equally popular with graduate physicians. This interest in the *Primer* reflects the central role of immunologic processes in health and disease, the rapidly changing database in the field, and the user-friendly format that we have tried to preserve in the third edition. Preface—deShazo RD ed, Smith RL associate ed. *Primer* (see also JAMA 258[20] November 27, 1987, and JAMA 248[20] November 26, 1982.)

Resources

American Academy of Allergy, Asthma, and Immunology
611 E Wells St, Milwaukee, WI 53202
414 272-6071
Web address: http://www.aaaai.org

American Academy of Allergy and Immunology
611 E Wells St, Milwaukee, WI 53202
414 272-6071   Fax 414 276-3349
Hotline: 800 822-2762
Web address: http://exeinc.com

American Academy of Otolaryngic Allergy
8455 Colesville Rd, Ste 745
Silver Spring, MD 20910-9998
301 588-1800   Fax 301 588-2454

American College of Allergy and Immunology
85 W Algonquin Rd, Ste 550
Arlington Heights, IL 60005
800 842-7777 847 427-1200   Fax 847 427-1294

American Board of Allergy and Immunology
University City Science Center
3624 Market St, Philadelphia, PA 19104
215 349-9466   Fax 215 222-8669

National Institute of Allergy and Infectious Diseases
Bldg 31, Rm 7A-32, 9000 Rockville Pike
Bethesda, MD 20892
301 496-5717
Web address: http://www.naiad.nih.gov

Wheat and Gluten Intolerance
Celiac Sprue Association/US of America
PO Box 31700, Omaha, NE 68131-0700
402 558-0600   402 553-3265   Fax 402 558-1347

Alternative Health

Eye opener

Wayne Hearn
AM News Oct 17, 1994 p17

In a 1990 survey, 34 percent of Americans had used at least one alternative therapy in the previous year.
- One-third had made an average of 19 visits a year to alternative providers.
- The highest users were better-educated, upper-income whites 25 to 49 years old.
- 72 percent did not inform their physicians of the visits.
- Most sought relief from chronic, non-life-threatening conditions, such as back pain, allergies, arthritis and insomnia.
- Estimated expenditures for the therapies totaled $13.7 billion, of which $10.3 billion was paid out-of-pocket.

Resource

Office on Alternative Health Clearinghouse
National Institutes of Health
PO Box 8218, Silver Spring, MD 20907-8218
888 644-6226 TTY/TDY: 888 644-6226
Fax 301 495-4957
Web address: http://altmed.od.nih.gov

Alzheimer's Disease

Poetry and Medicine

Memory harbor

Floyd Skloot
JAMA 1996 November 13; 276(18): 1452b

No one creates. The artist assembles memories.
　　　　　　　　　—Jack B. Yeats

The doctors say memory becomes
fragile in people with my disease.
The doctors say what memories
we do form are easily shattered.
The doctors say we are slow
to make decisions as the flow
of information swells. They say
we have great difficulty extracting
information from the environment.

I no longer know what to trust
when the past comes into view
like a harbor and the boat
my father pilots begins to swing
in one great arc toward the sea.
His face catches the grim
morning light and my mother
in the window of a shack turns
away from the view. Yet I know
my father was a butcher
in the city and my mother
never rose with morning light
in their whole life together.

Didn't we live by the sea
at the end and didn't we turn
away from one another morning
and night? I no longer know
where to turn when loss
like a gust of wind swings
me back again to open sea
where the sun that I knew
was a smooth disk rising
behind me grows edges now
as it sets and glows coral
and bittersweet, glows crimson
and scarlet in the moment it
sinks below the shimmering horizon.

JAMA Theme Issue: Alzheimer's Disease

JAMA 1997 Mar 12; 277(10)

Clinical, ethical, and genetic issues in relation to Alzheimer's disease are explored in this special, timely issue.

Resources

Alzheimer's Association
919 N Michigan Ave, Ste 1000
Chicago, IL 60611
800 272-3900   312 335-8700   312 335-1110
E-Mail: greenfld@alz.org
Web address: http://www.alz.org

Brain Tissue Donors:
McLean Hospital Brain Bank
115 Mill St, Belmont, MA 02178
800 272 4622   617 855-2400

THA (Tetrahydroaminocridine) Study
800 621-0379

Ambulances

American Ambulance Association (AAA)
3800 Auburn Blvd, Ste C
Sacramento, CA 95821
916 483-3827   Fax 916 482 5473

Ambulatory Care Organizations

Ambulatory health care accreditation

Unlike the requirements of state licensure laws, which must be met before a facility can operate, accreditation is voluntary. Facilities that seek accreditation are committed to providing the highest achievable quality of care for patients, a goal that is widely advocated and supported by organized medicine and encouraged by third-party payers.

Two organizations accredit freestanding ambulatory surgical centers: the Accreditation Association for Ambulatory Health Care, Inc, and the Joint Commission on Accreditation of Healthcare Organizations (JACHO), Division of Ambulatory Health Care. (The American Association for Accreditation of Ambulatory Plastic Surgery Facilities, Inc, inspects and accredits both office-based and freestanding plastic surgery facilities.) Both the AAAHC and the JCAHO have developed similar programs and standards with the technical assistance of recognized health care professionals active in ambulatory care. The underlying purpose and philosophy of both programs provides that:

1. surveys are conducted by a team that evaluates the operation of the facility and shares its experience and knowledge about techniques used by similar facilities that enhance patient care and efficiency of administrative systems;

2. standards are developed that reflect the state of the art and are surveyable; and

3. ongoing research in aspects of standards development and quality assurance is maintained.

Facilities must be operational for one year before being eligible for accreditation. The standards offer a systematic approach to designing organizational systems and establishing policies and procedures for the new facility. To date, the Accreditation Association for Ambulatory Health Care, Inc, has been more active than the JCAHO in working with freestanding ambulatory surgical centers. (EST-1982)

Resources

Accreditation Association for Ambulatory Health Care
9933 Lawler Ave, Skokie, IL 60077-3708
708 676-9610   Fax 708 676-9628

American Society of Outpatient Surgeons
401 N Michigan Ave, Chicago, IL 60611-4267
800 237-3768   Fax 312 321-6869

National Association for Ambulatory Care
18870 Rutledge Rd, Wayzata, MN 55391
612 476-0015   Fax 612 476-0646

Amputation

American Amputee Foundation, Inc
Box 250218, Hilcrest Station, Little Rock, AR 72225
501 666 2523   501 666 9540   Fax 501 666-8369

Amputee Services Association
3953 W Irving Park Rd, Chicago, IL 60618
773 583-3949

National Odd Shoe Exchange
7102 N 35th Ave, Ste 2, Phoenix, AZ 85015
602 841-6691   Fax 602 841-3349

Amyotrophic Lateral Sclerosis

Amyotrophic Lateral Sclerosis Association
(Lou Gehrig's Disease)
21021 Ventura Blvd, Ste 321
Woodland Hills, CA 91364
800 782-4747   818 340-7500   Fax 818 340-2060
ALS mailing list: bro@huey.met.fsu.edu

Anatomical Dolls

Eymann Anatomically Correct Dolls
3645 Scarsdale Ct, Sacramento, CA 95827
916 362-8503

Hal's Pals
Susan Anderson
PO Box 3490, Winter Park, CO 80482
303 726-8388

Patient Puppets
40 Home St, Winnipeg, Manitoba, Canada R3G 1W6
204 942-7291

Anesthesiologist's Assistant

History

Anesthesiologist assistant (AA) educational programs began in 1969 at Case Western University in Cleveland, Ohio, and at Emory University in Atlanta, Ga. The impetus for these new programs was task analysis studies showing the increased need for anesthetists with technical backgrounds. Although the Case Western curriculum was originally designed toward a baccalaureate degree, both programs currently award a master's degree for successful completion of their programs.

In 1975, the American Society of Anesthesiologists (ASA) took action in support of this new emerging profession, on the basis of its review of the educational and clinical objectives. In 1976, the ASA petitioned the American Medical Association (AMA) Council on Medical Education (CME) for recognition of the anesthesiologist assistant as an emerging health profession. The CME's recognition followed in 1978. This authorized the initiation of a collaborative activity between the AMA's Division of Allied Health Education and Accreditation and the ASA on the development of a body of educational *Standards*.

In 1981, ASA withdrew from this collaborative activity with the CME due to internal differences of opinion and the ASA's desire not to appear preferential to AAs over other members of the anesthesia care team. This action prompted members of the ASA who strongly supported the AA programs to establish a new physician sponsoring group called the Association for Anesthesiologists' Assistants Education (AAAE).

In 1983, the AAAE and the American Academy of Anesthesiologists' Assistants (AAAA) petitioned the CME to recognize them as collaborative sponsors for the programs designed to educate the anesthesiologist assistant. In 1984, the CME reinstated AMA's recognition of anesthesiologist assistants, and in 1987, *Standards* for the education of the AA were adopted by the AMA, the AAAE, and the AAAA. The Emory and Case Western programs were evaluated and initially accredited by CAHEA in 1988, and continue to be fully accredited by the Commission on Accreditation of Allied Health Education Programs, CAHEA's successor organization.

Occupational description

Anesthesiologist assistants function under the direction of a licensed and qualified anesthesiologist, principally in medical centers. The AA assists the anesthesiologist in developing and implementing the anesthesia care plan. This may include collecting preoperative data, such as taking an appropriate health history; performing various preoperative tasks, such as the insertion of intravenous and arterial catheters, and special catheters for central venous pressure monitoring if necessary; performing airway management and drug administration for induction and maintenance of anesthesia; assisting in the administering and monitoring of regional and peripheral nerve blockade; administering supportive therapy, for example, with intravenous fluids and cardiovascular

A drugs; adjusting anesthetic levels on a minute-to-minute basis; performing intraoperative monitoring; providing recovery room care; or functioning in the intensive care unit. The anesthesiologist assistant may also be utilized in pain clinics or participate in administrative and educational activities.

Job description

In addition to the duties described in the occupational description above, anesthesiologist assistants provide other support according to established protocols. Such activities may include pretesting anesthesia delivery systems and patient monitors and operating special monitors and support devices for critical cardiac, pulmonary, and neurological systems. Anesthesiologist assistants may be involved in the operation of bedside electronic computer-based monitors and have supervisory responsibilities for laboratory functions associated with anesthesia and operating room care. They provide cardiopulmonary resuscitation in association with other anesthesia care team members and in accordance with approved emergency protocols.

Employment characteristics

Anesthesiologist assistants work as members of the anesthesia care team in any locale where they may be appropriately directed by legally responsible anesthesiologists. AA anesthetists most often work within organizations that also employ nurse anesthetists, and their responsibilities are usually identical. Experience has shown the AAs are most commonly employed in larger facilities that perform procedures such as cardiac surgery, neurosurgery, transplant surgery, and trauma care, given the training in extensive patient monitoring devices and complex patients and procedures emphasized in AA educational programs. However, anesthesiologist assistants are utilized in hospitals of all sizes and assist anesthesiologists in a variety of settings and for a wide range of procedures. Starting salaries are in the $60,000 to $70,000 range for the 40-hour workweek plus benefits and consideration of on-call activity. (AHRP-1997)

Resources

AMA Allied Health Department
312 553-9355

Accreditation Review Committee for the Anesthesiologist's Assistant CAAHEP
515 N State St, Ste 7530, Chicago, IL 60610-4377
312 464-3636

American Academy of Anesthesiologists' Assistants
PO Box 33876, Decatur, GA 30033-0876
800 757-5858   404 727-5910

Anesthesiology

A Piece of My Mind

He lifted his eyes

Nancy Keene
JAMA 1997 May 21;277(19):1502

I felt sour nausea rise at my first glimpse of the flowering cherry trees that line the hospital driveway. I had made this trip so many times in the last two years, silent child by my side. That first night, Valentine's Day, 1992, she was a pale, bruised 3-year-old with a white blood cell count of 240,000. Michelle had unfortunately joined the ranks of children with the most common childhood cancer, acute lymphoblastic leukemia.

But today we had a different mission: port removal. Treatment had concluded, medically a rousing success. But the little girl huddled at my side, who didn't talk to most people and still had trouble with balance and sequential thought processes, wasn't feeling so lucky. She was scared.

Weeks before, she had threatened to "slice that thing out of me with a knife." She hated the port. She hated the way it made her chest look, hated the pokes into her breast, hated everything about it. I explained the reasons why it was better to leave it in until treatment was over, but I assured her that the surgeon would give it to her to do with as she wished. She talked of stomping it flat, tying it into knots, and cutting it into small pieces.

I had arranged for us to be the first surgical case of the day to avoid delays that might escalate her fears. As we sat in the waiting room, she wrapped her arms around herself and began to rock. I stroked her back. We were called into our cubicle and she changed into a child-sized flannel gown.

A tall, red-headed doctor walked in. He looked pale, exhausted, and had bags under his eyes. He shook my hand, introduced himself as the anesthesiologist, and mechanically began the series of questions we had heard many times before: Is she allergic to any medications? Has she had anything to eat or drink since midnight? Does she have any loose teeth? His eyes never left his clipboard. Michelle started rocking faster.

He lifted his eyes from his papers, and silently watched the tiny, hunched figure desperately trying to rock her fear away. He said, "Michelle, are you worried?" She remained silent. Then his eyes met mine and he asked, "Is your daughter worried about having her port accessed this last time?" I thought of saying, "Terrified would be a better term," but I merely replied, "Yes, she is." He looked at Michelle and gently said, "Would you rather have gas, with no pokes? I'll let you pick your favorite flavor." She nodded and stopped rocking. She chose bubble gum.

I explained to him that we wanted to take the port home with us. He said he didn't think it would be a problem. I looked him in the eyes and said, "I promised."

He asked me what Michelle's favorite bedtime story was and I said that she might enjoy The Three Bears since she had lately been calling herself a small bear. He let Michelle play with the bubble-gum mask, explained what was going to happen, and promised her the port. He put the mask on her face, leaned down, and whispered, Once there were three bears: Papa Bear, Mama Bear, and a beautiful small bear named Michelle. She drifted off with a smile on her face.

I found a quiet corner out in the corridor and wept. I wept for all of the tired residents who had been so tender with my fragile child; I wept for her stolen childhood; I wept thinking of the many times I carried her here to be hurt; I wept because I had recently learned that safe sedatives were often used to prevent children's pain and terror during procedures, but they were not offered at our clinic; and I wept with gratitude because she was alive and most probably would grow up, marry, and have her own babies some day.

Then I went into the bathroom, threw cold water on my face as I had done so many times before, and went back to meet her. A nurse brought Michelle out, still asleep but smiling, clutching a Baggie with the bloody port in it.

The next day, I wrote a note to that anesthesiologist, thanking him for not only practicing the mechanics but the art of medicine. He had noticed a little girl's unstated fears and transformed the last, dreaded procedure into a gentle triumph.

Anesthesiologist. Administers anesthetics to render patients insensible to pain during surgical, obstetrical, and other medical procedures: Examines patient to determine degree of surgical risk, and type of anesthetic and sedation to administer, and discusses findings with medical practitioner concerned with case. Positions patient on operating table and administers local, intravenous, spinal, caudal, or other anesthetic according to prescribed medical standards. Institutes remedial measures to counteract adverse reactions or complications. Records type and amount of anesthetic and sedation administered and condition of patient before, during, and after anesthesia. May instruct medical students and other personnel in characteristics and methods of administering various types of anesthetics, signs, and symptoms of reactions and complications, and emergency measures to employ. (DOT-1991)

Resources

American Board of Anesthesiology
410 Lake Boone Trail, Ste 510, Raleigh, NC 27607
919 881-2570   Fax 919 881-2575

American Society of Anesthesiologists
520 N Northwest Hwy, Park Ridge, IL 60068-2573
847 825-5586   Fax 847 825-1692

Anesthesiology, Ambulatory

Society of Ambulatory Anesthesiology
520 N Northwest Hwy, Park Ridge, IL 60068-2578
847 825-5586   Fax 847 825-5658
E-mail: Samba@asahg.org

Animal Rights

JAMA Article of Note: Human vs animal rights. In defense of animal research

JAMA Nov 17, 1989; 262(19): 2716-20

Abstract: For centuries, opposition has been directed against the use of animals for the benefit of humans. For more than four centuries in Europe, and for more than a century in the United States, this opposition has targeted scientific research that involves animals. More recent movements in support of animal rights have arisen in an attempt to impede, if not prohibit, the use of animals in scientific experimentation. These movements employ various means that range from information and media campaigns to destruction of property and threats against investigators. The latter efforts have resulted in the identification of more militant animal rights bands as terrorist groups. The American Medical Association has long been a defender of humane research that employs animals, and it is very concerned about the efforts of animal rights and welfare groups to interfere with research. Recently, the Association prepared a detailed analysis of the controversy over the use of animals in research, and the consequences for research and clinical medicine if the philosophy of animal rights activists were to prevail in society. This article is a condensation of the Association's analysis.

JAMA Article of Note: Use of animals in medical education

Council on Scientific Affairs, American Medical Association. *JAMA* 1991 Aug 14; 266(6): 836-7

Abstract: The use of animals in general medical education is essential. Although several adjuncts to the use of animals are available, none can completely replace the limited use of animals in the medical curriculum. Students should be made aware of an institution's policy on animal use in the curriculum before matriculation, and faculty should make clear to all students the learning objectives of any educational exercise that uses animals. The Council on Scientific Affairs recognizes the necessity for the responsible and humane treatment of animals and urges all medical school faculty members to discuss this moral and ethical imperative with their students.

Resources

American Association for Laboratory Animal Science
70 Timber Creek Dr, Ste 5, Cordova, TN 38018
901 754-8620   Fax 901 753-0046

Animal Resource Program Branch
Division of Research Resources
5335 Westbard Ave, Westwood Bldg, Rm 853
Bethesda, MD 20892
301 496-5175

The Center for Alternatives to Animal Testing
Johns Hopkins School of Hygiene and Public Health
615 N Wolfe St, Baltimore, MD 21205-2179
410 955-3540   Fax 410 955-0121

Foundation for Biomedical Research
818 Connecticut Ave NW, Ste 303
Washington, DC 20006
202 457-0654   Fax 202 457-0659
E-mail: nabr-fbr@access.digex.net

Animal Therapy

(Pets used for therapy)

Humane Society of the United States
2100 L St NW, Washington, DC 20037
202 452-1100   Fax 202 778-6132

Latham Foundation
Latham Plaza Bldg
Clement and Schiller Streets, Alameda, CA 94501
510 521-0920   510 621-0921   Fax 510 521-9861
E-mail: lath@aol.com

National Association for Humane and Environmental Education (NAHEE)
PO Box 362, East Haddam, CT 06423-0362
203 434-8666   Fax 203 434-9579

Anorexia Nervosa

National Association of Anorexia Nervosa and
Associated Disorders
Box 7, Highland Park, IL 60035
847 831-3438   Fax 847 433-4632

Anorexia Nervosa and Related Eating Disorders
PO Box 5102, Eugene, OR 97405
541 344-1144

BASH (Bulimia Anorexia Self-Help)
c/o Deaconess Hospital
6150 Oakland Ave, St Louis, MO 63139
800 762-3334
St Louis area 314 768-3838 or 768-3292 or 768-3800

Antitrust

Judge: No Marshfield Damages

AM News Apr 21, 1997 p2

Marshfield Clinic and its HMO this month chalked up
another win in their three-year antitrust slugfest with
Blue Cross & Blue Shield United of Wisconsin. On April
7, Federal District Judge Barbara Crabb dismissed the
Blues' suit against the doctor-owned clinic, ruling that
the insurer did not have sufficient evidence to support
any jury award of damages. The U.S. Seventh Circuit
Court of Appeals had ordered the trial to determine the
damages caused when Marshfield colluded with a competitor to illegally divide the Wausau market. The federal
appellate court also threw out a $17 million jury verdict
against Marshfield, cleared the rural Wisconsin clinic of
other antitrust charges and ordered the Blues plan to pay
all court costs.

* * * * *

The antitrust laws are a group of statutes that outline fair
trade practices in a competitive marketplace. The chief
enforcer of these laws is the Federal Trade Commission
(FTC). The FTC is a five-person administrative agency
that conducts investigations, announces rules and regulations, and enforces statutory provisions prohibiting
unfair trade and competitive practices (especially in the
instances of collaboration, merger, or acquisition). The
three pillars of US antitrust law are the Sherman Act of
1890, the Clayton Act of 1914, and the FTC Act of
1914. As many health systems move toward collaboration, combinations, and closer relations, the presence of
antitrust liability will have a definite impact on the future
of health care delivery. (MMCMP-1996)

Federal Trade Commission
Pennsylvania Ave at Sixth St NW, Washington, DC 20580
202 326-2222
E-mail: antitrust@ftc.gov
Web address: http://www.ftc.gov

Anxiety

NIMH spearheads new anxiety education campaign

Christina Kent
AM News Dec 2, 1996 p6

Armed with effective new treatments, the National Institute of Mental Health and various health organizations
are mounting a major campaign to educate the nation
about anxiety disorders.

Affecting an estimated 23 million Americans, anxiety
disorders—such as obsessive compulsive disorders, panic
disorder, hypochondriasis and eating disorders—are the
most common of all mental illnesses, said experts at an
AMA-hosted press briefing in November, sponsored by
Solvay Pharmaceuticals Inc. and Pharmacia & Upjohn.

The true number of sufferers may actually be much
higher, said AMA Trustee William E. Jacott, MD. That's
because few of the afflicted seek and receive treatment
because of widespread misunderstanding and stigma.

People with anxiety disorders may not seek treatment
because they feel ashamed of their symptoms; their physicians may fail to ask the questions that can lead to a
diagnosis; and their insurers may not pay for the necessary behavioral therapy and medication. The lack of
knowledge is such that, on average, 17 years pass between the onset of symptoms of OCD, for example, and
the start of treatment.

In an effort to change that, the NIMH in October
launched the Anxiety Disorders Education Program, a
raft of public education activities undertaken with the
assistance of voluntary and professional organizations,
including the AMA. "As we move to managed care, it is
absolutely critical that we educate consumers and health
care professionals that anxiety disorders are real, readily
diagnosable, and … readily treatable," NIMH Director
Steven E. Hyman, MD, said at the briefing.

Many people have habits that may seem compulsive to
casual observers, but in fact are not. Frequent hand
washing or organizing a desk in a certain way is not seen
as a symptom of OCD until it becomes pervasive and
destructive of the quality of the person's life. Affecting 5
million Americans, OCD is indicated by presence of
obsessive thoughts (such as fear of contracting AIDS)
and compulsive behavior (such as repeatedly checking a
locked door) to relieve anxiety caused by the obsession.

Physicians' role crucial

It's crucial that primary care physicians ask the right
screening questions to detect anxiety disorders, Dr.
Hyman said. While this will add yet another responsibility to already busy schedules, "not to make a diagnosis is
to condemn somebody" to a lifetime of unnecessary
difficulty and discomfort.

Eric Hollander, MD, a psychiatrist and director of the
Compulsive, Impulsive and Anxiety Disorders Program
at Mt. Sinai School of Medicine in New York City, suggested that primary care physicians watch for the physical
manifestations of anxiety disorders. For example, people
with extensively chapped hands can be asked how many
times a day they wash; patients who present with frequent phantom illnesses should be screened for
hypochondriasis.

Seda Ebrahimi-Keshishian, PhD, director of the Eating
Disorders Treatment Program at McLean Hospital in
Belmont, Mass., urged physicians to ask young, weight-
conscious women—the population most at risk for eating
disorders—about how they diet. The use of emetics,
diuretics, or laxatives, for example, are potential signs of
bulimia.

Children who are socially inhibited may have a biological predisposition to anxiety disorders, said NIMH Acting Scientific Director Susan E. Swedo, MD. Doctors should be on the lookout for early symptoms such as intense fear of school or repeatedly checking the answer to a single problem to the detriment of the entire test or assignment.

Adding another layer of complexity are comorbidities, such as substance abuse and depression, that often accompany anxiety disorders, the experts said.

Among the specialties, plastic surgeons may have the most practical reason to screen for OCD, especially body-dysmorphic disorder, in which a person perceives their physical appearance to be much worse than it is. Such patients may constantly check their appearance in the mirror and may go to plastic surgeons to have repetitive surgeries, all of which they perceive as unsuccessful. In fact, Dr. Hollander said, two plastic surgeons have been shot by displeased patients with body dysmorphic disorder.

"As a result of that, plastic surgeons are much more motivated to diagnose" the illness in prospective patients, Dr. Hollander said.

Advances in treatment
Dr. Hyman noted tremendous strides in understanding and treating anxiety disorders. Magnetic resonance imaging and PET scans have shown that OCD seems to be linked to the striatum portion of the brain, while panic disorder and posttraumatic stress disorder appear to be linked to the amygdala. Researchers are finding that medication, including antidepressants or benzodiazepines, can be used to effectively treat anxiety disorders. Dr. Swedo's research indicates that some cases of childhood OCD may be caused by an immunological reaction to streptococcal infection. She is examining penicillin prophylaxis to block recurrences of OCD in children. Dr. Hollander has found that compulsive shoppers and pathological gamblers can be helped by fluvoxamine.

Fully 90% of the 5 million to 10 million Americans with panic disorder can be helped through treatment, said David A. Spiegel, MD, medical director of the new Center for Anxiety and Related Disorders at Boston University. Managed care varies in terms of their willingness to cover such therapies, he added in an interview. He worked with one group, for example, that would pay for medication and for medical visits, but not for therapy sessions. He predicted more plans will be willing to pay for behavioral and other therapies as full capitation covers more lives, because it will create the financial incentive to keep people healthy.

Resources
National Institute of Mental Health, Rm 7-99
5600 Fishers Ln, Rockville, MD 20857
888 8-ANXIETY Fax 301 443-5158
Web address: http://www.nimh.nih.gov/

Pass Group (Panic Attack Sufferers' Support Group)
6 Mahogany Dr, Williamsville, NY 14221
716 689-4399

Art
American Physicians Art Association
c/o Ray Freeman, MD
502 W Stevenson St, Hale Center, TX 79041
806 839-2249

Art Therapy

History
Although visual expressions have been basic to humanity throughout history, art therapy did not emerge as a distinct profession until the 1930s. At the beginning of the 20th century, psychiatrists became interested in and began studying artwork done by patients to see if there might be a link between a patient's art and his or her illness. At this same time, art educators were discovering that the free and spontaneous art expression of children represented both emotional and symbolic communications.

Educator and psychotherapist Margaret Naumburg is considered the founder of art therapy as a separate profession in the United States. The profession's first journal, the *Bulletin of Art Therapy* (today the *American Journal of Art Therapy*), was published in 1961. The American Art Therapy Association (AATA) was founded in 1969. The AATA sponsors annual conferences and regional symposia, approves educational programs, and publishes *ART THERAPY: Journal of the American Art Therapy Association* (first published in 1983). In the 1970s, the first graduate degrees in art therapy were awarded; today, college curricula across the country include undergraduate introductory courses and preparatory programs in art therapy, as well as 27 masters degree programs approved by the AATA.

The AATA establishes and publishes standards for art therapy education, ethics, and practice. AATA committees actively work on governmental affairs, clinical issues, and professional development. The AATA's commitment to continuing education and research in art therapy is demonstrated by its annual national conferences and regional symposia, publications, videos, and awards.

Occupational description
Art therapy is a human service profession that uses art media, images, the creative art process, and patient/client responses to the artwork as reflections of an individual's development, abilities, personality, interests, concerns, and conflicts. Art therapy, through the nonverbal qualities of art media, can help individuals access and express memories, trauma, and intrapsychic conflict often not easily reached with words. Art therapy helps individuals reconcile their emotions, foster self-awareness and increase self-esteem, develop their social skills, manage behavior, solve problems, and reduce anxiety.

Job description
Art therapists use drawings and other art/media forms to assess, treat, and rehabilitate patients with mental, emotional, physical, and/or developmental disorders. Art therapists use and facilitate the art process, providing materials, instruction, and structuring of tasks tailored either to individuals or groups. Using their skills of assessment and interpretation, they understand and plan the appropriateness of materials applicable to the client's therapeutic needs.

With the growing acceptance of alternative therapies and increased scientific understanding of the link between mind, body, and spirit, art therapy is becoming more prevalent as a parallel and supportive therapy for almost any medical condition. For example, art therapists work with cancer, burn, pain, HIV-positive, asthma, and substance abuse patients, among others, in pediatric, geriatric, and other settings.

Art therapists also maintain appropriate charts, records, and periodic reports on patient progress as required by agency guidelines and professional standards; participate in professional staff meetings and conferences; and provide information and consultation regarding the client's clinical progress. They may also function as supervisors, administrators, consultants, and expert witnesses.

An art therapist must be sensitive to human needs and expressions and possess emotional stability, patience, a capacity for insight into psychological processes, and an understanding of art media. An art therapist must also be an attentive listener and keen observer and be able to develop a rapport with people. Flexibility and a sense of humor are important in adapting to changing circumstances, frustration, and disappointment.

Employment characteristics
Art therapists work in private offices, art rooms, or meeting rooms in facilities such as medical and psychiatric hospitals, outpatient facilities, clinics, residential treatment centers, day treatment centers, rehabilitation centers, halfway houses, shelters, schools and universities, correctional facilities, elder-care facilities, pain clinics, and art studios.

The art therapist may work as part of a team that includes physicians, psychologists, nurses, rehabilitation counselors, social workers, and teachers. Together, they determine and implement a client's therapeutic, school, or mental health program. Art therapists also work as primary therapists in private practice.

Earnings for art therapists vary depending on type of practice, job responsibilities, and practice location. Entry-level income is approximately $25,000, median income between $28,000 and $38,000, and top earning potential for salaried administrators between $40,000 and $60,000. Art therapists who possess doctoral degrees or state licensure or who qualify in their state to conduct a private practice can earn $75 to $90 per hour in private practice. (AHRP-1997)

Art therapist. Plans and conducts art therapy programs in public and private institutions to rehabilitate mentally and physically disabled clients: Confers with members of medically oriented team to determine physical and psychological needs of client. Devises art therapy program to fulfill physical and psychological needs. Instructs individuals and groups in use of various art materials, such as paint, clay, and yarn. Appraises client's art projection and recovery progress. Reports finding to other members of treatment team and counsels on client's response until art therapy is discontinued. Maintains and repairs art materials and equipment. (DOT-1991)

Resources
American Art Therapy Association
1202 Allanson Rd, Mundelein, IL 60060
847 949-6064   Fax 847 566-450
Web address: http://www.arttherapy.org

Art Therapy Credentials Board
401 N Michigan Ave, Chicago, IL 60611
312 527-6764   Fax 312 644-1815

Arthritis

The term *arthritis* refers to more than 100 different diseases that affect the joints (the places in the body where bones meet) and, sometimes, muscles and other soft tissues. These diseases fall into two general categories. One form of arthritis—called degenerative arthritis or osteoarthritis—results from the breakdown of the cushioning tissue inside joints called cartilage. The other form of arthritis—called inflammatory arthritis—results from inflammation (redness, warmth, and swelling) in the joints. Rheumatoid arthritis is a type of inflammatory arthritis.

Osteoarthritis is the most common form of arthritis. More than 16 million Americans have osteoarthritis to some degree. The disorder is the leading cause of disability in the United States. However, most people who have osteoarthritis are able to manage their symptoms and live productive lives. (ARTLIV-1996)

Arthritis Foundation
1314 Spring St NW, Atlanta, GA 30309
800 283-7800   404 872-7100   Fax 404 872-0457
Web address: http://www.arthritis.org

National Institute of Arthritis and Musculoskeletal
and Skin Diseases
9000 Rockville Pike, PO Box AMS, Bethesda, MD 20892
301 495-4484   Fax 301 587-4352

Arthroscopy

Arthroscopy Association of North America
6300 N River Rd, Ste 104, Rosemont, IL 60018
847 292-2262   Fax 847 292-2268

Artificial Organs

American Society for Artificial Internal Organs
PO Box C, Boca Raton, FL 33429-0468
407 391-8589

Asbestos

JAMA Article of Note: Asbestos removal, health hazards, and the EPA

Council on Scientific Affairs, American Medical Association. *JAMA* 1991 Aug 7; 266(5): 696-7

Resolution 193 (A-90), which was adopted by the House of Delegates of the American Medical Association, called on the Council on Scientific Affairs to study the situation regarding asbestos abatement, the risks to health, and the appropriateness of Environmental Protection Agency regulations, policies, and control measures. This report reviews the current status of asbestos abatement as applied to schools and public buildings, which currently accounts for the major expenditure of public funds.

Resources

Asbestos Information Association of North America
1745 Jefferson Davis Hwy, Ste 406
Arlington, VA 22202
703 412-1150   Fax 703 412-1152

Asbestos Victims of America
PO Box 66594, Scotts Valley, CA 95067-6594
408 438-5864   Fax 408 476-3646

Asthma

Asthma and Allergy Foundation of America
1125 15th St NW, Ste 502, Washington, DC 20005
800 7-ASTHMA   202 466-7643   Fax 202 466-8940

National Jewish Center for Immunology and
Respiratory Medicine
1400 Jackson St, Denver, CO 80206
303 388-4461   Fax 303 270-2165

Hotlines

American Academy of Allergy and Immunology
800 822-ASMA   414 272-6071 8am–5pm

Ataxia

The lack of coordination in body movements due to some form of nerve or brain damage. (FMG-1994)

National Ataxia Foundation
750 Twelve Oaks Center, Wayzata, MN 55391
612 473-7666   Fax 612 473-9289

Athletic Associations, Medical

Poetry and Medicine

Dear left knee

John Davis
JAMA 1997 April 2; 277(13): 1016h

Take this surgery as my apology,
my benediction to our ten thousand
running miles of charging pavement
and mountain hillsides, cushioning me over
boulders, frozen trails, and the all-night run over
Death Valley roads. Forgive me
for judging the world the way a knee bends.
By jolt, by jar, by quick jumps I
abused you. A man is killed for less.
Still, there was no sadness in shoes hitting
pavement. I admit I wanted my body
to be a guitar, scream high notes, float up
to rising dusk. I admit my knees were no
more than a clock's face in my mind, no brighter
than yappy dogs chasing us through downtown
streets on our runs to the mountains. Forgive me.
But damn we cursed those trails into blessings,
turned ourselves streetwise racing marathons
in American cities. No one passed us up
Heartbreak Hill. How you flexed and grinded.
You had more knee grind than winter had snow.
All your bruises spread like broken words no language

could accept. Until I watched the arthroscopic
screen, I never knew the pain that raced
through you like riptides. Sorry. You are numb tonight.
Call it Percoset holiday, knowing nothing
of polar bear-sized pain that pulses
inside your tendon. You'll like the incisions,
narrow as indigo leaves. In time we'll probe
the still earth, the reefs and volcanic ash
in our blood, in a pale gold summer,
in a moment, in a cloak of snow, in our running
world without end, Amen, Left Knee. Love, J.D.

Resources

American Medical Golf Association
38 Kemp Rd E, Greensboro, NC 27410
919 854-6463

American Medical Joggers Association
PO Box 4704, North Hollywood, CA 91607
818 706-2049

Surfer's Medical Association
2396 48th Ave, Great Highway
San Francisco, CA 94116
415 566-4687

American Medical Tennis Association
2301 Waleska Rd, Canton, GA 30114-2067
800 326-2682   404 479-8687   Fax 404 479-8687

Athletic Trainer

History

Work on establishing standards for athletic training educational programs was initiated in 1959 by the National Athletic Trainers' Association (NATA). In 1969, the NATA Committee on Curriculum Development approved the first two programs. By 1979, there were 23 undergraduate programs and two graduate programs approved by NATA. In 1982, the NATA Certification Committee completed a role delineation study that led to the NATA Professional Education Committee's development of an entry-level list of competencies. Another role delineation study was conducted in 1990, resulting in a 1990 revision of the athletic training entry-level competencies. A third role delineation study was completed in 1994. By 1996, NATA had approved 94 entry-level and 14 graduate athletic training educational programs.

During 1989, the NATA, through its Professional Education Committee, applied to the American Medical Association (AMA) Council on Medical Education (CME) for recognition of athletic training as an allied health occupation. Recognition was granted on June 22, 1990.

In October 1990, an initial meeting was conducted for the development of the *Standards (Essentials)* for accreditation of educational programs for athletic trainers. Individuals attending that meeting represented the AMA's Division of Allied Health Education and Accreditation (DAHEA), the American Academy of Pediatrics (AAP), the American Academy of Family Physicians (AAFP), the American Orthopaedic Society for Sports Medicine (AOSSM), and the NATA.

In late 1991, the *Standards* were adopted by the AMA CME and the sponsors of the Joint Review Committee on Educational Programs in Athletic Training (JRC-AT),

A including the AAFP, AAP, and NATA. In January 1995, the AOSSM also became a cosponsor of the JRC-AT. As of January 1997, all *Standards* will be adopted by the Commission on Accreditation of Allied Health Education Programs in conjunction with CAAHEP Committees on Accreditation and sponsoring organizations.

Occupational description
The athletic trainer, with the consultation and supervision of attending and/or consulting physicians, is an integral part of the healthcare system associated with physical activity and sports. Through preparation in both academic and practical experience, the athletic trainer provides a variety of services, including injury prevention, recognition, immediate care, treatment, and rehabilitation after physical trauma.

Job description
Role delineation studies conducted by the profession in 1982, 1990, and 1994 concluded that the role of an athletic trainer includes, but may not be limited to, six major domains: prevention, recognition and evaluation, management and treatment, rehabilitation, organization and administration, and education and counseling.

Employment characteristics
Athletic trainers typically provide their services in one or more of the following settings: secondary schools, colleges and universities, professional athletic organizations, industry, and private or hospital-based clinics.

According to the NATA, entry-level salaries in 1994 averaged $22,750. (AHRP-1997)

Resources
Joint Review Committee on Educational Programs in Athletic Training (JRC-AT)
School of Health and Human Performance
Rm C-33 Arena
Indiana State University
Terre Haute, IN 47809
812 237-3026   Fax 812 237-4338

National Athletic Trainers Association, Inc
2952 Stemmons, Ste 200, Dallas, TX 75247
800 879-6282   214 637-6282   Fax 214 637-2206

Audiovisuals, Medical

Anatomical Wall Chart Co
8221 N Kimball, Skokie, IL 60076
800 621-7500   708 679-4700

Audio Digest
1577 E Chevy Chase Dr, Glendale, CA 91206
213 245-8505

Medical Group Management Association
104 Inverness Terrace E, Englewood, CO 80112-5306
303 799-1111   303 397-7888   Fax 303 643-4427

International Communications Industries Association
3150 Spring St, Fairfax, VA 22031-2399
800 659-7469   703 273-7200   Fax 703 278-8082

National Library of Medicine, Audiovisual Section
8600 Rockville Pike, Bethesda, MD 20894
800 272-4787   301 496-5497   Fax 301 496-4450

Audiology

Audiologist
Accreditation. The following list of institutions of higher learning provides information on graduate degree programs in speech-language pathology and/or audiology accredited by the Council on Academic Accreditation (CAA) in Audiology and Speech-Language Pathology. CAA accreditation is sought voluntarily by educational programs that offer graduate degrees in speech-language pathology, audiology, or both. The CAA accreditation program is recognized by the Commission on Recognition of Postsecondary Accreditation (CORPA) and the US Department of Education.

CAA accreditation is awarded initially for a 5-year period and then for an 8-year period for reaccreditation. Programs seeking reaccreditation for the first time are reviewed by the CAA on the fourth anniversary of their accreditation period; those seeking reaccreditation for the second or subsequent times are reviewed on the seventh anniversary of their accreditation period.

CAA accreditation offers a graduate the assurance that the academic and clinical practicum experience obtained in an accredited program meets nationally established standards. CAA accreditation means that a program has:
- engaged in extensive self-study, often over a period of years;
- prepared and submitted a complex application, often 100 pages long;
- undergone an on-site visit by a team of specially trained peers;
- received, and responded to, a digest of the report submitted by the site visitors;
- had its application, the site visit report, and its response studied by the CAA;
- undergone final evaluation and approval by the CAA; and
- submitted annual reports during the period of its accreditation. (AHRP-1997)

Audiologist. Determines type and degree of hearing impairment and implements habilitation and rehabilitation services for patient: Administers and interprets variety of tests, such as air and bone conduction, and speech reception and discrimination tests, to determine type and degree of hearing impairment, site of damage, and effects on comprehension and speech. Evaluates test results in relation to behavioral, social, educational, and medical information obtained from patients, families, teachers, speech pathologists, and other professionals to determine communication problems related to hearing disability. Plans and implements prevention, habilitation, or rehabilitation services, including hearing aid selection and orientation, counseling, auditory training, lip reading, language habilitation, speech conservation, and other treatment programs developed in consultation with speech pathologists and other professionals. May refer patient to physician or surgeon if medical treatment is determined necessary. May conduct research in physiology, pathology, biophysics, or psychophysics of auditory systems, or design and develop clinical and research procedures and apparatus. May act as consultant to educational, medical, legal, and other professional groups. May teach art and science of audiology and direct scientific projects. (DOT-1991)

Resources

Academy of Rehabilitative Audiology (ARA)
c/o Dr Sharon Lesner, University of Akron
Department of Communication Disorders
Akron, OH 44325-3001
216 972-7883

The American Speech-Language-Hearing Association (ASHA)
10801 Rockville Pike, Rockville, MD 20852
301 897-5700   Fax 301 571-0457

Autism

Autism Society of America
7910 Woodmont Ave, Ste 650, Bethesda, MD 20814
800 3-AUTISM   301 657-0881   Fax 301 657-0869

Aviation

For referral to FAA authorized physician:
Federal Aviation Administration
Department of Transportation
800 Independence Ave SW, Washington, DC 20591
202 267-8521

Aviation Medicine

Aerospace Medical Association
320 S Henry St, Alexandria, VA 22314
703 739-2240   Fax 703 739-9652

Civil Aviation Medical Association
PO Box 23864, Oklahoma City, OK 73123-3864
405 840-0199   Fax 405 848-1053

Flying Physicians Association
PO Box 677427 Kansas City, MO 64134
816 763-9336 816 966-4003

Board Certification in Aerospace Medicine:
American Board of Preventive Medicine
9950 W Lawrence Ave, Ste 106
Schiller Park, IL 60176
847 671-1750

B

Baby Sitting

Baby Sitting Safety Kit
National Safety Council
1121 Spring Lake Dr, Itasca, IL 60143-3201
630 285-1121   Fax 630 285-1315
Web address: http://www.nsc.org

Back

American Back Society (interdisciplinary organization)
2647 E 14th St, Ste 401, Oakland, CA 94601
510 536-9929   Fax 510 536-1812
E-mail: Ambacksor@aol.com
Web address: http://www.americanback.soc.org/

Bell's Palsy

Facial Nerve Problems (booklet)
Send stamped, self-addressed envelope to:
American Academy of Otolaryngology-
Head & Neck Surgery
1 Prince St, Alexandria, VA 22314-3357
703 836-4444   Fax 703 683-5100

Better Business Bureau

Local Better Business Bureaus keep track of complaints
against businesses and may issue reports when many
people complain about a company (ie, clinics, imaging
centers). They can issue occasional pamphlets related to
health frauds and quackery. The Council that oversees
BBBs has also teamed with the FDA to issue educational
materials urging advertising managers to screen out
misleading ads for health products. (ALT-1993)

Resource

Council of Better Business Bureaus
4200 Wilson Blvd, Arlington, VA 22203-1804
703 276-0100   Fax 703 525-8277
Web address: http://www.bbb.org

Betty Ford Center

Betty Ford Center
39000 Bob Hope Dr, Rancho Mirage, CA 92270
800 854-9211
E-mail: Bfc@BettyFordCenter.org
Web address: http://www.bettyfordcenter.org/

Bibliographies, Medical

Current Bibliographies in Medicine from the National Library of Medicine

Series note

Current Bibliographies in Medicine (CBM) is a continuation in part of the National Library of Medicine's Literature Search Series, which ceased in 1987 with No. 87-15.
In 1989 it also subsumed the Specialized Bibliography
Series. Each bibliography in the new series covers a distinct subject area of biomedicine and is intended to fulfill
a current awareness function. Citations are usually derived from searching a variety of online databases. NLM
databases utilized include MEDLINE, AVLINE,
BIOETHICSLINE, CANCERLIT, CATLINE,
HEALTH, POPLINE, and TOXLINE. The only criterion for the inclusion of a particular published work is its
relevance to the topic being presented, not the format,
ownership, or location of the material.

Comments and suggestions on this series may be
addressed to:

Current Bibliographies in Medicine
Reference Section
National Library of Medicine
Bethesda, MD 20894
301 496-6097 Fax 301 402-1384
E-mail: ref@nlm.nih.gov
Web address: http://www.nlm.nih.gov/pubs/cbm

Ordering information

Current Bibliographies in Medicine is sold by the Superintendent of Documents, US Government Printing
Office, PO 371954, Pittsburgh, PA 15250-7954. To
order the entire CBM series for each calendar year since
1995 (approximately 10 bibliographies), send $47
($58.75 foreign) to the Superintendent of Documents
citing GPO List ID: CBM95. Orders for individual
bibliographies in the series ($5.50, $6.88 foreign) should
be sent to the Superintendent of Documents citing the
title, CBM number, and the GPO List ID given below.

Internet access

The *Current Bibliographies in Medicine* series is also
available at no cost to anyone through the library's web
page at http://www.nlm.nih.gov/pubs/resources.html.

B

1997

97-1 Management of hepatitis C: January 1989–January 1997—prepared by R. L. Gordner, T. S. Tralka; 2200 citations

The bibliography includes references that provide background for the main topics in the order they appear on the Conference agenda and other areas of interest. Included are selected journal articles, books, and conference proceedings, and meeting abstracts. The majority of selected references were published from 1993 through January 1997 and are in English. References within each subject category are listed alphabetically by author, and citations may be indexed to more than one category. Note that citations dealing with liver transplantation as the major focus of the article as a treatment option are listed under "liver transplantation," but if the major focus is the transmission of hepatitis C through liver transplantation the citations will appear in the "hepatitis C transmission through organ/tissue transplantation" category.

97-2 Genetic screening for cystic fibrosis: January 1989–February 1997—prepared by C. B. Love, E. J. Thomson; 2200 citations

This bibliography includes citations to medical journal articles in English published since the discovery of the cystic fibrosis gene in 1989. The bibliography addresses selected topics from the panel's questions: all aspects of genetic testing for cystic fibrosis; molecular biology of cystic fibrosis; genetic epidemiology of cystic fibrosis; genotype-phenotype correlations; and research on gene therapy. Articles are not included on the natural history of cystic fibrosis, clinical research, treatments other than gene therapy, animal research, or case reports of unique or rare cystic fibrosis gene mutations.

97-3 Domestic violence assessment by health care practitioners: January 1990–February 1997—prepared by A. Glazer, M. H. Glock, F. E. Page; 683 citations

Included in this bibliography are journal articles, monographs (books and proceedings of conferences), and audiovisuals from January 1990 through February 1997. All items are in English and focus on cases in the United States. Dissertations have been excluded. The bibliography has been broken down by subject as follows: child abuse; elder abuse; violence against women (including spouse abuse); and general domestic violence, where one of the previous subjects was not specifically mentioned. Journal articles, monographs, and audiovisuals are separated. The bibliography ends with a list of organizations, associations, and institutes that may be contacted for more information on or assistance with domestic violence issues.

1996

96-1 Cervical cancer: January 1993–March 1996—prepared by L. J. Klein, E. L.Trimble; 926 citations

This bibliography was prepared for the NIH Consensus Development Conference on Cervical Cancer held in Bethesda, Maryland, April 1–3, 1996. The conference focused on treatment and quality-of-life issues for women with cervical cancer. The bibliography concentrates on treatment issues in invasive disease. Included are journal articles, conference proceedings and papers, and dissertations related to the subject matter. The bibliography has been organized along the same lines as the conference,

with the first small section dealing with improving and strengthening efforts to prevent cervical cancer. The next sections cover the management of early-stage disease, then advanced-stage and recurrent cervical cancer. The last section includes references to new directions in research. Most references are included only under a single category.

96-2 Management of temporomandibular disorders: January 1990–December 1995—prepared by M. H. Glock, J. A. Lipton; 917 citations

This bibliography was prepared in support of the NIH Technology Assessment Conference on Management of Temporomandibular Disorders held in Bethesda, Maryland, April 29–May 1, 1996. It consists primarily of references to journal articles covering the following areas: history of diagnostic schema and management approaches to TMD; diagnosis, classification, assessment, and etiology (human and animal studies); health services and costs of care; psychosocial and behavioral studies; epidemiology; management approaches, including general considerations for care, occlusion and occlusal appliances, implants, and devices to replace or supplement the temporomandibular joint, surgery and other modalities; managing patients with failed implants, multiple surgeries, and chronic pain and dysfunction; and potential new approaches to care. All languages are considered. Each reference is cited under the heading(s) that describes the main topic of the article. In general, only articles that report clinical or basic science research studies or review comprehensively a particular topic are included; most letters and all editorials, textbooks, and theoretical or speculative articles have been omitted.

96-3 The role of dietary supplements for physically active people: January 1996–April 1996—prepared by K. M. Scannell, B. M. Marriott, R. B. Costello; 762 citations

This bibliography was prepared in support of the NIH Technology Assessment Conference on the Role of Dietary Supplements for Physically Active People, held in Bethesda, Maryland, June 3–4, 1996.

The bibliography provides a list of journals and books that contain information on the use of dietary supplements in humans for physical activity and recreational sports. It has been divided into five sections to include determining the metabolic basis of supplementation, macronutrients and amino acids, minerals, other supplements of potential interest for the physically active, and antioxidants. Because the literature is large, this bibliography is necessarily selective. Preference was given to references of original journal articles, technical reports, and books identified as of April 1996. The journal articles or publications have been limited to those in English that deal with human subjects.

96-4 Public health informatics: January 1980–December 1995—prepared by C. Selden et al; 471 selected citations

The bibliography focuses on the use of computers and communications to support population-based public health functions—excluding the primary care services often provided by public health authorities. In general, the large literature about primary care information systems has also been excluded, except as it relates to the transfer of data from primary care to public health information systems, to case management of individuals and families who rely on a range of social services, to home care services, or to care for the homeless. Outside the United States, in countries in which the national government provides personal health care services to the majority of citizens, the distinction between population-based public health and individual health care is less clear, but the bibliography attempts to maintain the focus on population-based health when citing non-US literature. The selected references in the bibliography include journal articles, books and book chapters, technical reports, and conference proceedings and papers. English and foreign language publications are cited. References are arranged by subject and appear under only one topic.

96-5 Breast cancer screening in women ages 40–49: January 1985–November 1996—prepared by J. P. Hunt, J. K. Gohagan; 334 selected citations

This bibliography was prepared in support of the NIH Consensus Development Conference on Breast Cancer Screening in Women Ages 40–49 held in Bethesda, Maryland, January 21–23, 1997.

This bibliography primarily includes journal articles within the defined year range with a few key articles from 1969 to 1984 and a few monographic references. Items were chosen for inclusion based on the following criteria: (1) they directly relate to the questions being addressed by the Conference; (2) they report the results of original research rather than speculation or commentary on the work of others; and (3) they report morbidity and mortality statistics and projections. Most letters and editorials have been excluded. The bibliography is organized into five major sections: Randomized Controlled Trials of Breast Cancer Screening; Incidence and Mortality of Breast Cancer; Technology for Breast Cancer Screening; Risks and Benefits of Breast Cancer Screening; and Supplemental References containing the journal articles published prior to 1985, monographic references, and other references selected by the Conference speakers. A citation may appear in more than one category. All citations are in English.

96-6 American Indian and Alaska Native health: January 1990–September 1996—prepared by M. E. Conway et al; 2050 citations

This publication is intended to serve as a useful resource for those interested in gaining a better understanding of health issues of special concern to American Indians and Alaska Natives. The bibliography lists selected references to journal articles, monographs, conference proceedings and abstracts, dissertations, technical reports, Congressional hearings, and audiovisuals, the majority in English. Some older monographs, dissertations, and audiovisual programs have been selected. References about Canadian populations of Eskimos and American Indians are included because they share the same ancestry and face many of the same health care challenges as American Indians in the US and Alaska Natives. Citations are organized in subject categories following the Healthy People 2000 priority areas with some modifications made to accommodate issues specific to American Indians and Alaska Natives. Citations may appear in more than one category.

B

96-7 Interventions to prevent HIV risk behaviors: January 1991–November 1996—prepared by P. S. Tillman, W. Pequegnat; 424 citations

This bibliography was prepared in support of an NIH Consensus Development Conference on Interventions to Prevent HIV Risk Behaviors held in Bethesda, Maryland, on February 11–13, 1997. This conference was timely because behavioral interventions are currently (and for the foreseeable future) the only effective way of containing the further spread of HIV infection. Citations to journal articles, books and book chapters, conference proceedings, conference papers, and meeting abstracts are included in the bibliography. Although the items selected are primarily in English, all languages were searched. The citations presented have been divided into seven sections to permit researchers and service providers to access the relevant literature: (1) Epidemiology of HIV/AIDS; (2) Behavioral Epidemiology of Risk Behaviors for HIV/AIDS; (3) Behavioral Issues in Vertical Transmission of HIV/AIDS; (4) At Risk Populations for HIV/AIDS; (5) Modeling of HIV Infection; (6) Theories in AIDS Prevention Research; and (7) Prevention Programs for HIV/AIDS.

96-8 Unified Medical Language System (UMLS): January 1986–December 1996—prepared by C. R. Selden, B. L. Humphreys; 280 citations

This bibliography marks the 10th anniversary of the National Library of Medicine's Unified Medical Language System® (UMLS®) project, a long-term research and development effort with the ambitious goal of enabling computer systems to "understand" medical meaning. The project was proposed to Congress as essential to the development of advanced health information systems—and as requiring an initial 5- to 10-year development phase that would cost $1–$3 million per year. The Congress responded with generous and faithful support.

1995

95-1 Gaucher disease: January 1984–January 1995, plus selected earlier citations — prepared by M. E. Beratan, E. Sidransky; 594 citations

This bibliography was prepared in support of the NIH Technology Assessment Conference on Gaucher Disease: Current Issues in Diagnosis and Treatment, held in Bethesda, Maryland, February 27–March 1, 1995.

95-2 Cochlear implants, April 1988–March 1995— prepared by P. S. Tillman, A. Donahue, L. Shotland; 881 citations

This bibliography was prepared in support of the National Institutes of Health Consensus Development Conference on Cochlear Implants in Adults and Children convened in Bethesda, Maryland, May 15–17, 1995. The literature from April 1988 forward was searched. Journal articles, monographs, conference papers and proceedings, and dissertations are cited; editorials and letters are not included. Arrangement is by 14 subject categories, and alphabetically by author within each category. Citations appear in only one category. Readers interested in the literature from January 1983 through March 1988 are referred to CBM 88-3.

B

95-3 Asian/Pacific Islander American health: January 1990–March 1995—prepared by L. D. Ulincy, Fu-Sen Hu, A. Lock, R. Liu, J. S. Lin-Fu, G. A. Alexander; 1197 citations

This bibliography lists selected references to monographs, journal articles, conference proceedings and abstracts, dissertations, and audiovisuals published from January 1990 through March 1995. Foreign language material is included. Several of the items chosen for this bibliography discuss other minority groups in addition to Asian/Pacific Islander Americans (APIA). These references were included whenever the Asian/Pacific Islander American community formed a part of the study population. This bibliography is intended to serve as a handy and useful resource for health professionals, including policymakers, administrators, researchers, and health service providers. It is designed for those who are interested in gaining a better understanding of health issues of special concern to APIAs through published medical literature. It is a joint project of the NIH APIA Advisory Committee and the National Library of Medicine.

95-4 Telemedicine: past, present, future: January 1985–July 1995—prepared by K. M. Scannell, D. A. Perednia, H. M. Kissman; 1634 citations

The concept of telemedicine is not new. Articles on telemedicine projects can be found in the literature over the past 25 to 30 years. To gain historical perspective, this bibliography covers the literature on all three aspects of telemedicine described above going back to 1966 and written in the English language. Each of the three areas is limited to aspects of medical diagnosis, patient care, and education. It includes human as well as veterinary medicine, and includes the technical aspects as well as the clinical concerns. Areas of patient record storage or shared hospital and computer resources are not addressed since they do not relate directly to patient care. Several related issues, such as the Unified Medical Language System, Integrated Advanced Information Management Systems, and communications technology infrastructures, are addressed but only as they relate to telemedicine. Arrangement is by subject, and items may appear in more than one category. Within each category, arrangement is alphabetical by author.

95-5 Whole-body irradiation: January 1944–December 1974—prepared by L. J. Klein, P. J. Perentesis; 229 citations

A literature search was performed to identify all English language publications from 1944 through 1974, possibly involving whole-body irradiation. A review of this literature was then made by the Advisory Committee on Human Radiation Experiments, and experiments were categorized into human, animal, instrumentation, and theory. All of the publications involved whole-body irradiation of humans, reports of accidents and therapy, as well as experiments, were then compiled into this bibliography.

95-6 Integration of behavioral and relaxation approaches into the treatment of chronic pain and insomnia: January 1985–July 1995—prepared by M. H. Glock, R. Friedman, P. Myers; 1147 citations

This bibliography was prepared in support of the National Institutes of Health Technology Assessment Conference on the Integration of Behavioral and Relaxation Approaches into the Treatment of Chronic Pain and Insomnia, held in Bethesda, Maryland, October 16–18, 1995. Because the literature is large, the bibliography is necessarily selective. It emphasizes monographs and journal articles published in English from January 1985 through July 1995. Preference was given to articles dealing with adult human subjects. The bibliography is arranged with categories devoted to assessment, psychological and behavioral interventions, and somatic treatments. Also included is a section on methods and policy issues. Within each category, arrangement is alphabetical by author.

95-7 Physical activity and cardiovascular health, January 1990–September 1995—prepared by J. P. Hunt, K. A. Donato, C. J. Crespo; 1966 citations

This bibliography was produced in support of the National Institutes of Health Consensus Development Conference on Physical Activity and Cardiovascular Health held in Bethesda, Maryland, December 18–20, 1995. It provides a list of journals and books that contain information on physical activity or physical fitness and cardiovascular health. The bibliography has been divided into four sections: physical activity and health, physical activity and primary prevention of CVD, physical activity and secondary prevention of CVD, and physical activity in special populations or situations.

95-8 Critical pathways; January 1988–December 1995—prepared by R. L. Gordner, P. Moritz; 753 citations

95-9 Viral hemorrhagic fever; January 1990–June 1996—prepared by C. B. Love, P. B. Jahrling; 1723 citations

95-10 Confidentiality of electronic health data; Methods for Protecting Personally Identifiable Information; January 1990–March 1996—prepared by I. Auston, et al; 448 selected citations

1994

94-1 Effect of corticosteroids for fetal maturation on perinatal outcomes: January 1985–December 1993, plus selected earlier citations — prepared by K. Patrias, et al

94-2 Ovarian cancer: January 1990–January 1994, plus selected earlier references — prepared by M. E. Conway, E. L. Trimble; 1908 citations

This bibliography was prepared in support of the National Institutes of Health Consensus Development Conference titled "Ovarian Cancer: Screening, Treatment and Follow-up" convened in Bethesda, Maryland, April 5–7, 1994. Subject categories include screening and prevention; management of early stage ovarian cancer; management of advanced epithelial ovarian cancer; follow-up and primary therapy; and new directions for research.

94-3 Persian Gulf experience and health: January 1971–March 1994 — prepared by J. van de Kamp, J. H. Ferguson; 594 selected citations

Prepared in support of a National Institutes of Health Technology Assessment Workshop on the Persian Gulf Experience and Health held in Bethesda, Maryland, April 27–29, 1994, this bibliography includes various health situations, including the Persian Gulf and Vietnam. Arranged in 10 subject sections.

94-4 Optimal calcium intake: January 1990–April 1994, plus selected earlier citations — prepared by L. D. Ulincy, J. A. McGowan, L. E. Shulman; 775 citations

This bibliography lists references in English on calcium intake and health status published as monographs, journal articles, audiovisuals, bibliographies, and pamphlets from January 1990 through April 1994, plus selected earlier journal citations included for their importance or unique coverage.

94-5 Total hip replacement: January 1991–April 1994 — prepared by C. B. Love, S. L. Gordon; 1095 citations

Prepared in support of the National Institutes of Health Consensus Development Conference on Total Hip Replacement held September 12–14, 1994, in Bethesda, Maryland, this bibliography is limited to human studies with the exception of animal studies articles written by Conference speakers. It is arranged in 17 subject categories.

94-6 Hispanic-American health: January 1990–July 1994 — prepared by J. P. Hunt, G. E. Tello, E. E. Huerta; 1799 citations

This presents a bibliography of publications materials on Hispanic-American health from the National Library of Medicine's MEDLINE file and other appropriate databases from January 1990 through July 1994. Includes journal articles, books, dissertations, technical reports, conference papers, meeting abstracts, and audiovisual material.

94-7 Psychosocial aspects of AIDS: January 1992–May 1994 — prepared by P. S. Tillman, E. R. Turner; 1275 citations

This bibliography of literature published between January 1992 and May 1994, contains 1275 citations including journal articles, monographs, book chapters, audiovisuals, and the meeting abstracts from the International Conferences on AIDS. It is divided into 10 sections: adjustment; at-risk populations; diagnosis; ethical and policy issues; knowledge and attitudes; legal issues; occupational stress; psychological stress; social support; and treatment and counseling.

94-8 Silicone implants: January 1989–August 1994 — prepared by J. van de Kamp, J. P. Hunt; 1810 citations

This bibliography updates and includes all the citations from an earlier bibliography of the same name published in 1992. It contains selected references to English and foreign language publications on silicone implants, including articles on technique as well as articles on adverse effects. It is limited to human studies and includes journal articles, conference papers, editorials, letters to the editor, books, and audiovisuals.

94-9 Bioelectric impedance analysis in body composition measurement: January 1989–December 1994 — prepared by R. L. Gordner, C. R. Selden, W. R. Foster; 627 citations

This bibliography represents the clinical and research literature on Bioelectric impedance analysis for the 5-year period ending with December 1994. It includes citations to journal articles, books, conference proceedings and papers, government publications, and dissertations and is arranged by subject. Within each category, arrangement is alphabetical by author. Citations are to English and foreign language publications.

94-10 Infectious disease testing for blood transfusions: January 1975–October 1994 — prepared by M. H. Glock, P. R. McCurdy, 30 citations.

Prepared in support of the Consensus Development Conference on Infectious Disease Testing of Blood Transfusions, held January 9–11, 1995, at the National Institutes of Health in Bethesda, Maryland, this bibliography attempts to include key articles and papers back to 1975. Includes selected articles that address infectious disease testing of donated blood. It consists primarily of journal articles, conference papers, and abstracts arranged by disease or virus tested for.

1993

93-1 Laboratory animal welfare: January 1992–December 1992 — prepared by F. P. Gluckstein; 87 citations

This is the ninth supplement to a selective annotated bibliography issued in January 1984.

93-2 Orthotics, prosthetics, & mobility aids: January 1989–June 1993 — prepared by R. L. Gordner, L. A. Quatrano, C. M. Chanaud; 2316 citations

This bibliography provides citations to English and foreign language literature discussing artificial limbs, orthotic devices, neuroprostheses, wheelchairs, walkers, canes, crutches, and other devices or technologies such as computers, robotics, functional electrical stimulation, and myoelectric devices to aid in mobility. It provides an appendix of national organizations. Orthotics is misspelled on the cover.

93-3 Disease prevention research at NIH: January 1990–August 1993 — prepared by R. L. Gordner; 2326 citations

Citations are to English language publications on disease prevention. Included are such topics as: maternal and child health; adolescents and young adults; older adults; DHHS initiative "Healthy People 2000"; vaccines; cancer chemoprevention; cardiovascular and periodontal disease prevention; prevention of violent behavior and substance abuse; the prevention of AIDS; physical health and activity; obesity; and diet and nutrition.

93-4 Morbidity and mortality of dialysis: January 1991–August 1993 — prepared by M. H. Glock et al; 2115 citations

93-5 Health care for women: access, utilization, outcomes: January 1990–July 1993 — prepared by L. D. Ulincy, S. J. Simmons; 580 citations

Citations restricted to the English language. This bibliography addresses a number of issues influencing health care for women in the United States. Arranged in nine major categories, it includes sections on underserved populations; financial access barriers; life stage considerations; health care provider concerns; and a broad range of issues pertaining to maternal-infant health, reproductive health, and health behaviors and health conditions (eg, cancer and HIV/AIDS).

93-6 Helicobacter pylori in peptic ulcer disease: January 1988–November 1993 — prepared by M. E. Beratan, F. A. Hamilton; 1191 citations

93-7 Community-based health care models: January 1987–August 1993 — prepared by C. R. Selden, N. Wiederhorn; 113 citations

B

This bibliography contains citations to very selective models of community-based health care. They are grouped by subject area, including access to health care; community health; community health models; health promotion; models of care delivery; nursing centers; primary care; transitional care; rural and urban health; and vulnerable populations. Most citations concern some facet of nursing.

1992

92-1 Methods for voluntary weight loss and control: January 1985–December 1991 — prepared by K. M. Scannell, S. M. Pilch; 1119 citations

92-2 Laboratory animal welfare: January 1991–December 1991 — prepared by F. P. Gluckstein; 86 citations

92-3 Adolescent alcoholism: January 1986–April 1992 — prepared by P. Tillman; 928 citations

Citations cover subjects such as prevention and control; genetics; psychology; social factors; health services; rehabilitation; complications; and statistics.

92-4 Gallstones and laparoscopic cholecystetomy: January 1989–August 1992 — prepared by P. S. Tillman, S. C. Kalser; 683 citations

Citations consist of journal articles published from 1989 to the present and monographs and audiovisuals from 1986. It includes English language citations only, arranged by type of material. Subject matter includes open cholecystectomy, laparoscopic cholecystectomy, dissolution therapy, lithotripsy, other gallbladder stone treatments, and treatments of nongallbladder stones.

92-5 Saliva as a diagnostic fluid: January 1982–April 1992 — prepared by M. H. Glock, P. A. Heller, D. Malamud; 2298 citations

This bibliography was compiled in conjunction with a conference sponsored by the New York Academy of Sciences and held in Panama City, Florida, October 21–24, 1992. The concept for the meeting was initiated by the National Institute of Dental Research. Cited are journal articles, books, and patents. The introduction states that "saliva is a readily obtainable fluid that can be used to monitor the presence and concentration of a wide variety of drugs, hormones, antibodies, and other molecules present in the body." Also provided is an alphabetical index to the journal articles.

92-6 "Silicone implants:" January 1989–July 1992 — prepared by J. Hunt, J. van de Kamp; 985 citations

92-7 Seafood safety: January 1990–July 1992 — prepared by F.P. Gluckenstein; 961 citations

This bibliography deals with the safety of fish, including freshwater fish and shellfish. Arranged in 16 subject categories, it excludes items dealing strictly with the use of fish and shellfish in environmental monitoring and those dealing solely with the physical and sensory quality of seafood.

92-8 Impotence: January 1986–September 1992 — prepared by M. E. Beratan; 956 citations

92-9 Multidrug resistance: January 1988–September 1992 — prepared by L. D. Ulincy, M. M. Gottesman; 2250 citations

92-10 Early identification of hearing impairment in infants and young children: January 1988–December 1992 — prepared by L. J. Klein, L. E. Huerta; 861 citations

92-11 Off-label use of prescription drugs: January 1986–December 1992 — prepared by J. van de Kamp; 103 citations

92-12 Audiovisuals in dermatology: January 1970–September 1992, plus selected earlier citations— prepared by D. T. Lukas; 645 citations

This is a comprehensive bibliography of commercially available audiovisual programs in dermatology. It includes productions from NLM's AVLINE database and Research Libraries Information Group's RLIN entered through September 1992. Arranged by subject, primarily by disease, it excludes material on plastic surgery.

92-13 Meta-analysis: January 1980–December 1992 — prepared by C. R. Selden; 337 citations

92-14 Practice guidelines: January 1985–December 1992 — prepared by K. M. Scannell, N. Miller, M. Glock; 533 citations

This bibliography includes selected references to articles containing practice guidelines published in the professional journal literature for the years 1985 through 1992. Citations cover all aspects of practice guidelines and are arranged by 26 broad subject categories. Emphasis is on English language articles, but non-English references indexed to the publication type "practice guideline," which started in 1992, are included.

1991

91-1 Laboratory animal welfare: January 1990–December 1990 — prepared by F. P. Gluckstein; 89 citations

91-2 Therapy-related second cancers: January 1986–March 1991 — prepared by N. Miller; 880 citations

91-3 Nutrition and AIDS: January 1986–April 1991 — prepared by R. L. Fordner, S. Evans; 668 citations

91-4 Medical waste disposal: January 1986–January 1991 — prepared by J. van de Kamp; 629 citations

91-5 Transmissible subacute spongiform encephalopathies: transmission between animals and man: January 1986–May 1991 — prepared by F. P. Gluckstein; 148 citations

91-6 Dental restorative materials: January 1986–June 1991 — prepared by L. D. Ulincy; 779 citations

91-7 Adverse effects of fluoxetine (Prozac): January 1987–June 1991 — prepared by J. S. Martyniuk; 270 citations

91-8 Treatment of panic disorder with and without agoraphobia: January 1985–July 1991 — prepared by K. Patrias, B. E. Wolfe; 1448 citations

91-9 Pain, anesthesia, and analgesia in common laboratory animals: June 1988–October 1991 — prepared by F. P. Gluckstein; 474 citations

91-10 Diagnosis and treatment of depression in later life: January 1980–September 1991 — prepared by M. H. Glock, L. S. Schneider: 886 citations

91-11 Acoustic neuroma: January 1986–October 1991 — prepared by R. L. Gordner, R. Eldridge, D. M. Parry; 1112 citations

91-12 Regional medical programs: January 1964– December 1977 — prepared by M. H. Glock; 602 citations

91-13 Diagnosis and treatment of early melanoma: January 1983–November 1991 — prepared by K. Patrias, A. N. Moshell; 447 citations

91-14 Postpartum depression: January 1984– December 1991 — prepared by J. P. Hunt; 729 citations

This bibliography contains references about depression or the "baby blues" after a normal pregnancy and the birth of a normal, healthy infant.

91-15 Electromagnetic fields: January 1989–October 1991 — prepared by M. E. Beratan; 733 citations

This focuses on the nonthermal effects of electromagnetic fields. Cited are materials on electromagnetic fields from low-frequency electromagnetic waves; microwaves, radio waves, and other high-frequency electromagnetic waves; radar; and magnetic resonance imaging and nuclear magnetic resonance.

91-16 Triglyceride, high density lipoprotein, and coronary heart disease: January 1989–February 1992 — prepared by N. Miller, P. T. Einhorn; 1636 citations

91-17 Health effects of global warming: January 1986– December 1991 — prepared by J. van de Kamp; 175 citations

91-18 Seasonal affective disorder: January 1986– December 1991 — prepared by L. J. Klein; 402 citations

Seasonal affective disorder, or SAD, is a syndrome characterized by depressions that occur annually at the same time of year. It is most frequently associated with winter depression but can occur in summer as well. Other frequent symptoms include anxiety, irritability, decreased energy, increased appetite, increased duration of sleep, and weight gain.

91-19 Biomedical effects of volcanoes: January 1980– September 1991 — prepared by C. B. Love; 697 citations

1990

90-1 Surgery for epilepsy: January 1985–February 1990 — prepared by K. Patrias, W. H. Theodore; 681 citations

90-2 Sleep disorders of older people: January 1985– March 1990 — prepared by L. J. Klein, L. D. Ulincy, A. A. Monjan; 725 citations

90-3 Adjuvant therapy for colon and rectum cancer: January 1985–April 1990 — prepared by K. Patrias, J. M. Hamilton; 491 citations

90-4 Intravenous immunoglobulin: prevention and treatment of disease: January 1986–April 1990 — prepared by M. E. Beratan, H. B. Dickler; 888 citations

90-5 Laboratory animal welfare: December 1988– December 1989 — prepared by F. P. Gluckstein; 86 citations

90-6 Treatment of early-stage breast cancer: January 1985–May 1990 — prepared by N. Miller, F. A. Dorr; 668 citations

90-7 Cocaine, pregnancy, and the newborn: January 1988–March 1990 — prepared by C. B. Love; 468 citations

90-8 Fish oils: January 1989–July 1990 — prepared by J. van de Kamp; 653 citations

90-9 Alzheimer's disease and the family: January 1986– July 1990 — prepared by J. S. Martyniuk; 343 citations

90-10 "Clinical Use of botulinum toxin: January 1987– September 1990 — prepared by F. P. Gluckstein, M. Hallett; 318 citations

90-11 Diagnosis and management of asymptomatic primary hyperparathyroidism: January 1986–September 1990 — prepared by K. Patrias, J. E. Fradkin; 1057 citations

90-12 Prison health care: January 1986–September 1990 — prepared by R. L. Gordner; 1132 citations

90-13 Bovine somatotropin: January 1985–October 1990 — prepared by F. P. Gluckstein, M. Glock, J. G. Hill; 1097 citations

90-14 Adverse effects of aspartame: January 1986– December 1990 — prepared by J. van de Kamp; 167 citations

90-15 Patient education for self-care: the role of nurses: January 1983–November 1990 — prepared by P. S. Tillman; 468 citations

90-16 Blood substitutes: January 1986–December 1990 — prepared by J. van de Kamp; 744 citations

90-17 Hospital technology assessment: January 1984– December 1990 — prepared by A. Carbery-Fox, L. J. Klein, T. Meikle; 784 citations

90-18 Gastrointestinal surgery for severe obesity: January 1986–December 1990 — prepared by M. H. Glock, W. R. Foster; 548 citations

90-19 Human-pet relations: January 1983–December 1990 — prepared by J. Hunt; 385 citations

Billing, Electronic

American Medical Informatics Association
4915 St Elmo Ave, Ste 302, Bethesda, MD 20814
301 657-1291   Fax 301 657-1296
Web address: http://amia2.amia.org

Bioethics

Hastings Center
255 Elm Rd, Briarcliff Manor, NY 10510
914 762-8500   Fax 914 762-2124

Joseph and Rose Kennedy Institute of Ethics
National Reference Center for Bioethics Literature
Georgetown University, Washington, DC 20057
800 633-3849
Web address: http://quwels.georgetown.edu

President's Commission for the Study of Ethical Problems in Medicine and Biomedicine Behavioral Research Report
Government Printing Office
Washington, DC 20402
202 783-3238

B

Biofeedback

A technique in which a person uses information about a normally unconscious body function, such as blood pressure, to gain conscious control over that function. Biofeedback training may help in the treatment of stress-related conditions, including certain types of hypertension, anxiety, and migraine. (ENC-1989)

Resource
Association of Applied Psychophysiology and Biofeedback
10200 W 44th Ave, Ste 304, Wheat Ridge, CO 80033
800 477-8892   303 422-8436   Fax 303 422-8894
E-mail: aapb@resourcecenter.com

Biomedical Engineering

Biomedical Engineering Society
PO Box 2399, Culver City, CA 90231
310 618-9322
E-mail: bmes@netcom.com
Web address: http://isdl.ee.washington.edu/ABME/bmes.html

Birth Control

Free pamphlet on contraception:
American College of Obstetricians and Gynecologists
409 12th St SW, Washington, DC 20024-2188
202 638-5577   Fax 202 488-8107

Planned Parenthood Federation of America
810 Seventh Ave, New York, NY 10019
212 541-7800 . Fax 212 245-1845
Web address: http://www.igc.apc.org/ppfa

Birth Defects

Association of Birth Defect Children
Orlando Executive Park
827 Irma Ave, Orlando, FL 32803
800 313-ABDC   407 245-7035   Fax 407 245-7087

March of Dimes Birth Defects Foundation
1275 Mamaroneck Ave, White Plains, NY 10605
914 428-7100   Fax 914 428-8203

National Easter Seal Society
230 W Monroe, Chicago, IL 60606
800 221-6827   312 726-6200   Fax 312 726-1494
E-mail: nessinfo@seals.com

Blind

American Council of the Blind
1155 15th St NW, Ste 720, Washington, DC 20005
800 424-8666   202 467-5081   Fax 202 467-5085
Web address: http://www.acb.org

Council of Families With Visual Impairment
26616 Rouge River Dr, Dearborn Heights, MI 48127
800 424-8666

Eye Bank Association of America
1001 Connecticut Ave NW, Ste 601
Washington, DC 20036-5504
202 775-4999   Fax 202 429-6036

Guide Dog Foundation for the Blind Training Center
371 E Jericho Turnpike, Smithtown, NY 11787
800 548-4337   516 265-2121   Fax 516 361-5192

Helen Keller National Center for Deaf Blind Youths and Adults
111 Middle Neck Rd, Sands Point, NY 11050
516 944-8900   516 944-7302

Leader Dogs for the Blind
1039 S Rochester Rd, Rochester Hills, MI 48307
810 651-9011   Fax 810 651-5812

Lion's Club International
300 22nd St, Oak Brook, IL 60521
630 571-5466   Fax 630 571-8890

National Alliance of Blind Students
c/o American Council of the Blind
1155 15th St NW, Ste 720, Washington, DC 20005
800 424-8666   202 467-5081   Fax 202 467-5085
E-mail: jbeach@acess.digex.net

National Library Service for the Blind and Physically Handicapped
Library of Congress
1291 Taylor St NW, Washington, DC 20542
800 424-8567 (in DC) 202 707-5100
Web address: http://cwed.loc.gov/nls/nls.html

Prevent Blindness America
500 E Remington Rd, Schaumburg, IL 60173
800 331-2020   847 843-2020   Fax 847 843-8458

Blindness, Societies to Prevent, Statewide

Arkansas Prevent Blindness
400 W Capitol, Little Rock, AR 72201
501 376-6217

Prevent Blindness America Southern California Division
3702 Ruffin Rd, Ste 201
San Diego, CA 92123-1812
619 576-2122   Fax 619 576-2122

Prevent Blindness America Northern California Affiliate
4200 California St, San Francisco, CA 94118
800 338-3041   415 387-0934   Fax 415 387-1689

Colorado Prevent Blindness
3500 E 12th Ave, Denver, CO 80206
303 399-8090

Connecticut Affiliate Prevent Blindness
1275 Washington St, Middletown, CT 06457
800 850-2020   203 347-2020   Fax 203 347-0613

Prevent Blindness Florida Affiliate
711 E Kennedy Blvd, PO Box 172418, Tampa, FL 33672
800 226-6772   813 874-2020   Fax 813 225-2048

Prevent Blindness America Georgia Affiliate
455 E Paces Terry Rd, #222, Atlanta, GA 30305
404 266-0071   Fax 404 266-0860

Prevent Blindness America Indiana Affiliate
911 E 86th St, Indianapolis, IN 46204
317 259-8163   Fax 317 259-8175

Prevent Blindness America Iowa Affiliate
1111 9th St, Ste 250, Des Moines, IA 50314
515 244-4341   Fax 515 224-4718

Prevent Blindness America Kentucky Affiliate
101 W Chestnut St, Louisville, KY 40202
800 828-1179   502 584-6127   Fax 502 584-0828

Prevent Blindness America Massachusetts Affiliate
375 Concord Ave, Belmont, MA 02178
617 489-0007

Prevent Blindness America Mississippi Affiliate
115 Broadmoor Dr, Jackson, MS 39206
601 362-6985

Prevent Blindness America Nebraska Affiliate
7101 Newport Ave, Ste 308
Omaha, NE 68132-2172
402 572-3520   Fax 402 572-3522

Prevent Blindness America New Jersey Affiliate
200 Centennial Ave, Ste 203
Piscataway, NJ 08854-3910
908 844-2020   Fax 908 980-0011

Prevent Blindness America New York Division
160 E 56th St, 8th Fl, New York, NY 10022
212 980-2020   Fax 212 688-9641

Prevent Blindness North Carolina Affiliate
3801 Lake Boone Trails, Ste 410
Raleigh, NC 27607
919 832-2020   Fax 919 571-1502

Prevent Blindness America Ohio Affiliate
1500 W Third St, Ste 200
Columbus, OH 43212-2874
614 464-2020   Fax 614 481-9670

Prevent Blindness America Oklahoma Affiliate
6 NE 63rd St, Ste 150, Oklahoma City, OK 73105
405 848-7123   Fax 405 848-6935

Prevent Blindness America Puerto Rico Affiliate
PO Box 3232, San Juan, PR 00904
809 722-3531   Fax 809 725-0809

Prevent Blindness America Rhode Island Affiliate
1800 17th Post Rd, Warwick, RI 02886
401 738-1150

Prevent Blindness America Tennessee Affiliate
95 White Bridge Rd, Ste 513
Nashville, TN 37205
615 352-0450   Fax 615 352-5750

Prevent Blindness America Texas Affiliate
3211 W Dallas, Houston, TX 77019
713 526-2559   Fax 713 529-8310

Prevent Blindness America Utah Affiliate
661 S 200 East, Salt Lake City, UT 84111
800 675-5065   801 524-2020   Fax 801 322-3647

Prevent Blindness America Virginia Affiliate
3820 Augusta Ave, Richmond, VA 23230
804 355-0773   Fax 804 355-3142

Prevent Blindness America Wisconsin Affiliate
759 N Milwaukee St, Milwaukee, WI 53202
414 765-0505   Fax 414 765-0377

Blood

American Red Cross
431 18th St NW, Washington, DC 20006
202 737-8300
Web address: http://www.redcross.org

American Society of Hematology
1200 19th St NW, Ste 300
Washington, DC 20036-2412
202 857-1118   Fax 202 857-1164

Blood Banks

American Association of Blood Banks
8101 Glenbrook Rd, Bethesda, MD 20814-2749
301 907-6977   Fax 301 907-6895

National Phlebotomy Association
5615 Landoner Rd, Hyattsville, MD 20784
301 699-3846   Fax 301 699-5766

Blood Bank Technologist

History
In 1954, the first examination for blood bank technologists was administered by the American Society of Clinical Pathologists' Board of Registry. It is significant that both the examination and the process for approving blood bank schools were the result of a cooperative effort between the Board of Registry and the American Association of Blood Banks (AABB). Technologists working for 5 years in blood banking were eligible to take the examination.

After 1960, individuals could attend a 12-month educational program at an accredited school in lieu of the 5-year experience route. Levels of competency were established, and the scope of knowledge pertinent to the field was prescribed to ensure that the institutions would maintain acceptable standards of practice; would follow a curriculum that included all phases of blood bank technology, laboratory management, and transfusion services; and would support a faculty adequate to assume teaching responsibilities. To date, more than 4000 individuals have been certified as specialists in blood bank technology.

Because the number of programs had increased by 1969, *Standards (Essentials)* were prepared by the Committee on Education of the AABB and were adopted by the House of Delegates of the American Medical Association (AMA) in 1971. Subsequently, the *Standards* underwent major revisions in 1977, 1983, and 1991 and were adopted by the AMA Council on Medical Education and the AABB.

Occupational description
Specialists in blood bank technology perform both routine and specialized tests in blood bank immunohematology in technical areas of the modern blood bank and perform transfusion services, using methodology that conforms to the Standards for Blood Banks and Transfusion Services of the AABB.

Job description
Specialists in blood bank technology demonstrate a superior level of technical proficiency and problem-solving ability in such areas as (1) testing for blood group antigens, compatibility, and antibody identification; (2) investigating abnormalities such as hemolytic diseases of the newborn, hemolytic anemias, and adverse responses to transfusion; (3) supporting physicians in transfusion therapy, including patients with coagulopathies or candidates for organ transplant; and (4) performing blood

B collection and processing, including selecting donors, drawing and typing blood, and performing pretransfusion tests to ensure the safety of the patient. Supervision, management, and/or teaching make up a considerable part of the responsibilities of the specialist in blood bank technology.

Employment characteristics

Specialists in blood banking work in many types of facilities, including community blood centers, private hospital blood banks, university-affiliated blood banks, transfusion services, and independent laboratories; they also may be part of a university faculty. Specialists may work some weekend and night duty, including emergency calls. Qualified specialists may advance to supervisory or administrative positions, or move into teaching or research activities. The criteria for advancement in this field are experience, technical expertise, and completion of advanced education courses.

Entry-level salaries for specialists in blood banking average between $32,000 and $42,000, depending on previous experience. (AHRP-1997)

Resources

AMA Department of Allied Health
312 553-9355

American Association of Blood Banks
8101 Glenbrook Rd, Bethesda, MD 20814-2749
301 907-6977

Accreditation:
AABB Committee on Accreditation of SBB Schools
American Association of Blood Banks
8101 Glenbrook Rd, Bethesda, MD 20814-2749
301 907-6977   Fax 301 907-6895
Web address: http://www.aabb.org

*Board Certification in Blood Banking
Transfusion Medicine:*
American Board of Pathology
5401 W Kennedy Blvd, PO Box 25915
Tampa, FL 33622
813 286-2444   Fax 813 289-5279

Blood Pressure

What is high blood pressure and what causes it?

High blood pressure is the most common health problem in the United States. The American Heart Association estimates that more than 50 million Americans have high blood pressure and that most of them do not get treatment for it.

High blood pressure, or hypertension, occurs when the blood exerts too much force against the walls of the heart and blood vessels as it circulates around the body. The heart works harder than normal to pump blood, causing the person to have abnormally high blood pressure at all times, even when at rest. Hypertension is usually detected by a doctor during a routine physical exam. As we shall see, many factors can play a part in hypertension.

There are two types of hypertension:

Essential (or primary) hypertension is high blood pressure that has no obvious cause. Most people who have high blood pressure (90% to 95%) have essential hypertension.

Secondary hypertension is high blood pressure that is caused by a specific disease or condition.

Only about 5% to 10% of people who have high blood pressure have secondary hypertension.

Some diseases that can cause secondary hypertension are:
- Kidney disease—The kidneys are the main regulators of blood pressure; hypertension frequently develops if the kidneys are not functioning properly.
- Adrenal gland disease—The adrenal glands produce hormones (epinephrine and norepinephrine) that play an important role in regulating the blood pressure and heart rate; too little or too much of these hormones in the bloodstream can lead to high blood pressure.
- Thyroid gland disease—An overactive thyroid gland (hyperthyroidism) speeds up the heart and increases the demands on the circulatory system; the extra strain increases the risk of hypertension and serious complications, such as heart failure.

Other causes of secondary hypertension include:
- Oral contraceptives—Using the pill slightly raises the blood pressure of any woman who uses it; for women who have hypertension, this increases the risk of stroke. Women with high blood pressure may have to quit taking the pill and switch to an alternative method of birth control.
- Pregnancy—A pregnant woman's blood pressure will tend to rise during pregnancy but will usually return to normal after the baby is born. Preeclampsia, a condition that causes a dangerous rise in blood pressure, may develop in some pregnant women (preeclampsia can be treated with bed rest, decreased sodium intake, and blood pressure medication).
- Alcohol and other drug abuse—Heavy drinking and repeated use of certain illegal drugs (for example, cocaine) can cause a condition called cardiomyopathy, in which the heart muscle becomes weak and damaged.

In many (but not all) people who have secondary hypertension, the blood pressure returns to normal after the underlying disease or condition has been successfully treated. (DX-HBP-1996)

Citizens for Public Action on Blood Pressure and Cholesterol
PO Box 30374, Bethesda, MD 20824
301 770-1711   Fax 301 770-1113

High Blood Pressure Information Center
National Institutes of Health
Bethesda, MD 20205
301 951-3260

Contact local state department of health for testing information or local heart association for consumer information.

Blood Tests

Contact local state department of health for testing information.

Book Donations

American Overseas Medical Aid Association
(medical books and journals)
4433 W Montana St, Chicago, IL 60639
312 486-4809

Darien Book Aid Plan, Inc
(books and journals)
1926 Post Rd, Darien, CT 06820
203 655-2777

The Foundation for Books to China
5337 College Ave, Ste 314, Oakland, CA 94618-1416
415 392-1080

International Book Project, Inc.
(professional books and journals)
1440 Delaware Ave, Lexington, KY 40505
606 254-6771

Medical Books for China
13021 E Florence Ave, Santa Fe Springs, CA 90670
213 946-8774

Book(s), Medical

Recommended Books

Frisse ME, Florance V. A Library for internists.
Recommendations from the American College of
Physicians.
Ann Intern Med. 1997 May 15; 126(10)836-46

Brandon AN, Hill DR. Selected List of books and journals
in allied health. *Bull Med Lib Assoc.* 1996: 84(3): 289-309

Brandon AN, Hill DR. Selected list of books and journals
for the small medical library. *Bull Med Lib Assoc.* 1997:
85(2): 111-135; published in 2- or 3-year intervals

AMA Book Source
(Selection includes any medical book
currently published)
1851 Diplomat Ave, Dallas, TX 75234
800 451-2262

Boxing

JAMA Theme Issue: Boxing

JAMA 1986 May 9; 255(18)

Five articles discuss various medical aspects of boxing and
its danger to the athlete. A clinical presentation of retinal
detachment, a review of boxing and health listing 43
citations, comments on the liberty of choosing one's
sport no matter how dangerous, a prototype program to
help boxing evolve into a safer sport, and an editorial
listing both the pros and cons against boxing make up
this theme issue.

Brain Bank

Alzheimer's Association
919 N Michigan Ave, Ste 1000, Chicago, IL 60611
800 272-3900   312 225-8700   Fax 312 335-1110
E-mail: greenfld@alz.org
Web address: http://www.alz.org

Brain Donors:
McLean Hospital Brain Bank
115 Mill St, Belmont, MA 02178
617 855-2400

Brain Disorders, Pediatrics

National Brain Research Association
1439 Rhode Island Ave NW, Washington, DC 20005
202 483-6272
(Also provides support groups for parents)

Brain Injuries

National Institute of Neurological Disorders and Stroke
900 Rockville Pike, Bethesda, MD 20892
301 496-5751

Brain Tumor

National Brain Tumor Foundation
785 Market St, Ste 1600, San Francisco, CA 94103
800 934-CURE   415 284-0208   415 284-0209

American Brain Tumor Association
2720 River Rd, Ste 146, Des Plaines, IL 60018
800 886-2282   847 827-9910   847 827-9918
E-mail: abta@aol.com
Web address: http://pubweb.nwu.edu/~/berko/
abta_html/abta1.htm

Breast Cancer

AMA Policy

Silicone Gel Breast Implants. (H-525.983) CSA Rep. C,
I-92; Amended by CSA Rep. 8, I-96

The AMA (1) continues to support the establishment of
a registry of all patients with breast implants so that data
pertaining to health outcomes can be regularly reviewed
and reported to physicians and patients; (2) supports the
position that women have the right to choose silicone
gel-filled or saline-filled breast implants for both aug-
mentation and reconstruction after being fully informed
about the risks and benefits; (3) urges physicians to be
informed of the current scientific data available in order
to recognize and address the considerable public anxiety
concerning the safety of breast implants. Patients can be
reassured that, to date, there is no conclusive or convincing evidence that relates silicone breast implants to human autoimmune disease; (4) supports appropriate data
collection and follow-up in all cases in which such implants are utilized, and that clinical trials as proposed by
the FDA do not limit the woman's right to choose; (5)
will monitor the process of decision making by the FDA
on the use of not only silicone gel breast implants but
also all silicone-based devices, with particular attention to
use of expert medical judgment and to issues of conflict
of interest; (6) requests that specific FDA policies regarding the process of evaluation of devices be publicized to
the medical profession and the public, and that the process be sensitive to the emotional impact on the patient;
and (7) condemns the inappropriate use of laboratory
tests that purport to measure the dissemination of silicone through a patient's body and that are used to make
unsubstantiated diagnoses of silicone-related illness.

B

B

Poetry and Medicine

Mastectomy

Sarah Singer
JAMA 1993 Oct 13; 270(14): 1754

No epitaph, no measured requiem
Marks this small death that so diminishes
The verities of mind and heart and limb;
But there is need for grief, for obsequies
Defined anew by roses. Though the sun
Attains horizon still, and seasons flare,
I wake and sleep where seasons are undone,
And thoughts are spent like leaves the winds impair.
Yet somehow breath endures but does not grace
Nor counter circumstance; what dreams intrude,
Soon lost. Beyond affinity to place
and reel of time, beyond solicitude
Professed by lips and outstretched hands, I all
But founder, light itself inimical.

Resources

Food and Drug Administration Implant Hotline
800 532-4440

Food and Drug Administration
Office of Device Evaluation
5600 Fishers Ln, Rockville, MD 20857
301 443-3170
Web address: http://www.fda.gov

National Alliance of Breast Cancer Organizations
9 E 37th St, 10th Fl, New York, NY 10016
800 719-9154   212 719-0154   Fax 212 689-1213
E-mail: NABCOinfo@aol.com

Y-Me Breast Cancer Support Program
c/o Sharon Green
212 W Van Buren, Chicago, IL 60607
800 221-2141   312 986-8338   312 986-8228
Fax 312 294-8597
E-mail: YMEONE@aol.com
Web address: http://www.nabco.org

Breast Feeding

La Leche League International
1400 Meacham, Schaumburg, IL 60173
800 LA-LECHE   847 519-7730   847 519-0035

Broadcasters, Physicians

National Association of Physician Broadcasters
515 N State St, Chicago, IL 60610
312 464-6659

Bureau of Health Professions

The Bureau provides national leadership in coordinating, evaluating, and supporting the development and utilization of the nation's health personnel.

To accomplish this goal, the Bureau:
- serves as a focus for health care quality assurance activities, issues related to malpractice, and the operation of the National Practitioner Data Bank, and the Vaccine Injury Compensation Program;
- supports through grants health professions and nurse training institutions, targeting resources to areas of high national priority such as disease prevention, health promotion, bedside nursing, care of the elderly, and HIV/AIDS;
- funds regional centers that provide educational services and multidisciplinary training for health professions faculty and practitioners in geriatric health care;
- supports programs to increase the supply of primary care practitioners and to improve the distribution of health professionals;
- develops, tests, and demonstrates new and improved approaches to the development and utilization of health personnel within various patterns of health care delivery and financing systems;
- provides leadership for promoting equity in access to health services and health careers for the disadvantaged;
- administers several loan programs supporting students training for careers in the health profession and nursing;
- funds regional centers to train faculty and practicing health professionals in the counseling, diagnosis, and management of HIV/AIDS-infected individuals;
- collects and analyzes data and disseminates information on the characteristics and capacities of US health training systems;
- assesses the nation's health personnel force and forecasts supply and requirements; and
- in coordination with the Office of the Administrator, Health Resources and Services Administration, serves as a focus for technical assistance activities in the international projects relevant to domestic health personnel problems. (USG-1996)

Resource

Bureau of Health Professions
Park Lawn Bldg, 5000 Fishers Ln
Rockville, MD 20857
301 443-1173

Burn Centers

Medical and Health Information Directory, 9th edition (Detroit: Gale Publishing Company, 1998); ISBN 0-7876-1559-5; three-volume set. Volume three, chapter 5, lists alphabetically by state the US hospitals that provide specialized burn care services.

Burns

American Burn Association
c/o Cleon W. Goodwin, MD
New York Hospital—Cornell Medical Center
525 E 68th St, Rm L-706, New York, NY 10021
800 548-2876   212 746-5078   212 746-8991

Cancer

Black lung

Eric L. Dyer, MD
JAMA 1997 May 14; 277(18): 1420r

Cancer is a loud word
spilling over the sea like an alarm
that will not stop clanging no matter
how much water is tossed onto the blaze,
an intricate word stretching, repeating
its crude syllables like waves of oil
slicking from the coast near Durham,
near Winston-Salem, past Tampa and Havana,
through the filter tip of the Panama Canal,
then curling all the way to Valdez
and the last end-expiratory wheeze.

Cancer is a plot
told in disorganized paragraphs of run-on sentences
and awkward conjunctions, a sea story
describing a a split hull bleeding
offshore toward gaping avocets and pelicans
and heavy, dripping cormorants
too far down the beach
for any government clean-up crew to reach.

Cancer is one syllable, a cough
rattling a thin figure perched on his coastal rock,
watching his own massive stern upend,
listening to the waves pound his cliff
as busy sand crabs chew dead fish,
admiring one more sunset
through the bank of his own blue smoke,
dredging one more black breath,
in no particular hurry to extinguish his fire,
to quit his stained finger play
or to reach the end of his day.

Resources

American Cancer Society
1599 Clifton Rd, NE, Atlanta, GA 30329
800 ACS-2345   404 320-3333
404 329-7648   Fax 404 325-0230
Web address: http://www.cancer.org

Cancer Information Clearinghouse (NCI/OCC)
9000 Rockville Pike, Bldg 31, Rm 10A07
Bethesda, MD 20892-2580
800 4-CANCER   Fax 301 402-0555

Candlelighters Childhood Cancer Foundation
7910 Woodmont Ave, Ste 460
Bethesda, MD 20814-3015
800 366-2223   301 657-8401   Fax 301 718-2686

National Cancer Institute
9000 Rockville Pike, Bethesda, MD 20892
800 4CANCER (800 422-6237) 301 496-5583
Web address: http://www.nci.nih.gov

Insurance Problems:
Cancer treatments your insurance should cover
Association of Community Cancer Centers
11600 Nebel St, Ste 201, Rockville, MD 20852
301 984-9496   Fax 301 770-1949

Cancer Research

In general, these institutions provide research grants to health professionals:

Philanthropic Association of Virginia
Council of Better Business Bureaus
1515 Wilson Blvd, Arlington, VA 22209
703 276-0133

Sloan-Kettering Institute for Cancer Research
1275 York Ave, New York, NY 10021
212 639-2000

Contact the state or local office of the American Cancer Society for a local affiliate of the American Institute of Cancer Research.

Cancer Societies, Statewide

American Cancer Society Alabama Division
504 Brookwood Blvd, Homewood, AL 35209
205 879-2242   Fax 205 870-7436

American Cancer Society Alaska Division
406 W Fireweed Ln, Ste 204
Anchorage, AK 99503
907 277-8696   Fax 907 263-2073

American Cancer Society Arizona Division
2929 E Thomas Rd, Phoenix, AZ 85016
602 224-0524   Fax 602 381-3096

American Cancer Society Arkansas Division
901 N University, Little Rock, AR 72207
501 664-3480   Fax 501 666-0068

American Cancer Society California Division
1710 Webster St, Oakland, CA 94612
510 893-7900   Fax 510 835-8656

American Cancer Society Colorado Division
2255 S Oneida, Denver, CO 80224
303 758-2030   Fax 303 758-7006

American Cancer Society Connecticut Division
Barnes Park S, 14 Village Ln, Wallingford, CT 06492
203 265-7161   Fax 203 265-0281

American Cancer Society Delaware Division
92 Read's Way, New Castle, DE 19720
302 324-4227   Fax 302 324-4233

American Cancer Society
District of Columbia Division
1875 Connecticut Ave NW, Ste 315
Washington, DC 20009
202 483-2600   Fax 202 483-1174

American Cancer Society Florida Division
3709 W Jetton Ave, Tampa, FL 33629-5146
813 253-0541   Fax 813 254-5857

American Cancer Society Georgia Division Lenox Park
2200 Lake Blvd, Atlanta, GA 30319
404 816-7800   Fax 816-9443

American Cancer Society Hawaii Pacific Division
200 N Vineyard Blvd, Ste 100-A
Honolulu, HI 96817
808 531-1662   Fax 808 526-9729

American Cancer Society Idaho Division
2676 Vista Ave, PO Box 5386, Boise, ID 83705
208 343-4609   Fax 208 343-9922

American Cancer Society Illinois Division
77 E Monroe, Chicago, IL 60603
312 641-6150   Fax 312 641-6588

American Cancer Society Indiana Division
8730 Commerce Park Pl, Indianapolis, IN 46268
317 872-4432   Fax 317 879-4114

American Cancer Society Iowa Division
8364 Hickman Rd, Ste D
Des Moines, IA 50325-4300
515 253-0147   Fax 515 253-0806

American Cancer Society Kansas Division
1315 SW Arrowhead Rd, Topeka, KS 66604-4020
913 273-4114   Fax 913 273-1503

American Cancer Society Kentucky Division
701 W Muhammad Ali Blvd, PO Box 1807
Louisville, KY 40203-1909
502 584-6782   Fax 502 584-8946

American Cancer Society Louisiana Division
2200 Veterans Memorial Blvd, Ste 214
Kenner, LA 70062
504 469-0021   Fax 504 469-0033

American Cancer Society Maine Division
52 Federal St, Brunswick, ME 04011
207 729-3339   Fax 207 729-0635

American Cancer Society Maryland Division
8219 Town Center Dr, Baltimore, MD 21162-0026
410 931-6850   Fax 410 931-6875

American Cancer Society Massachusetts Division
247 Commonwealth Ave, Boston, MA 02116
617 267-2650   Fax 617 536-3163

American Cancer Society Michigan Division
1205 E Saginaw St, Lansing, MI 48906
517 371-2920   Fax 517 371-2605

American Cancer Society Minnesota Division
3316 W 66th St, Minneapolis, MN 55435
612 925-2772   Fax 612 925-6333

American Cancer Society Mississippi Division
1380 Livingston Ln, Jackson, MS 39213
601 362-8874   Fax 601 362-8876

American Cancer Society Missouri Division
3322 American Ave, PO Box 1066
Jefferson City, MO 65102
314 893-4800   Fax 314 893-2017

American Cancer Society Montana Division
17 N 26th St, Billings, MT 59101
406 252-7111   Fax 406 252-7112

American Cancer Society Nebraska Division
8502 W Center Rd, Omaha, NE 68124-5255
402 393-5800   Fax 402 393-7790

American Cancer Society Nevada Division
1325 E Harmon Ave, Las Vegas, NV 89119
702 798-6877   Fax 702 798-0530

American Cancer Society New Hampshire Division
Gail Singer Memorial Bldg
360 State Rd Ste 501, Bedford, NH 03110-5032
603 472-8899   Fax 603 472-7093

American Cancer Society New Jersey Division
2600 US Hwy 1, North Brunswick, NJ 08902-0803
908 297-8000   Fax 908 297-9043

American Cancer Society New Mexico Division
5800 Lomas Blvd NE, Albuquerque, NM 87110
505 260-2105   505 266-9513

American Cancer Society New York State Division
6725 Lyons St, East Syracuse, NY 13057
315 437-7025   315 437-0540

American Cancer Society Queens Division
112-25 Queens Blvd, Forest Hills, NY 11375
718 263-2224   Fax 718 261-0758

American Cancer Society Long Island Division
75 Davids Dr, Hauppauge, NY 11788
516 436-7070   516 436-5380

American Cancer Society New York City Division
19 W 56th St, New York, NY 10019
212 586-8700   Fax 212 237-3852

American Cancer Society Westchester Division
30 Glenn St, White Plains, NY 10603
914 949-4800   Fax 914 949-4279

American Cancer Society North Carolina Division
11 S Boylan Ave, Ste 221, Raleigh, NC 27603
919 834-8463   919 839-0551

American Cancer Society North Dakota Division
123 Roberts St, Fargo, ND 58102
701 232-1385   701 232-1109

American Cancer Society Ohio Division
5555 Frantz Rd, Dublin, OH 43017
614 889-9565   Fax 614 889-6578

American Cancer Society Oklahoma Division
4323 NW 63rd, Ste 110, Oklahoma City, OK 73116
405 843-9888   Fax 405 848-0795

American Cancer Society Oregon Division
0330 SW Curry, Portland, OR 97201
503 295-6422   Fax 503 228-1062

American Cancer Society Pennsylvania Division
Route 422 Sipe Ave, PO Box 897
Hershey, PA 17033-0897
717 533-6144   717 534-1075

American Cancer Society Philadelphia Division
1626 Locust St, Philadelphia, PA 19103
215 985-5400   Fax 215 985-5406

American Cancer Society Puerto Rico Division
Calle Alverio, #577, Hato Rey, PR 00918
809 764-2295   Fax 809 764-0553

American Cancer Society Rhode Island Division
400 Main St, Pawtucket, RI 02860
401 722-8480   Fax 401 727-9449

American Cancer Society South Carolina Division
128 Stonemark Ln, Columbia, SC 29210-3855
803 750-1693   Fax 803 750-4000

American Cancer Society South Dakota Division
4101 Carnegie Pl, Sioux Falls, SD 57106-2322
605 361-8277   Fax 605 361-8537

American Cancer Society Tennessee Division
1315 8th Ave S, Nashville, TN 37203
615 255-1227   Fax 615 255-1230

American Cancer Society Texas Division
2433 Ridgepoint Dr, Austin, TX 78754
512 928-2262   Fax 512 298-2262

American Cancer Society Utah Division
941 E 3300 S, Salt Lake City, UT 84106
801 483-1500   801 483-1558

American Cancer Society Vermont Division
13 Loomis St, Drawer C, PO Box 1452
Montpelier, VT 05601-1452
802 223-2348   Fax 802 223-4818

American Cancer Society Virginia Division
4240 Park Pl, Glen Allen, VA 23060
804 527-3700   804 527-3797

American Cancer Society Washington Division
2120 1st Ave N, Seattle, WA 98109-1140
206 283-1152   Fax 206 285-3469

American Cancer Society West Virginia Division
2428 Kanawha Blvd E, Charleston, WV 25311
304 344-3611   304 343-6549

American Cancer Society Wisconsin Division
N 19 W 24350 Riverwood Dr, Waukesha, WI 53188
414 523-5500   414 523-5533

American Cancer Society Wyoming Division
4202 Ridge Rd, Cheyenne, WY 82001
307 638-3331   Fax 307 638-1199

Candida Albicans (Yeast Theory of Disease)

Candida Research and Information Foundation
Box 2719, Castro Valley, CA 94546
415 582-2179

Capitation

A method of reimbursement where organizations receive a fixed per-month premium for each of their plan's covered lives. In return for this stream of revenue premiums, their plan provides a full range of health care services to its plan members. The organization bears the risk for the utilization of health care services and costs. An alternative to fee-for-service, this method is used primarily for HMO members but can be extended to EPO and POS plans. Although capitation payments can be based on a number of criteria, such as the age and gender mix of the group, previous group experience, etc, the general structure is a flat rate per member per month (pm/pm). (MMCMP-1996)

Do your homework before jumping into capitation

Judy Capko
AM News June 13, 1994 p43-4

There is a frenzy to restructure health care delivery through the integration of physicians, hospitals and insurance plans. The integrated delivery system brings about shared risk and capitation for many physicians.

As they begin to tread in these new waters, physicians are beginning to understand the significance capitation will play in their future. They sometimes lack a clear understanding of what it will mean to them. They aren't sure if taking it on is prudent for them.

Often a practice has not done the necessary homework and is not prepared for the transition to capitation. In fact, they have not evaluated whether they can really deliver care at the rate being offered, and what patient care responsibility they would have to assume.

Physicians need to plan for capitation—to look before they leap. In addition to examining the actuarial bases used to determine the cap rates, what should they look at and how can they prepare? The considerations for primary care and specialties may be different. Regardless, it would be prudent to examine how different issues could apply to your particular practice and specialty.

The contract
Scrutinize it. It is important to read the detail of the contract and be perfectly clear on what responsibility you are assuming in return for the cap rate being offered. What other factors exist? You need to understand the patient's co-pay, and what responsibility you have when this is not met.

What is the financial responsibility of the plan or IPA issuing the contract? Know when you are going to get paid, and what happens if there is a delay in payment.

Find out what you are obligating yourself for and for how long. Is it reasonable, and do you have the resources to meet this responsibility? This can include a broad range of considerations: availability, coverage, emergency services, quality-of-care issues, record retention, etc. What is the length of your agreement, and what are the terms for opting out and terminating the agreement?

There are myriad other considerations that make it essential to seek legal counsel to understand and protect your position now and in the future. There is always a potential for unexpected personal, professional and financial consequences if you are not well-protected in the contract. In addition, you will want your malpractice carrier to take a look at the contract to be sure you are covered for the liability you will be assuming.

Utilization patterns
To anticipate the future, look at the delivery of care you have provided in the past. This will give you a thumbnail sketch of your utilization patterns and the cost of those services based on your past reimbursement rate. If you

are not involved in managed care, you can examine your cost of services based on your standard billing fees.

If all aspects of the contract are agreeable, you will still have some mechanics to deal with. Preparing and organizing in advance will make the transition far easier.

Tracking enrollees
The next step is having an effective tracking mechanism in place to monitor the enrollees you are responsible for.

You will need to be assured that you will be provided with an "accurate" list of each enrollee you are being paid for. Establish a procedure to audit this report every month against the patients you have entered into your system as enrollees for the plan. You will need to keep accurate records of those that transfer in or out to be assured you are being paid appropriately.

Remember, you will be paid for enrollees, not individual services rendered to patients. This means you will receive a capitated payment each month — on a pre-paid basis — whether or not the patient is actually seen. The payment should discontinue when the patient is no longer covered by the plan or transfers their care. Once this occurs, you will want to be sure the plan is not compensating you for those patients.

By the same token, it will be important to cross-reference your patient list to be sure payment is received for every patient appearing on your system.

Screening
If you are a primary care practice you will need to be clear on what preliminary services you are required to provide before referring on to a specialist. For example, if carpal tunnel syndrome is suspected, is it the primary care physician's responsibility to provide x-rays and splint for the patient, or is the orthopedic surgeon assuming this responsibility?

Tracking
Don't make the mistake of thinking that it is not important to use a routing slip and track services rendered on your computer. This provides a record for the plan, the patient and yourself of all services rendered. The plan will want to know that you are delivering the same quality of care for cap patients as for fee-for-service patients.

You will want to get an HMO tracking module on your accounts receivable system. You will need to know what you would receive from this same patient base if they were fee-for-service patients. It will help you establish your utilization patterns and costs for care. After all, when it comes time to renew or renegotiate your contract, you will need to know if your cap rate is adequate to provide quality care to the enrollees. At the same time, this becomes a management tool to ensure you are providing services prudently. You certainly don't want to deny a patient needed services, but at the same time it is important to see if lab studies or testing have been duplicated, and to determine where utilization differs from your norm and why. The emphasis on early access and preventive care can play an important role in improving utilization and quality outcomes—getting patients better quicker.

Be flexible
Adjusting to this new method of payment may take you out of your comfort zone. It is a shift in paradigms, and will take some getting used to. A flexible attitude and approach will help. It may be time to seek some professional assistance in preparing your practice to succeed in this new health care economy. With capitation, it is important to look before you leap. You can increase your odds for success.

Resource
Capitation: The Physician's Guide, Second Edition. 1997 American Medical Association, Chicago. 104pp. ISBN 0-89970-867-6 OP601597

Captioning
Captioned Films for the Deaf:
Modern Talking Picture Service
5000 Park St N, St Petersburg, FL 33709
800 237-6213 813 541-7571 Fax 800 237-7143

National Captioning Institute, Inc
1900 Gallows Rd, Ste 3000, Vienna, VA 22182
703 917-7600 Fax 703 917-9878

Cardiology

Poetry and Medicine

Learning to hear

Neil Scheurich
JAMA 1992 Jul 1; 268(1): 39

Son, the stethoscope is a tool
connecting man to man, man
to world, for science is society.
Withdraw from cacophony into
the chamber of an interview.
Just as you might tear apart
the clouds at night to see
the burning stars, painfully bright,
so you hear the heart, the secret
of a body's architecture.
Auscultate—to the body's heartfelt
speech. A rhythm bound to vessel
bone and blood that voices huge
cries, echoed to mute whisperings
in the cleverness of a wrist.
Hearken—to the throb, the code
of earth's ancient persistence,
the soul of smile, of rage
and careless laughter, the slight
unsuspected continuum of life.
Listen—to that which speaks
just above and behind you
in the depths of restless time,
and yet to you alone
the axis of the spinning sky.

A Piece of My Mind

A thin green line

Scott Waters
JAMA 1994 Oct 12; 272(14): 1086

Today I saw my father's heart.

It was a glowing green line on a monitor in the naval air station hospital intensive care unit. Early this morning his prostate had been removed, along with a battalion of adventurous cells that had dared to become cancerous without his permission.

The tiny line squiggled along, dropped to a narrow notch, then zoomed back up to resume formation. After a dozen repetitions, the line disappeared and began again, marching across the screen from left to right in a stubbornly consistent procession of green phosphors.

On the bed, a thin, gray man slept, pierced by transparent tubes and wrapped in clean, white linen. His thin, gray hair stood in disarray. Pale flesh and slack muscles hung from diminished bones. Each soft breath moved the sheet so little that I had to look closely to detect the motion.

I inched around to see his face, a face driven deep into my heart through years and decades. There was no anger there, no scorn or praise. The eyes that had watched me turn, one day at a time, into another person were closed. The ears that had heard me cry and sing and laugh rested unhearing. I wanted to brush his hair back with my hand; he'd be concerned about that. Instead, I looked up at the thin green trace progressing across the monitor. Minor detours appeared, subtle changes moved the pace along, but the overall pattern remained consistent.

He stirred. Some hidden dream rose close enough to the surface that he shifted his hips, flexed his jaw, then settled back into the steady dip and beep of postoperative sleep. Was he dreaming about B-17s over Texas? Or cargo planes in the dark skies of the South Pacific? I hoped he was someplace where small kids jumped into his lap, or cold beers formed bridges between young airmen who leaned laughing against shiny American cars.

My heart assumed that slow rhythm advancing across the screen. For just one second, the small, gray man in the cold steel bed was large and strong again. Dry hospital winds turned warm. Again I missed the baseball he tossed, felt the disappointment, felt the pain, touched the cool green grass of one distant summer. Saw the smile and sparkling blue eyes as he shook his head and clapped his hands for me to throw it back.

Instead, I sank into a cloudy day, where one old sergeant lay sleeping, surrounded by his son and two hearts drawn together across the flickering screen.

Cardiologist. Alternate title: heart specialist. Diagnoses and treats diseases of heart disorders, using medical instruments and equipment: Studies diagnostic images and electrocardiograph recordings to aid in making diagnoses. Prescribes medications and recommends dietary and activity program as indicated. Refers patient to surgeon specializing in cardiac cases when need for corrective surgery is indicated. May engage in research to study anatomy of and diseases peculiar to heart. (DOT-1991)

Resources

American College of Angiology
1044 Northern Blvd, Ste 103, Roslyn, NY 11576
516 484-6880   Fax 516 625-1174

American College of Cardiology
9111 Old Georgetown Rd, Bethesda, MD 20814-1699
800 253-4636   301 897-5400   Fax 301 897-9745
Web address: http://www.acc.org

Board Certification in Cardiovascular Disease:
American Board of Internal Medicine
3624 Market St, Philadelphia, PA 19104
800 441-ABIM (800 441-2246)   215 243-1500
Fax 215 382-4702

Cardiopulmonary Resuscitation
A historical perspective

JAMA 1992 Oct 28; 268(16): 2172

In the past thirty years, since the introduction of modern techniques of CPR, there have been dramatic advances in ECC of victims of profound circulatory collapse and cardiac arrest. These techniques have restored the lives of many people when breathing has ceased and the heart has stopped beating. For those with spared neurological function and treatable cardiopulmonary disease, prolonged and vigorous life may ensue.

Sporadic accounts of attempted resuscitation are recorded since antiquity[1-3] but until 1960 successful resuscitation was largely limited to occasional victims of respiratory arrest. Emergency thoracotomy with "open chest massage" was described in the 1950s and was often successful if definitive therapy was readily available.[4] Electric reversal of ventricular fibrillation by externally applied electrodes was described in 1956.[5] The ability to reverse a fatal arrhythmia without opening the chest challenged the medical community to develop a method of sustaining ventilation and circulation long enough to bring the defibrillator to the patient's aid. In 1958 adequate rescue ventilation with mouth-to-mouth technique was described.[6,7] In 1960 "closed-chest" compression was described, ushering in the modern era of CPR.[8] The simplicity of this technique has led to its widespread dissemination: "All that is needed are two hands."[8] The interaction of closed-chest compression with mouth-to-mouth ventilation was developed as basic CPR, which offered the hope for substantially reducing the nearly 1000 sudden deaths that occurred each day in the United States before the patients reached the hospital.

References

1. Standards for cardiopulmonary resuscitation (CPR) and emergency cardiac care (ECC). *JAMA* 1974;227(suppl):833-868

2. Safar P. History of cardiopulmonary-cerebral resuscitation. In: Kaye W, Bircherr N, eds. *Cardiopulmonary Resuscitation.* New York, NY: Churchill-Livingstone Inc; 1989:1-9

3. Paraskos JA. Biblical accounts of resuscitation. *J Hist Med Allied Sci.* 1992;47:310-321.

4. Stephenson HE Jr, Reid LC, Hinton JW. Some common denominators in 1200 cases of cardiac arrest. *Ann Surg.* 1953;137:731-744.

C

5. Zoll PM, Linenthal AJ, Gibson W, Paul MH, Norman LR. Termination of ventricular fibrillation in man by externally applied electric countershock. *N Engl J Med*. 1956;254:727-732.

6. Safar P, Escarraga L, Elam JO. A comparison of the mouth-to-mouth and mouth-to-airway methods of artificial respiration with the chest-pressure arm-lift method. *N Engl J Med* 1958;258:671-777.

7. Elam JO, Greene DG, Brown ES, Clements JA. Oxygen and carbon dioxide exchange and energy cost of expired air resuscitation. *JAMA* 1958;167:328-334.

8. Kouwenhoven WB, Jude JR, Knickerbocker GG. Closed-chest cardiac massage. *JAMA* 1960;173:1064-1067.

JAMA Theme Issue: Emergency Cardiac Care (CPR)

JAMA 1992 Oct 28: 268(16)

The Guidelines for Cardiopulmonary Resuscitation and Emergency Cardiac Care are printed here in nine detailed sections. A full listing of those individuals participating in the revision of these guidelines (see June 6, 1986 JAMA for previous version), editorials, conference news, and book reviews round out this current treatment of the status of emergency cardiac care.

Standards and Guidelines for Cardiopulmonary Resuscitation and Emergency Care available through:
American Heart Association
7220 Greenville Ave, Dallas, TX 75231-4596
800 242-1793   214 373-6300   Fax 214 706-1341
Web address: http://www.amht.org

Contact local heart association for CPR courses.

Cardiovascular Technologist

History
In December 1981, the American Medical Association (AMA) Council on Medical Education (CME) officially recognized cardiovascular technology as an allied health profession. Subsequently, organizations that had indicated an interest in sponsoring accreditation activities for the cardiovascular technologist were invited to appoint a representative to an ad hoc committee to develop *Standards (Essentials)*. Interested individuals were also invited to join the committee.

The ad hoc committee on development of *Standards* for the cardiovascular technologist held its first meeting on April 29, 1982, in Atlanta, Georgia. Twenty-one individuals attended the first meeting representing the following organizations: American College of Cardiology; AMA; American Society of Echocardiography; American College of Radiology; American Registry of Diagnostic Medical Sonographers; Grossmont College, El Cajon, Calif; American Society of Radiologic Technologists; Society of Diagnostic Medical Sonographers; National Alliance of Cardiovascular Technologists; Society of Non-Invasive Vascular Technology; American College of Chest Physicians; American Cardiology Technologists Association; Santa Fe Community College, Gainesville, Florida; and National Society for Cardiopulmonary Technology.

An initial draft of the proposed *Standards and Guidelines of an Accredited Educational Program in Cardiovascular Technology* was developed as a result of this meeting.

Subsequent meetings were held to refine and polish the *Standards*. In September 1983, the committee members reached agreement on the *Standards*. The Joint Review Committee on Education in Cardiovascular Technology (JRC-CVT) held its first meeting in November 1985 in preparation for its ongoing review of programs seeking accreditation in cardiovascular technology.

The *Standards* are adopted by the Commission on Accreditation of Allied Health Education Programs and the following sponsor organizations of the JRC-CVT: the American College of Cardiology, American College of Chest Physicians, American College of Radiology, American Society of Echocardiography, American Society of Cardiovascular Professionals, and Society of Vascular Technology (formerly the Society of Non-Invasive Vascular Technology).

Occupational description
The cardiovascular technologist performs diagnostic examinations at the request or direction of a physician in one or more of the following three areas: (1) invasive cardiology, (2) noninvasive cardiology, and (3) noninvasive peripheral vascular study. Through subjective sampling and/or recording, the technologist creates an easily definable foundation of data from which a correct anatomic and physiologic diagnosis may be established for each patient.

Job description
The cardiovascular technologist is qualified by specific technological education to perform various cardiovascular/peripheral vascular diagnostic procedures. The role of the cardiovascular technologist may include but is not limited to (1) reviewing and/or recording pertinent patient history and supporting clinical data; (2) performing appropriate procedures and obtaining a record of anatomic, pathologic, and/or physiologic data for interpretation by a physician; and (3) exercising discretion and judgment in the performance of cardiovascular diagnostic services.

Employment characteristics
Cardiovascular technologists may provide their services to patients in any medical setting, under the supervision of a doctor of medicine or osteopathy. The procedures performed by the cardiovascular technologist may be found in, but are not limited to, one of the following general settings: (1) invasive cardiovascular laboratories, including cardiac catheterization, blood gas, and electrophysiology laboratories; (2) noninvasive cardiovascular laboratories, including echocardiography, exercise stress test, and electrocardiography laboratories; and (3) noninvasive peripheral vascular studies laboratories, including Doppler ultrasound, thermography, and plethysmography laboratories.

According to the 1992 CAHEA Annual Supplemental Survey, entry-level salaries average $28,490. (AHRP-1997)

Resources
AMA Division of Allied Health
312 553-9355

American Registry of Diagnostic Medical Sonographers
600 Jefferson Plaza, Ste 360
Rockville, MD 20852-1150
800 541-9754   301 738-8401   Fax 301 738-0312
E-mail: bricksin-Rajev@msn.com

American Society of Cardiovascular Professionals/
Society for Cardiovascular Management
120 Falcon Dr, Unit #3
Fredericksburg, VA 22408
800 683-NSCT   703 891-0079   Fax 703 898-2393
E-mail: scanmce@aol.com

American Society of Echocardiography
4101 Lake Boone Trail, Ste 201, Raleigh, NC 27607
919 787-5181   Fax 919 787-4916
E-mail: ase@mercury.interpath.com

Cardiovascular Credentialing International
4456 Corporation Ln, Ste 120
Virginia Beach, VA 23462
800 326-0268   804 497-3380   Fax 804 497-3491

Joint Review Committee on Education in
Cardiovascular Technology
3525 Ellicott Mills Dr, Ste N
Ellicott City, MD 21043-4547
410 418-4800   Fax 410 418-4805
E-mail: assnhdqtrs@aol.com

Society of Vascular Technology
4601 President Dr, Ste 260, Lanham, MD 20706
800 SVT-VEIN   301 459-7550   Fax 301 459-5651

Careers, Medical (Physician)

Thinking about a career change? Take it step by step

Celia Paul
AM News Feb 25, 1995 p18-9

In the past five years, increasing numbers of physicians have grown dissatisfied with clinical practice and developed an interest in pursuing other careers. Yet determining which nonclinical options are appropriate can seem like an overwhelming task.

Below is a brief outline of an effective decision-making process, and suggestions of careers that have provided challenging opportunities for doctors.

The process
To focus on which nonclinical career might work for you, several steps are critical:

• *Examine your priorities.* What do you want from life? Is it more leisure time, including more control over your schedule? Do you want to develop an interest in an area that you now enjoy as an avocation? Are you willing to give up other factors to gain what you want? For example, are you interested in working regular hours, even if it means sacrificing high income?

• *Assess your skills.* There are many skills you have developed as a doctor that can be applied to different fields. These include: managing, persuading, thinking on your feet, research, quick decision-making and problem solving. They can all be utilized in careers as diverse as advertising and investment banking. As with your values, the question becomes one of focusing on your desires—that is, what skills do you now possess that you enjoy using most?

The careers
Let's look at some of the areas that might interest you. The actual choices are up to you, but this information can stimulate your thinking about options.

• *Entrepreneur.* Doctors have many of the necessary skills to become successful entrepreneurs. They know how to organize their time and determine priorities. They learn new skills quickly, think independently and follow through on plans. They also know how to promote—or even sell—which they use with patients to convince them to follow a course of treatment. Physicians' professionalism, however, often prevents them from accepting their selling abilities.

A wide variety of businesses interest doctors. Sometimes the choice is based on the individual's medical background. But a business also can be based on a side interest such as following the stock market, or a creative field, such as art dealership.

• *Hospital or private health care administration.* If you have strong organizational skills and an interest in staying closer to medicine, becoming a hospital administrator may be an attractive new career. Opportunities in private health care use these skills as well as entrepreneurial talents.

• *Corporate work.* Corporations, particularly those in the pharmaceutical and medical-equipment areas, have opportunities for doctors interested in working in a more structured setting. But some doctors become concerned about the loss of the autonomy that they have in private practice. Salaried corporate positions might be corporate medical departments or nonclinical positions in research and marketing.

• *Consulting.* If you would like to maintain autonomy, consulting may answer your needs. Media firms hire doctors to work on medical shows. Law firms hire medical consultants to advise on personal-injury and disability cases. Insurers use doctors for assessments, although this is a role increasingly filled by nurses. Besides knowledge of medicine, your analytical abilities combined with your communication skills enable you to make a contribution to these fields. You can provide consultation services independently or create your own business with a team of diverse colleagues.

• *Writing.* A growing field is medical public relations. Your responsibility is to obtain publicity for the client or company you are representing—which could be a private health care program, a medical product or a new drug. Some doctors also work for advertising agencies, writing copy that appeals to the medical market.

Another writing career is medical publishing for trade journals, books and newsletters. Your investigative skills, as well as written communication, are utilized extensively here. Opportunities here are much more limited, however, than in public relations.

Get guidance
Individual professional guidance can be extremely helpful in developing a career plan. Counselors who have worked with a number of doctors will be particularly tuned in to your situation and your options. Although no one can provide you with magical solutions, a counselor can guide you through the process, and help focus on what options will work best for you. Career testing will also help.

Whatever you do, think of the process of career change as an exciting opportunity to discover who you are, and fulfill your dreams.

How wide is the nonclinical universe?

The short answer to that question is this: It's wide—and getting wider. Although the vast majority (79 percent) of today's physicians are involved in patient care, more than 111,000 are not.

What are all those nonclinicians doing? The AMA gathered ideas gleaned from anecdotes offered by career consultants and search firms, and from the research of others. Career counselors report that physicians are finding nonclinical employment in the following fields/areas/roles:

Public relations. Many PR firms serve the field of medicine or its allied industries.

Medical publishing. Trade journals, books, abstracts, newsletters.

Media consultants on medical issues. Appearing on radio and TV talk shows is an effective way for a physician to build his or her medical practice; some doctors, however, are able to make a full-time career out of medical education for the public.

Copywriting for advertising agencies. Many ad agencies need people who can write copy that appeals to doctors and others in the medical community. The ad agencies' client includes HMOs, private health care, pharmaceutical manufacturers, and so on.

Heading up corporate medical departments.

Consultants. Law firms, insurance companies, and so on need experts. Performed on a per diem basis or through a retainer arrangement, part-time consulting can be a low-risk way of exploring other work environments and broadening one's network.

Program analyst or policy planner. At a private foundation or for a government group, such as the National Institutes of Health.

Investment banking. One physician banker's job is to analyze companies that produce high-tech medical products. According to a career consultant, this is a hot area, one in which tremendous amounts of money can be made.

Securities analysts. Physicians evaluate pharmaceutical firms or hospital chains for stock firms.

Hospital administration/private health care administration.

Sales of medical equipment. As employees of large medical-wares suppliers, like Baxter, physicians sell very sophisticated technical equipment to other physicians.

Sales of private health care programs.

Quality assurance. This is a good area for doctors who want to cut back on their schedules, because they can work at it part-time.

Accreditation. Being part of the team that evaluates hospitals.

Peer-review panelists.

Disability determination. A psychiatrist who works part-time for the federal government reviewing charts for people applying for disability benefits enjoys the flexible hours and "relaxing" work atmosphere. And if she ever decides to quit her regular full-time job, she knows she'll have at least some income while she is looking.

Computer-system developers.

Deans of medical schools.

Staff physicians to advertising agencies. The physician's job is to watch for potential problems with the Food and Drug Administration (FDA) and offer advice on specific medical problems.

Doctor-turned-writer. There are dozens of these, including the novelist-filmmaker Michael Crichton and psychiatrists Robert Coles and Oliver Sacks.

Real-estate developers. Many physicians are doing this. They work with hospitals first and see the opportunity to develop medical-office buildings and research facilities. Physicians can develop ophthalmological surgical centers, magnetic resonance imaging and ENT surgical centers.

Speculation that many of today's dissatisfied physicians suffered as medical students or residents from a lack of good career information does exist. Martin D. Keller, MD, PhD, chairman of the Department of Preventive Medicine at Ohio State University, reports that the information medical students receive today about their career options is still woefully inadequate. "In residency, they're exposed to only a very narrow band of clinical specialties and to virtually nothing nonclinical," he told us. "This restricts their horizons terribly."

In response to this need, Keller and his colleague, T. Donald Rucker, PhD, published *Careers in Medicine*[2] in 1986, which included a study of nonclinical job titles. How wide was the nonclinical universe in 1986? Keller and Rucker unearthed more than 900 job titles—a number that has certainly risen in the ensuing years.

They discovered some of what might be expected: MDs working as executive VPs of quality control (in pharmaceuticals manufacturing), associate deans of alumni affairs (in medical schools), directors of ethics advisory boards (at NIH), and health officers (for USAID)—and others were not: members of the US House of Representatives, commanders in chief (for the Pacific Fleet), and mayors (of Coos Bay, Oregon). They also found numerous presidents (of a major oil company, a publishing company, the Flying Physicians Association, and baseball's American League). They even found a magician (part-time).

The recent rapid changes in medicine, and the many organizations that have sprung up around the nonclinical fields, have given Keller and his colleagues an idea. "Perhaps it's time for an offshoot of the American Board of Medical Specialties," he said recently, "one that addresses the many nonclinical medical specialties. Perhaps an 'American Board of Nonclinical Medical Specialties'?"

Rucker and Keller did a multipage study on the diversity of the nonclinical options physicians have to choose from. The job titles, divided into 14 categories, "all...depict positions that differ significantly from those of traditional medical practice," Rucker and Keller note. Their search focused on jobs "where at least 80% of the physician's time was probably devoted to duties other than direct patient care."

Rucker and Keller complied their information through a process Rucker describes as "haphazard incrementalism": for two and a half years he saved everything that crossed his desk that mentioned an MD in a nonclinical role. The sources included numerous periodicals, newsletters, directories, and related references. "Since the source material did not cover the entire universe, or purport to be representative," Rucker and Keller caution, "our examples should be approached as guideposts for career exploration and not as a road map that specifies every choice that may appear on your journey. Moreover, additional career options may be found as doctors create their own businesses and assume positions never held previously by a physician."

Rucker and Keller note the study's limitations, which include a bias toward executive positions and some duplications of titles with similar responsibilities. "In cases where minimum numbers could be established, a figure is reported as a suffix to the entry, viz, 'Publishing, Editor.'"

"Finally," they add, "certain positions may require special experience and or additional training beyond the standard medical residency program"; for example, a dual doctorate (MD/PhD) may be required for some teaching or research positions, and "a master's degree in public health or business administration may be mandated by some employers."

Reference

1. Rucker TD, Keller, MD, eds. *Careers in Medicine: Traditional and Alternative Opportunities.* Garrett Park, Md: Garrett Park Press; 1986:223-245. Also see 1990 version.

(BED-1996; Adapted from)

Resources

Leaving the Bedside: The Search for a Nonclinical Medical Career, rev ed. Chicago, Ill: American Medical Association; 1996, 139 pp.
ISBN 0-88870-808-0 OP392096

American College of Physician Executives
4890 W Kennedy Blvd, Ste 200, Tampa, FL 33609
800 562-8088   813 287-2000   Fax 813 287-8993

Association of American Medical Colleges
2450 N Street NW, Washington, DC 20037
202 828-0400   Fax 202 828-1125
E-mail: webmaster@aamc.org

National Association of Advisors for the Health Professions, Inc.
PO Box 1518, Champaign, IL 61824-1518
217 355-0063   Fax 217 355-1287

National Health Council
1730 M St NW, Ste 500, Washington, DC 20036
202 785-3910   Fax 202 785-5923

Careers, medical, undergraduate

Medicine: A chance to make a difference and *Got that healing feeling;* brochures available from the American Medical Association.

Cataract

American Society of Cataract and Refractive Surgery
4000 Legato Rd, #850, Fairfax, VA 22033
800 451-1339   703 591-2220   Fax 703 591-0614
Web address: http://gwww.ascrs.org

Census

US Bureau of Census, Public Information Office
Department of Commerce, Washington, DC 20033
301 457-3670   Fax 301 547-3670
Web address: http://www.census.gov

Centers for Disease Control and Prevention

The Centers for Disease Control and Prevention (CDC), established as an operating health agency within the Public Health Service by the Secretary of Health, Education, and Welfare in 1973, is the federal agency charged with protecting the public health of the nation by providing leadership and direction in the prevention and control of diseases and other preventable conditions and responding to public health emergencies. It is composed of 11 major operating components: Epidemiology Program Office, International Health Program Office, National Immunization Program Office, Public Health Practice Program Office, National Center for Prevention Services, Center for Environmental Health, National Center for Injury Prevention and Control, National Institute for Occupational Safety and Health, National Center for Chronic Disease Prevention and Health Promotion, National Center for Infectious Diseases, and the National Center for Health Statistics.

The Agency administers national programs for the prevention and control of communicable and vector-borne diseases and other preventable conditions. It develops and implements programs in chronic disease prevention and control, including consultation with state and local health departments. It develops and implements programs to deal with environmental health problems, including responding to environmental, chemical, and radiation emergencies.

The Agency directs and enforces foreign quarantine activities and regulations; provides consultation and assistance in upgrading the performance of public health and clinical laboratories; organizes and implements a National Health Promotion Program, including a nationwide program of research, information, and education in the field of smoking and health. It also collects, maintains, analyzes, and disseminates national data on health status and health services.

To ensure safe and healthful working conditions for all working people, occupational safety and health standards are developed, and research and other activities are carried out, through the National Institute for Occupational Safety and Health.

The Agency also provides consultation to other nations in the control of preventable diseases, and participates with national and international agencies in the eradication or control of communicable diseases and other preventable conditions. (USG-1996)

C

Resources

Centers for Disease Control and Prevention
1600 Clifton Rd, NE, Atlanta, GA 30333
404 639-3311
Public Inquiry: 404 639-3286
Web address: http://www.cdc.gov

Center for Health Promotion and Education
Centers for Disease Control and Prevention
Bldg 1 South, Rm SSB249
1600 Clifton Rd NE, Atlanta, GA 30333
404 639-3492 404 639-3698

CDC Voice Information System and Disease
Information Hotline
404 332-4555
(Provides information on the *Morbidity and Mortality
Weekly Report* and public health topics with an option to
speak to a public health professional)

Cerebral Palsy

American Academy for Cerebral Palsy and
Developmental Medicine
6300 N River Rd, Ste 727, Rosemont, IL 60018-4226
847 698-1635   Fax 847 823-0536

United Cerebral Palsy Associations
71522 K St NW, Ste 1112, Washington, DC 20005
800 872-5827 202 842-1266   Fax 202 842-3519
Web address: http://www.ucpa.org/UCPA2.HTM

CHAMPUS — Military Dependents Care

The Office of Civilian Health and Medical Program of
the Uniformed Services (CHAMPUS) was established as
a field activity in 1974 under the policy guidance and
operational direction of the Assistant Secretary of Defense (Health Affairs). The Office is responsible for
administering a civilian health and medical care program
for retirees and the spouses and dependent children of
active duty, retired, and deceased service members. Also
included are spouses and dependent children of totally
disabled veterans. CHAMPUS also administers, for the
Uniformed Services, a program for payment of emergency medical and dental services provided to active duty
service members by civilian medical personnel.
(USG-1996)

Civilian Health and Medical Program
Office of CHAMPUS
Aurora, CO 80045-6900
303 361-1313

Charity

National Charities Information Bureau
19 Union Square West, New York, NY 10003-3395
212 929-6300   Fax 212 463-7083
(Evaluations of charitable groups)

Chemotherapy

The treatment of infections or malignant diseases by
drugs that act selectively on the cause of the disorder, but
that may have substantial effects on normal tissue.
(ENC-1989)

Resources

Chemotherapy Foundation
183 Madison Ave, Rm 403, New York, NY 10016
212 213-9292   Fax 212 689-5164

Child Abuse

JAMA Article of Note: AMA diagnostic and
treatment guidelines concerning child abuse and
neglect. Council on Scientific Affairs.

JAMA 1985 Aug 9; 254(6): 796-800

Child maltreatment is a serious and pervasive problem.
Every year, more than a million children in the United
States are abused, and between 2000 and 5000 die as a
result of their injuries. Physicians are in a unique position
to detect child abuse and neglect and are mandated by
law to report such cases. These guidelines were developed to assist primary care physicians in the identification
and management of the various forms of child maltreatment. A brief historical introduction and specific information about vulnerable families and children are presented. The physical and behavioral diagnostic signs of
physical abuse, physical neglect, sexual abuse, and emotional maltreatment are delineated. Information about
specific techniques for interviewing the abused child and
family, case management objectives, reporting requirements, and trends in treatment and prevention are also
provided.

*AMA diagnostic and treatment guidelines concerning
child abuse and neglect are available from:*

American Medical Association
Department of Mental Health
312 464-5066

Resources

Clearinghouse on Child Abuse and
Neglect Information
PO Box 1182, Washington, DC 20013-1182
800 394-3366   703 385-7565   Fax 703 385-3206
E-mail: nccanch@clark.net

National Child Abuse Hotline: Childhelps
PO Box 630, Hollywoood, CA 90028
800 422-4453
(24-hour number)
(For calls expressing concern about and suspect of
child abuse)

National Coalition Against Domestic Violence
PO Box 18749, Denver, CO 80218
303 839-1852   Fax 303 831-9251

National Committee for Prevention of Child Abuse
332 S Michigan Ave, Ste 1600, Chicago, IL 60604-4357
312 663-3520   Fax 312 939-8962

National Council on Child Abuse and Family Violence
1155 Connecticut Ave NW, Ste 400
Washington, DC 20036
800 222-2000   202 429-6695   Fax 818 914-3616
E-mail: nccafv@compuserve.com

Parents Anonymous
675 W Foothill Blvd, Ste 220
Claremont, CA 91711-3416
909 621-6184   Fax 909 625-6304

*Contact state Department of Child and Youth Services
for information on local programs and protective
initiatives.*

Children, Hospitalized

Children in Hospitals
300 Longwood Ave, Boston, MA 02115
617 355-6000   Fax 617 355-7429

Children and Youth Services, State Government Offices

Alabama Bureau of Family and Children's Services
64 N Union St, Montgomery, AL 36130
205 242-9500

Alaska Division of Family and Youth Services
PO Box H, Juneau, AK 99811
907 465-3170

Arizona Children, Youth and Families
1717 W Jefferson, Phoenix, AZ 85007
602 542-3981

Arkansas Children and Family Services
PO Box 1437, Little Rock, AR 72203
501 682-8770

California Office of Child Abuse Prevention
744 P St, MS 9-100, Sacramento, CA 95814
916 323-2888

Colorado Division of Family and Children's Service
1575 Sherman St, 2nd Fl, Denver, CO 80203
303 866-3672

Connecticut Department of Children and Youth Services
170 Sigourney St, Hartford, CT 06105
203 566-3536

Delaware Department of Services for Children,
Youth and their Families
1825 Faulkland Rd, Wilmington, DE 19805
302 633-2500

District of Columbia Family Services Administration
First and I St SW, Rm 215
Washington, DC 20024
202 727-5947

Florida Children, Youth and Families
1317 Winewood, Building 8, 3rd Fl
Tallahassee, FL 32399
904 488-8762

Georgia Family and Children Services
878 Peachtree St, 4th Fl, Atlanta, GA 30309
404 894-6389

Hawaii Child Protective Services
810 Richards St, Ste 400, Honolulu, HI 96813
808 548-6123

Idaho Division of Family and Children Services
450 W State St, Boise, ID 83720
208 334-5700

Illinois Department of Children and Family Services
406 E Monroe, Springfield, IL 62701
217 785-2509
800 252-2873 (24-hour number to report child abuse)

Indiana Division of Families and Children
302 W Washington, IGC-S, E414
Indianapolis, IN 46204
317 233-4451

Iowa Adult, Children and Family Services
Hoover State Office Bldg, Des Moines, IA 50319
515 281-5521

Kansas Youth Services Social and
Rehabilitations Department
Smith-Wilson Building
300 SW Oakley, Topeka, KS 66606
913 296-3284

Kentucky Division of Family Services
275 E Main St, Frankfort, KY 40601
502 564-6852

Louisiana Office of Community Services
PO Box 44367, Baton Rouge, LA 70804
504 342-4000

Maine Child and Family Services
State House Station #11, Augusta, ME 04333
207 289-5060

Maryland Child Welfare Services Office
300 W Preston St, Baltimore, MD 04333
301 333-0208

Massachusetts Department of Social Services
150 Causeway St, Boston, MA 02114
617 727-0900

Michigan Office of Children and Youth Services
300 S Capitol, PO Box 30037, Lansing, MI 48909
517 373-4506

Minnesota Community Social Services Division
658 Cedar St, 4th Fl, St. Paul, MN 55155
612 297-2673

Mississippi Division of Family and Children's Services
PO Box 352, Jackson, MS 39205
601 354-6661

Missouri Children's Services
Broadway Building, Box 88
Jefferson City, MO 65103
314 751-2882

Montana Department of Family Services
48 N Last Chance Gulch, Helena, MT 59601
406 444-5902

Nebraska Division of Human Services
PO Box 95026, Lincoln, NE 68509
402 471-9308

Nevada Children and Family Services
505 E King St, Carson City, NV 89710
702 687-4400

New Hampshire Children and Youth Services
Hazen Dr, Concord, NH 03301
603 271-4451

New Jersey Division of Economic Assistance
Quakerbridge Rd, CN 716, Trenton, NJ 08625
609 588-2361

New Mexico Children's Bureau
PO Box 2348, Santa Fe, NM 87504
505 827-8439

New York Department of Social Services
40 N Pearl St, Albany, NY 12243
518 474-9475

North Carolina Division of Social Services
325 N Salisbury St, Raleigh, NC 27603
919 733-3055

North Dakota Children and Family Services
State Capitol, Judicial Wing
600 E Blvd, Bismarck, ND 58505
701 224-4811

Ohio Family and Children's Services Division
51 N High St, 3rd Fl, Columbus, OH 43266
614 466-8783

Oklahoma Department of Human Services
PO Box 25352, Oklahoma City, OK 73125
405 232-1942

Oregon Children's Services Division
198 Commercial St SE, Salem, OR 97310
503 378-4374

Pennsylvania Children, Youth and Families
PO Box 2675, Harrisburg, PA 17105
717 787-4756

Rhode Island Department of Children and Families
610 Mt Pleasant Ave, Providence, RI 02908
401 861-6000

South Carolina Children and Families Services Division
PO Box 1520, Columbia, SC 29202
803 734-5670

South Dakota Child Protection Services Division
Knelp Bldg, Pierre, SD 57501
605 773-3227

Tennessee Department of Human Services
111 Seventh Ave N, Nashville, TN 37243
615 741-1820

Texas Department of Human Services
PO Box 149030, Austin, TX 78714
512 450-3080

Utah Division of Family Services
120 N 200 W, 4th Fl, Salt Lake City, UT 84103
801 538-4004

Vermont Department of Social and
Rehabilitation Services
103 S Main St, Osgood Bldg, Waterbury, VT 05671
802 241-2131

Virginia Department of Social Services
8007 Discovery Dr, Richmond, VA 23229
804 662-9236

Washington Children and Family Services Division
Office Building #2 M S: OB-41, Olympia, WA 98504
206 586-8654

West Virginia Social Services Bureau
1900 Washington E, Building 6
Charleston, WV 25305
304 348-7980

Wisconsin Children Youth and Services
PO Box 7851, Madison, WI 53707
608 266-6946

Wyoming Division of Youth Services
Hathaway Bldg, 3rd Fl, Cheyenne, WY 82002
307 777-6095

American Samoa Child Abuse Commission
Pago Pago, AS 96799
684 633-4485

Guam Department of Public Health and Social Services
PO Box 2816, Agana, GU 96910
671 734-7399

Northern Mariana Islands Youth Services Division
Office of the Governor, Saipan, MP 96950
670 322-9366

Puerto Rico Fernandez Juncos Station
PO Box 3349, Santurce, PR 00904
809 725-0753

US Virgin Islands Department of Human Services
Barbel Plaza S, St Thomas, VI 00802
809 774-0930

Childbirth, Natural

American Society for Psychoprophylaxis in Obstetrics
(ASPO Lamaze)
1200 19th St NW, Ste 300
Washington, DC 20036-2422
800 368-4404   202 857-1128   Fax 202 223-4579
E-mail: aspo@sba.com

International Childbirth Education Association (ICEA)
PO Box 20048, Minneapolis, MN 55420
612 854-8660

Children, Missing

Childfind Hotline
800 426-5678

Missing Child Hotline
800 843-5678 9 am-Midnight

MEDWATCH
800 I-AM-LOST (800 426-5678)
(Sponsored by Wyeth Laboratories)

National Center for Missing and Exploited Children
201 Wilson Blvd, Ste 550, Arlington, VA 22201
703 235-3900

Runaway Hotline
800 231-6946

Children's Health

Association for the Care of Children's Health
7910 Woodmont Ave, Ste 300
Bethesda, MD 20814
301 654-6549   Fax 301 986-4553

Children's Defense Fund
25 E St NW, Washington, DC 20001
800 CDF-1200   202 628-8787   Fax 202 662-3530

National Institute of Child Health and
Human Development
9000 Rockville Pike, Bethesda, MD 20892
301 496-5133

Chiropractic Medicine

Chiropractor. Alternate titles: Chiropractic; doctor, chiropractic. Diagnoses and treats musculoskeletal conditions of spinal column and extremities to prevent disease and correct body abnormalities believed to be caused by interference with nervous system: Examines patient to determine nature and extent of disorder. Performs diagnostic procedures including physical, neurologic, and orthopedic examinations, laboratory tests, and other procedures, using x-ray machine, proctoscope, electrocardiograph, otoscope, and other instruments and equipment. Manipulates spinal column and other extremities to adjust, align, or correct abnormalities caused by neurologic and kinetic articular dysfunction. Utilizes supplementary measures, such as exercise, rest, water, light, heat, and nutritional therapy. (DOT-1991)

Chiropractor Assistant. Aids chiropractor during physical examination of patients, gives specified office treatments, and keeps patient's records: Writes history of patient's accident or illness, and shows patient to examining room. Aids chiropractor in lifting and turning patient under treatment. Gives physiotherapy treatment, such as diathermy, galvanics, or hydrotherapy, following directions of chiropractor. Takes and records patient's temperature and blood pressure, assists in x-ray procedures, and gives first aid. Answers telephone, schedules appointments, records treatment information on patient's chart, and fills out insurance forms. Prepares and mails patient's bills. (DOT-1991)

JAMA Article of Note: Chiropractic decision and general counsel's statement.

JAMA 1988 Jan 1; 259(1): 81-3.

Resource
American Chiropractic Association
1701 Clarendon Blvd, Arlington, VA 22209
800 986-4636   703 276-8800   Fax 703 243-2593

Chiropractic Schools

California
Cleveland Chiropractic College
590 N Vermont Ave, Los Angeles, CA 90004
213 660-6166   Fax 213 665-5387

Life Chiropractic College, West
2005 Via Barrett, PO Box 367, San Lorenzo, CA 94580
510 276-9013   510 276-6798

Palmer College of Chiropractic, West
90 E Tasman Dr, San Jose, CA 95134
408 944-6000   Fax 408 944-6111

Los Angeles College of Chiropractic
PO Box 1166, Whittier, CA 90609-1166
310 902-3330   Fax 310 947-7863

Georgia
Life College
1269 Barclay Circle, Marietta, GA 30060
404 424-0554   Fax 404 429-8359

Illinois
National College of Chiropractic
200 E Roosevelt Rd, Lombard, IL 60148
630 629-2000   Fax 630 268-6600

Iowa
Palmer College of Chiropractic, West
1000 Brady St, Davenport, IA 52803
319 326-9656

Minnesota
Northwestern College of Chiropractic
2501 W 84th St, Bloomington, MN 55431
612 888-4777   Fax 612 888-6713

Missouri
Logan College of Chiropractic
PO Box 1065, Chesterfield, MO 63006-1065
314 227-2100   Fax 314 227-3832

Cleveland Chiropractic College
6401 Rockhill Rd, Kansas City, MO 64131
816 333-8230   Fax 816 361-0272

New York
New York Chiropractic College
PO Box 800, 2360 State Route 89
Seneca Falls, NY 13148-0800
315 568-3000   Fax 315 568-3015

Oregon
Western States Chiropractic College
2900 NE 132nd Ave, Portland, OR 97230
503 256-3180   Fax 503 251-5723

Texas
Parker College of Chiropractic
2500 Walnut Hill Ln, Dallas, TX 75229
214 438-6932   Fax 214 357-3620

Texas Chiropractic College
5912 Spenser Hwy, Pasadena, TX 77505
713 487-1170   Fax 713 487-1170

Christian Medical Society

Christian Medical and Dental Society
PO Box 5
Bristal, TN 37621-0005
423 844-1000   432 844-1005
E-mail: 75364.331@compuserve.com

Chronic Fatigue

CFIDS Association
PO Box 220398, Charlotte, NC 28222-0398
800 442-3437   704 365-9755

National Chronic Fatigue Syndrome and
Fibromyalgia Association
PO Box 18426, Kansas City, MO 64133
816 313-2000   Fax 816 313-2001
(Recorded message on publications—
about 3 minutes long)
E-mail: keal55A@prodigy.com

Cleft Palate

Cleft Palate Foundation
1218 Grandview Ave, Pittsburgh, PA 15211
800 24-CLEFT   412 481-1376   Fax 412 481-0847

American Cleft Palate Craniofacial Association
1218 Grandview, Pittsburgh, PA 15211
412 481-1376   Fax 412 481-0847

Cleveland Clinic

Obituary

George Washington Crile (1864-1943)
JAMA 1943 Jan 16; 209(121): 209

George Crile, cofounder of the Cleveland Clinic, died, January 7, 1943, at the Clinic, aged 78, of subacute bacterial endocarditis.

Dr. Crile was born in Chili, Ohio, November 11, 1864. He graduated from Ohio Northern University and in 1887 at the University of Wooster Medical Department, Cleveland, now Western Reserve University School of Medicine. Early in his career Dr. Crile studied in Vienna, London, and Paris. He served at Wooster University first as lecturer and demonstrator in histology and professor of the principles and practice of surgery. He was professor of clinical surgery at Western Reserve University from 1900 to 1911 and professor of surgery from 1911 to 1924. He was also director of research at the Cleveland Clinic Foundation, of which in 1921 he was a cofounder.

Research conducted by Dr. Crile included the basic factors concerned in circulation, respiration, blood chemistry and the body's source of energy. He was perhaps first to make a direct blood transfusion, performed in 1905.

Dr. Crile was awarded the Alvarenga prize by the College of Physicians of Philadelphia in 1901, the Cartwright prize by Columbia University in 1897 and 1903, the Senn prize by the American Medical Association in 1898, the American Medicine medal for service to humanity in 1914, the National Institute Society Sciences medal in 1917 and the Trimble Lecture medal in 1921. In 1925 the Lannelongue International Medal of Surgery was presented to him by the Societe internationale de chirurgie de Paris, in 1931 the Cleveland medal for public service and in 1940 the distinguished service gold key of the American Congress of Physical Therapy. He was a member of the founders' group of the American Board of Surgery. In 1923 he served as president of the American Surgical Association.

A member of the board of regents of the American College of Surgeons since 1913, Dr. Crile was chairman of the board from 1917 to 1939 and president of the college in 1916. In 1907 he was third vice president of the American Medical Association and chairman of its Section on Surgery, 1910-1911. He was also an honorary or corresponding fellow or member of many American and European societies.

In 1898 Dr. Crile was brigade surgeon in the volunteers with the rank of major, serving in Cuba and Puerto Rico. He was a major in the Officers' Reserve Corps, and professional director of the U.S. Army Base Hospital number 4, Lakeside Unit (British Expeditionary Force number 9) in service in France for one year beginning May 1917, subsequently serving as senior consultant in surgical research, lieutenant colonel and, in November, 1918, colonel. He was brigadier general in the Medical Officers' Reserve Corps in 1921, holding the same rank in the auxiliary reserve corps since 1929. In 1919 he was awarded the Distinguished Service Medal and in the same year became an honorary member of the Military Division, third class, Companion of Bath (British). In 1922 he was made a Chevalier in the French Legion of Honor.

Dr. Crile was a prolific contributor to scientific literature. Among numerous articles and textbooks are *Surgical Shock*, 1897: *Surgery of the Respiratory System*, 1899; *Certain Problems Relating to Surgical Operations*, 1901; *On the Blood Pressure in Surgery*, 1903; *Hemorrhage and Transfusion*, 1909; *Anemia and Resuscitation*, 1914; *Anoci-Association* (with Lower), 1914; second edition, *Surgical Shock and the Shockless Operation through Anoci-Association*, 1920; *Origin and Nature of the Emotions*, 1915; *A Mechanistic View of War and Peace*, 1915; *Man, an Adaptive Mechanism*, 1916; *The Kinetic Drive*, 1916; *The Fallacy of the German State Philosophy*, 1918; *A Physical Interpretation of Shock Exhaustion and Restoration*, 1921; *The Thyroid Gland* (with others), 1922; *Notes on Military Surgery*, 1924; *A Bipolar Theory of Living Processes*, 1926; *Problems in Surgery*, 1928; *Diagnoses and Treatment of Diseases of the Thyroid Gland* (with others), 1932; *Diseases Peculiar to Civilized Man*, 1934; *The Phenomena of Life*, 1936; *The Surgical Treatment of Hypertension*, 1938; and *Intelligence, Power and Personality*, 1941.

Dr. Crile's contributions to experimental work through the years resulted in many improvements in surgery and medical practice. He traveled widely; his charm and his forceful personality marked him for leadership early in his career. The contributions of his active and curious mind are a lasting monument.

Resource

Cleveland Clinic Hospital
9500 Euclid Ave, Cleveland, OH 44195
216 444-2200

Clinical Investigation

American Society for Clinical Investigation
6900 Grove Rd, Thorofare, NJ 08086
800 257-8290   609 848-1000   Fax 609 848-5274

Clinical Laboratories

AMA Policy

Clinical Laboratory Improvement Act of 1988 (260.980). Sub. Res. 46, A-90

It is the policy of the AMA to (1) continue and intensify its efforts to seek appropriate and reasonable modifications in the proposed rules for implementation of the CLIA 88; (2) communicate to Congress and to HCFA the positive contribution of physician office laboratory testing to high quality, cost effective care so that through administrative revision of the regulations, clarification of Congressional intent and, if necessary, additional legislation, the negative impact of these proposed regulations on patient care and access can be eliminated; (3) continue to work with Congress, HFCA, the Commission on Laboratory Assessment, and other medical and laboratory groups for the purposes of making the regulations for physicians' office laboratories reasonable, based on scientific data, and responsive to the goal of improving access to quality services to patients; (4) protest the reported high costs being considered for certification of laboratories and the limited number of laboratory categories proposed; (5) encourage all components of the federation to express to HFCA and members of Congress their concerns about the effect of the proposed rules on access and cost of laboratory services; and (6) protest the very limited list of waivered tests.

Clinical Laboratory Improvement Amendment
Public Law #101-578 enacted October 31, 1988

JAMA Article of Note: S.I. (Systeme International) Units

JAMA 1988 Jul 1; 260(1): 73-8

Guide for conversion from conventional units to Systeme International (S.I.) Units (Catalog #35-9-001-00), from:

American Society of Clinical Pathologists
2100 W Harrison St, Chicago, IL 60612-3798
800 621-4142   312 738-4890   Fax 312 738-1619

Resources
Commission on Office Laboratory Assessment (COLA)
9881 Broken Land Pkwy, Ste 200
Columbia, MD 21045
800 298-8044

Contact CLIA Hotline or Regional HCFA Office for applications of current law within each state.

Clinical Laboratory Sciences

History
The American Society of Clinical Pathologists (ASCP) began program accreditation review as one of the functions of its Board of Registry of Medical Technologists in 1933, working with the American Medical Association (AMA) Council on Medical Education (CME). The first set of Essentials of an Acceptable School for Clinical Laboratory Technicians was prepared by the ASCP Board of Registry and subsequently adopted by the AMA House of Delegates in 1937. The first list of 211 accredited programs was issued by the ASCP Board of Registry in 1933. The program title was changed to medical technology in 1947 with that year's revised *Essentials.*

The American Society for Clinical Laboratory Sciences (ASCLS) was organized in 1932. ASCLS joined ASCP in periodically revising the *Essentials* and was represented on the ASCP Board of Registry and the ASCP Board of Schools (established in 1949). ASCLS was recognized by the CME as one of the organizations collaborating with the AMA in accrediting educational programs.

In 1972, representatives of ASCLS and ASCP began talks that culminated in the incorporation of the National Accrediting Agency for Clinical Laboratory Sciences (NAACLS), in October 1973, as an organization independent of the professional organizations to which the authority to approve *Essentials* was delegated. NAACLS is the first agency of its kind to conduct the processes of detailed program review and recommendations through which the Committee on Allied Health Education and Accreditation (CAHEA) accredited programs. NAACLS is now an independent agency recognized by the US Department of Education.

Units within NAACLS include the Board of Directors, the Clinical Laboratory Sciences Programs Review Committee, and the executive office staff. The Board of Directors is the governing unit. The bylaws provide for sponsoring and participating organization representation on the board. ASCP and ASCLS are sponsoring organizations. Current participating organizations are the National Society for Histotechnology and the Association of Genetic Technologists. In addition to representatives from these professional organizations, the membership of the board includes two college educators, two public members, and a technician practitioner. The programs review committee includes technologist and pathologist program officials and educators/practitioners.

The American Association of Pathologists' Assistants is an affiliating organization and cooperates in the accreditation of training programs for pathologists' assistants.

In addition to the work associated with conducting program reviews, NAACLS provides workshops and publishes a periodic newsletter, as well as publications related to clinical laboratory scientist/medical technologist, clinical laboratory technician/medical laboratory technician, histologic technician/technologist, pathologists' assistant, phlebotomy, and cytogenetic technology programs. (AHRP-1997)

Clinical Laboratory Scientist/Medical Technologist

Occupational description

Laboratory tests play an important role in the detection, diagnosis, and treatment of many diseases. Clinical laboratory scientists/medical technologists perform these tests in conjunction with pathologists (physicians who diagnose the causes and nature of disease) and other physicians or scientists who specialize in clinical chemistry, microbiology, or the other biological sciences. Clinical laboratory scientists/medical technologists develop data on the blood, tissues, and fluids of the human body by using a variety of precision instruments.

Job description
In addition to possessing the skills of clinical laboratory technicians/medical laboratory technicians, clinical laboratory scientists/medical technologists perform complex analyses, fine-line discrimination, and error correction. They are able to recognize interdependency of tests and have knowledge of physiologic conditions affecting test results so that they can confirm these results and develop data that may be used by a physician in determining the presence, extent, and, as far as possible, cause of disease.

Clinical laboratory scientists/medical technologists assume responsibility and are held accountable for accurate results. They establish and monitor quality control and quality assurance programs and design or modify procedures as necessary. Tests and procedures performed or supervised by clinical laboratory scientists/medical technologists in the clinical laboratory focus on major areas of hematology, microbiology, immunohematology, immunology, clinical chemistry, and urinalysis.

Employment characteristics
Most clinical laboratory scientists/medical technologists are employed in hospital laboratories. The remainder are employed chiefly in physicians' private laboratories and

clinics; by the armed forces; by city, state, and federal health agencies; in industrial medical laboratories; in pharmaceutical houses; in numerous public and private research programs dedicated to the study of specific diseases; and as faculty of accredited programs preparing medical laboratory personnel. Salaries vary depending on the employer and geographic location.

Based on a 1994 survey by the American Society of Clinical Pathologists' Board of Registry, the median entry-level salary was $25,126, and the supervisor entry-level salary was $30,680. (AHRP-1997)

Clinical Laboratory Technician

Occupational description
Laboratory tests play an important role in the detection, diagnosis, and treatment of many diseases and in the promotion of health. Clinical laboratory technicians or medical laboratory technicians perform these tests under the supervision or direction of pathologists (physicians who diagnose the causes and nature of disease) and other physicians, clinical laboratory scientists/medical technologists, or other scientists who specialize in clinical chemistry, microbiology, or the other biological sciences. Clinical laboratory technicians/medical laboratory technicians (associate degree) develop data on the blood, tissues, and fluids of the human body by using a variety of precision instruments.

Job description
Clinical laboratory technicians/medical laboratory technicians (associate degree) perform all of the routine tests in an up-to-date medical laboratory and can demonstrate discrimination between closely similar items and correction of errors by use of preset strategies. The technician has knowledge of specific techniques and instruments and is able to recognize factors that directly affect procedures and results. The technician also monitors quality control programs within predetermined parameters.

Employment characteristics
Most clinical laboratory technicians/medical laboratory technicians (associate degree) work in hospital laboratories, averaging a 40-hour week. Salaries vary, depending on the employer and geographic location. Based on a 1994 survey by the American Society of Clinical Pathologists' Board of Registry, the median entry-level salary was $20,176, and the average salary was $24,544. (AHRP-1997)

Clinical Laboratory Technician/Medical Laboratory Technician (Certificate)

Occupational Description
Laboratory tests play an important role in the detection, diagnosis, and treatment of many diseases and in the promotion of health. Clinical laboratory technicians/ medical laboratory technicians perform these tests under the supervision or direction of pathologists (physicians who diagnose the causes and nature of disease) and other physicians, clinical laboratory scientists/medical technologists, or other scientists who specialize in clinical chemistry, microbiology, or biological sciences. Clinical laboratory technicians/medical laboratory technicians (certificate) perform many routine procedures in the clinical laboratory under the direction of a qualified physician and/or clinical laboratory scientist/medical technologist.

Job description
Clinical laboratory technicians/medical laboratory technicians (certificate) perform routine, uncomplicated procedures in the medical laboratory. These procedures involve the use of common laboratory instruments in processes where discrimination is clear, errors are few and easily corrected, and results of the procedures can be confirmed with a reference test or source within the working area.

Employment characteristics
Most clinical laboratory technicians/medical laboratory technicians (certificate) work in hospital laboratories, averaging a 40-hour week. Based on a 1994 survey by the American Society of Clinical Pathologists' Board of Registry, the median entry-level salary was $20,176, and the average salary was $24,544. (AHRP-1997)

Resources
American Society for Clinical Laboratory Sciences
7910 Woodmont Ave, Ste 1301
Bethesda, MD 20814
301 657-2768   Fax 301 657-2909

American Society of Clinical Pathologists
2100 W Harrison St, Chicago, IL 60612
800 621-4142   312 738-1336   Fax 312 738-1619
E-mail: info@asco.org or info@ascp.org
Web address: http://www.ascp.org

National Accrediting Agency for Clinical
Laboratory Sciences
8410 W Bryn Mawr Ave, Ste 670
Chicago, IL 60631-3415
773 714-8880   Fax 773 714-8886
E-mail: naacls@gnn.com

National Certification Agency for Medical
Laboratory Personnel
PO Box 15945-289, Lenexa, KS 66285
913 438-5110

Clinics
Contact state or local Department of Health for credentials on free clinics. Keep in mind that each state may vary as to what type of information they provide.

Closing a Medical Practice
Time to close

Greg Borzo
AM News Jan 1, 1995 p19-21

Closing a practice doesn't take as much work as building one, but it's more complex, expensive, and time-consuming than physicians may realize.

"There's a lot more to it than just locking the door on your way out," says Joan Damsey, president of Damsey & Associates in Portsmouth, Va.

Of course, rather than paying close attention to their soon-to-be former patients, payers, colleagues, and employees, many physicians find it more appealing to look ahead—whether that calls for retiring to a tropical island or joining a dynamic practice in a big city.

"With so much to look forward to, it's easy to overlook the mundane, sometimes painstaking details of closing a practice," says Robert Clausen, consultant with Medical Business Consultants-Midwest in Northbrook, Ill.

In fact, closing up shop takes careful planning and a lot of hard work.

"You should approach it like a military campaign and map out every step of the way," says J. Robert McGhee, DO, who recently closed his solo practice in Narragansett, RI, and moved to Ocala, Fla.

Although no statistics are available, consultants say physicians are closing their practices in record numbers due to the growth of group practice, managed care and vertical integration.

But not adequately tying up loose ends can lead to liability, tax, and professional problems soon after or years later, physicians say. Patients can suffer, too.

What to watch out for
One of the most important but often overlooked steps in closing a practice is properly preserving medical records. This is important to protect both you and your patients.

Some consultants say it's best to keep original records and give copies to whoever is taking responsibility for your patients. Others say it's OK to hand over the originals, as long as the new physician signs a legal agreement to maintain those records for a set number of years and make them available to anyone who needs them, including government agencies, professional associations and yourself.

"Just handing over the records is insufficient," Damsey says. "You need to protect yourself legally down the road."

Make sure the agreement covers anyone the physician may turn the records over to and the physician's heirs. In one case, a doctor died and his widow threw out all his records, including hundreds he got from another doctor, Damsey says. "This created legal problems for the original doctor and hurt the continuity of care for his patients."

Many states specify how long physicians must keep records. Where there are no requirements, such as in Virginia, keep records indefinitely, Damsey advises.

Others recommend keeping records for as long as the statute of limitations for professional liability, which varies by state and is usually less than 10 years.

For children, the statue of limitations does not begin running until they are 18 or 21 years old. As a result, obstetricians and pediatricians in some states may be required to keep records for more than 30 years.

To ease copying and storage expenses, purge your records by removing the ones of patients you saw only once for a routine checkup or procedure, the AMA suggests. Generally, it's safe to toss records of patients with uncomplicated problems that you haven't seen for several years.

Of course, business records are handled differently. Internal Revenue Service (IRS) guidelines suggest keeping those at least seven years.

Notify appropriate parties
Another crucial step is notifying patients, employees, agencies, and medical groups.

Start with employees to give them a chance to find another job. Don't expect all employees to take the news well, says *Closing Your Practice*, an AMA publication. Terminated employees have been known to sue physicians for back wages covering years of uncompensated overtime.

Try to alleviate hard feelings by helping employees find new jobs with colleagues, through pharmaceutical and supply sales representatives, or with the physician taking over your patients. But give at least one employee an incentive to stay on to handle accounts receivable and other loose ends after your practice closes.

In terms of patients, write to the active ones about 90 days before you plan to close, consultants say. Double that in rural or underserved areas. Send high-risk patients a registered letter; for inactive ones, run a notice in the paper.

Letters should include the reason you are leaving, your departure date and suggestions or resources for finding a new doctor. Include a form authorizing you to transfer their records.

Don't notify the patients too far in advance, however. They will start leaving you, which will hurt your cash flow, consultants and physicians advise. In addition, early notification prolongs the often unpleasant separation process.

"I was very close to my patients and the community, so the last month before I left felt like a month-long wake," Dr. McGhee says. "You don't want to drag that out."

Several agencies and organizations should be notified, too. These include hospitals, state licensing boards, Medicare, Medicaid, Blue Shield, major insurers, the IRS, state medical societies, specialty associations and the AMA.

Notify the Drug Enforcement Administration and state drug controllers early to give these typically overworked agencies extra time to respond with instructions on and clearance for disposing of narcotics and other controlled substances.

Finally, don't forget to notify everyone—from HMOs to janitorial services—with whom you have a contract, Damsey says. "It's very important to review all your contracts. Some of them could restrict your options."

One Virginia family physician, for instance, made plans to close his solo practice and join a group. After finalizing his plans, he notified his HMO 90 days in advance. The HMO reminded him, however, that his contract required him to give 180 days notice. As a result, his new group had to cover more than 1,000 HMO patients for three months.

Secretaries, nurses, and physicians at the new group resented this because they had no experience with managed care and had to learn a whole new set of rules and forms for dealing with these patients, Damsey says. "To say the least, this doctor did not start off on the right foot."

C

Other issues:

- *Professional liability insurance.* Be sure to get "tail" coverage for your liability exposure from work performed in the past. Physicians with occurrence coverage don't need to worry about tail coverage because their policies protect them regardless of when a claim is filed. Most physicians, however, have claims-made coverage, which provides protection for claims filed only while the policy is in effect.

Tail coverage can be very expensive. If you're going out of active practice, lifelong tail coverage can cost two to three times your annual medical professional liability premium, consultants say.

"Many physicians think they're going to retire with this huge chunk of cash, but tail coverage ends up taking a big bite out of that," Clausen says.

If you're moving rather than going out of practice, you still need tail coverage, but it will probably be offered as a relatively affordable rider on your new policy.

- *Consulting services.* Don't assume that your accountant, attorney, or practice management consultant knows enough about closing a practice to guide you through the process. Consider supplementing their skills with others who have more experience in this area. If you're joining a new group, hospital or employer, ask them to cover the expense as part of your incentive package.
- *Cash flow.* Giving up an established practice with a healthy cash flow for a new one with a a weak cash flow can be tenuous at best. Ease the transition by asking current patients to pay at the time of service. That way you get your money up front, you reduce the cost of billing and collecting, and you can clear the old books sooner.

In addition, don't hesitate to go after overdue bills, aggressively if necessary. Letters should get progressively tougher as the bills age. Telephoning is the next step, followed by turning over the old accounts to a collection agency.

If you're incorporated, consider letting the corporation continue to exist into the next tax year, Clausen says. As an asset, accounts receivable count as income and are taxed in the year a corporation dissolves.

In any event, cope with the drop in cash flow by securing a line of credit, looking for an income guarantee at your new practice setting or being prepared to dip into savings.

Despite such hurdles, those who have closed their practices say that it's not so bad. If there are good reasons to move on, don't shy away from the prospect.

"Closing up and moving to another state was a difficult decision because I was afraid it might turn out to be more trouble than it was worth," Dr. McGhee says. "Now I can say that if you don't like where you are, it pays to consider moving rather than grumbling about your situation or just letting inertia keep you where you are."

Cocaine

Cocaine Baby Helpline
800 662-4357
Operated by Northwestern University Memorial Hospital-Chicago

Cocaine Baby Helpline
800 821-4351
Operated by National Association for Prenatal Addiction and Education

Cocaine Hotline
800 662-4357 (800 662-HELP)
Operated by the National Institute on Drug Abuse

Information About Cocaine
800 262-2463 (800 COCAINE)
Operated by Fair Oaks Hospital, Summit, NJ

National Clearinghouse for Drug Abuse Information
PO Box 416, Kensington, MD 20795
301 443-6500

College Health

American College Health Association
PO Box 28937, Baltimore, MD, 21240-8937
410 859-1500   Fax 410 859-1510

Colon Disease

Crohn's and Colitis Foundation of America
386 Park Ave S, New York, NY 10016-7374
800 932-2423   212 685-3440   212 779-4098

Colon and Rectal Surgery
American Board of Colon and Rectal Surgery
20600 Eureka Rd, Ste 713, Taylor, MI 48180
313 282-9400   Fax 313 282-9402
E-mail: AdmnABCRS@aol.com

American Society of Colon and Rectal Surgeons
85 W Algonquin Rd, Ste 550
Arlington Heights, IL 60005
847 290-9184   Fax 847 290-9203

Competency Assurance

National Organization for Competency Assurance
1200 19th NW, Ste 300
Washington, DC 20036-2401
202 857-1165   202 223-4579

Complaints

Introduction

Physicians have long recognized that enforcement of their code of ethics is one of the fundamental responsibilities of the medical profession. As Principle II of the American Medical Association's *Principles of Medical Ethics* instructs, "A physician shall deal honestly with patients and colleagues, and strive to expose those physicians deficient in character or competence, or who engage in fraud or deception."

Enforcement of ethical guidelines has traditionally been conducted at several levels, including hospitals, county and state medical societies, and state licensing boards. Many state and county societies have met their responsibilities in this regard. Others have been deterred by the threat of expensive litigation. The purpose of this book is to provide direction to county and state medical societies for their enforcement activities, and by so doing increase the effectiveness of this essential form of professional self-regulation.

Following the procedures described herein will not eliminate the threat of litigation, but it should reduce the threat to an acceptable level of risk. The AMA will stand behind, and assist in the defense of, any medical society that follows these procedures in a good faith effort to enforce the AMA's *Current Opinions and Principles of Medical Ethics.*

This essay is not intended to preempt all other guidelines; the AMA recognizes that there are other acceptable approaches to enforcement.

General considerations

A program to enforce professional conduct has both substantive and procedural components. That is, the program must include (1) standards for what constitutes professional misconduct and (2) guidelines for processing an allegation that professional misconduct has occurred.

Substantive standards

Substantive standards for what constitutes professional misconduct must satisfy a number of criteria. First, they must be directly related to the purpose of ensuring competent, honest, and lawful medical care and not act as unreasonable restraints on competition among physicians. Thus, for example, it is permissible to prohibit the alteration of a patient's medical records with fraudulent intent, the breaching of a professional confidence, or the practicing of medicine while impaired by alcohol, drugs, physical disability, or mental instability. On the other hand, it would not be permissible to prohibit all advertising of medical services by physicians.

The difference between appropriate ethical canons and inappropriate restraints on competition can be further illustrated by the following example. It would not be permissible for a medical society to issue a fee schedule for its members on the ground that price competition leads to deceptive advertising of prices. However, it would be permissible for a medical society to prohibit the deceptive advertising of prices.

Substantive standards must also meet a requirement of specificity. If a professional conduct standard is characterized by vague language, then it can be applied in an arbitrary fashion. For instance, it would not be permissible to require simply that a physician have the ability "to get along with others" since it is uncertain how such an ability would be determined. On the other hand, it probably would be acceptable to impose sanctions for an inability to work with professional colleagues such that patient care is compromised.

Substantive standards should cover the full range of potential misconduct, including those that are commonly the subject of complaints. For example, medical societies should process allegations of excessive fees, substandard care, sexual misconduct, discourteous service, improper withholding of medical records, and impairment by alcohol or other drug use. Other examples of appropriate substantive standards can be found in the AMA's ethics code and the standards for disciplinary action of state licensing boards.

Procedural guidelines

Complaints against physicians that allege professional misconduct should be processed through two independent committees, a grievance committee and a disciplinary committee. The grievance committee screens, reviews, and/or refers complaints. In addition, it educates physicians and their patients about the professional obligations of physicians and decides whether disciplinary proceedings should be pursued.

When disciplinary proceedings are appropriate, they are conducted by a separate committee, the disciplinary committee. By maintaining the independence of the two committees, the disciplinary committee members undertake their responsibilities without any prior exposure to the case. This helps ensure that the ultimate judgment is rendered by an impartial decision maker.

The establishment of enforcement activities is an important public service, but such activities cannot succeed unless the public knows their existence and understands how to use them. The availability and the method of operation of the grievance and disciplinary committees should be continually publicized through appropriate channels of lay communication to the extent feasible. Concurrently, the profession should be kept informed of the committees' work by utilizing professional media such as medical journals, newsletters, secretary's letters, and president's pages.

The cooperation of the members of the medical societies, both in serving as committee members and in subjecting themselves to the jurisdiction of the committees when charged with misconduct, is essential if the enforcement activities are to be a success. The committees cannot function effectively unless the committee members have the full and complete cooperation of all member-physicians. In order to help ensure cooperation, the society may define as a ground for discipline the failure of a physician to cooperate with the proceedings of grievance and disciplinary committees. In addition, if a physician does not respond to a complaint after receiving notice, then the committees should process the complaint on the basis of the information that is presented by the complainant and that is discovered in the process of the committees' review.

Jurisdiction

Ordinarily, a medical society can exercise jurisdiction over its members only. However, it is in the interest of the public and the profession for patients to be able to pursue complaints against any physician. Consequently, non-member physicians should be encouraged to subject themselves to the jurisdiction of the committees. Some societies will accept a complaint against a nonmember physician only if the nonmember agrees to abide by the grievance and disciplinary procedures and to accept the decision of the grievance and disciplinary committees. In the absence of an agreement, these societies will refer the complaint to the state licensing board or another appropriate institution. Other societies will process a complaint against a nonmember without the nonmember's consent, although it may be difficult to do so without the nonmember's cooperation.

Medical societies often ask nonmember physicians to sign a consent form to demonstrate their willingness to abide by the grievance and disciplinary procedures. Other

C medical societies find a consent form unnecessary on the basis that nonmember physicians demonstrate their willingness to cooperate by responding to the complaints against them. In some cases, the signing of a consent form may deter a nonmember physician from pulling out of the process in midstream.

Bylaws and rules and regulations

All enforcement activities should be codified in the medical society's bylaws or the rules and regulations of the grievance and disciplinary committees to ensure that there is appropriate authority for the activities. Because amending bylaws is a cumbersome process, medical societies typically include much of the procedural information for grievance and disciplinary committees in their rules and regulations.

Some information should ordinarily be codified in the bylaws, including a statement of the authority of the grievance and disciplinary committees, the grounds for discipline, the size and general responsibilities of the committees, and the jurisdiction of the committees. Information that is not incorporated in the bylaws must still be provided to the medical society's membership, for example, in a policy manual.

Provisions for temporary committee members should be included for cases in which there is an insufficient number of committee members who qualify as impartial decision makers. Committee members will not meet the requirement of impartiality if they have prior involvement in the matter of if they have a conflict of interest.

Complaints

The handling of all complaints should include prompt acknowledgment, immediate review, impartial hearings, and transmittal of the decisions to those concerned.

Complaints may be filed by any person, professional or lay. While complaints are commonly filed by patients, they may also be filed by family or friends of patients or by colleagues of the physician. Ordinarily, complaints should be submitted in writing, and a simple form may be developed for the filing of complaints. The form should include places for the person making the complaint (the "complainant") to state his/her name and address, the name and address of the physician against whom the complaint is being filed, the names and addresses of any other persons who have knowledge of the facts involved, and a brief description of the reasons why the complaint is being filed. In addition, the medical society should ask for permission from the complainant, or the patient if the complainant is not the patient, to review the medical records that are relevant to the complaint. If permission is not received, then the complainant should be informed that it may not be possible to process the complaint. It may be appropriate to require that the complainant's signature be notarized to limit the possibility of abuse of the complaint process and to ensure that there is authority for the release of the patient's medical records.

When it is not feasible for the complaint to be submitted in writing, some societies permit the complaint to be presented orally, and the society's staff prepares a verbatim transcript of the complaint. Other societies find that a requirement of a written complaint does not present problems. If the patient is impaired, for example, a family member or friend can prepare the complaint. Because of the difficulties with accepting oral complaints, it may make sense to take them only in the exceptional cases in which it is not reasonable to require a written complaint.

Once a complaint has been received, it should be acknowledged promptly. The complainant should be informed of the procedures that the medical society will follow in response to the complaint. A simple brochure may be printed for this purpose. In particular, the complainant should be given a sense of the time that may be required before the complaint can be resolved. If the complainant understands that the process may be a lengthy one, then a good deal of impatience, frustration, and anger may be avoided.

In some cases, because of fear of reprisal, the complainant may desire that his or her name be kept confidential. If possible, a request for confidentiality should be honored. However, the complainant's desire for anonymity may conflict with the physician's right to confront or respond to any testimony or evidence that is used against him/her. While in some cases, the physician may not need to know who filed the complaint in order to respond to the charges, in other cases, the physician will need to know the name of the complainant. In such cases, the complainant should be notified that further proceedings may not be possible if the complainant is unwilling to have his/her name disclosed. (Adapted from GRE-1991)

Resource

Guidebook for Medical Society Grievance Committees and Disciplinary Committees. Chicago, Ill: American Medical Association; 1991 pp36. OP632891

To complain about:

Advertisements in newspapers:

Contact regional Federal Trade Commission.

Advertisements on TV and radio:

Federal Trade Commission
Sixth St and Pennsylvania Ave NW
Washington, DC 20580
202 326-2222
Web address: http://www.ftc.gov

Hospitals:

Contact appropriate state or local hospital council.

Physicians:

Contact appropriate county or state society.

Poor or questionable business practice:

Council of Better Business Bureaus
4200 Wilson Blvd, Ste 800, Arlington, VA 22203-1804
703 276-0100   Fax 703 525-8277

Contact local Better Business Bureau.

Distribution of Groups by Computer Use for Selected Applications

Computer Applications	Computer Use					
	Own/Lease		No		Total	
	%	N	%	N	%	N
Automated medical records	14.8	2327	85.2	13,443	100.0	15,770[a]
Search of medical information libraries	20.1	3158	79.9	12,548	100.0	15,706[b]
Drug utilization review	5.7	881	94.3	14,640	100.0	15,521[c]
CD-ROM drive	26.0	4031	74.0	11,475	100.0	15,506[d]

a. Excludes 1797 long-form respondents for whom computer use for medical records is unknown.

b. Excludes 1861 long-form respondents for whom computer use for online medical information is unknown.

c. Excludes 2046 long-form respondents for whom computer use for drug utilization review is unknown.

d. Excludes 2061 long-form respondents for whom computer use for ordering and inventory is unknown.

(MDG-1996)

Computers

References

American Association for Medical Systems and Informatics
1101 Connecticut Ave NW, Ste 700
Washington, DC 20036
202 857-1189

American Medical Informatics Association
4915 St Elmo Ave, Ste 302, Bethesda, MD 20814
301 657-1291   Fax 301 657-1296
E-mail: amia@camis.stanford.edu
Web address: http://amia2.amia.org

Medical computer journals:

Computers and Medicine
PO Box 36, Glencoe, IL 60022
708 446-3100 ISSN 0163-0547

MD Computing
Springer-Verlag, 175 Fifth Ave, New York, NY 10010
212 460-1500 ISSN 0724-6811

Physicians and Computers
Physicians Publications, Limited Partnership
2333 Waukegan Rd, Ste S-280, Bannockburn, IL 60015
847 940-8333

Consultants and Consulting Organizations

How to choose an advisor

Defining goals

The first step in achieving a goal is identification of that goal. This maxim is obvious but too easily overlooked, especially by physicians who are anxious about their futures. They may not identify the source of their anxiety —whether a shrinking patient base, loss of clinical autonomy, or fear of losing all options—or the specific goals they might establish to address those problems. Instead, their impulse may be to hire an expert immediately to find a "quick fix," without first fully analyzing the situation.

Before retaining an expert, physicians must clearly identify the specific goals to be accomplished. In a multiphysician practice, the physicians should discuss their individual concerns and goals as a group. Open discussion will prompt thoughtful evaluation and may reveal that individual concerns and goals vary among the group. Concerns and objectives should be committed to writing to assist in moving all parties in the same direction and, subsequently, in evaluating the progress and results of the project.

The attorney or consultant selected should also be capable of providing strategic analysis on an ongoing basis, especially when the project goal is creation of a physician hospital organization, a physician network, an individual practice association, or some other entity. It is essential to determine whether the proposed structure will meet the physicians' objectives. Otherwise, the physicians may invest substantial resources in an entity that is doomed to fail. *Just as diagnosis precedes treatment in medicine, strategic analysis must precede creation of a business venture.*

Screening candidates

The first step in screening potential candidates is to identify the training, skill, and experience that the consultant or attorney should possess. This job description will serve as an objective yardstick against which to evaluate candidates.

To begin narrowing the search, qualifications related to education and experience can be checked against the criteria outlined in the job description. Then, depending on the nature of the work to be performed, there are many other factors to consider, such as:

- whether the consultant or attorney has particular expertise, as demonstrated by training and experience, and whether that expertise is directly applicable to the job requirements;
- how long and for how many clients the candidate has provided the particular services that are required;
- whether there are any possible conflicts of interest; and
- whether consulting is a full-time occupation, or something that supplements other work.

Understanding important differences

Physicians also must understand the variations that exist among consultants and attorneys, and consider how those differences may impact the advisor's ability to complete the project successfully. Consulting and legal services come in many packages. They may be provided by those who work independently, in small groups or as members of large firms. No particular arrangement is necessarily better than another, but physicians must understand exactly with whom they will be working once a contract is signed and how accessible that party will be.

For example, those retaining a sizable firm may discover after a contract is signed that junior staffers have been assigned to their account. Physicians working with individual practitioners or small firms could find them too overcommitted to give full attention to every client. While none of these problems necessarily will occur, it is important to understand the nature of the consultant or attorney under consideration and carefully evaluate the possible advantages and disadvantages of each.

Reviewing responses

How candidates reply to the request for information may be as important as the content of their reply.

- Is the response prompt? A consultant or attorney may be unable to reply promptly because his or her services are in great demand. However, no matter how competent, an advisor will be of little value if he or she is stretched too thin to accommodate the physician's needs. On the other hand, a generic glossy brochure that can be sent out in immediate reply to an inquiry does not necessarily indicate quality or responsiveness.
- Does the response directly address the questions and issues raised in the request for information, or does it consist of "boiler plate" culled from the computer? The amount of attention paid to the inquiry is a good indicator of the attention the project will receive.

Checking references

Reviewing a candidate's references is one of the most important parts of the screening process.

- Are timely and relevant references provided? Providing relevant references, and not just those of satisfied clients, probably indicates that the advisor clearly understands the nature of the work to be performed. It is also important to determine if there is a consistent pattern of satisfactory performance in the advisor's background.
- Do the references check out? References are of no use unless verified, but surprisingly few people take this step. The basic questions to ask are obvious:
  1. Was the work satisfactorily completed?
  2. Was it completed on time and on budget?
  3. Did the advisor work comfortably and well with physicians and staff members?
  4. Would the practice hire the advisor again?

You can probably anticipate the answers—no one is likely to provide references to dissatisfied clients. What is more valuable, then, is not to ask only these questions, but to ask "Why?" and "In what way?" to gain real insight into how the candidate operates.

Draft a structured questionnaire and end each interview with an open-ended question to encourage spontaneous answers, such as "What did you like most about this consultant?" "What did you like least?" It's also worth asking whether the client knows of others who have used the advisor; that may lead you to sources of information beyond those screened by the advisor.

Finding the right fit

The final test is purely subjective: Is the chemistry right? Objective analysis may eliminate many candidates, but final selection requires the subjective assessment of compatibility that only face-to-face encounters can provide. An advisor who must work with the physician can determine whether the fit in personalities, values, and working styles is right. (CON-1993)

Resources

American Association of Healthcare Consultants
11208 Waples Mill Rd, Ste 109, Fairfax, VA 22030
800 362-4674   703 691-2242   Fax 703 691-2247
E-mail: consultahc@aol.com

Doctors Advisory Network
American Medical Association
515 N State St, Chicago, IL 60610
800 AMA-1066 press #2

Society of Medical-Dental Management
Consultants (SMD)
6215 Larson, Kansas City, MO 64133
800 826-2264   Fax 816 353-3137
In Missouri: 816 353-8488

Consumer Health Information Centers

A Piece of My Mind

Encourage information therapy

Katherine Lindner
JAMA 1992 May 20; 267(19): 2592

About eight years ago, all health professionals and the public had unrestricted access to the medical library where I was then employed, but patients were required to "ask their doctor" for information from the library. When patients themselves came in or called the library directly, many situations arose that required delicate handling and resulted in rather embarrassing situations. I would have to say, "Our policy requires that I consult with your physician. Sometimes he or she likes to help us select material for you. This arrangement can help you communicate better with your physician." Some patients who became perturbed by this policy might try sending a relative to the public library or might send their family member to get the materials from us later. We could give the materials to family members since they were "members of the public," but if we knew they were going to give the information to a patient, we had to explain and deal with the "doctor-approval policy."

As I became more distraught by the manner in which I had to handle patient requests for information, I began to investigate the ethics of restricting access to any information. The mandate to open medical libraries to health consumers has been with us since 1982, as stated in the President's Commission on Ethical Practices in Medicine. The Library Bill of Rights states that libraries should challenge censorship, and the American Library Association Statement of Professional Ethics states that librarians should protect each user's right to privacy.

The Office of Intellectual Freedom of the American Library Association also pointed out that there are state laws that guarantee confidentiality for library patrons (for example, New Jersey statute a:73-43.2 entitled "Confidentiality of Library Users' Records"). According to the administrators in the Intellectual Freedom Office, the policy of giving information to a patient only through his or her physician both breaches the patient's confidentiality and breaks the law by revealing the question to a third party, the physician.

The Medical Library Association has formulated standards for certain-sized hospital libraries recommending reference services to patients and the public. At the Medical Library Association's annual convention in Washington, DC, this week the membership will be voting to adopt the MLA Code of Ethics, which includes an ethical obligation "to advocate access to health information for all." There is a Consumer and Patient Health Information Section of the Medical Library Association with about 300 members, but there are still many medical libraries that are closed to consumers and many physicians who think it is inappropriate for health consumers to use them.

After becoming aware of the ethical standards and recommendations, the Englewood Hospital Library staff developed guidelines for providing information to patients and the public. We explain that questions are kept confidential. We include a disclaimer letter with the material we send to health consumers at home or in the hospital. We state that we are not recommending any particular treatment; that this material might not represent all that is available on the subject; that the information might not apply specifically to the patient's own condition; and that the material should be used to formulate questions for discussion with his or her physician.

The following represent typical questions at our state-funded Regional Consumer Health Information Center. We received a phone call from a health consumer who wanted information on phrenic nerve paralysis secondary to the use of a Hickman catheter for chemotherapy. A man called whose wife was scheduled to have knee replacement surgery: "Can I stop in to pick up some information? She has to make up her mind." A public librarian called: "I have a patron who is interested in the latest research on amyotrophic lateral sclerosis." Consumers also request PDQ (Physician Data Query) computer searches on cancer treatment and protocols around the United States. Often a patient will find an alternative procedure or therapy in another area of the country, call the researcher, and ask for advice. Sometimes surgery is avoided; sometimes treatments are found that the patient's physician had not discussed. Some physicians wonder how we handle providing information on a disease with a probable fatal outcome. We always ask the person what he or she already knows. In 100 percent of the cases, the person already knew the prognosis and was presently looking for any new therapies.

Every scrap of information leading patients in the direction of discovering more about their disease becomes "information therapy." We have found that the physician-patient relationship is greatly enhanced when the physi-

cian says to the patient, "Go to the library, read about your disease, let me know what you find, and we'll discuss it." The process of finding information gives the patient a sense of control and empowerment. It is also a challenge for today's physicians to keep up with the great volume of medical literature by reading current journals, making information requests to libraries, and taking advantage of the new on-line and CD-ROM technologies that enable users to search Medline from their office computers.

All the information gathered by the patient and the physician is beneficial for continued care and treatment decisions.

Physicians and health professionals should continue on the path of sending their patients through the doors of medical libraries. Judging from the questions we librarians receive, there may be an information gap between what physicians are providing to patients and what patients want to know. Physicians can take advantage of consumer health library collections to build their own medical office resources. At the June 1991 meeting of the American Medical Association House of Delegates, a resolution (No. 237) was proposed that encouraged hospitals and medical schools to make their libraries accessible for use by patients and their families. As the AMA Board of Trustees continues to study this resolution, we hope it will also encourage funding for consumer health resources and library staffing and medical school libraries.

At a conference in June 1991, Dr. Bernie Siegel said, "The word patient means a submissive sufferer. If you have an illness, please just get the word uncooperative into your medical record. You do that and your statistics improve dramatically." We assume "uncooperative" means asking millions of questions, being persistent, examining one's own medical records, and so on. I am hoping that patients will get in their charts that they have "researched their disease [or procedure] in the medical library." Patients will be more satisfied with their care as they become more knowledgeable and participate in the decision-making process.

Resources

Center for Medical Consumers and
Health Care Information
237 Thompson St, New York, NY 10012
212 674-7105   Fax 212 674-7100

Community Health Information Library
Hamady Health Sciences Library
Hurley Medical Center
1 Hurley Plaza, Flint, MI 48502
810 257-9427   Fax 810 257-4257

Consumer Health Information Network
Mary Lou Himes Burton
The College of Physicians of Philadelphia
19 S 22nd St, Philadelphia, PA 19103
215 561-6050

Consumer Health Protection
Center for Science in the Public Interest
1875 Connecticut Ave NW, #300
Washington, DC 20009-5728
202 332-9110   Fax 202 265-4954

Consumer Information Center
18 F St NW, Rm G-142, Washington, DC 20405
202 501-1794   Fax 202 501-4281

Health Education Center
5th Avenue Pl, Ste 313, Pittsburgh, PA 15222-3099
412 392-3160

Medical Library, Kaiser Permanente Medical Center
280 W MacArthur Blvd, 12th Fl, Oakland, CA 94611
510 596-6158   Fax 510 595-7522

National Center for Health Education
72 Spring St, Ste 208, New York, NY 10012-1273
212 334-9470   212 334-9845

National Health Information Center
PO Box 1133, Washington, DC 20013-1133
800 336-4797   301 565-4167   Fax 301 984-4256
E-mail: nhicinfo@health.org
Web address: http://nhic-nt.health.org

Office of Disease Prevention and Health Promotion
US Department of Health and Human Services
800 336-4797   301 565-4167

Consumer Protection Hotline

Contact state Attorney General's office.

Contact local state Department of Public Health.

Consumer Price Index

Bureau of Labor Statistics
441 G St NW, Washington, DC 20212
202 523-1221
Web address: http://www.stats.bls.gov

Contact Lenses

Contact Lens Association of Ophthalmologists, Inc
523 Decatur St, Ste 1
New Orleans, LA 70130-1027
504 581-4000   Fax 504 581-5884

Continuing Medical Education

When a physician makes a life-long commitment to serving others through the profession of medicine, he or she must also make a commitment to continuous learning. Medical knowledge, science, and technology advance so quickly and so dramatically that it is impossible to offer competent medical care without ongoing medical education.

As a result, one of the great challenges physicians face is how to integrate ongoing education into a daily life already filled with other equally important professional and personal commitments. Physicians who want to realize the goals articulated by Manning and DeBakey in their book *Medicine, Preserving the Passion*, must attend to their personal as well as their professional needs.

They must be self-directed and look for learning opportunities in every dimension of their practices. This means reflecting on the patient care they provide; determining precisely what they need and want to learn; choosing the learning activities that will most effectively help them reach their learning goals; and finding the time and place for the experience.

Reflection on patient care
Continuous learning in medicine is grounded in patient care and the active process of reflecting on the decision made. Every time a physician asks, "Why?" and then goes on to find the right answer, learning occurs. It happens each time a physician reviews a patient's chart and questions: "Do I really know this patient? Did I relate and communicate effectively? Would I do anything differently today in diagnosis and management?"

Needs and objectives
Physicians should work to discover, on their own, where their educational needs lie by conducting a personal "needs assessment" and then setting specific learning objectives. Their objectives will vary. Some may want simply to confirm that they have the critical content knowledge needed in a particular area; others may want to learn the latest new developments or master advanced techniques; still others may need knowledge in a new content area in order to provide the best possible patient care.

Planning
Once a physician has established his or her learning objectives, the next step is to develop an educational plan for accomplishing them. The more precise the objectives, the easier and more effective the planning will be. The planning process should include consideration of different learning strategies and opportunities as well as a combination of educational methods and formats.

Reading
Reading the medical literature provides the foundation of continuous learning for most physicians. A literature search can quickly identify the total body of knowledge on a specific subject, but physicians must be selective in their reading.

Consultation
Consulting with another physician who has special expertise in a particular area provides a rewarding learning experience, especially when the consultant explains his or her approach to clinical problem solving. Some organizations now offer consultations by telephone, computer, or other electronic media to physicians who may be in more isolated areas. Computerized databases offer access to extensive data sources at the physician's convenience and computer technology will have an increasingly important impact on medical education.

Discussions with colleagues
Studies have shown that many physicians bridge the gap between learning and changing how they practice through discussions with colleagues, either individually or in small groups. Such opportunities are numerous in medical settings—on rounds, at meals, in the staff lounge. Discussions about specific patients should, of course, always take place in a setting that ensures confidentiality.

Teaching
Teaching, because it requires preparing subject matter and communicating to others, often leads to increased knowledge for the instructor. Teaching well is not easy and demands considerable insight, concentration, and organization so that the subject matter is clearly and effectively communicated to the individual learner.

Formal education programs

Many institutions and organizations sponsor educational conferences, seminars, and workshops, at both the national and local level. Those who have demonstrated that they meet the basic standards for planning, presenting, and evaluating quality continuing medical education (CME) are accredited. While most physicians can easily identify a wide variety of accredited CME activities, selecting those that best meet their individual needs presents a greater challenge. (LIFE-1993)

Continuing Medical Education Learning Assessment Form

The Continuing Medical Education Learning Assessment Form (CLAF) is designed for use by a sponsor of continuing medical education courses to provide information about training in new procedures for which the physician will request new or expanded privileges. CLAF is not intended to document competency in a specific procedure. It is not designed for sponsors to use in all CME activities or for sponsors to use in CME courses on procedures that will not support a physician's request for new or expanded hospital privileges. It may be useful to hospital credentialing committees as part of the evidence considered in their privileging decisions.

This form is available from The American Hosptial Association or the Continuing Medical Education Division of the American Medical Association.

Resources
Association of CME Professionals
Alliance for Continuing Medical Education
60 Revere Dr, Ste 500, Northbrook, IL 60062

Accreditation:
Accreditation Council for Continuing Medical Education
515 N State St, Ste 7340, Chicago, IL 60610
312 464-2500   Fax 312 464-2586

Accreditation, intrastate:
Contact state medical association to apply.

Cooley's Anemia

Cooley's Anemia Foundation
129-09 26th Ave, Flushing, NY 11354
800 221-3571 718 321-2873   Fax 718 321-3340

Correctional Health Care

National Commission on Correctional Health Care
2105 N Southport, Ste 200, Chicago, IL 60614
312 528-0818   Fax 312 528-4915

Credentialing

For professional:
Data Bank (Information prior to 1990)
Federation of State Medical Boards of the United States
6000 Western Pl, Ste 707
Fort Worth, TX 76107
817 735-8445   Fax 817 738-6629

National Practitioner Data Bank
(Established under the Health Care Quality Improvement Act)
UNISYS Corporation
8301 Greensboro Dr, Ste 1100
McLean, VA 22102
800 767-6732

For public:
Directory of Physicians in the United States,
35th ed Chicago, Ill. American Medical Association; 1996; 4 volumes hardbound. ISBN 0-89970-618-5 (found in many public and university libraries); on CD-ROM, ISBN 0-89970-830-7.

Physician Select
Web address: http://www.ama-assn.org

American Board of Medical Specialties
1007 Church St, Ste 404
Evanston, IL 60201-5913
800 776-2378 847 491-9091   Fax 847 328-3596
(information on board certification)
Web address: http://www.certifieddoctor.com

Critical Care

American Board of Internal Medicine
U. City Science Ctr, 3624 Market St
Philadelphia, PA 19104
800 441-2246   215 243-1500   Fax 215 382-4702

American Board of Neurological Surgery
Smith Tower, Ste 2139, 6550 Fannin St
Houston, TX 77030-2701
713 790-6015

American Board of Obstetrics and Gynecology
2915 Vine St, Dallas, TX 75204-1069
214 871-1619   Fax 214 871-1943

Society of Critical Care Medicine
8101 Kaiser Blvd, Anaheim, CA 92808-2214
714 282-6000   Fax 714 282-6050
Web address: http://execpc.com/sccm

Board Certification:
American Board of Anesthesiology
4101 Lake Boone Trail, Ste 510, Raleigh, NC 27607
919 881-2570   Fax 919 881-2575

Pediatric Critical Care:
American Board of Pediatrics
111 Silver Cedar Ct, Chapel Hill, NC 27514
919 929-0461   Fax 919 929-9255

Surgical Critical Care:
American Board of Surgery
1617 John F. Kennedy Blvd, Ste 860
Philadelphia, PA 19103
215 568-4000   Fax 212 563-5718

Cults

Cult Hotline and Clinic
1651 Third Ave, New York, NY 10028
212 860-8533

Task Force on Cults
711 Third Ave, 12th Fl, New York, NY 10017
212 983-4977

Current Procedural Terminology

Poetry and Medicine

Terms

Bruce A. Noll
JAMA 1993 July 7; 270(1): 10

Come to terms
with terminology
biopsy, hematology,
phlebotomy,
cirrhosis, hemochromatosis,
venipuncture, platelets, CBC,
ferritin, hemoglobin,
weekly bleeding,
barber tradition.
Feel it in your veins,
it's in your blood line,
the good news—it's treatable,
the bad news—the treatment,
blood bags, skim off the slag,
this is a sticky one,
it's a stickler all right,
better than leeches,
take a cotton to this,
take a little sample here,
there'll be a little stick,
need a little blood,
needle him a bit.
Come to terms
with terms like
mortal after all,
nothing lives forever,
lease on life, life is short,
hang by a thread,
end of the rope,
end of the trail,
this too will pass,
pass this way but once,
can't pass this by,
I'll pass, thank you.

How was the Current Procedural Terminology developed?

Current Procedural Terminology (CPT) was first developed and published by the American Medical Association in 1966. This first edition was designed to serve as a method to cultivate the use of standard terms and descriptors for documentation of procedures in the medical record; to facilitate the communication of accurate information on procedures and services to agencies concerned with insurance claims; to provide the basis for a computer-oriented system for the evaluation of operative procedures; and to contribute basic information for actuarial and statistical purposes.

The first edition of CPT was a preliminary document that included primarily surgical procedures, with limited sections on medicine, radiology, and laboratory procedures. In 1970, the second edition was published and was presented as an expanded system of terms and codes for the designation of diagnostic and therapeutic procedures in surgery, medicine, and the specialties. At this time, a five-digit coding system was introduced, to re-place the former four-digit classification. Another significant change in the second edition was a listing of procedures relating to internal medicine.

In the mid- to late 1970s, the third and fourth editions of CPT were introduced. The fourth edition, published in 1977, represented significant updates in medical technology. In this edition, a system of periodic updating was introduced to keep pace with the rapidly changing medical environment.

In 1983, CPT was adopted as part of the Health Care Financing Administration's (HCFA) Common Procedure Coding System (HCPCS). With this adoption, HCFA mandated the use of HCPCS for the reporting of services for Part B of the Medicare Program. By October 1986, HCFA had also required the use of HCPCS by state medical agencies for use in the Medical Management Information System. In July 1987, as part of the Omnibus Budget Reconciliation Act, HCFA mandated the use of CPT for reporting outpatient hospital surgical procedures.

Today, in addition to use in federal programs (Medicare and Medicaid), CPT is used extensively throughout the United States as the preferred system of coding and describing physicians' services. (CPT-1993)

The CPT process

Many inquiries about the CPT process are received by the AMA. For example, how does a code get assigned for a service or a procedure performed by a physician? The following essay presents an overview of the CPT process.

Who maintains CPT?

The CPT Editorial Panel has the responsibility for the maintenance of CPT. This panel is made up of 12 physicians, eight nominated by the AMA and one each nominated by the Blue Cross and Blue Shield Association, the Health Insurance Association of America, the Health Care Financing Administration, and the American Hospital Association. This panel of physicians has the authority to revise, update, or modify CPT.

The American Medical Association provides staff support for the CPT Editorial Panel. The AMA appoints a staff secretary who is responsible for recording the minutes of the meetings and keeping records as necessary for the work of the panel.

Supporting the Editorial Panel in its work is the CPT Advisory Committee. The Advisory Committee is made up primarily of physicians nominated by the National Medical Specialty Societies represented in the AMA House of Delegates. The primary objectives are (1) to serve as a resource to the Editorial Panel, by advising them on procedure coding and nomenclature as relevant to the member's specialty; (2) to provide documentation to staff and the Editorial Panel regarding the medical appropriateness of various medical and surgical procedures; and (3) to suggest revisions to CPT. Most of the work of the Advisory Committee is conducted through AMA staff by letter and telephone. The Advisory Committee meets annually to discuss items of mutual concern and to keep abreast of current issues in coding and nomenclature.

How are suggestions for changes to CPT reviewed?

A very specific pathway is followed when a suggestion is

received for a revision of CPT, whether it be an addition or deletion of a code or modification of existing nomenclature.

First, AMA staff reviews all correspondence to evaluate coding suggestions. If it is determined that the question has already been addressed by the panel, the requestor is informed of the Panel's interpretation. However, if it is determined that the request is a new issue or *significant* new information is received on an item that has been previously reviewed by the Panel, it is referred to the appropriate members of the Advisory Committee. If the advisors who have been contacted agree that no new code or revision is needed, then AMA staff responds to the requestor, providing information on how existing codes should be used to report the procedure.

However, if all advisors concur that a change should be made, or if two or more advisors disagree or give conflicting information, then the issue is referred to the Editorial Panel for resolution.

In addition to the Advisory Committee opinions, current medical periodicals and textbooks are used to provide up-to-date information about the procedure or service. Further data are also obtained about the efficacy and clinical utility of procedures from other sources, such as the AMA's Diagnostic and Therapeutic Technology Assessment Program (DATTA) and various other technology assessment panels.

Agenda materials for each panel meeting are prepared by AMA staff. The topics for the agenda are gathered from several sources. Medical specialty societies, individual physicians, hospitals, third-party payers, and other interested parties may submit material for consideration by the Editorial Panel. Agenda materials are sent to panel members at least 30 days in advance of each meeting. This gives each panel member time to review the material and to confer with experts on each subject, as appropriate.

The CPT Editorial Panel meets quarterly and regularly faces complex problems associated with new and emerging technologies, as well as the difficulties encountered with outmoded procedures. The panel addresses nearly 150 major topics a year, which typically involves over 2000 votes on individual items.

The final meeting prior to publication of a new volume of CPT is held in August. For example, the August 1990 Panel meeting was the final meeting for changes to be made in CPT 1991.

How can I submit a suggestion for changes to CPT?

The effectiveness of CPT is dependent on constant updating to reflect changes in medical practice. This can only be accomplished through the interest and timely suggestions of practicing physicians, medical specialty societies, state medical associations, and those who deal regularly with medical records. Accordingly, the AMA welcomes correspondence, inquiries, and suggestions concerning old and new procedures. (CPT-1993)

Resource

Current Procedural Terminology (CPT 1997). Chicago, Ill: American Medical Association; 1997 ISBN 0-89970-651-7 Available in several editions and formats.

Curriculum Vitae

Preparing a Curriculum Vitae

Content

A CV says who you are, summarizes your experience, and reveals personal information, special talents, and skills. It is a chronological summary of your background; your CV also is a self-marketing tool to help you maintain continued career satisfaction and rewarding life/work planning. In addition, it is important for you to see your accomplishments on paper and plan your future objectives.

As you prepare your CV, you may want to keep the following comments in mind.

Name: List your full "legal" name. This is particularly important if you were single when you received your MD degree and have since married, or if you have changed your name for other reasons. This allows prospective employers to verify that the information you provided is accurate.

Address: Provide home and office/hospital addresses. If you do not want to receive correspondence at your work address, do not list it. Make sure that the addresses are current.

Telephone/Fax/Pager: Make it easy for a potential employer to contact you: give home and office/hospital telephone, fax and/or pager numbers. Do not provide numbers where you do not want to be reached. Verify that you have listed a current area code, since many frequently change.

Certification and Licensure: List applicable board certification(s), national board examination, and licensure data [year and state(s)]. Give dates of completion for each. If you are in the "board certification pipeline" but have not yet taken the final boards, you may want to state just where in the process you are (written boards, oral boards, awaiting results, board "eligible" [only if your specialty board recognizes this designation], etc).

Education: List in descending order, with most recent first. Note name of the institution, degree received, and dates.

Postgraduate Training: Cite all training, such as internship, residency, and fellowship, with name of institution and dates. List the most recent training experience first.

Practice Experience: Again, begin with the most recent experience and work backward. This makes the CV much more practicably usable.

Professional or Teaching Appointments: Include academic and professional appointments, fellowships, and other unique training experiences. Also mention special expertise in a certain medical procedure, administrative experience, and fluency in foreign language.

Professional Society Memberships: List the societies to which you belong. Here also is the place to list those societies in which you hold leadership positions. Indicate the name of the committee, the position held, and the time period in which it occurred.

Personal and Professional References: Decide on several references that can be used. Include physicians who can comment on the quality of your clinical skills

C and on your personality within the last several years. You may also want to consider as references hospital administrators, residency training directors, nurses, and referring physicians. Also, be sure to inform those whom you would like to list as references that you are seeking a new practice opportunity and would like to list their names.

State on your CV that references will be furnished on request. This protects your references from being inconvenienced by many unsolicited telephone calls and allows you to evaluate a potential practice opportunity before you release your references.

Bibliography: Cite presentations and publications. If this listing is lengthy, you may want to tailor this section to the position being sought.

If you have a "track record" for getting results, you may want to add a category to your CV called "Accomplishments." Here you can provide concise results from committees on which you served and projects and task forces you directed or managed, or highlight your clinical and nonclinical administrative or managerial skills. Adopting a "bullet" format here will make your accomplishments stand out, and make them easier to read. It also will help you prepare brief statements.

When listing the above information, do not go into great detail, as this tends to clutter and lengthen the CV unnecessarily.

What Not to Include
Never include the following types of information on a CV: race, religion, anticipated compensations, reasons for leaving previous positions, personal health problems or disabilities, examination scores, and license and DEA numbers (these could be used by an impostor). It is also permissible to omit references to age, place of birth, citizenship, and marital status. (PREP-1997)

Cystic Fibrosis
Cystic Fibrosis Foundation
6931 Arlington Rd, Bethesda, MD 20814
800 344-4823   301 951-4422   Fax 301 951-6378

Cytotechnology

History
In the pioneer days of clinical pathology, it was the rare pathologist who did not have an assistant. These first technical "assistants," some of whom were trained by George N. Papanicolaou, MD, famed American anatomist and cytologist, were always the product of an apprentice-type training. As their number and the number of "apprentice programs" grew, there was a need to certify that the "apprentices" had indeed learned their tasks well. The Board of Registry of the American Society of Clinical Pathologists (ASCP) offered the examination for the cytology technician for the first time in 1957.

Five years later, in 1962, the *Standards (Essentials) of an Acceptable School for the Cytotechnologist* were developed by the Cytology Committee of the ASCP and the ASCP Board of Schools and were adopted by the House of Delegates of the American Medical Association (AMA). Until 1975, representatives of the ASCP served on the Cytotechnology Review Committee of the National Accrediting Agency for Clinical Laboratory Sciences

(NAACLS), which replaced the ASCP Board of Schools in 1974. In 1975, the American Society of Cytopathology (ASC) was recognized as the organization that would collaborate with the AMA Council on Medical Education (CME), and the ASC formed the Cytotechnology Programs Review Committee, which assumed the responsibilities formerly handled by NAACLS. In 1977, 1983, and 1992, the cytotechnology *Standards and Guidelines* were revised and adopted by the AMA CME and the ASC. In 1996, the *Essentials* were renamed *Standards* and adopted by the Committee on Accreditation of Allied Health Education Programs in conjunction with the Committees on Accreditation and sponsoring organizations.

Occupational description
Cytology is the study of the structure and the function of cells. Cytotechnologists are specially trained technologists who work with pathologists to detect changes in body cells that may be important in the early diagnosis of cancer and other diseases. This is done primarily with the microscope to evaluate slide preparations of body cells for abnormalities in structure, indicating either benign or malignant conditions.

Job description
Using special techniques, cytotechnologists prepare cellular samples for study under the microscope and assist in the diagnosis of disease by examining the samples. Cell specimens may be obtained from various body sites, such as the female reproductive tract, the oral cavity, the lung, or any body cavity shedding cells. Using the findings of cytotechnologists, the physician is then able in many instances to diagnose cancer and other diseases long before they can be detected by other methods. Cytologic techniques can also be used to detect diseases involving hormonal abnormalities and other pathologic disease processes. In recent years, fine needles have been used to aspirate lesions, often deeply seated in the body, thus greatly enhancing the ability to diagnose tumors located in otherwise inaccessible sites.

Employment characteristics
Most cytotechnologists work in hospitals or in commercial laboratories, while some prefer to work on research projects or to teach. Employment opportunities vary, depending on geographic location, experience, and ability. The demand for trained cytotechnologists varies by geographic area. According to the 1994 ASCP Wage and Vacancy Survey, entry-level salaries average $28,579. (AHRP-1997)

Resources
AMA Division of Allied Health
312 553-9355

Cytotechnology Programs Review Committee
American Society of Cytopathology
400 W 9th St, Ste 201, Wilmington, DE 19801
302 429-8802   Fax 302 429-8807

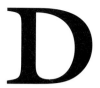

Dance Medicine

Dance Therapist. Plans, organizes, and leads dance and body movement activities to improve patients' mental outlook and physical well-being. Observes and evaluates patient's mental and physical disabilities to determine dance and body movement treatment. Confers with patient and medical personnel to develop dance therapy program. Conducts individual and group dance sessions to improve patient's mental and physical well-being. Makes changes in patient's program based on observation and evaluation of progress. Attends and participates in professional conferences and workshops to enhance efficiency and knowledge. (DOT-1991)

Resources

American Dance Therapy Association
2000 Century Plaza, Ste 108
Columbia, MO 21044-3263
410 997-4040

Center for Dance Medicine
41 E 42nd St, Rm 200, New York, NY, 10017
212 661-8401

Dental Assistant

Miscellaneous facts

- The 237 dental assisting education programs in the US accredited by the American Dental Association's Commission on Dental Accreditation enrolled 7210 students in 1995–1996.
- Approximately 98% of the students enrolled in dental assisting programs were women in 1995–1996.
- Minority students represented approximately 22% of enrollees in dental assisting programs in 1995–1996.
- Excellent career opportunities exist for "nontraditional" dental assisting students, including those over 23 years of age, seeking career change or job reentry after a period of unemployment, or from a culturally diverse background. Many dental assisting education programs offer more flexible program designs that meet the needs of nontraditional students by offering a variety of educational options, such as part-time or evening hours.

History

In 1957, the Council on Dental Education sponsored the first national workshop on dental assisting. Practicing dentists, dental educators, and dental assistants made recommendations for the education and certification of dental assistants. These recommendations were considered in developing the first Requirements for an Accredited Program in Dental Assisting Education, which were approved by the House of Delegates of the American Dental Association in 1960.

Prior to 1960, the American Dental Assistants Association (ADAA) approved courses of training for dental assistants, varying in length from 104 clock hours to 2 academic years. Subsequent to the adoption in 1960 of the first accreditation standards, the Council on Dental Education granted "provisional approval" to those programs approved by the ADAA that were at least 1 academic year in length until site visits could be conducted. Thus, 26 programs appeared on the first list of accredited dental assisting programs published in 1961.

The accreditation standards have been revised four times—in 1969, 1973, 1979, and 1991—to reflect the dental profession's changing needs and educational trends. The communities of interest provided input into the latest revision of the standards through an ad hoc committee, open hearings, and review of and comment on two drafts of the proposed revision of the standards. Prior to approving the revised standards in December 1991, the Commission carefully considered comments received from all sources. The revised accreditation standards were implemented in January 1993.

Occupational description

The dental assistant increases the efficiency of the dental care team by aiding the dentist in the delivery of oral health care. The dental assistant performs a wide range of tasks requiring both interpersonal and technical skills. Routine duties range from aiding and educating patients to preparing dental instruments and performing administrative work.

Job description

Dental assistants are responsible for helping patients feel comfortable before, during, and after treatment; assisting the dentist during treatment; taking and developing dental radiographs (X rays); recording the patient's medical history and taking blood pressure, pulse, and temperature readings; preparing and sterilizing instruments and equipment for the dentist's use; providing patients with oral care instructions after such procedures as surgery or placement of a restoration (filling); teaching patients proper brushing and flossing techniques; making impressions of patients' teeth for study casts; and performing routine administrative and scheduling tasks, including using a personal computer, answering the telephone, and ordering supplies.

Employment characteristics

Most of the more than 200,000 active dental assistants are employed by general dentists. In addition, dental specialists—such as orthodontists or oral and maxillofacial surgeons—employ dental assistants. Most assistants work chairside, although they may also participate in the business aspects of the practice. Besides dental offices, other practice settings available to dental assistants include schools and clinics (public health dentistry); hospitals (assisting dentists who are treating bedridden patients or in more elaborate dental procedures performed only in hospitals); dental school clinics; insurance companies (processing dental insurance claims); and vocational schools, technical institutes, community colleges, and universities (teaching others to be dental assistants).

The number of dental assistants, dental hygienists, and dental laboratory technicians employed by general dentists has risen from an average of 3.3 positions per practice in 1986 to 4.0 positions in 1994. Since many dentists employ two or three dental assistants, employment opportunities in this field are excellent.

Dental assisting also offers both flexibility and stability. Approximately 27% of dental assistants work on a part-time basis, sometimes in more than one dental office, so assistants have considerable freedom to choose their own hours. As of 1996, dental assistants had been working in their current practices for an average of 6 years.

The salary of a dental assistant varies, depending upon the responsibilities associated with the specific position, the individual training, and the geographic location of employment. The average national wage of a dental assistant in 1994 was $9.90 per hour. In addition to salary, many dental assistants receive benefit packages from their employers that may include health and disability insurance coverage, dues for membership in professional organizations, allowance for uniforms, and paid vacations.

Employment outlook
According to the 1993–1994 edition of the *Occupational Outlook Handbook,* published by the US Department of Labor's Bureau of Labor Statistics, employment of dental assistants is expected to grow at the average rate for all occupations through the year 2000. Most areas of the country are currently reporting shortages of dental assistants. Due to the success of preventive dentistry in reducing the incidence of oral disease, senior citizens—a growing population—will retain their teeth longer and will be even more aware of the importance of regular dental care. (AHRP-1997)

Resources
American Dental Assistants Association
203 N LaSalle St, Ste 1340, Chicago, IL 60601-1225
312 541-1550   Fax 312 541-1496

Dental Assisting National Board, Inc
216 E Ontario St, Chicago, IL 60611
312 642-3368

Dental Hygienist

Miscellaneous facts
- The US has approximately 223 dental hygiene education programs accredited by the American Dental Association's Commission on Dental Accreditation.
- Approximately 97% of the students enrolled in dental hygiene programs in 1995–1996 were women.
- Minority students represented approximately 11% of enrollees in dental hygiene programs in 1995–1996.
- Excellent career opportunities exist for "nontraditional" dental hygiene students, who might meet one or more of the following criteria: over 23 years of age, seeking career change or job reentry after a period of unemployment, or from a culturally diverse background. Some dental hygiene education programs offer more flexible program designs that meet the needs of nontraditional students by offering a variety of educational options, such as part-time or evening hours.

History
The first dental hygiene accreditation standards were developed by three groups: the American Dental Hygienists' Association, the National Association of Dental Examiners, and the American Dental Association's Council on Dental Education. The standards were submitted to and approved by the American Dental Association House of Delegates in 1947, 5 years prior to the launching of the dental hygiene accreditation program in 1952. The first list of accredited dental hygiene programs was published in 1953, with 21 programs. Since then the standards for accreditation have been revised four times—in 1969, 1973, 1979, and 1991.

The communities of interest provided input into the latest revision of the standards through an ad hoc committee, open hearings, and review of and comment on two drafts of the proposed revised standards. Prior to approving the revised standards in December 1991, the Commission carefully considered comments received from all sources. The revised accreditation standards were implemented in January 1993.

Occupational description
Dental hygienists work with dentists in the delivery of dental care to patients. Hygienists use their knowledge and clinical skills to provide dental care to patients and their interpersonal skills to motivate and instruct patients on methods to prevent oral disease and maintain oral health.

Job description
Although the range of services performed by dental hygienists varies from state to state, patient services rendered by dental hygienists frequently include:
- performing patient screening procedures, such as reviewing health and dental history and taking blood pressure, pulse, and temperature;
- taking and developing dental radiographs (X rays);
- removing calculus and plaque (hard and soft deposits) from teeth;
- applying preventive materials to teeth (eg, sealants and fluorides);
- teaching patients appropriate oral hygiene techniques;
- counseling patients regarding good nutrition and its impact on oral health;
- making impressions of patients' teeth for study casts; and
- performing office management activities.

Employment characteristics
Most of the approximately 100,000 active dental hygienists in the US today are employed by general dentists. Additionally, dental specialists (such as periodontists or pediatric dentists) employ dental hygienists. Most hy-

gienists work chairside, although they often participate in the business aspects of the practice.

Dental hygienists may also be employed to provide dental hygiene services for patients in hospitals, nursing homes, and public health clinics. Depending on the level of education and experience they have achieved, dental hygienists can also apply their skills and knowledge to other career activities, such as teaching hygiene students. Research, office management, and business administration are other options. In addition, employment opportunities may be available with companies that market dentistry-related materials and equipment.

The total number of dental hygienists, dental assistants, and dental laboratory technicians employed by general dentists has risen from an average of 3.3 positions per practice in 1986 to 4.0 positions in 1994. Because approximately 63% of general dentists employ at least one dental hygienist, and 37% employ two or more hygienists, employment opportunities in this field are excellent.

As a career, dental hygiene also offers both stability and flexibility. As of 1996, for example, dental hygienists had been working in their current practices for an average of 6.2 years. Many hygienists also have considerable freedom to choose their own hours and to undertake a full- or part-time schedule with evening or weekend hours.

The salary of a dental hygienist varies, depending upon the responsibilities associated with the specific position, the geographic location of employment, and the type of practice or other setting in which the hygienist works. The average national wage of a full-time dental hygienist in 1994 was $19.80 per hour. Hygienists who work part-time averaged $23.70 per hour. In addition, many dental hygienists receive benefit packages from their dentist/employers, which may include health insurance coverage, dues for membership in professional organizations, paid vacations and sick leave, and tuition assistance for continuing education.

Employment outlook

According to the 1993–1994 edition of the *Occupational Outlook Handbook* and the *Monthly Labor Review*, published by the US Department of Labor's Bureau of Labor Statistics, dental hygiene will continue to be among the top 10 growth disciplines in the health care professions through the year 2005. Some areas of the country are currently reporting shortages of dental hygienists.

Due to the success of preventive dentistry in reducing the incidence of oral disease, senior citizens—a growing population—will retain their teeth longer and will be even more aware of the importance of regular dental care. (AHRP-1997)

Resource

American Dental Hygienists Association
444 N Michigan Ave, Ste 3400, Chicago, IL 60611
800 243-ADHA   312 440-8929   Fax 312 440-8929

Dental Laboratory Technician

Miscellaneous facts

- In 1995, 798 first-year dental laboratory technician students were enrolled in the approximately 40 dental technology education programs in the US accredited by the American Dental Association's Commission on Dental Accreditation.
- Dental technology presents equal career opportunities for women and men. In 1995–1996, 46% of the students enrolled in dental technology programs were women and 54% were men.
- Minority students represented approximately 38% of enrollees in dental technology programs in 1995–1996.
- Excellent career opportunities exist for "nontraditional" dental technology students, who might meet one or more of the following criteria: over 23 years of age; seeking career change or job reentry after a period of unemployment; or from a culturally diverse background.

History

The first educational standards for the education of dental laboratory technicians, adopted by the American Dental Association House of Delegates in 1946, were rescinded and revised in 1957. Since then the accreditation standards have been revised four times—in 1967, 1973, 1979, and 1991—to reflect the changing needs and educational trends of the dental profession and laboratory industry.

The communities of interest provided input into the latest revision of the standards through an ad hoc committee, open hearings at annual meetings of the National Association of Dental Laboratories and American Association of Dental Schools, and review of and comment on drafts of the proposed revision of the standards. Prior to approving the revised standards in December 1991, the Commission carefully considered comments received from all sources. The revised accreditation standards were implemented in January 1993.

Occupational description

Dental laboratory technicians make dental prostheses replacements for natural teeth, including dentures and crowns. The hallmarks of the qualified dental laboratory technician are skill in using small hand instruments, accuracy, artistic ability, and attention to detail to create practical, esthetically pleasing teeth replacements.

Job description

Dental laboratory technicians seldom interact directly with patients; rather, they work with dentists by following detailed written instructions to make dental prostheses, which are replacements for natural teeth that enable people who have lost some or all of their teeth to eat, chew, talk, and smile in a manner similar to the way they did before. The dental technician uses impressions (molds) of the patient's teeth or oral soft tissues to create full dentures, removable partial dentures or fixed bridges, crowns, caps, and orthodontic appliances and splints.

Dental technicians use sophisticated instruments and equipment and work with a variety of materials for replacing damaged or missing tooth structure, including waxes, plastics, precious and nonprecious alloys, stainless steel, and porcelain.

Employment characteristics

Most of the more than 60,000 active dental laboratory technicians in the US today work in commercial dental laboratories, which on average employ between three and five technicians. In addition, some dentists employ dental technicians in their private dental offices. Other employment opportunities for dental technicians include dental

D schools, hospitals, the military, and companies that manufacture dental prosthetic materials. Dental laboratory technician education programs also offer teaching positions for qualified technicians.

The starting salary of a dental technician is approximately $20,000, and varies depending upon the responsibilities associated with the specific position and the geographic location of employment. In addition to salary, many dental technicians receive benefit packages from their employers, which may include health and disability insurance coverage, reimbursement for continuing education programs, and paid vacations and holidays.

Employment outlook

Since most dentists use laboratory services, employment opportunities in this field are excellent. Due to the success of preventive dentistry in reducing the incidence of oral disease, senior citizens—a growing population—will retain their teeth longer and will require more sophisticated prostheses for longer periods, thus increasing demand for dental laboratory services. (AHRP-1997)

Resources

National Board for Certification in Dental Laboratory Technology
555 Braddock Rd, Alexandria, VA 22314-2106
703 683-5263

National Association of Dental Laboratories
555 E Braddock Rd, Alexandria, VA 22314-2106
703 683-5263

Laboratory Conference Section Board of the American Dental Trade Association
4222 King St W, Alexandria, VA 22302
703 379-7755

Dentist

Job description

Diagnoses and treats diseases, injuries, and malformations of teeth and gums, and related oral structures. Examines patient to determine nature of condition, utilizing X rays, dental instruments, and other diagnostic procedures. Cleans, fills, extracts, and replaces teeth using rotary and hand instruments, dental appliances, medication, and surgical implements. Provides preventive dental services to patient, such as applications of fluoride and sealants to teeth, and education in oral and dental hygiene. (DOT-1991)

Resources

American Association of Dental Schools
1625 Massachusetts Ave NW, Washington, DC 20036
202 667-9433

American Dental Association
211 E Chicago Ave, Chicago, IL 60611
312 440-2500   Fax 312 440-7494
Web address: http://www.ada.org
Library open to public 8:30am-5:00pm

National Institute of Dental Research
9000 Rockville Pike, Bethesda, MD 20892
301 496-6621

Dental Associations, Statewide

Alabama Dental Association
836 Washington Ave, Montgomery, AL 36104
205 265-1684   Fax 205 262-6218

Alaska Dental Society
3400 Spenard Rd, Ste 10, Anchorage, AK 99503
907 277-4675   Fax 907 274-2960

Arizona State Dental Association
4131 N 36th St, Phoenix, AZ 85018
602 957-4777   Fax 602 957-1342

Arkansas State Dental Association
2501 Crestwood Dr, Ste 205
North Little Rock, AR 72116
501 771-7650   Fax 501 771-1016

California Dental Association
PO Box 13749, Sacramento, CA 95853-4749
916 443-3382   Fax 916 443-2943

Colorado Dental Association
3690 S Yosemite, Ste 100, Denver, CO 80237-1808
303 740-6900   Fax 303 740-7989

Connecticut State Dental Association
62 Russ St, Hartford, CT 06106-1589
203 278-5550   Fax 203 522-6587

Delaware State Dental Society
1925 Lovering Ave, Wilmington, DE 19806-2147
302 654-4335   Fax 302 427-9412

District of Columbia Dental Society
502 C St NE, Washington, DC 20002-5810
202 547-7613   Fax 202 546-1482

Florida Dental Association
1111 E Tennessee St, Ste 102
Tallahassee, FL 32308-6913
904 681-3629   904 561-0504

Georgia Dental Association
2801 Buford Hwy, Ste T-60
Atlanta, GA 30329-2137
404 636-7553   404 633-3943

Hawaii Dental Association
1000 Bishop St, Ste 805
Honolulu, HI 96813-4281
808 536-2135   808 536-2137

Idaho State Dental Association
1220 W Hays, Boise, ID 83702-5315
208 343-7543   208 343-0775

Illinois State Dental Society
524 S Fifth St, PO Box 376, Springfield, IL 62705-0376
217 525-1406   Fax 217 525-8872

Indiana Dental Association
PO Box 2467, Virginia Ave
Indianapolis, IN 46204-2467
317 634-2610   Fax 317 634-2612

Iowa Dental Association
333 Insurance Exchange Bldg
Des Moines, IA 50309-2322
515 282-7250   Fax 515 282-7256

Kansas Dental Association
5200 Huntoon, Topeka, KS 66604-2398
913 272-7360   Fax 913 272-2301

Kentucky Dental Association
1940 Princeton Dr, Louisville, KY 40205-1873
502 459-5373   Fax 502 458-5915

Louisiana Dental Association
320 3rd St, Ste 201, Baton Rouge, LA 70801
504 336-1692   Fax 504 334-9215

Maine Dental Association
Association Dr, PO Box 215
Manchester, ME 04351-0215
207 622-7900   Fax 207 622-6210

Maryland State Dental Association
6450 Dobbin Rd, Columbia, MD 21045-5824
301 964-2880   Fax 410 964-0583

Massachusetts Dental Society
83 Speen St, Natick, MA 01760-4125
508 651-7511   Fax 508 653-7115

Michigan Dental Association
230 N Washington Sq, #208, Lansing, MI 48933-1392
517 372-9070   517 372-0008

Minnesota Dental Association
2236 Marshall Ave, St Paul, MN 55104-5758
612 646-7454   612 646-8246

Mississippi Dental Association
2630 Ridgewood Rd, Jackson, MS 39216-4920
601 982-0442   601 366-3050

Missouri Dental Association
PO Box 1707, Jefferson City, MO 65102-1701
314 634-3436   Fax 314 635-0764

Montana Dental Association
PO Box 1154, Helena, MT 59624-1154
406 443-2061   Fax 406 443-1546

Nebraska Dental Association
3120 O St, Lincoln, NE 68510-1599
402 476-1704   Fax 402 476-2641

Nevada Dental Association
6889 W Charleston Boulevard, Ste B
Las Vegas, NV 89117
702 255-4211   Fax 702 255-3302

New Hampshire Dental Society
PO Box 2229, Concord, NH 03302-2229
603 225-5961   603 226-4880

New Jersey Dental Association
1 Dental Plaza, North Brunswick, NJ 08902-4311
908 821-9400   Fax 908 821-1082

New Mexico Dental Association
3736 Eubank Blvd NE, Ste 1A
Albuquerque, NM 87111-3556
505 294-1368   Fax 505 294-9958

Dental Society of the State of New York
7 Elk St, Albany, NY 12207-1023
518 465-0044   Fax 518 427-0461

North Carolina Dental Society
PO Box 12047, Raleigh, NC 27605-2047
919 832-1222   Fax 919 833-7666

North Dakota Dental Association
PO Box 1332, Bismarck, ND 58502-1332
701 223-8870   Fax 701 223-0855

Ohio Dental Association
1370 Dublin Rd, Columbus, OH 43215-1098
614 486-2700   Fax 614 486-0381

Oklahoma Dental Association
629 W Interstate 44, Service Rd
Oklahoma City, OK 73118-6832
405 848-8873   Fax 405 848-8875

Oregon Dental Association
17898 SW McEwan Rd, Portland, OR 97224-7798
503 620-3230   Fax 503 620-4169

Pennsylvania Dental Association
PO Box 3341, Harrisburg, PA 17105-3341
717 234-5941   Fax 717 232-7169

Colegio de Cirujanos Dentistas de Puerto Rico
Avenue Domenech #200, Hato Rey, PR 00918-3507
809 764-1969   Fax 809 763-6335

Rhode Island Dental Association
200 Centerville Pl, Warwick, RI 02886-0204
401 732-6833   Fax 401 732-9351

South Carolina Dental Association
120 Stonemark Ln, Columbia, SC 29210-3841
803 750-2277   Fax 803 750-1644

South Dakota Dental Association
PO Box 1194, Pierre, SD 57501-1194
605 224-9133   Fax 605 224-9168

Tennessee Dental Association
PO Box 120188, Nashville, TN 37212-0188
615 383-8962   Fax 615 383-0214

Texas Dental Association
PO Box 3358, Austin, TX 78764-3358
512 443-3675   Fax 512 443-3031

Utah Dental Association
1151 E 3900 S, Ste B-160
Salt Lake City, UT 84124-1216
801 261-5315   Fax 801 261-1235

Vermont State Dental Society
132 Church St, Burlington, VT 05401-8401
802 864-0115   Fax 802 646-0116

Virgin Islands Dental Association
PO Box 10422, St Thomas, VI 00801-3422
809 775-9110   809 779-8326

Virginia Dental Association
5006 Monument Ave, PO Box 6906
Richmond, VA 23230
804 358-4927   804 353-7342

Washington State Dental Association
2033 Sixth Ave, #333, Seattle, WA 98121-2514
206 448-1914   206 443-9266

West Virginia Dental Association
300 Capitol St, #1002
Charleston, WV 25301-1794
304 344-5246   Fax 304 344-5316

Wisconsin Dental Association
111 E Wisconsin Ave, Ste 1300
Milwaukee, WI 53202-4811
414 276-4520   Fax 414 276-8431

Wyoming Dental Association
33 S Center St, Ste 322, Casper, WY 82601-2875
307 234-0777   Fax 307 234-6040

Depression

Poetry and Medicine

Depression

Joseph Geskey
JAMA 1996 Sept 11; 276(10): 778g

On good days
he could sift through limestone
a quarry of tombstones,
and parse out soil with his pen
fertilizing poems with verbs
like *rise* and *soar*, gliding
on the wings of a whooping crane
in air so pure the wind burned
flames across his face,
or walk through copper mines
in heat-furnace summer days
scraping off patina,
turning everything he touched
into a bright silver penny.

But on bad days,
when he would relapse
into addiction to old memories,
when the calligraphy of her signature
signed away from him,
nouns like pronouncements
waked over his body.
It was enough just
to take a shower and put on new clothes,
resisting the urge
of even this simple task,
when all he wanted
was to follow that crane into the sky
for as long as his wings could carry him.

Resources

National Foundation for Depressive Illness, Inc
(NAFDI maintains a referral list of doctors and support groups by state.)
PO Box 2257, New York, NY 10116-2257
800 245-4306

National Depressive and Manic-Depressive Association
730 N Franklin Street, Chicago, IL 60610
800 826-3632

National Alliance for the Mentally Ill
200 N Glebe Rd, #1015, Arlington, VA 22203
800 950-NAMI
Web address: http://www.cais.com/vikings/nami/index.html

National Mental Health Association
1201 Prince St, Alexandria, VA 22314-2971
800 969-6942
NMHA Public Education Campaign on Clinical Depression
800 228-1114
Web address: http://www.worldcorp.com/dc-online/nmha

Recovery Inc
(a national self-help group with local chapters and groups throughout the country)
802 N Dearborn St, Chicago, IL 60610
312 337-5661

Dermatology

Dermatologist. Alternate title: skin specialist. Diagnoses and treats diseases of human skin. Examines skin to determine nature of disease, taking blood samples and smears for affected areas, and performing other laboratory procedures. Examines specimens under microscope, and makes various chemical and biological analyses and performs other tests to identify disease-causing organisms or pathological conditions. Prescribes and administers medications, and applies superficial radiotherapy and other localized treatments. Treats abscesses, skin injuries, and other skin infections, and surgically excises cutaneous malignancies, cysts, birthmarks, and other growths. Treats scars, using dermabrasion. (DOT-1991)

Resources

American Academy of Dermatology
930 N Meacham Rd, Schaumburg, IL 60172-4965
847 330-0230 Fax 847 330-0050
Web address: http://www.derm-infonet.com

American Board of Dermatology
Henry Ford Hospital
Detroit, MI 48202-3450
313 874-1088 Fax 313 872-3221

American Society for Dermatologic Surgery
PO Box 4014, Schaumburg, IL 60173
800 441-2737
847 330-0230 Fax 847 330-0050

DEBRA of America, Inc
(Dystrophic Epidermolysis Bullosa Research Association of America)
40 Rector St, New York, NY 10006
212 693-6610

National Foundation for Ectodermal Dysplasia
219 E Main St, Box 114, Mascoutah, IL 62258
618 566-2020 Fax 618 566-4718
E-mail: nfedl@aol.com

Society for Investigative Dermatology, Inc
c/o David R. Bickers MD
Cleveland, OH 44106
216 844-6859 Fax 216 844-6810
E-mail: sid@halcyon.com
Web address: http://www.telemedicine.oeg/sidhome

Xeroderma Pigmentosum Registry
c/o Dept of Pathology
Medical Science Bldg, Rm C 520
NJ Medical School
185 S Orange Ave, Newark, NJ 07103-2757
201 456-6255

Devices, Medical

Medical Device Register: United States and Canada: *Official Directory of Medical Suppliers.* 1997.
2 vol, sold as set, ISBN 1-563-63-225-X

International volume also available from:
Medical Device Register, Inc
Medical Economics Data Inc
5 Paragon Dr, Montvale, NJ 07645-1725
800 222-3045 201 358-7603

Resources

Association for the Advancement of Medical Instrumentation
3330 Washington Blvd, Ste 400
Arlington, VA 22201-4598
800 332-2264   703 525-4890   Fax 703 276-0793

For health care professional to report malfunction:
USP 800 638-6725 (24 hours)
FDA 301 881-0256 (7 am to 4:30 pm EST)

ECRI (to evaluate health care technology)
5200 Butler Pike, Plymouth Meeting, PA 19462
215 825-6700 or 6000

Health Industry Distributors Association
225 Reinekers Ln, #650, Alexandria, VA 22314-2875
703 549-4432   Fax 703 549-6495

Health Industry Manufacturers Association
1200 G St NW, Ste 4000, Washington, DC 20005
202 783-8700   Fax 202 783-8750

National Association of Medical Equipment Suppliers
625 Slaters Ln, Ste 200, Alexandria, VA 22314-1171
703 836-6263   Fax 703 836-6730
E-mail: info@names.org

Diabetes

Type II diabetes

What is type II diabetes?

Diabetes is a disorder of metabolism—the way in which the body converts food that is eaten into energy. Most of the food that is eaten is broken down by digestive juices into chemicals, including a simple sugar called glucose. Glucose is the body's main source of energy. After digestion, glucose passes into the bloodstream, where it is available for cells to take in and use or store for later use.

In order for cells to take in glucose, a hormone called insulin must be present in the blood. Insulin acts as a "key" that unlocks "doors" on cell surfaces to allow glucose to enter the cells. Insulin is produced by special cells (called islet cells) in an organ called the pancreas, which is about 6 inches long and lies behind the stomach.

In healthy people, the pancreas automatically produces the right amount of insulin to enable glucose to enter cells. In people who have diabetes, cells do not respond to the effects of the insulin that the pancreas produces. If glucose cannot get inside cells, it builds up in the bloodstream. The buildup of glucose in the blood—sometimes referred to as high blood sugar or hyperglycemia (which means "too much glucose in the blood")—is the hallmark of diabetes.

When the glucose level in the blood goes above a certain level, the excess glucose flows out from the kidneys (two organs that filter wastes from the bloodstream) into the urine. The glucose takes water with it, which causes frequent urination and extreme thirst. These two conditions—frequent urination and unusual thirst—are usually the first noticeable signs of diabetes. Another symptom is weight loss, which results from the loss of calories and water in the urine.

Type I diabetes: the other form

Diabetes has two forms—type I and type II. Nine out of 10 people with diabetes have type II diabetes. But to give you an idea of how the two are related—their similarities and differences—type I will be briefly described here.

Type I diabetes is, at least initially, much more serious than type II. Type I diabetes is sometimes referred to as insulin-dependent diabetes. It used to be known as juvenile diabetes because most people develop it when they are children or teenagers. Type II diabetes is also known as non–insulin-dependent diabetes. In the past it was often referred to as adult-onset diabetes because it usually occurs after age 40. Unlike type II diabetes, there is no known way to prevent type I diabetes.

A person has type I diabetes if his or her pancreas cannot make enough insulin to help glucose get inside the cells. This type of diabetes occurs when the cells in the pancreas that make insulin are attacked by the body's own immune defense system, which mistakes these insulin-producing cells for germs and tries to destroy them. Doctors do not know exactly what makes the immune system attack healthy tissue; they think a virus may be the cause.

Type I diabetes will make a person feel very sick very quickly because the human body cannot survive for long without insulin. People who have type I diabetes must give themselves shots of insulin every day just to stay alive. In addition to taking shots of insulin to help regulate the level of glucose in their blood, people with type I diabetes work very closely with their doctor, nurses, and a dietitian (a person who is trained to provide education and counseling about nutrition) to establish an individualized treatment program. This program will include a meal plan designed just for them, which they must carefully follow to control their diabetes. (DX-D-1996)

Resources

American Diabetes Association
National Service Center, 1660 Duke St
PO Box 25757, Alexandria, VA 22314
800 ADA-DISC   703 549-1500   Fax 703 836-7439
Web address: http://www.diabetes.org

Juvenile Diabetes Foundation
120 Wall St, New York, NY 10005-3904
800 JDF-CURE   212 889-7575   Fax 212 725-7259
E-mail: jbroch@jdf.usa.com

National Diabetes Information Clearinghouse
Box NDIC, Bethesda, MD 20892
301 468-2162

Diabetes Associations, Statewide

American Diabetes Association Alabama Affiliate
200 Office Park Circle, Ste 303, Birmingham, AL 35223
800 824-7891   205 870-5172

American Diabetes Association Alaska Affiliate
The Diamond Center, 800 E Diamond Blvd, Ste 3-218
Anchorage, AK 99515
907 344-4459

American Diabetes Association Arizona Affiliate
2328 W Royal Palm Rd, Ste D, PO Box 37579
Phoenix, AZ 85021
800 824-7891   602 995-1515

D

American Diabetes Association Arkansas Affiliate
11500 N Rodney Parham, Ste 19-20
Little Rock, AR 72212
501 221-7444

American Diabetes Association California Affiliate
10445 Old Placerville Rd, Sacramento, CA 95827
800 828-8293   916 369-0999

American Diabetes Association Colorado Affiliate
2450 S Downing St, Denver, CO 80210
800 782-2873   303 778-7556

American Diabetes Association Connecticut Affiliate
300 Research Pkwy, Meridan, CT 06450
800 842-6323   203 639-0385

American Diabetes Association Delaware Affiliate
110 S French St, Wilmington, DE 19801
800 734-5030   302 656-0030

American Diabetes Association
District of Columbia Affiliate
1211 Connecticut Ave NW, #501
Washington, DC 20036
202 331-8303

American Diabetes Association Florida Affiliate
1101 N Lake Destiny Rd, Ste 415, Maitland, FL 32751
800 741-5698   407 660-1926

American Diabetes Association Georgia Affiliate
1 Corporate Sq, Ste 127, Atlanta, GA 30329
800 241-4556   404 320-7100

American Diabetes Association Hawaii Affiliate
310 Paoakalani Ave, Bldg E, Rm 204
Honolulu, HI 96815
808 924-7755

American Diabetes Association Idaho Affiliate
1528 Vista Ave, Boise, ID 83705
208 342-2774

American Diabetes Association
Northern Illinois Affiliate
6 N Michigan Ave, Ste 1202, Chicago, IL 60602
800 433-4966   312 346-1805

American Diabetes Association
Downstate Illinois Affiliate
2580 Federal Dr, Ste 403, Decatur, IL 62526
800 445-1667   217 875-9011

American Diabetes Association Indiana Affiliate
7363 E 21st St, Indianapolis, IN 46219
800 228-2897   317 352-9226

American Diabetes Association Iowa Affiliate
6200 Aurora Ave, Ste 504W, Des Moines, IA 50322
800 678-4232   515 276-2237

American Diabetes Association Kansas Affiliate
3210 E Douglas, Wichita, KS 67208
800 362-1355   316 684-6091

American Diabetes Association Kentucky Affiliate
721 W Main St, Ste 102, Louisville, KY 40202
800 766-1698   502 589-3837

American Diabetes Association Louisiana Affiliate
9420 Lindale Ave, Ste B, Baton Rouge, LA 70815
800 960-7732   504 927-7732

American Diabetes Association Maine Affiliate
9 Church St, PO Box 2208, Augusta, ME 04338
800 870-8000   207 623-2232

American Diabetes Association Maryland Affiliate
407 Central Ave, Reisterstown, MD 21136
800 232-3662   410 526-2900

American Diabetes Association
Massachusetts Affiliate
PO Box 968, Farmingham, MA 01701
800 229-2559   508 879-1776

American Diabetes Association Michigan Affiliate
30600 Telegraph Rd, Ste 2255
Bingham Farms, MI 48025
800 525-9292   810 433-3830

American Diabetes Association Minnesota Affiliate
715 Florida Ave S, Ste 307, Minneapolis, MN 55426
800 232-4044   612 593-5333

American Diabetes Association Mississippi Affiliate
16 Northtown Dr, Ste 100, Jackson, MS 39211
800 232-8393   601 957-7878

American Diabetes Association Missouri Affiliate
PO Box 1013, Columbia, MO 65205
800 404-2873   314 443-8611

American Diabetes Association Montana Affiliate
600 Central Plaza, Ste 201, Box 2411
Great Falls, MT 59403
800 232-6668   406 761-0908

American Diabetes Association Nebraska Affiliate
12838 Augusta Ave, Omaha, NE 68144
800 852-0386   402 333-5556

American Diabetes Association Nevada Affiliate
2785 E Desert Inn Rd, Ste 140
Las Vegas, NV 89121
800 800-4232   702 369-9995

American Diabetes Association New Hampshire Affiliate
132 Middle St, Manchester, NH 03105
800 477-9579   603 627-9579

American Diabetes Association New Jersey Affiliate
Vantage Ct N, 200 Cottontail Ln, Somerset, NJ 08873
800 562-2063   908 469-7979

American Diabetes Association New Mexico Affiliate
525 San Pedro NE, Ste 101, Albuquerque, NM 87108
800 992-5142   505 266-5716

American Diabetes Association New York
Downstate Affiliate
149 Madison Ave, 7th Fl, New York, NY 10016
800 281-4925   212 725-4925

American Diabetes Association New York
Upstate Affiliate
1603 Genesee St, Syracuse, NY 13204-1949
800 724-3060   315 488-9464

American Diabetes Association
North Carolina Affiliate
3109 Poplarwood Ct, Ste 125
Raleigh, NC 27604-1043
800 682-9692   919 872-6006

American Diabetes Association
North Dakota Affiliate
PO Box 5234, Grand Forks, ND 58206-5234
800 666-6709   701 746-4426

American Diabetes Association Ohio Affiliate
937 N High St, Worthington, OH 43085
800 232-6366   614 436-1917

American Diabetes Association Oklahoma Affiliate
6465 S Yale Ave, Ste 519, Tulsa, OK 74136
800 259-6553   918 492-3839

American Diabetes Association Oregon Affiliate
6915 SW Macadam, Ste 130, Portland, OR 97219
800 234-0849   503 245-2010

American Diabetes Association
Pennsylvania Affiliate
5020 Ritter Rd, Ste 106, Mechanicsburg, PA 17055
800 351-5800   717 691-6170

American Diabetes Association Puerto Rico Affiliate
PO Box 4525, San Juan, PR 00919
809 766-4644

American Diabetes Association
Rhode Island Affiliate
107 Waterman Ave, East Providence, RI 02914
401 431-1900

American Diabetes Association
South Carolina Affiliate
2711 Middleburg Dr, Ste 311, Columbia, SC 29204
800 354-5292   803 799-4246

American Diabetes Association
South Dakota Affiliate
PO Box 659, Sioux Falls, SD 57101
800 658-4502   605 335-7670

American Diabetes Association Tennessee Affiliate
4205 Hillsboro Rd, Ste B-216, Nashville, TN 37215
800 627-1152   615 298-3066

American Diabetes Association Texas Affiliate
9430 Research, Echelon II, Ste 300
Austin, TX 78759
800 252-8233   512 343-6981

American Diabetes Association Utah Affiliate
340 E 400 South, Salt Lake City, UT 84111-2909
800 888-1734   801 363-3024

American Diabetes Association Vermont Affiliate
431 Pine St, Burlington, VT 05401
800 639-2105   802 862-3882

American Diabetes Association Virginia Affiliate
1290 Seminole Trail, Ste 2
Charlottesville, VA 22901
800 582-8323 804 974-9905

American Diabetes Association Washington Affiliate
557 Roy St, LL, Seattle, WA 98103
800 628-8808   206 282-4616

American Diabetes Association
West Virginia Affiliate
121-A Ohio Ave, Dunbar, WV 25064
800 232-9824   304 768-2596

American Diabetes Association Wisconsin Affiliate
2949 N Mayfair Rd, #306, Wauwatosa, WI 53222
800 776-7118   414 778-5500

American Diabetes Association Wyoming Affiliate
Enterprise Center, 400 E 1st St, Ste 205C
Casper, WY 82601
800 877-0106   307 265-2725

Diagnostic and Statistical Manual of Mental Disorders

American Psychiatric Association
1400 K St NW, Washington, DC 20005
202 682-6000   Fax 202 682-6114
Web address: http://www.psych.org

D

Diagnostic Medical Sonographer

History

In 1972, the American Society of Ultrasound Technical Specialists (ASUTS) appointed a committee to explore the mechanism of accreditation of educational programs for the ultrasound technical specialist through the American Medical Association (AMA) Council on Medical Education (CME). In October 1973, members of ASUTS (now known as the Society of Diagnostic Medical Sonographers) met with a representative from the AMA Department of Health Manpower and initiated activities to receive formal recognition as an occupation. One year later the occupation of diagnostic medical sonography received recognition by the AMA.

From 1974 to 1979, the *Standards (Essentials) of an Accredited Educational Program for the Diagnostic Medical Sonographer* were developed. Because of the multidisciplinary nature of diagnostic ultrasound, many interested medical and allied health organizations collaborated in drafting the *Standards,* which were formally adopted by the following organizations: the American College of Cardiology (withdrew as a sponsoring organization in 1983; resumed sponsorship in 1986), American College of Radiology, American Institute of Ultrasound in Medicine, AMA, American Society of Echocardiography, American Society of Radiologic Technologists, Society of Diagnostic Medical Sonographers, and Society of Nuclear Medicine (withdrew as a sponsoring organization in 1981). These organizations, with the exception of the AMA and the Society of Nuclear Medicine, and the addition of the Society of Vascular Technology in 1993, currently sponsor the Joint Review Committee on Education in Diagnostic Medical Sonography. New *Standards* were adopted in 1996 and will be used exclusively beginning January 1, 1998. Programs undergoing evaluation prior to January 1, 1998, may continue to use the 1987 *Standards* if they choose. Educational programs were first accredited in January 1982.

Occupational description

The diagnostic medical sonographer provides patient services using medical ultrasound under the supervision of a physician responsible for the use and interpretation of ultrasound procedures. The sonographer assists the physician in gathering sonographic data necessary to diagnose a variety of conditions and diseases.

Job description

The sonographer provides patient services in a variety of medical settings in which the physician is responsible for the use and interpretation of ultrasound procedures. In assisting physicians in gathering sonographic data, the diagnostic medical sonographer is able to obtain, review, and integrate pertinent patient history and supporting clinical data to facilitate optimum diagnostic results; perform appropriate procedures and record anatomical, pathological, and/or physiological data for interpretation by a physician; record and process sonographic data and other pertinent observations made during the procedure for presentation to the interpreting physician; exercise discretion and judgment in the performance of sonographic services; provide patient education related to medical ultrasound; and promote principles of good health.

Employment characteristics

Diagnostic medical sonographers may be employed in hospitals, clinics, private offices, and industry. There is also a need for suitably qualified educators, researchers, and administrators. The demand for sonographers continues to exceed the supply. The supply and demand ratio affects salaries, depending on experience and responsibilities.

According to the Society of Diagnostic Medical Sonographers, the current (1995) salary for diagnostic medical sonographers with less than 1 year of experience is $29,800. (AHRP-1997)

Resources

AMA Allied Health Department
312 553-9355

American Registry of Diagnostic
Medical Sonographers
600 Jefferson Plz, Ste 360, Rockville, MD 20852-1150
800 541-9754   301 738-8401   Fax 301 738-0312
E-mail: Bricksin_Rajev@msn.com

Joint Review Committee on Education in Diagnostic
Medical Sonography
7108-C S Alton Way, Englewood, CO 80112
303 741-3533   Fax 303 741-3655

Society of Diagnostic Medical Sonographers
12770 Coit Rd, Ste 508, Dallas, TX 75251
800 229-9506   214 239-7367   212 239-7378

Dialysis Technician

Alternate title: hemodialysis technician. Sets up and operates hemodialysis machine to provide dialysis treatment for patients with kidney failure. Attaches dialyzer and tubing to machine to assemble for use. Mixes dialysate, according to formula. Primes dialyzer with saline or heparinized solution to prepare machine for use. Transports patient to dialysis room and positions patient on lounge chair at hemodialysis machine. Takes and records patient's predialysis weight, temperature, blood pressure, pulse rate, and respiration rate. Explains dialysis procedure and operation of hemodialysis machine to patient before treatment to allay anxieties. Cleans area of access (fistula, graft, or catheter), using antiseptic solution. Connects hemodialysis machine to access in patient's forearm or catheter site to start blood circulating through dialyzer. Inspects equipment settings, including pressures conductivity (proportion of chemical to water), and temperature to ensure conformance to safety standards. Starts blood flow pump at prescribed rate. Inspects venous and arterial pressures as registered on equipment to ensure pressures are within established limits. Calculates fluid removal or replacement to be achieved during dialysis procedure. Monitors patient for adverse reaction and hemodialysis machine for malfunction. Takes and records patient's postdialysis weight, temperature, blood pressure, pulse rate. May fabricate

parts, such as cannulas, tubing, catheters, connectors, and fittings, using handtools. (DOT-1991)

Resource

American Nephrology Nurses Association
PO Box 56, E Holly Ave, Pitman, NJ 08071
609 256-2320   609 589-7463

Diet

JAMA Article of Note: Report of the Council on Scientific Affairs: Diet and cancer: Where do matters stand? *Arch Intern Med* 1993 Jan 11; 153(1): 50-6

During the past decade, the scientific literature base on the putative but elusive relationship between diet and cancer expanded enormously. Increased emphasis by funding agencies, fueled in turn by broadening public interest in the topic, led to this growth. The laboratory and epidemiologic research conducted in the past decade has shown that a simple solution does not exist. The key to the diet/cancer puzzle may lie in nutrient interactions and in individual response to dietary factors, determined in turn by genetic, physiological and lifestyle factors. Given the rapid strides being made in furthering the understanding of the biochemistry and molecular biology of cancer, it may be possible to look forward to the day when optimal dietary and lifestyle guidelines can be tailored to a specific individualized basis.

JAMA Theme Issue: Cholesterol

Dec 19 1990; 264(23)

This theme issue of JAMA presents several clinical articles discussing specific relationships of disease with and treatments for cholesterol problems. Two review articles, editorials, Centers for Disease Control and Prevention reports, and various medical perspectives on cholesterol round out what is printed here.

Dietetics

History

Founded in 1917, The American Dietetic Association (ADA) is the largest organization of food and nutrition professionals promoting optimal nutrition to improve public health and well-being. The early leaders laid a strong foundation for dietetics education. In 1923, the first plans for courses for student dietitians were discussed. By 1928, a list of hospitals with the approved course for student dietitians in hospitals was published. The approved course required that students have a baccalaureate degree with a major in foods and nutrition and receive at least 6 months' training in a hospital under the supervision of a dietitian.

As the number of programs increased, the need for evaluating the quality of the course became evident. In 1929, it was determined that a committee of three association members would conduct site visits every 2 years.

From 1932 until 1987, recommended academic requirements for entering dietetic internships were published and periodically revised to reflect practice needs. In 1987, the Knowledge Requirements for Dietitians were implemented under the Standards of Education, the minimum criteria to be met by all dietetics education programs.

In 1991 and 1994, the Standards of Education were updated to reflect Role Delineation Studies and environmental changes affecting dietetics practice and to clarify and streamline the criteria and documentation required for accreditation and approval. Programs approved as meeting the Knowledge Requirements for Entry-Level Dietitians were designated Didactic Programs in Dietetics (DPD). Programs were encouraged to continually update their curricula based on current practice in dietetics.

As academic requirements changed, so did the types of programs offered. In 1962, the first Coordinated Undergraduate Program was developed. As an accredited program, it integrated experiential and academic components in an undergraduate curriculum. In 1987, the Standards of Education allowed for the approval of Preprofessional Practice Programs (AP4s) as an alternative to Dietetic Internships.

In the early 1970s, the ADA membership voiced a need for support personnel at the associate degree level. In 1974, *Essentials* were published for approving dietetic technician programs for food service management and nutrition care dietetic technicians.

In an effort to maintain appropriate standards for program review, the ADA became involved in program accreditation. In 1974, the ADA was first recognized by the US Department of Health, Education, and Welfare, now the US Department of Education (ED), as the accrediting agency for Dietetic Internships and Coordinated Undergraduate Programs. At the same time, COPA, now the Commission on Recognition of Postsecondary Accreditation (CORPA), also recognized the ADA as an accrediting agency for Coordinated Undergraduate Programs, and later Dietetic Internships. In 1988, postbaccalaureate Coordinated Programs were recognized as accredited by COPA.

In 1994, accreditation of Dietetic Technician and Preprofessional Practice Programs (AP4s), in addition to Coordinated Programs and Dietetic Internships, was implemented. As AP4s are phased into the accreditation process, they are designated Dietetic Internships.

In 1994, the ADA Bylaws were amended to demonstrate the administrative autonomy of the body charged with accreditation. ADA's accrediting body is now the Commission on Accreditation/Approval for Dietetics Education (AHRP-1997).

Dietitian, Clinical

Alternate title: dietitian, therapeutic. Plans therapeutic diets and implements preparation and service of meals for patients in hospital, clinic, or other health care facility Consults with physician and other health care personnel to determine nutritional needs and diet restrictions of patients, such as low fat or salt free. Formulates menus for therapeutic diets based on medical and physical condition of patients and integrates patients' menus with basic institutional menus. Inspects meals served for conformance to prescribed diets and for standards of palat-

ability and appearance. Instructs patients and their families in nutritional principles, dietary plans, food selection, and preparation. May supervise activities of workers engaged in food. May teach nutrition and diet therapy to medical students and hospital personnel. (DOT-1991)

Dietetic Technician

Occupational/job description
Dietetic technicians assist in shaping the public's food choices and provide nutrition assessment and counseling to persons with illnesses or injuries. Technicians often screen patients to identify nutrition problems, provide patient education and counseling to individuals and groups, develop menus and recipes, supervise food service personnel, purchase food, and monitor inventory and food quality. Dietetic technicians also use computer skills for tasks ranging from inputting inventory and payroll to charting patients' nutritional progress.

Employment characteristics
As an integral part of the nutrition care team, dietetic technicians work together with registered dietitians in a number of different settings, such as hospitals, public health nutrition programs, and long-term care facilities. Technicians also work in child nutrition and school lunch programs, community wellness centers, health clubs, nutrition programs for the elderly, food companies, restaurants, and food-service management.

According to the American Dietetic Association's 1995 membership database, of those registered dietetic technicians who have been employed full-time in their current primary position for 1 to 5 years, 23% report annual gross incomes of less than $20,000, 62% report incomes between $20,000 and $30,000, and 12% report incomes between $30,000 and $40,000. Salary levels may vary based on location, scope of responsibility, and supply of job applicants. (AHRP-1997)

Dietitian/Nutritionist

Occupational/job description
Dietetics is the science of applying food and nutrition to health. Dietitians and nutritionists integrate and apply the principles derived from the sciences of food, nutrition, biochemistry, physiology, food management, and behavior to achieve and maintain the health status of the public they serve.

Employment characteristics
Dietitians and nutritionists work in a variety of settings:

- Clinical dietitians are a vital part of the medical team in hospitals, nursing homes, health maintenance organizations, and other health care facilities. As a key member of the health care team, the clinical dietitian provides medical nutrition therapy, the use of specific nutrition services to treat chronic conditions, illnesses, or injuries. Opportunities for advancement are available by choosing a particular area of nutrition practice, such as diabetes, heart disease, or pediatrics, or by expanding into hospital administration.
- Community dietitians work in public and home health agencies, day care centers, and health and recreation clubs, and in government-funded programs that feed and counsel families, the elderly, pregnant women,

D

children, and individuals with special needs. Wherever proper nutrition can help improve quality of life, community dietitians reach out to the public to teach, monitor, and advise.

- Educator dietitians work in colleges, universities, and community or technical schools, teaching future doctors, nurses, dietitians, and dietetic technicians the sophisticated science of foods and nutrition.
- Research dietitians work in government agencies, food and pharmaceutical companies, and major universities and medical centers. They conduct or direct experiments to answer critical nutrition questions, study alternative foods, and help modify dietary recommendations for the public.
- Consultant dietitians work full- or part-time, usually under contract with a health care facility or in their own private practice. Consultant dietitians in private practice perform nutrition screening and assessment of their own clients and those referred to them by physicians. They offer advice on weight loss, cholesterol reduction, and a variety of other diet-related concerns. Those under contract with health care facilities often consult with food service managers, providing expertise on sanitation and safety procedures, budgeting, and portion control. Other clients include athletes and nursing home residents.
- Management dietitians work in health care institutions, schools, cafeterias, and restaurants, playing a key role where food is served. They are responsible for personnel management, menu planning, budgeting, and purchasing.
- Business dietitians work in food- and nutrition-related industries. They work in such areas as product development, sales, marketing, advertising, public relations, and purchasing.

According to the ADA's 1995 membership database, of those registered dietitians who have been employed full-time in dietetics for 1 to 5 years after registration, 63% report annual gross incomes between $25,000 and $35,000 and 24% report incomes between $35,000 and $45,000. Salary levels may vary with location, scope of responsibility, and supply of job applicants.

Employment outlook
According to the US Bureau of Labor Statistics, employment of dietitians is expected to grow faster than the average profession through the year 2000, especially in the community, consulting, and business areas. (AHRP-1997)

Resource
American Dietetic Association
216 W Jackson Blvd, Chicago, IL 60606-6995
312 899-0040
Web address: http://www.eatright.org

Diethylstibestrol (DES)

DES Action-USA
1615 Broadway, Ste 510, Oakland, CA 94612
800 DES-9288 510 465-4011 Fax 510 465-4815
E-mail: desact@well.com

Digestive Diseases

National Digestive Diseases Information Clearinghouse
2 Information Way, Bethesda, MD 20892-3570
301 654-3810 Fax 301 907-8906

The Disabled

What is the ADA?
On July 26, 1990, President George Bush signed the Americans With Disabilities Act, one of the most sweeping civil rights measures enacted in decades. The ADA prohibits discrimination against people with disabilities in the areas of employment, public services, public accommodations and commercial facilities run by private entities, and telecommunications. The law's objective is to ensure people with disabilities equal opportunity and access to jobs, goods, and services.

Although, in some instances, the ADA's requirements are specifically outlined, the law also contains a number of vaguely defined terms. Lawmakers purposefully used these terms to make the law flexible. The problem with this approach is that in some instances the law provides limited guidance for those trying to comply with its requirements. As a result, the meanings of some of these terms will not be clear until resolved by courts.

The AMA supports the intent of the ADA and other efforts to eliminate discrimination against individuals with disabilities. The AMA is concerned that the vagueness of many requirements makes litigation inevitable. The AMA is seeking to improve the requirements of the Act concerning the provision of auxiliary aids and services, and to expand existing tax credits and tax deductions related to compliance. The AMA is seeking to clarify the application of the ADA to hospital medical staff credentialing procedures.

Although there are many vague terms in the ADA, the definition of the term disability is set forth quite clearly in the law and its regulations.

Disability
Under the ADA a disabled person is someone who:

1. has a physical or mental impairment that substantially limits that person in a major life activity; or
2. has a record of such a physical or mental impairment; or
3. is regarded as having such an impairment.

Physical and mental impairments include, but are not limited to, contagious and noncontagious diseases and conditions such as tuberculosis, HIV infection, cancer, alcoholism, and drug addiction, and orthopedic, visual, speech, and hearing impairments. The phrase physical or mental impairments does not include homosexuality or bisexuality. The term disability does not include transvestism, pedophilia, kleptomania, or compulsive gambling.

Major life activities are functions such as caring for oneself, performing manual tasks, seeing, speaking, breathing, and working.

The three-part definition makes it illegal to discriminate against:

1. a person with a disability—someone who has an **actual physical or mental impairment**—not simply

a physical condition such as hair or eye color, left-handedness, or advanced age; or

2. **a person with a record of impairment**—such as a person with a history of cancer or mental illness—who no longer has the disease but is discriminated against because of his or her record of an impairment; or

3. a person who **is regarded as having an impairment**—such as a person with a visible scar which does not actually limit the person in any major life activity, but the person is nonetheless discriminated against because of the scar.

Physicians and the ADA

Three sections of the ADA may apply to physicians. All physicians are affected by Title III of the ADA, which concerns public accommodations and applies to virtually all businesses open to the public; fewer physicians will be impacted by Title I, which applies only to businesses with more than 15 employees; and some physicians in the public sector will be affected by Title II of the ADA, which prohibits discrimination in public services provided by state or local governments. (ADA-1992)

Americans With Disabilities Act
Pub L No. 101-336 enacted on July 26, 1990

Resources

Architectural and Transportation Barriers
Compliance Board
1331 F St NW, Ste 1000, Washington, DC 20004-1111
800 872-2253 202-272-5434

Department of Justice
Tenth St and Constitution Ave NW
Washington, DC 20530
202 514-0301
Web address: http://www.doj.gov

Mobility International
(Assistance to handicapped people when traveling)
228 Borough High St, London SEI 1JX, England
171 4035688 Fax 171 3781292

Mobility International, USA
(North American affiliate of Mobility International)
PO Box 10767, Eugene, OR 97440
541 343-1284 Fax 541 343-6812
E-mail: miusa@iqc.apc.org

National Foundation of Dentistry for the Handicapped
1800 Glenarm Pl, Ste 500, Denver, CO 80202
303 298-9650 Fax 303 573-0267

National Information Center for Children
and Youth With Disabilities
PO Box 1492, Washington, DC 20013
800 695-0285 202 884-8200 Fax 202 884-8441
E-mail: nichcy@aed.org

Disabled Physicians

AMA Policy

Provisions for Physicians With Handicaps (H-90-989).
Council on Medical Education Rpt E, A-91.

The AMA encourages all medical schools, residency programs, state licensing boards, and medical specialty boards to establish written policies governing the education, licensure, and certification of physicians with handi-

caps, and to establish procedures for the examination of physicians with handicaps.

Resources

American Society of Handicapped Physicians
105 Morris Dr, Bastrop, LA 71220
318 281-4436

Department of Veteran Affairs
Technology Information Center
Rm 237, 810 Vermont Ave NW, Washington DC 20420
202 233-5524

Disability Evaluation

One way in which a physician can provide high-quality care is to ensure that his or her opinion is substantiated by clear, concise, and well-reasoned reports of initial impairment and follow-up treatment. The reports must contain sufficient information to allow a knowledgeable reviewer to understand the initial impairment, and the degree and speed of recovery. The physician must allot a sufficient amount of time to examine the patient thoroughly and to prepare such reports.

The following is an outline of the kinds of information that should be found in each report:

Medical evaluation

1. A narrative history of the medical condition(s) with specific reference to onset and course of the condition, findings on previous examinations, treatment, and responses to treatment.
2. The results of the most recent clinical evaluation, including any of the following that were obtained:
   a. Physical examination findings
   b. Laboratory test results
   c. Electrocardiogram
   d. X rays
   e. Rehabilitation evaluation
   f. Other specific tests or diagnostic procedures and, in the case of psychiatric disease, the results of mental status examination and psychological tests.
3. Assessment of the current clinical status and plans for future treatment, rehabilitation, and reevaluation.
4. Diagnoses and clinical impressions.
5. Estimate of the expected date of full or partial recovery.

Analysis of the findings

1. Explanation of the impact of the medical condition(s) on life activities.
2. Narrative explanation of the medical basis for any conclusion that the medical condition has, or has not, become static or well stabilized.
3. Narrative explanation of the medical basis for any conclusion that the individual is, or is not, likely to suffer sudden or subtle incapacitation as a result of the medical condition.
4. Narrative explanation of the medical basis for any conclusion that the individual is, or is not, likely to suffer injury or harm or further medical impairment by engaging in activities of daily living or any other activity necessary to meet personal, social, occupational, or legal demands.
5. Narrative explanation of any conclusion that restrictions or accommodations are, or are not, warranted with respect to activities of daily living or any other

D activities required to meet personal, social, occupational or legal demands, and if they are, an explanation of the therapeutic or risk-avoiding value of the restrictions or accommodations.

If the examiner elects to use the American Medical Association's *Guides to the Evaluation of Permanent Impairment*, then the following should also be included in the report:

Comparison of the results of analysis with the impairment criteria:

1. Description of specific clinical findings related to each impairment with reference to the relevance of the finding to the criteria of the chapter. Reference to the absence of, or inability to obtain, particular findings is essential.
2. Comparison of the clinical findings with the criteria for the particular body system contained in the Guides.
3. Explanation of the basis for each quantitative impairment rating with reference to the criteria.
4. Summary list of all impairments with ratings.
5. Combined "whole person" rating when more than one impairment is present. (WOR-1983)

The fourth edition of the *Guides to the Evaluation of Permanent Impairment (Guides)* continues an activity begun by the AMA almost four decades ago, the purpose of which was to bring greater objectivity to estimating the degree of long-standing or "permanent" impairments. The rationale for the new edition is that the pace of progress and advances in medicine continues to be rapid, and that a new look at the impairment criteria for all organ systems is advisable. This edition has been prepared under that auspices of the AMA's Council on Scientific Affairs. (EVL-1993)

Doege TC, ed. *Guides to the Evaluation of Permanent Impairment.* 4th ed. Revised. Chicago, Ill: American Medical Association; 1993.
ISBN 0-89970-553-7 0P025493

Resources
American Academy of Disability Evaluating Physicians
150 N Wacker Dr, Ste 920, Chicago, IL 60606-1605
800 456-6095   312 658-1171   Fax 312 658-1175

National Association of Disability Examiners
PO Box 4188, Frankfort, KY 40603
502 875-8388   Fax 502 825-8388

Disaster Medical Care
American Red Cross
431 18th St, Washington, DC 20006
202 737-8300
Web address: http://redcross.org

Medecins Sans Frontieres
(Doctors Without Borders)
8, rue St Sabin, F-75544 Paris Cedex 11, France 1
1 40212929   TX214360F   Fax 1 48066868

New York Office
11 E 26th St, Ste 1904, New York, NY 10112
212 679-6800   212 679-7016

Diving
Undersea and Hyperbaric Medical Society, Inc
10531 Metropolitan Ave, Kensington, MD 20895
301 942-2980   Fax 301 942-7804
E-mail: uhms@radix.net

DAN (Divers Alert Network)
Hall Laboratory for Environmental Science
Duke University Medical Center, Durham, NC 27710
919 684-8111

Doctors' Day, National

Observed March 30

US (officially) honors physicians with first 'National Doctors' Day'

JAMA 1991 Mar 6; 265(9): 1069

This national observance is authorized by the US Congress and the president. In signing the proclamation, President George Bush noted that the March 30 special day honors physicians for what he and Congress call their "invaluable contributions" to the welfare of the nation.

Actually, Doctors' Day began 58 years ago when Eudora B. Almond of the Barrow County (Ga) Medical Society Auxiliary suggested that her auxiliary set aside March 30 to recognize the contributions of local physicians. March 30 was selected because it was on that day in 1842 that Crawford W. Long, MD, a Georgian, became the first physician to use ether anesthesia in surgery.

Well received
The Barrow County auxiliary immediately approved the suggestion. Members agreed that this could be an "observance demanding some act of kindness, gift, or tribute in remembrance of the doctors."

The idea quickly gained wider acceptance. Doctors' Day became a regional observance on March 30, 1935, when the Southern Medical Association Auxiliary, Birmingham, Ala, adopted a similar resolution.

Since then, an increasing number of communities have used this day to express appreciation for the care physicians have provided the sick, for the advances they have made in medical knowledge, and for their leadership in improving public health. In fact, through the nationwide network of medical auxiliaries, Doctors' Day became a national project long before Congress and the President established it as a national day, says Norma Skoglund, Roseburg, Ore, president of the American Medical Association Auxiliary.

Cards, flowers, and more
Those observing that first Doctors' Day in 1933 did so by mailing cards to the doctors (and their spouses) of Winder, Ga, and by placing flowers on the graves of deceased physicians. Since then, Doctors' Day has been celebrated in many communities across the country by diverse activities that include the donation of medical equipment and furniture to hospitals and nursing homes, delivering meals to the elderly, blood donation drives, health fairs, the awarding of scholarships for studies in health-related fields, and numerous other generous acts, Skoglund says.

Sometimes, physicians are the recipients of needed services, as on Doctors' Day in 1988, when the Greensboro, NC, auxiliary arranged for the busy physicians themselves to receive free physical examinations from colleagues. Since 1935, the traditional tribute for physicians on this day, however, has been a gift of red carnations.

For each annual Doctors' Day, the American Medical Association Auxiliary urges its members to honor their physicians by supporting medical education through contributions to the AMA Education and Research Foundation.

"From the rural doctor to the most highly trained specialist, physicians touch the lives of almost every person in the community. We must promote this caring, involved image to our fellow citizens," says Roberta Barnett, president of the Southern Medical Association Auxiliary.

"On Doctors' Day, it is important for auxiliary members to become involved in community service projects on a local basis," she adds. "Our involvement shows the public that physicians are interested in and contribute to their local communities."

"The AMA auxiliary has a national clearinghouse for medical auxiliary programs," says Skoglund. "We have a catalog that lists more than 800 projects developed by auxiliaries. Approximately 30 of these are projects by which communities can recognize the contributions of their physicians."

Do-Not-Resuscitate Orders

Current Opinions of the Council of Ethical and Judicial Affairs 1996-1997. Section 2.22 p56-61.

Efforts should be made to resuscitate patients who suffer cardiac or respiratory arrest except when circumstances indicate that cardiopulmonary resuscitation (CPR) would be inappropriate or not in accord with the desires or best interests of the patient.

Patients at risk of cardiac or respiratory failure should be encouraged to express in advance their preferences regarding the use of CPR and this should be documented in the patient's medical record. These discussions should include a description of the procedures encompassed by CPR and, when possible, should occur in an outpatient setting when general treatment preferences are discussed, or as early as possible during hospitalization. The physician has an ethical obligation to honor the resuscitation preferences expressed by the patient. Physicians should not permit their personal value judgments about quality of life to obstruct the implementation of a patient's preferences regarding the use of CPR.

If a patient is incapable of rendering a decision regarding the use of CPR, a decision may be made by a surrogate decision maker, based upon the previously expressed preferences of the patient or, if such preferences are unknown, in accordance with the patient's best interests.

If, in the judgment of the attending physician, it would be inappropriate to pursue CPR, the attending physician may enter a do-not-resuscitate (DNR) order into the patient's record. Resuscitative efforts should be considered inappropriate by the attending physician only if they cannot be expected either to restore cardiac or respiratory function to the patient or to meet established ethical criteria, as defined in the *Principles of Medical Ethics and Opinions* 2.03 and 2.095. When there is adequate time to do so, the physician must first inform the patient, or the incompetent patient's surrogate, of the content of the DNR order, as well as the basis for its implementation. The physician also should be prepared to discuss appropriate alternative, such as obtaining a second opinion (eg, consulting a biothics committee) or arranging for transfer of care to another physician.

Do-not-resuscitate orders, as well as the basis for their implementation, should be entered by the attending physician in the patient's medical record.

DNR orders only preclude resuscitative efforts in the event of cardiopulmonary arrest and should not influence other therapeutic interventions that may be appropriate for the patient.

Note: Issued March 1992, based on the report Guidelines for the Appropriate Use of Do-not-resuscitate Orders, issued December 1990. (*JAMA* 1991;265: 1868-71)

Donations, Books

American Overseas Medical Aid Association
(medical books and journals)
4433 W Montana St, Chicago, IL 60639
312 486-4809

Darien Book Aid Plan, Inc
(books and journals)
1926 Post Rd, Darien, CT 06820
203 655-2777

The Foundation for Books to China
5337 College Ave, Ste 314, Oakland, CA 94618-1416
415 392-1080

International Book Project, Inc
(professional books and journals)
1440 Delaware Ave, Lexington, KY 40505
606 254-6771

Medical Books for China
13021 E Florence Ave, Santa Fe Springs, CA 90670
213 946-8774

Donations, Medical Supplies

American Near East Refuge Aid, Inc
(pharmaceutical and medical supplies)
1522 K St NW, #202, Washington, DC 20005
202 347-2558   Fax 202 682-1637

American Overseas Medical Aid Association
(surgical and diagnostic equipment, pharmaceutical)
4433 W Montana St, Chicago, IL 60639
312 486-4809

Catholic Medical Mission Board, Inc
(pharmaceutical and medical equipment)
10 W 17th St, New York, NY 10011-5765
212 242-7757   Fax 212 807-9161

Direct Relief International
(pharmaceutical, medical equipment and supplies)
27 S LaPatrea Ln, Santa Barbara, CA 93117
805 964-4767   Fax 805 681-4838

Focus, Inc
(ophthalmologic supplies)
Department of Ophthalmology
Loyola University Medical Center
2160 S First Ave, Maywood, IL 60153
708 216-9408   Fax 708 216-3557

Interchurch Medical Assistance, Inc
(pharmaceutical and hospital supplies)
College Ave at Blue Ridge, PO Box 429
New Windsor, MD 21776
410 635-8720   Fax 410 635-8726

Pan American Development Foundation
(medical equipment and supplies)
2600 16th St NW, Washington, DC 20009-4202
202 458-3969   202 458-6347   Fax 202 458-6316

Plenty International
(medical equipment and supplies, pharmaceutical)
PO Box 394, Summertown, TN 38483
615 964-4864   615 964-4391   615 964-4864

Rescue Now
(medical equipment and supplies, pharmaceutical)
870 Market St, Rm 1050, San Francisco, CA 94102
415 894-6365

World Medical Relief, Inc
(pharmaceutical, medical equipment and supplies)
11745 Rosa Parks Blvd, Detroit, MI 48206
313 866-5333   Fax 313 866-5599

World Opportunities International
(medical supplies)
1415 N Cahuangua Blvd, Hollywood, CA 90028
213 466-7187   Fax 213 871-1546

Drug Abuse

Anti-drug czar Gen. McCaffrey: Make treatment key weapon

Wayne Hearn
AM News Jul 15, 1996 p27

The nation's top drug-policy official called on America's physicians to help "establish the credibility" of treatment programs as a major weapon in the antidrug campaign. "You have to help me persuade legislators and state leaders and the Congress that treatment programs can help and that education and prevention pays off," Gen. Barry R. McCaffrey, director of the Office of National Drug Policy, told the AMA delegates. "We now know more about drug running in Bolivia than we do about the effectiveness of treatment programs and education," he said during a brief dialogue with Michael M. Miller, MD, delegate from the American Society of Addiction Medicine, who told the general that many physicians suffer "therapeutic pessimism" in treating patients who abuse substances.

"Let's get the scientific data, subject to peer review, so we can argue [from] a set of facts and a set of hypotheses—that's what we lack right now," said McCaffrey, a Vietnam veteran and an infantry commander during Operation Desert Storm.

His nomination as the Clinton administration's chief drug policy strategist was confirmed in February.

Millions of dollars at stake

At stake, he said, are millions of federal dollars that can easily be diverted from treatment programs unless lawmakers can be convinced that treatment is a cost-effective approach to the drug problem.

For example, he told delegates that the budget for the federal Substance Abuse and Mental Health Administration was slashed by 40% last year, and $540 million for the Safe and Drug-Free Schools program almost was lost.

He also urged physicians to participate in the approximately 3,000 community-based antidrug alliances nationwide.

"They would benefit not only from your knowledge, but from your leadership," he said. "You have to educate yourselves on drug addiction, pay attention to your patients, and see the people who are suffering ... and do something about it. Your judgment, example, and influence are enormous."

Top goal: youth prevention

McCaffrey said that the No. 1 goal of his $15.1 billion national drug-control strategy, which was just unveiled in April, is "to motivate young people to reject the abuse of drugs, alcohol and tobacco."

"I don't need to tell this group that we have a national emergency in drug abuse among children," he said, citing data showing more youths are experimenting with tobacco, alcohol and drugs—from marijuana to inhalants to Rohypnol, the so-called "date-rape drug"—at younger ages than ever before.

"Sixth grade is the onset of serious exposure to drugs in America," he said. "We understand that if you can get from age 10 to 20 without smoking cigarettes, abusing alcohol, or using drugs, the chances of you having an addictive problem during your lifetime drops, statistically, to zero."

But while his plan stresses education and prevention to cut demand, McCaffrey said law enforcement efforts that are aimed at drug dealers, especially international distribution cartels, must continue.

"We'll never stop drugs from coming into America ... but we can reduce the amount of drugs floating around this country," he said.

"We are aware that if there is less drugs in America, fewer people try them and less become addicted. So we have to do the foreign interdictions. We have to defend America's air, land, and sea frontiers."

Asked his opinions of drug legalization, McCaffrey responded: "Some of them are unprintable. One of the things I am sure of is, we ain't legalizing drugs in America." His adamant stand against legalization elicited sustained applause from the delegates, this three days after published news accounts about an early draft of a Council on Scientific Affairs report said to recommend the decriminalization of marijuana and the easing of penalties on other drugs as part of a harm-reduction approach to the drug problem.

Association officials stressed that the draft, which was written by an outside author, was a work in progress and would undergo considerable revision before it is submitted for approval, possibly at the December AMA Interim Meeting.

In pledging AMA support for the government's antidrug policy, House Speaker Richard F. Corlin, MD, referred to McCaffrey's military success in Operation Desert Storm, where he led the successful "left hook" strike against the elite Iraqi Republican Guard.

"We'd like to be your battalion to help deliver the right hook in this battle," Dr. Corlin said.

Resources

National Directory of Alcoholism, Drug Abuse Treatment Programs
Available from *US Journal of Drug and Alcohol Dependence*
1721 Blount Rd, Ste 1, Pompano Beach, FL 33069
800 851-9100

American Council for Drug Education
c/o Phoenix House, 164 W 74th St
New York, NY 10023
800 488-DRUG   Fax 212 721-2164

Drug and Alcohol Hotline Information
and Referral Service
800 252-6465

National Clearinghouse for Drug Abuse Information
PO Box 416, Kensington, MD 20795
301 468-2600

National Family Partnership
11159-B, S Town Square, St Louis, MO 63123
314 845-1933
Web address: http://www.nfp.org

National Institute on Drug Abuse
800 843-4971
(hotline to assist medical departments of business and industry in establishing programs to deal with drug-related problems in work force)
Web address: http://www.nida.nih.gov

National Institute on Drug Abuse
800 662-HELP (treatment and referral hotline)
Office of Drug Control Policy
Executive Office of the President
Washington, DC 20500
202 467-9800
Web address: http://www.nida.nih.gov

Pregnancy and drug abuse
800 327-BABE (800-327-2223) or
800 638-BABY (800 638-2229)

Drug Compliance

Drug compliance (excerpt)

Larry Stevens
AM News Feb 21, 1994 p19-23

A few years ago, Peter Rudd, MD, an internist at Stanford University Medical Center, examined a 29-year-old man. The severely hypertensive patient had been referred by another doctor who said he was not responding to standard therapies.

An extensive conversation with the patient told Dr. Rudd why: "He admitted he didn't like taking medication, and he didn't have much motivation to do so. His compliance was sporadic at best."

Unfortunately, the revelation came too late. The patient was suffering from complications that soon resulted in renal failure. He entered a dialysis program and, the last Dr. Rudd heard, was waiting for a donated kidney.

The lesson, the physician said, is that "motivating patients to take medications is part of treatment. A doctor can't assume when he writes out a prescription that the medicine will be taken. He or she has to take extra steps in order to ensure that it is."

Resist clairvoyance

The first step toward boosting patient compliance is to realize how difficult it is to know which patients are taking their pills correctly. In one recent study, doctors were able to identify only 53 percent of patients' adherence problems, and 13 percent of the time the patients had volunteered information about the problem before the clinician asked.

This is not to say it is impossible to gauge noncompliance risk. Patients who are unreliable in other areas of their lives are most likely to have problems maintaining a treatment regimen. Therefore, patients who often miss appointments, have trouble keeping jobs or bounce checks should be scrutinized carefully. But you'll miss cases if you don't assume all patients are at risk for noncompliance.

Watch what you say

The most direct way to determine if patients are taking medications correctly is to ask. But getting the information you need takes some skill. Keep in mind that a major problem is that patients often are afraid or ashamed to admit their noncompliance.

Know that pill counting has limits

Many physicians ask patients to bring their medications with them, and then count the pills. Physical evidence is a strong tool for detectives, and it can help doctors sleuth out some difficulties. But it has drawbacks. Patients embarrassed about their noncompliance may simply discard the number of pills they think they've missed. Second, a pill count, even if accurate, doesn't determine if the patient is taking the pills on time or in the right dosage.

Consider high-tech helpers

One high-tech alternative to the pill count is an electronic monitoring system, such as MEMS, manufactured by Aprex Corp. The lids of these pill vials contain microprocessors that record each date and time a bottle is opened.

Until recently, such systems were used exclusively to ensure compliance in clinical drug trials.

Be ready for surprises

If the first step to solving compliance problems is identifying at-risk patients, the second step is finding out why they didn't follow instructions. The reason may be surprising. One possibility: They misunderstand the expected outcome. Patients who think the medicine isn't working are less likely to continue taking it. Another cause of noncompliance: financial barriers that keep patients from filling prescriptions. Even insured patients may feel unable to meet deductibles or copayments. In addition, a patient legitimately may conclude that the regimen offering optimal outcome isn't worth the expense, side effects or inconvenience it causes.

Dig into your bag of tricks

There are dozens of tricks to help patients remember to take their meds. They can place the morning pills near the coffeemaker; leave a pill bottle at work in the desk drawer; reverse the position of the bottle (upside down, then right side up), or move it from pocket to pocket, each time a pill is taken; use an electronic reminder to signal pill-taking time; associate pill-taking with a regularly watched TV show.

Put it in writing

It is also helpful to give patients written instructions.

Reinforce verbal counseling by putting in writing: the name of the medicine and what it is being prescribed for; how and when it should be taken and for how long; any precautions (such as foods or activities to avoid); and potential side effects.

Keep it simple

One of the most helpful things a physician can do is simplify the therapy. Avoid the confusion of regimens involving one set of pills twice a day and another set three times a day. And when possible, avoid pills that must be scheduled around food intake.

Get thee to a (good) pharmacy

Once you write a prescription, make sure your patient takes it to a good pharmacy. Many patients choose a pharmacy on no more rational basis than that it is along the route taken to the doctor's office. Physicians should advise against such behavior.

You can't win 'em all

Most noncompliant patients miss no more than one out of every three or four doses.

But, no matter how heroic a doctor's efforts, some patients still will deviate wildly from the treatment plan and, as a result, suffer poor outcomes. Don't give up on these patients, but realize they will be difficult, and in most cases, impossible to help.

Drug Enforcement Administration

The Drug Enforcement Administration (DEA) is the lead federal agency in enforcing narcotics and controlled substances laws and regulations. It was created in 1973, by Reorganization Plan No. 2 of 1973 (5 USC app), which merged four separate drug law enforcement agencies.

DEA's responsibilities include:
- investigation of major narcotic violators who operate at interstate and international levels;
- seizure and forfeiture of assets derived from, traceable to, or intended to be used for, illicit drug trafficking;
- enforcement of regulations governing the legal manufacture, distribution, and dispensing of controlled substances;
- management of a national narcotics intelligence system;
- coordination with federal, state, and local law enforcement authorities and cooperation with counterpart agencies abroad; and
- training, scientific research, and information exchange in support of drug traffic prevention and control. (USG-1996)

Resources

US Dept of Justice
Drug Enforcement Administration
600-700 Army-Navy Dr, Arlington, VA 22202
202 307-1000

Public Affairs Section
Drug Enforcement Administration
Department of Justice, Washington, DC 20537
202 307-7977
Obtain a DEA registration number by calling
202 254-8255 or 8259

Drug Information

Drug Information Association
PO Box 3113, Maple Glen, PA 19002
215 628-2288   Fax 215 641-1229

Medical Economics Co
5 Paragon Dr, PO Box 430
Montvale, NJ 07645-1742
800 232-7379

Patient Medication Instruction Sheets (PMI)
Information sheets by the USPC on particular drugs, available at two educational levels, prepared especially for the consumer.

USP DI System 14th edition; USPC, Rockville, MD 1995
3 vols in 4 pieces, ISBN 0-91359-551-9
Updated by "USP DI Update" both available from:
United States Pharmacopeial Convention (USPC)
Order Department
PO Box 5367, Twinbrook Station
Rockville, MD 20851
800 227-8772 (Visa and Mastercard orders only)
301 881-0666
800 877-6209 (Publications)

Drug Program, Indigent

Report listing pharmaceutical companies and the prescription drugs they provide for the needy. May be requested in writing from Senate Special Committee on Aging, Room G-31, Dirksen Senate Office Building, Washington, DC 20510-6400.

A program to aid physicians in locating drug companies offering free prescription drugs to indigent patients. The directory and hot line for this information is for use by physicians only.

For the directory, please write to:

1997 Pharmaceutical Industry Patient Assistance Directory
PMA, 1100 15th St NW
Washington, DC 20005
Hotline 800 762-4636   Local 202 393-5200

Contact your state Department of Aging for local programs.

Drug Testing

AMA Policy

Issues in Employee Drug Testing (H-95.984) CSA Rep A, A-87; Reaffirmed: Sub Res 39, A-90, CSA Rep D, I-90; BOT Rep I, A-90; CSA Rep 2, I-95

The AMA (1) reaffirms its commitment to educate physicians and the public about the scientific issues of drug testing; (2) supports monitoring the evolving legal issues in drug testing of employee groups, especially the issues of positive drug tests as a measure of health status and potential employment discrimination resulting therefrom; (3) takes the position that urine drug and alcohol testing of employees should be limited to (*a*) preemployment examinations of those persons whose jobs affect the health and safety of others, (*b*) situations in which there is reasonable suspicion that an employee's (or physician's) job performance is impaired by drug and/or alcohol use, (*c*) monitoring as part of a comprehensive program of treatment and rehabilitation of alcohol and drug abuse or dependence, and (*d*) urine, drug and alcohol testing of all physicians and appropriate employees of health care institutions may be appropriate under these same conditions; and (4) urges employers who choose to establish drug testing programs to use confirmed, positive test results in employees primarily to motivate those employees to seek appropriate assistance with their alcohol or drug problems, preferably through employee assistance programs.

JAMA Article of Note: The efficacy of preemployment drug screening for marijuana and cocaine in predicting employment outcome.

JAMA 1990 Nov 28; 264(20): 2639-43 (see also *JAMA* 1985 Apr 26).

Resources
Guidelines:
American College of Occupational Medicine
55 W Seegers Rd, Arlington Heights, IL 60005
847 228-6850   Fax 847 228-1856

College of American Pathologists
325 Waukegan Rd, Northfield, IL 60095
847 446-8800

Drunk Driving

A Piece of My Mind

Waste

George D. Lundberg, MD
JAMA 1986 Sept 19; 256(11): 1493

He was the best pathology resident I had ever known, before or since that day nine years ago. And that includes hundreds of residents at seven institutions where I have had direct responsibility. He has entered medical school later in life than most, having first become a cytotechnologist, thus acquiring a skill that helped him work his way through medical school. Only three months into his internship, he made a pathology presentation to medical grand rounds at the largest teaching hospital in the United States and received a standing ovation from the usually cynical crowd. In addition to excelling in every standard rotation in anatomic and clinical pathology, he ran a major course in general and systemic pathology for 150 sophomore pharmacy students as an add-on to his second-year residency duties.

He was also an exceptional human being on a personal level. I remember a softball game at a fund-raising Medical Olympics where he made a spectacular catch in centerfield. His wife was a flight attendant, so even though he was a resident they were able to take long trips from time to time. He told me that the thing he liked best was fly-fishing for trout in New Zealand lakes at high altitudes.

When I left to become a departmental chair, I tried hard to recruit him. Despite the fact that he was still in training, he was first on the list of those people I wanted most to bring along from my prior institution to help revitalize my new organization.

The last time I saw him was at a national professional meeting in Las Vegas in 1977, where I took him to dinner to continue my efforts to recruit him. He was grappling with the common problem of whether he should stay in academia, which he loved, or go into private practice with its more immediate tangible rewards, especially since he had by then a number of children to support as well. Obviously, he had many professional opportunities.

The next time I heard about him, he was dead. While he was going home from work one evening, an oncoming car swerved over the center divider and smashed his small sports car head on. An embankment to his right had prevented any evasive action. The next morning in the medical examiner's office his resident colleague did not even recognize him, so severely was he damaged. Both the driver and the passenger in the offending car were drunk. But Lynn was a devout Mormon. He had recently told me that he had never tasted a drop of alcohol in his life.

Resources
Mothers Against Drunk Driving
511 E John Carpenter Fwy, #700, Irving, TX 75062
800 GET-MADD   214 744-6233   Fax 214 869-2206

National Commission Against Drunk Driving
1900 L St NW, Ste 705
Washington, DC 20036
202 452-6004   Fax 202 223-7012

National Safety Council
1121 Spring Lake Dr, Itasca, IL 60143-3201
630 285-1121 (brochure available)   Fax 630 285-1315
Web address: http://www.nsc.org

Dyslexia
Orton Dyslexia Society
8600 La Salle Rd, Ste 382, Baltimore, MD 21286-2044
800 ABCD-123   410 296-0232   Fax 410 321-5069
E-Mail: ods@pie.org

E

Easter Seals

The National Easter Seal Society
230 W Monroe, Chicago, IL 60606
800 221-6827   312 726-6200   Fax 312 726-1494
E-mail: nessinfo@seals.com

Eating Disorders

People who have anorexia nervosa have an intense fear of gaining weight or becoming fat, and often claim to feel fat regardless of how thin they become. They say "no" to the normal food demands of their bodies, doing anything to avoid eating. Bulimia nervosa patients often have normal body weights. However, they are dissatisfied with their bodies and are overly concerned with body shape and weight. These people binge on huge quantities of high-caloric food and then purge their bodies of calories through self-induced vomiting and the use of laxatives. Most anorexics and bulimics are female. Estimates are that as many as one out of every 100 females aged 12 to 18 suffers from anorexia nervosa, and an estimated 2 million women aged 19 to 39 suffer from bulimia. (SHAPE-1993)

Resources

Anorexia Nervosa and Associated Disorders
Box 7, Highland Park, IL 60035
847 831-3438   Fax 847 433-4632

Anorexia Nervosa and Related Eating Disorders
PO Box 5102, Eugene, OR 97405
503 344-1144

BASH (Bulimia Anorexia Self-Help)
c/o Deaconess Hospital
6150 Oakland Ave, St Louis, MO 63139
St Louis area 314 768-3838 or 768-3292

Echocardiography

Echocardiograph Technician. Alternate title: diagnostic cardiac sonographer. Produces two-dimensional ultrasonic recordings and Doppler flow analyses of heart and related structures, using ultrasound equipment, for use by physician in diagnosis of heart disease and study of heart. Explains procedures to patient to obtain cooperation and reduce anxiety. Attaches electrodes to patient's chest to monitor heart rhythm and connects electrodes to leads of ultrasound equipment. Adjusts equipment controls to areas of heart to be examined according to physician's orders. Keys patient information into computer keyboard on equipment to record information on video cassette and strip printout of test. Starts ultrasound equipment that produces images of real-time tomo-graphic cardiac anatomy and adjusts equipment to obtain quality images. Moves transducer, by hand, over patient's heart areas, observes ultrasound display screen, and listens to Doppler signals to acquire data for measurement of blood flow velocities. Prints pictures of graphic analysis recordings and removes video cassette for permanent record of internal examination. Measures heart wall thicknesses and chamber sizes recorded on strip printout, using calipers and ruler, or keys commands into video tape, and compares measurement to standard norms to identify abnormalities in heart. Measures blood flow velocities and calculates data, such as cardiac physiology and valve areas, for evaluation of cardiac function by physician. Reviews test results with interpreting physician. (DOT-1991)

Resources

American Society of Echocardiography
4101 Lake Boone Trl, Ste 201, Raleigh, NC 27607
919 787-5181   Fax 919 784-4916
E-mail: ase@mercury.interpath.com

National Society for Cardiovascular Technology/
Pulmonary Technology
1133 15th St NW, Ste 1000, Washington, DC 20005
202 293-5933

Ecology

Citizens for a Better Environment Reference Center
407 S Dearborn, Ste 1775, Chicago, IL 60605
312 939-1530

Pesticides and Related Medical Treatment Hotline
EPA Hotline 800 858-7378

National Institute of Environmental Health Sciences
PO Box 12233, Research Triangle Park, NC 27709
919 541-3345

Electrocardiography

EKG

Paula Tatarunis
JAMA Oct 23/30 1996, 276(18): 1280x

A bit of sagging on your tracing, he called to say,
the STs to be specific, oh, inferolaterally,
about half a millimeter in 2, 3, F and V3-6,
terribly nonspecific, as a doctor you must
see it all the time yourself; I ran it past
the cardiologist, he said don't worry —
absent symptoms, it's most likely nothing.
You *will* call, though, won't you, for any squeezing
in the chest, short breath, skips or faintness?
Good. We'll do another in a year. Just to be safe.

E

Take care, he said, and then hung up and left me
alone with a half millimeter of deviant electricity
sagging like crepe down my sad sack left ventricle.
Damn! I always thought my Apocalypso Now
would be announced by mammogram or Papanicolaou,
as an errant constellation stippling the webby
gamma space inside my tit, or some queer mitoses
among the exfoliated eosinophilic roses
of my cervix. If not the when, I thought I knew the how:
languishing through a long grim reaper foreplay —

long enough, at least, to see it coming,
le grand *petit mort*, the *coitam* post whose drumming
there is no *tristesse*, ever, nor cigarette.
But no, it could be a simple hydraulic glitch
that delivers me straight from *media res* to ditch
with no chance for confession or even for hamming
it up a bit! *Et tu, Brute!* You seditious chunk of meat!
You pull the heist and I take the heat?
Well, lub dub to you too, bub. You bet I'm gonna
snitch!
We'll both fry together when they pull the switch.

Electrocardiograph Technician. Alternate titles: ECG
technician; EKG technician. Produces recordings of
electromotive variations on patient's heart muscle, using
electrocardiograph (ECG), to provide data for diagnosis
of heart ailments. Attaches electrodes to chest, arms, and
legs of patient. Connects electrode leads to electrocardiograph and starts machine. Moves electrodes along specified area of chest to produce electrocardiogram that
records electromotive variations occurring in different
areas of heart muscle. Monitors electrocardiogram for
abnormal patterns. Keys information into machine or
marks tracing to indicate positions of chest electrodes.
Replenishes supply of paper and ink in machine and
reports malfunctions. Edits and forwards final test results
to attending physician for analysis and interpretation.
May attach electrodes of Holter monitor (electrocardiograph) to patient to record data over extended period of
time. (DOT-1991)

Resource

National Society for Cardiovascular Technology/
Pulmonary Technology
1133 15th St, Ste 1000, Washington, DC 20005
202 293-5933

Electroencephalography

Electroencephalographic Technician. Alternate title:
EEG technologist. Measures electrical activity of brain
waves, using electroencephalograph (EEG) instrument,
and conducts evoked potential response tests for use in
diagnosis of brain and nervous system disorders: Measures patient's head and other body parts, using tape
measure, and marks points where electrodes are to be
placed. Attaches electrodes to predetermined locations,
and verifies functioning of electrodes and recording
instrument. Operates recording instruments (EEG and
evoked potentials) and supplemental equipment and
chooses settings for optimal viewing of nervous system.
Records montage (electrode combination) and instrument settings, and observes and notes patient's behavior
during test. Conducts visual, auditory, and somatosen-
sory evoked potential response tests to measure latency

of response to stimuli. Writes technical reports summarizing test results to assist physician in diagnosis of brain
disorders. May perform other physiological tests, such as
electrocardiogram, electro-oculogram, and ambulatory
electroencephalogram. May perform video monitoring of
patient's actions during test. May monitor patient during
surgery, using EEG or evoked potential instrument. May
supervise other technologists and be known as chief
electroencephalographic technologist. (DOT-1991)

Resource

American Medical Electroencephalographic Association
850 Elm Grove Rd, Elm Grove, WI 53122
414 797-7800   Fax 414 782-8788

Electromyography

Electromyographic Technician. Alternate title: EMG
technician. Measures electrical activity in peripheral
nerves, using electromyograph (EMG) instrument, for
use by physician in diagnosing neuromuscular disorders:
Explains procedures to patient to obtain cooperation and
relieve anxieties during test. Rubs electrode paste on
patient's skin to ensure contact of electrodes. Attaches
surface recording electrodes to extremity in which activity is being measured to detect electrical impulse. Attaches electrodes to electrode cables or leads connected
to EMG instrument and selects nerve conduction mode
on EMG. Operates EMG instrument to record electrical
activity in peripheral nerves. Presses button on manually
held surface stimulator electrode to deliver pulse and
send electrical charge along peripheral nerve. Monitors
response on oscilloscope and presses button to record
nerve conduction velocity. Measures and records time
and distance between stimulus and response, manually or
using computer, and calculates velocity of electrical impulse in peripheral nerve. Removes electrodes from
patient upon conclusion of test and cleans electrode paste
from skin, using alcohol and cotton. (DOT-1991)

Resource

American Association of Electrodiagnostic Medicine
21 Second St SW, Ste 103, Rochester, MN 55902
507 288-0100   Fax 507 288-1225
E-mail: AAEM@aol.com
Web address: http://www.pitt.edu/~nab4/aaem.html

Electroneurodiagnostic Technologist

History
The American Medical Association's (AMA) involvement
in the evaluation and accreditation of educational programs in electroencephalographic (EEG) technology
began in 1972 with the recognition of EEG technology
as an allied health profession by the AMA Council on
Health Manpower. Subsequently, AMA staff worked with
representatives of the professional organizations representing this clinical discipline to develop a draft of the
*Standards (Essentials) of an Accredited Educational Pro-
gram for the Electroencephalographic Technologist.*

In 1973, representatives of the American EEG Society,
the American Medical EEG Association, and the American Society of Electroneurodiagnostic Technologists

(then the American Society of EEG Technologists) presented statements supporting the *Standards*. These organizations and the AMA House of Delegates then considered and adopted the *Standards* for entry-level educational programs for the electroencephalographic technologist.

The Joint Review Committee on Education in Electroencephalographic Technology was established and held its initial meeting in September 1973. In 1988, the name of the committee was changed to the Joint Review Committee on Education in Electroneurodiagnostic Technology.

This review body is composed of six members—four members appointed by the American Society of Electroneurodiagnostic Technologists and two members appointed by the American Electroencephalographic Society. Meetings are held twice annually. The committee develops recommendations on accreditation status of programs, which are subsequently forwarded to the Commission on Accreditation of Allied Health Education Programs for final action. The *Standards* were revised in 1980, 1987, and 1995. In 1987, evoked potential (EP) techniques were included in *Standards* for programs desiring recognition in both electroencephalograpy and EP techniques. In 1995, polysomnography (PSG) techniques were included for programs desiring recognition in EEG, EP, and PSG techniques.

Occupational description
Electroneurodiagnostic technology is the scientific field devoted to recording and studying the electrical activity of the brain and nervous system. Electroneurodiagnostic technologists possess the knowledge, attributes, and skills to obtain interpretable recordings of patients' nervous system function. They work in collaboration with the electroencephalographer.

Job description
The electroneurodiagnostic technologist is skilled in the following functions: communicating with patients, family, and other health care personnel; taking and abstracting histories; applying adequate recording electrodes and using EEG, EP, and PSG techniques; documenting the clinical condition of patients; and understanding and employing the optimal utilization of EEG, EP, and PSG equipment. Among other duties, the electroneurodiagnostic technologist also understands the interface between EEG, EP, and PSG equipment and other electrophysiological devices, recognizes and understands EEG and EP and sleep activity displayed, manages medical emergencies in the laboratory, and prepares a descriptive report of recorded activity for the electroencephalographer. The responsibilities of the technologist may also include laboratory management and the supervision of EEG technicians.

Employment characteristics
Although electroneurodiagnostic personnel work primarily in the neurology departments of hospitals, many work in private offices of neurologists and neurosurgeons. Growth in employment in the profession is expected to be greater than the average for all occupations owing to the increased use of EEG and EP techniques in surgery, in diagnosing and monitoring patients with epilepsy, and in diagnosing sleep disorders. Technologists generally work a 40-hour week. According to

the American Society of Electroneurodiagnostic Technologists, 1995 entry-level salaries averaged $25,000. (AHRP-1997)

Resources
AMA Department of Allied Health
312 553-9355

Executive Director
American Board of Registration of
Electroencephalographic and Evoked Potential
Technologists
PO Box 916633, Longwood, FL 32791-6633
Web address: www.stats.bls.gov

American Society of
Electroneurodiagnostic Technologists
204 W Seventh St, Carroll, IA 51401-2317
712 792-2978   Fax 712 792-6962

Joint Review Committee in
Electroneurodiagnostic Technology
Rte 1 Box 63A, Genoa, WI 54632
608 689-2058

Electronic Dissemination of Information

AMA Policy

National Clearinghouse for Health Care Claims
(H-190.978) BOT Rep 9, A-96; Amended by CMS Rep 11,
I-96

(1) The AMA adopts the following policy principles to encourage greater use of electronic data interchange (EDI) by physicians and improve the efficiency of electronic claims processing: (*a*) public and private payors who do not currently do so should cover the processing costs of physician electronic claims and remittance advice; (*b*) vendors, claims clearinghouses, and payors should offer physicians a full complement of EDI transactions (eg, claims submission; remittance advice; and eligibility, coverage, and benefit inquiry); (*c*) vendors, clearinghouses, and payors should adopt American National Standards Institute (ANSI) Accredited Standard's Committee (ASC) Insurance Subcommittee (X12N) standards for electronic health care transactions and recommendations of the National Uniform Claim Committee (NUCC) on a uniform data set for a physician claim; (*d*) all clearinghouses should act as all-payor clearinghouses (ie, accept claims intended for all public and private payors); (*e*) practice management systems developers should incorporate EDI capabilities, including electronic claims submission; remittance advice; and eligibility, coverage, and benefit inquiry into all of their physician office-based products; (*f*) states should be encouraged to adopt AMA model legislation concerning turnaround time for "clean" paper and electronic claims; and (*g*) federal legislation should call for the acceptance of the Medicare National Standard Format (NSF) and ANSI ASC X12N standards for electronic transactions and NUCC recommendations on a uniform data set for a physician claim. This legislation should also require that (i) any resulting conversions, including maintenance and technical updates, be fully clarified to physicians and their office staffs by vendors, billing agencies, or health insur-

E ers through educational demonstrations and (ii) that all costs for such services based on the NSF and ANSI formats, including educational efforts, be fully explained to physicians and/or their office staffs during negotiations for such contracted services.

(2) The AMA continues to encourage physicians to develop electronic data interchange (EDI) capabilities and to contract with vendors and payors who accept American National Standards Institute (ANSI) standards and who provide electronic remittance advice as well as claims processing.

(3) The AMA will continue to explore EDI-related business opportunities.

(4) The AMA continues to facilitate the rapid development of uniform, industrywide, easy-to-use, low-cost means for physicians to exchange electronically claims and eligibility information and remittance advice with payors and others in a manner that protects confidentiality of medical information and to assist physicians in the transition to electronic data interchange.

(5) The AMA will continue its leadership roles in the NUCC and WEDI.

Emergency Medical Technician—Paramedic

History
The emergency medical technician-paramedic (EMT-Paramedic) was first recognized as an allied health occupation in 1975 by the American Medical Association (AMA) for the purpose of accrediting entry-level educational programs in the profession. Beginning in 1976, a concerted effort by many organizations was begun to develop the educational *Standards (Essentials)* that would be used to evaluate EMT-paramedic programs seeking accreditation. Following several drafts of the proposed *Standards,* with wide distribution to the appropriate communities of interest, the *Standards* were adopted in 1978. Adoption was by the AMA Council on Medical Education (CME) on behalf of the AMA and by the organizations collaborating with the AMA in this accreditation process and sponsoring the newly formed Joint Review Committee on Educational Programs for the EMT-Paramedic (JRC/EMT-P): the American College of Emergency Physicians, American College of Surgeons, American Psychiatric Association, American Society of Anesthesiologists, National Association of Emergency Medical Technicians, and National Registry of Emergency Medical Technicians. The AMA's role of adopting *Standards* is now the responsibility of the Commission on Accreditation of Allied Health Education Programs and the collaborating agencies.

The JRC/EMT-P is currently sponsored by the American Academy of Pediatrics, American College of Cardiology, American College of Emergency Physicians, American College of Surgeons, American Society of Anesthesiologists, National Association of Emergency Medical Technicians, National Council of State Emergency Medical Services Training Coordinators, and National Registry of Emergency Medical Technicians.

Occupational description
Emergency medical technician-paramedics, working under the direction of a physician (often through radio communication), recognize, assess, and manage medical emergencies of acutely ill or injured patients in prehospital care settings. EMT-paramedics work principally in advanced life-support units and ambulance services under medical supervision and direction.

Job description
To fulfill the role of the EMT-paramedic, an individual must be able to:
1. Recognize a medical emergency; assess the situation; manage emergency care and, if needed, extricate the patient; coordinate efforts with those of other agencies that may be involved in the care and transportation of the patient; and establish rapport with the patient and significant others to decrease their state of anxiety.
2. Assign priorities to emergency treatment data for the designated medical command authority or assign priorities of emergency treatment.
3. Record and communicate pertinent data to the designated medical command authority.
4. Initiate and continue emergency medical care under medical control, including the recognition of presenting conditions and initiation of appropriate treatments—for example, traumatic and medical emergencies, airway and ventilation problems, cardiac dysrhythmias, cardiac standstill, and psychological crises—and assess the response of the patient to that treatment, modifying medical therapy as directed.
5. Exercise personal judgment and provide such emergency care as has been specifically authorized in advance in cases where medical direction is interrupted by communication failure or in cases of immediate life-threatening conditions.
6. Direct and coordinate the transport of the patient by selecting the best available method(s) in conjunction with medical command authority.
7. Record in writing or dictate the details related to the patient's emergency care and the incident.
8. Direct the maintenance and preparation of emergency care equipment and supplies.

Employment characteristics
Variations in geographic, sociologic, and economic factors have an impact on emergency medical services and subsequently on the type of practice engaged in by EMT-paramedics. Some EMT-paramedics are employed by community fire and police departments and have related responsibilities in those fields; some serve as community volunteers. Not only are these individuals being employed in the prehospital phase of acute care provided by fire departments, police departments, public services, and private purveyors, but there also is an increased demand for their skills in hospital emergency departments and private industry.

According to the 1992 CAHEA Annual Supplemental Survey, entry-level salaries average $21,672. (AHRP-1997)

Resources

AMA Allied Health Department
312 553-9355

Accreditation Review Committee on Educational and
Surgical Technology for the EMT-Paramedic
7108-C S Alton Way, Ste 150
Englewood, CO 80112-2106
303 694-6191   Fax 303 741-3655

National Association of Emergency Medical Technicians
102 W Leake St, Clinton, MS 39056
800 34-NAEMT   601 924-7744   Fax 601 924-7325

National Registry of Emergency Medical Technicians
PO Box 29233, Columbus, OH 43229
614 888-4484

Emergency Medicine

AMA Policy

Access to Emergency Services. (H-130.970) CMS Rep A,
A-89; Modified by CMS Rep 6, I-95

The AMA supports the following principles regarding
access to emergency services; and these principles will
form the basis for continued AMA legislative and private
sector advocacy efforts to assure appropriate patient
access to emergency services: (1) Emergency services
should be defined as those health care services that are
provided in a hospital emergency facility after the sudden
onset of a medical condition that manifests itself by
symptoms of sufficient severity, including severe pain,
that the absence of immediate medical attention could
reasonably be expected by a prudent layperson, who
possesses an average knowledge of health and medicine,
to result in: (*a*) placing the patient's health in serious
jeopardy; (*b*) serious impairment to bodily function; or
(*c*) serious dysfunction of any bodily organ or part. (2)
All physicians and health care facilities have an ethical
obligation and moral responsibility to provide needed
emergency services to all patients, regardless of their
ability to pay. (Reaffirmed by CMS Rep 1, I-96) (3) All
health plans should be prohibited from requiring prior
authorization for emergency services. (4) Health plans
may require patients, when able, to notify the plan or
primary physician at the time of presentation for emergency services, as long as such notification does not delay
the initiation of appropriate assessment and medical
treatment. (5) All health plans should be required to
cover emergency services provided by physicians and
hospitals to plan enrollees, as required under Section
1867 of the Social Security Act (ie, medical screening
examination and further examination and treatment
needed to stabilize an "emergency medical condition" as
defined in the Act). (6) Failure to obtain prior authorization for emergency services should never constitute a
basis for denial of payment by any health plan or third-
party payor whether it is retrospectively determined that
an emergency existed or not. (7) States should be encouraged to enact legislation holding health plans and
third-party payors liable for patient harm resulting from
unreasonable application of prior authorization requirements or any restrictions on the provision of emergency
services. (8) Health plans should educate enrollees regarding the appropriate use of emergency facilities and
the availability of community-wide 911 and other emergency access systems that can be utilized when for any
reason plan resources are not readily available. (9) In
instances in which no private or public third party coverage is applicable, the individual who seeks emergency
services is responsible for payment for such services.

Resources

American Board of Emergency Medicine
3000 Coolidge Rd, East Lansing, MI 48823-6319
517 332-4800   Fax 517 332-2234

American College of Emergency Physicians
PO Box 619911, Dallas, TX 75261-9911
214 550-0911   Fax 214 580-2816

Wilderness Medical Society
PO Box 2463, Indianapolis, IN 46206
317 631-1745   Fax 317 259-8150
E-mail: wms@indy.net

Employee Health

Adapted from **Employee assistance programs**
Beth Bengston, *AMA Reporter*, Sept 1989

A major change has occurred in corporate America since
the middle 1900s. In the past, employees' personal problems were ignored or covered up, or if they affected
one's work employees might have been disciplined or
fired. Today, more and more companies help troubled
employees regain their health and productivity rather
than discipline them.

A major tool for employers is employee assistance programs (EAPs). An EAP is a confidential, professional way
to help employees tackle personal problems. Most current EAPs are considered "broadbrush" programs, because they help employees deal with a wide range of
problems, including job stress, single parenting, financial,
or legal problems, marital and family relations, alcohol
and drug dependency, emotional problems, gambling
addiction, and eating disorders. More emphasis is being
placed on problem prevention and on catching problems
early, before they become crises.

Employee Assistance Programs have experienced phe-
nomenal growth in the US in the past 40 years. Their
scope has also changed dramatically, from a focus mainly
on alcohol and drug problems to a more comprehensive
approach. Interestingly, the initial EAP boom coincided
with the AMA's recognizing, and the public's beginning
to accept, alcoholism as a disease rather than a personal
deficiency. There were fewer than 100 EAPs operating in
1950, compared to [approximately 6000 in 1989.]

How do EAPs work?
Through an EAP, employees can obtain confidential
assistance for a personal problem from a trained professional. Typically, an EAP is a starting point to help
people help themselves. Some EAPs are internal—staffed
and run by counselors who are employed by the company. But many employers use an independent professional assistance agency to implement a program.

The process begins when an employee voluntarily calls
the EAP. The next step is a professional assessment of his
or her situation. Sometimes a problem can be resolved in
just a few sessions with an EAP professional. Other cases
may require more specialized help, and the client is

E referred to an outside resource—a hospital program, a counselor, an agency, or a self-help group specializing in the individual's particular problem. The EAP counselor then stays in touch with the client to see how he or she is progressing and to offer support and encouragement. Clients are advised to follow through with the program, but have the option to leave or re-enter it at any time.

Confidentiality
Confidentiality and privacy are essential elements of any EAP. Counselors are required to maintain a client's privacy and confidentiality within strict state and federal guidelines. There are stiff penalties for a person who discloses confidential information to anyone without the client's written permission, except in rare cases of extreme danger to self or others, or in cases of unreported child abuse.

EAPs away from the worksite are conducive to confidentiality—employees can meet a counselor after working hours, and away from coworkers and managers. In some cases an independent auditor evaluates the EAP to ensure confidentiality.

Management training
Since managing a problem employee can be fraught with uncertainty, an ongoing management education and training function is part of most EAPs. This training is invaluable to supervisors. It is crucial that a supervisor know how to talk with an employee and encourage him or her to contact the EAP.

This type of discussion between a manager and employee does not hinder confidentiality since participation in the EAP is voluntary. The employee alone is responsible for calling the EAP, seeing the counselor, and following through with the prescribed course. A counselor can disclose no information to the manager or anyone else at the workplace unless the employee consents. Job security and promotional opportunities are based on work performance and attendance, and are not affected by participation or nonparticipation in the EAP.

The success of any EAP hinges on the employees who utilize it. For a program to be effective, employees must understand it, know how it works, and feel comfortable using it. To encourage this, most employers conduct employee orientation sessions. Situations in which an EAP may help, how the procedure works, how confidentiality is maintained, and who is eligible to participate are generally discussed. The orientation is also an important time for employees to ask questions about the program.

The employee/employer partnership
An employee assistance program is obviously meant to benefit employees, but the employer also comes out a winner. By helping the employee, the company also benefits as the employee becomes more productive. Studies have shown decreased absenteeism and accidents, lower turnover, better morale, and greater job satisfaction after the introduction of an EAP.

Resources
Employee Assistance Professionals Association
2101 Wilson Blvd, Ste 500, Arlington, VA 22201-3062
703 522-6272   Fax 703 522-4585

Employee Assistance Society of North America
2728 Phillips, Berkely, MI 48072
810 545-3888   Fax 810 545-5528

Endocrinology
Endocrine Society
4350 E West Hwy, Ste 500
Bethesda, MD 20814-4410
301 941-0200   Fax 301 941-0259

Board Certification in Endocrinology and Metabolism
American Board of Internal Medicine
3624 Market St, Philadelphia, PA 19104
800 441-ABIM (800 441-2246)   215 243-1500
Fax 215 382-4702

Board Certification in Reproductive Endocrinology
American Board of Obstetrics and Gynecology
2915 Vine St, Dallas, TX 78504-1069
214 871-1619   Fax 214 871-1943

End-of-life Care

AMA Policy

Medical Futility in End-of-Life Care. H-140.948 CEJA Rep 2, I-96

Policy of the AMA states that: health care institutions, whether large or small, should adopt a policy on medical futility; and that policies on medical futility follow a due process approach. The following seven steps should be included in such a due process approach to declaring futility in specific cases.

1. Earnest attempts should be made in advance to deliberate over and negotiate prior understandings between patient, proxy, and physician on what constitutes futile care for the patient, and what falls within acceptable limits for the physician, family, and possibly also the institution.
2. Joint decision making should occur between patient or proxy and physician to the maximum extent possible.
3. Attempts should be made to negotiate disagreements if they arise, and to reach resolution within all parties' acceptable limits, with the assistance of consultants as appropriate.
4. Involvement of an institutional committee such as the ethics committee should be requested if disagreements are irresolvable.
5. If the institutional review supports the patient's position and the physician remains unpersuaded, transfer of care to another physician within the institution may be arranged.
6. If the process supports the physician's position and the patient/proxy remains unpersuaded, transfer to another institution may be sought and if done should be supported by the transferring and receiving institution.
7. If transfer is not possible, the intervention need not be offered.

The machine

Don Lewis
JAMA Sept 24, 1994; 272(12): 970

The machine
always perfect
without any flaw
performing all functions
cares nothing at all.
It never grows weary
no reason to rest
compression is constant
while moving the chest
of Mr. Montgomery
who lies in his bed.
His eyes stare
relentlessly
out of his head;
onto the ceiling
dark shadows fall
upward and downward
they drift on the wall.
Oxygen flows through
valves more alive
than Mr. Montgomery
whose breathing they drive.
Inhaling, exhaling
his color is gray
the machine washes wasted
corpuscles away.
His muscles lie flaccid
red lips are now blue
while no one is noting
both eyes are askew.
The machine knows no limit
no visible goal;
pistons slide silently
out of control
forever recycling
but no word is said.
With nobody knowing
Montgomery is dead.

End-of-life care

Daniel P. Sulmasy, OFM, MD, PhD, and Joanne Lynn, MD
JAMA 1997 Jun 18, 277(3): 1854-5

Hippocrates wrote that the art of medicine consisted of relieving the sufferings of the sick, lessening the violence of their diseases, and refraining from attempts at cure when patients were overmastered by disease.[1] Physicians, unfortunately, seemed to interpret this as advice to avoid those who are dying. By 1505, Francis Bacon was urging physicians to treat patients' symptoms not only when they might recover, "but also when, all hope of recovery gone, it serves only to make a fair and easy passage from life."[2] Five centuries later, the profession is beginning to address Bacon's challenge.

Professionals and the public are troubled by current patterns of inadequate care and are seeking improvements. Almost every type of health care professional and organization treat dying patients, so responsibility is broad and myriad changes are needed. Reform requires broad interdisciplinary collaboration and depends primarily on better use of existing therapeutic knowledge and continued expansion of the research base. Searching the Medical Subject Heading key word "terminal care" yielded 124 articles per year in the early 1970s. That figure for the last three years averages 543. The World Health Organization, the Agency for Health Care Policy and Research (AHCPR), and the American Pain Society have promulgated guidelines for treating cancer pain within the past few years.

Most of us now die of progressive chronic illness, mostly in old age (average age at death is 77 years[3]) and mostly after a substantial period of disability. Thus, most people know someone whose dying seemed to go awry, whether through injudicious overtreatment or inadequate supportive care services. The limited data available support the pervasiveness of these anecdotes. The Study to Understand Prognoses and Preferences for Outcomes and Risks of Treatment (SUPPORT) found that half of conscious patients suffered severe pain near death.[4] Serious chronic illness threatens almost everyone with impoverishment.[5] Most oncologists report feeling unskilled at pain management[6] and few care systems ensure continuity. Advance care planning remains the exception rather than the rule, even for predictable decisions like resuscitation.

In response, the Open Society Institute initiated the Project on Death in America, which is funding an array of research and demonstration projects and a few dozen scholars in medical centers. The biennial palliative care conference in Montreal (the International Congress on the Care of the Terminally Ill, September 7-11, 1996) and various hospice providers' meetings were joined this past year by four prominent meetings focused on reform agendas: The Robert Wood Johnson Foundation brought together public and professional organizations to share information and set agendas; the Center to Improve Care of the Dying convened policymakers; the American Medical Association convened professional society representatives to focus on education and practice reform; and the Milbank Memorial Fund convened professional society representatives to consider policy statements and practice guidelines. The American Medical Association's Council on Scientific Affairs called for improvements in education, research, and services for the dying.[7]

Forty professional and lay organizations have signed a statement that advocates that health care organizations and clinicians be held accountable for quality of care at the end of life and presents a list of 10 areas that should be measured: symptoms, function, advance planning, aggressive life-extending treatments, satisfaction (patient and family), quality of life, family burden, survival time, provider continuity and skill, and bereavement support.[8] A collaborative effort to develop measures of quality of care was initiated at a meeting of survey researchers in August (Toolkit Conference, Woods Hole, Mass, August 27-28, 1996).

The movement to legalize physician-assisted suicide has made legislative and judicial gains. As of January 1, 1997, Jack Kevorkian, MD, an unlicensed pathologist, has acknowledged assisting at least 44 patients with suicide, though several attempted prosecutions have failed. Oregon passed a statute legalizing physician-assisted suicide, but legal challenges have blocked implementation. In the spring of 1996, two US district courts declared state bans

E

E on assisted suicide to be unconstitutional, invoking the liberty/due process and the equal protection clauses of the Fourteenth Amendment.[9] Both states appealed. The US Supreme Court heard oral arguments on January 8, 1997, and is likely to rule this summer. The American Medical Association and most established health care professional groups are opposed to constitutionalizing the question and to legalizing the practice, but the public[10,11] and physicians[12,13] are divided.

The suicide debate might galvanize medical and social forces to effect real improvement in the care of the dying.[14] In Oregon, for example, most physicians have received continuing education on good care of the dying in the past two years, and the site of death is shifting from hospitals to nursing homes, hospices, and homes. Regardless of the Supreme Court decision, health care has a moral imperative and a political mandate to provide better care for the dying.

Federal funding to improve care of the dying through research or education is hard to discern, especially at the National Institutes of Health. Current funding for health professionals' education does not require attention to end-of-life care. The Agency for Health Care Policy and Research has sponsored an array of projects on advance care planning and now on the measurement of quality. The Robert Wood Johnson Foundation, which funded the SUPPORT project, is following up with a major public information campaign and a research and demonstration initiative. Congress required the US Department of Veterans Affairs to evaluate their hospice services, though this will be a very limited study.

Educators are also beginning to respond. Initiatives for medical students are under way at multiple medical schools, with one collaborative project being coordinated by the consumer group Choice in Dying in New York City. Representatives from several specialty boards recently met to incorporate curricular requirements into the reviews of the Residency Review Committees and to develop board examination questions.[15] The American Board of Internal Medicine has produced an educational resource on care of the dying,[16] and new recommendations of the Federated Council for Internal Medicine require classroom and hands-on clinical experiences.[17]

Care at the end of life probably cannot improve dramatically without major changes in financing and organization of care. At present, supportive services and palliative care are inadequately compensated, especially in comparison with technological interventions. Incentives also discourage continuity. Dying patients are undesirable to enroll or retain in capitated health plans since they incur major expenses without bringing additional income. One small improvement may be the current experiment with an *International Classification of Diseases* code for palliative care.[18] More fundamental reform is also gathering support. "MediCaring," for example, proposes hospice-like comprehensive service programs on a salary or capitation basis for those who are seriously ill with an eventually fatal illness, even if survival time is relatively unpredictable.[19]

We are now poised to respond to Bacon's 500-year-old plea to make the care of the dying an integral part of medical research, teaching, and practice. The truism that all of us will die means that all of us have an interest in being confident that our suffering and pain will be compassionately addressed, and that we will find our time at the end of life conducive to the experiences of being loved and finding meaning. Clinicians will need improved skills and more appropriate care systems in order to improve care at the end of life.

References

1. Hippocrates. The art, iii. In: Jones WHS, trans. *Hippocrates.* Cambridge, Mass: Harvard University Press; 1992;2:193.

2. Bacon F; Spedding E, Spedding J, trans. *De dignitatae et augmentis scientiarum.* In: Robertson JM, ed. *The Philosophical Works of Francis Bacon.* New York, NY: EP Dutton; 1905;2:487.

3. *Statistical Abstract of the United States.* 115th ed. Washington, DC: US Bureau of the Census; 1995:86.

4. The SUPPORT Investigators. A controlled trial to improve care for seriously ill hospitalized patients: The Study to Understand Prognoses and Preferences for Outcomes and Risks of Treatments (SUPPORT). *JAMA.* 1995;274:1591-1598. Correction: *JAMA.* 1996;275:1232.

5. Covinsky KE, Goldman L, Cook EF, et al. The impact of serious illness on patients' families. *JAMA.* 1994;272:1839-1844.

6. Von Roenn JH, Cleeland CS, Gonin R, et al. Physician attitudes and practice in cancer pain management: a survey from the Eastern Cooperative Oncology Group. *Ann Intern Med.* 1993;119:121-126.

7. Council on Scientific Affairs, American Medical Association. Good care of the dying patient. *JAMA.* 1996;275:474-478.

8. Vitez M. Coalition sets standards for care of the dying. *Philadelphia Inquirer.* January 8, 1997:3.

9. Lynn J, Cohn F, Pickering JH, et al. The American Geriatric Society on physician assisted suicide: brief to the US Supreme Court. *J Am Geriatr Soc.* 1997;45:489-499.

10. Blendon RJ, Szalay US, Knox RA. Should physicians aid their patients in dying? The public perspective. *JAMA.* 1992;267:2658-2662.

11. AMA poll: the more patients know, the less they want suicide aid. *Am Med News.* January 13, 1997;40:3, 56.

12. Bachman JG, Alcser KH, Doukas DJ, Lichtenstein RL, Corning AD, Brody H. Attitudes of Michigan physicians and the public toward legalizing physician-assisted suicide and voluntary euthanasia. *N Engl J Med.* 1996;334:303-309.

13. Back AL, Wallace JI, Starks HE, Pearlman RA. Physician-assisted suicide and euthanasia in Washington State. *JAMA.* 1996;275:919-925.

14. Lee MA, Tolle SW. Oregon's assisted suicide vote: the silver lining. *Ann Intern Med.* 1996;124:267-269.

15. Conference: Education of Physicians About Dying, Hackensack University Medical Center; April 19, 1996; Hackensack, NJ. Sponsored by the Open Society Institute Project on Death in America.

16. The American Board of Internal Medicine End-of-Life Care Project Committee. *Caring for the Dying: Identification and Promotion of Physician Competency.* Philadelphia, Pa: American Board of Internal Medicine; 1996.

17. Ende J, Kelley M, Ramsey P, Sox H, eds. *Graduate Education in Internal Medicine: A Resource Guide: Report of the FICM Task Force on the Internal Medicine Curriculum.* Philadelphia, Pa: American College of Physicians; 1997.

18. Cassel CK, Vladeck BC. ICD-9 code for palliative or terminal care. *N Engl J Med*. 1996;335:1232-1234.

19. Lynn J. Caring at the end of our lives. *N Engl J Med*. 1996;335:201-202.

Endodontics

Endodontist. Examines, diagnoses, and treats diseases of nerve, pulp, and other dental tissues affecting vitality of teeth. He or she examines teeth, gums, and related tissues to determine the condition, using dental instruments, and x-ray and other diagnostic equipment. Endodontists diagnose conditions and plan treatment, treat exposure of pulp by pulp capping or removal of pulp from pulp chamber and root canal, using dental instruments, perform partial or total removal of pulp using surgical instruments, treat infected root canal and related tissues and fill pulp chamber and canal with endodontic materials, surgically remove pathologic tissue at apex of tooth, reinsert teeth that have been knocked out of mouth by accident, and bleach discolored teeth to restore natural color. (DOT-1991)

Endometriosis

Endometriosis is a condition in which fragments of the endometrium (lining of the uterus) are found in other parts of (or on organs within) the pelvic cavity.

Incidence and cause

Endometriosis is most prevalent between the ages of 25 and 40 and is a common cause of infertility. About 10 to 15 percent of infertility patients have endometriosis and about 30 to 40 percent of women suffering from endometriosis are infertile.

The exact cause of endometriosis is uncertain, but in some cases it is thought to occur because fragments of the endometrium that are shed during menstruation do not leave the body with the menstrual flow. Instead, they travel up the fallopian tubes and into the pelvic cavity. There, they may adhere to and grow on any of the pelvic organs.

These displaced patches of endometrium continue to respond to the menstrual cycle as if they were still inside the uterus, so each month they bleed. This blood cannot escape, however, and causes the formation of slowly growing cysts from the size of a pinhead to the size of a grapefruit. The growth and swelling of the cysts are responsible for much of the pain associated with endometriosis.

Symptoms and signs

The symptoms of endometriosis vary widely, with abnormal or heavy menstrual bleeding being most common. There may be severe abdominal and or lower back pain during menstruation, which is often most severe toward the end of a period. Other possible symptoms include dyspareunia and digestive tract symptoms such as diarrhea, constipation, or painful defecation. Rectal bleeding that happens only at the time of the menses may occur. In some cases, however, endometriosis causes no symptoms. (ENC-1989)

Resource

Endometriosis Association
8585 N 76th Pl, Milwaukee, WI 53223
800 992-3636
414 355-2200 (in WI)   Fax 414 355-6065

Environmental Protection Agency

The Environmental Protection Agency (EPA) protects and enhances the environment today and for future generations to the fullest extent possible under the laws enacted by the US Congress. The agency's mission is to control and abate pollution of air, water, solid waste, pesticides, radiation, and toxic substances. Its mandate is to mount an integrated, coordinated attack on environmental pollution in cooperation with state and local governments.

The Environmental Protection Agency was established in the executive branch as an independent agency pursuant to Reorganization Plan No. 3 of 1970 (5 USC app), effective December 2, 1970.

The agency was created to permit coordinated and effective government action on behalf of the environment. It endeavors to abate and control pollution systematically, by proper integration of a variety of research, monitoring, standard setting, and enforcement activities. As a complement to its other activities, the Agency coordinates and supports research and antipollution activities by state and local governments, private and public groups, individuals, and educational institutions. It also reinforces efforts among other federal agencies with respect to the impact of their operations on the environment, and it is specifically charged with publishing its determinations when those hold that a proposal is unsatisfactory from the standpoint of public health or welfare or environmental quality. In all, the Environmental Protection Agency is designed to serve as the public's advocate for a livable environment. (USG-1996)

Resource

Environmental Protection Agency
401 M St SW, Rm 211B, Washington, DC 20460
Public Information 202 260-4700
Web address: http://www.epa.gov

Environmental Health

American Academy of Environmental Medicine
4510 W 89th St, Ste 110, Prairie Village, KS 66207
913 642-6062   Fax 913 341-6912

Citizens for a Better Environment
33 E Congress Pkwy, Ste 523, Chicago, IL 60605
312 939-1530

National Institute of Environmental Health Sciences
PO Box 12233, Research Triangle Park, NC 27709
919 541-3345

Pesticides and Related Medical Treatment Hotline
EPA Hotline 800 858-7378

E Epilepsy

American Epilepsy Society
638 Prospect Ave, Hartford, CT 06105-4298
203 586-7565   Fax 203 586-7550

Epilepsy Foundation of America
4351 Garden City Dr, Ste 406
Landover, MD 20785
800 EFA-1000   301 459-3700   Fax 301 577-2684

Epilepsy Information Line 800 332-1000

Equipment, Medical

Association for the Advancement of Medical
Instrumentation
3330 Washington Blvd, Ste 400
Arlington, VA 22201-4598
800 332-2264   703 525-4890   Fax 703 276-0783

ECRI (to evaluate health care technology)
c/o Ed Stevenson, Communications Dept
5200 Butler Pike, Plymouth Meeting, PA 19462
215 825-6000   Fax 610 834-1275

Health Industry Distributors Association
225 Reinekers Ln, #650, Alexandria, VA 22314 -2875
703 549-4432   Fax 703 549-6495

Health Industry Manufacturers Association
1200 G St NW, Ste 400, Washington, DC 20005
202 783-8700   Fax 202 783-8750

National Association of Medical Equipment Suppliers
625 Slaters Ln, Ste 200, Alexandria, VA 22314-2875
703 836-6263   Fax 703 836-6730
E-mail: info@names.org

*Contact (for Health Care Professionals) to report
malfunction:*
US Pharmacopeial Convention
800 638-6725 (24-hour) or
Food and Drug Administration 301 881-0256
(7 am to 4:30 pm EST)

ERISA

AMA Policy

ERISA (H-165.883) CMS Rep 6, I-96

The AMA will seek, through amendment of the ERISA
statute, through enactment of separate federal patient
protection legislation, through enactment of similar state
patient protection legislation that is uniform across states,
and through targeted elimination of the ERISA preemption of self-insured health benefits plans from state regulation, to require that such self-insured plans: *a*) Ensure
that plan enrollees have access to all needed health care
services; *b*) Clearly disclose to present and prospective
enrollees any provisions restricting patient access to or
choice of physicians, or imposing financial incentives
concerning the provision of services on such physicians;
c) Be regulated in regard to plan policies and practices
regarding utilization management, claims submission and
review, and appeals and grievance procedures; *d*) Conduct scientifically based and physician-directed quality
assurance programs; *e*) Be legally accountable for harm to
patients resulting from negligent utilization management
policies or patient treatment decisions through all avail-

able means, including proportionate or comparative
liability, depending on state liability rules; *f*) Participate
proportionately in state high-risk insurance pools that are
financed through participation by carriers in that jurisdiction; *g*) Be prohibited from indemnifying beneficiaries
against actions brought by physicians or other providers
to recover charges in excess of the amounts allowed by
the plan, in the absence of any provider contractual
agreement to accept those amounts as full payment; *h*)
Inform beneficiaries of any discounted payment arrangements secured by the plan, and base beneficiary coinsurance and deductibles on these discounted amounts when
providers have agreed to accept these discounted
amounts as full payment; *i*) Be subject to breach of contract actions by providers against their administrators;
and *j*) Adopt coordination of benefits provisions applying
to enrollees covered under two or more plans.

Court rulings chip away at managed care's ERISA shield

Julie Johnsson
AM News Oct. 14, 1996 pp 3, 68–69

Managed care plans now face unprecedented state oversight, thanks to a barrage of new laws following a landmark 1995 US Supreme Court decision that broadened
states' authority to regulate employee benefit plans.

But experts predict that the mother of all legal battles in
this arena lies ahead, as states and insurers struggle over
how to apply a new generation of managed care legislation to self-funded plans.

During the 1996 legislative session, 33 states enacted
laws regulating managed care plans, while state assemblies nationwide considered more than 1,000 anti-man-
aged care bills.

This avalanche of activity was largely the result of well-
orchestrated campaigns by consumer and provider
groups to mandate quality and access standards for
health plans.

But state lawmakers also responded to the first opening
granted them by the courts to establish rules for an
industry that remains largely unregulated.

Historically, state health insurance coverage mandates
often have proved to be little more than symbolic gestures. That's because the courts have long interpreted the
federal Employee Retirement Security Act of 1974 to
nullify or preempt any state law that "relates to" a qualified self-insured plan in any way.

Roughly 65% of the private health insurance market is
controlled by self-insured plans and their contracting
partners. This means that most managed care players
long have been immune from any-willing-provider requirements, physician deselection bans, and other state
laws.

But this immunity also has freed employers to spur competition in their markets through cutting-edge contracting arrangements with providers.

"ERISA is the legal cornerstone of all the innovative
work we've done up here," says Steve Wetzel, executive
director of the Buyers Health Care Action Group. The
coalition of 24 Minneapolis businesses attracted national
acclaim by working with area doctors to create compet-

ing provider-sponsored organizations for its 100,000 covered lives.

Legal free-for-all

But other health plans' ability to claim similar exemption from state oversight may be narrowed by a spate of appellate court decisions following the Supreme Court's unanimous—and surprising—ruling in the 1995 *Travelers v. Cuomo*.

Reversing 20 years of ERISA case law, the high court found that self-funded plans and contracting agents of employer plans have no absolute guarantee of preemption from state laws.

The Supreme Court held that plans couldn't use ERISA as a shield from state health reform efforts that carried only an indirect economic effect. But it also forbade states from mandating employee benefits or regulating key benefit administration functions (*AMNews,* May 15, 1995).

"The *Travelers* case made clear that ERISA was not intended to preempt the whole panoply of state tort law," says Carol O'Brien, senior AMA attorney.

Now, legal experts foresee a litigation free-for-all, as insurers contest both the precedent set by *Travelers* and the new generation of managed care laws created in its wake.

"It certainly is going to be a battleground with those laws," says James Jacobson, an attorney with the Washington, DC, office of Gardner, Carton & Douglas. Prime targets for litigation include statutes mandating plans contract with "any willing provider," due process requirements, mandated access to certain specialists, direct contracting, and capitation, he adds.

"It's going to be a very fertile area for legal battles and legal maneuvering," O'Brien adds. "It's going to be one of the most exciting new areas of law to emerge over the next few years."

"Gag clause" restrictions and other patient protection legislation should survive courtroom ambushes, she predicts. "Under the *Travelers* case, states are going to have a lot more room to make a convincing argument that these patient protection laws are exactly the types of quality, health and welfare laws that have traditionally been within their purview."

But nothing is certain at this point. That's because the state and federal appellate courts have already issued conflicting interpretations of *Travelers* in cases contesting any-willing-provider requirements and HMOs' vicarious liability for malpractice committed by their physicians.

The problem is that the Supreme Court based its opinion narrowly upon the facts of that case, leaving lower courts little guidance on how to apply this doctrine to other managed care laws.

"The courts are in total disarray on this," Jacobson says. "They have already ruled on both sides of the any-willing-provider issue."

Narrowing preemption

But at least one trend is emerging from this confusion. So far, the courts seem much less willing to quickly assume that state insurance requirements are preempted by the federal law.

"This definitely has opened up the opportunity for the courts to get into the preemption issue more deeply than before," says Gary Howell, an attorney with the Chicago law office of Gardner, Carton & Douglas.

"Before *Travelers,* courts just performed a knee-jerk, 'relates to' analysis."

Organized medicine scored victories this summer in Connecticut and Michigan after state appeals courts overturned lower court findings that ERISA preempted insurers from complying with new state laws on provider selection.

"A win in one state impacts all of us," says Tim Norbeck, executive director of the Connecticut State Medical Society. "A win on ERISA impacts the whole country."

His state medical society joined the AMA in filing an amicus brief asking the state Supreme Court to consider whether Cigna Healthcare of Connecticut should be preempted from a state law requiring insurers to list all physicians in their network, as well as the criteria used to fire or hire them.

In 1994, a lower court dismissed a suit brought against Cigna by Robert Napoletano, MD, who claimed he was unjustly deselected by the health plan. The Hartford Superior court threw out the case, agreeing with Cigna that the health plan was shielded by federal law from the claims in the lawsuit.

But this July, the state high court decided that preemption was no longer appropriate, given the *Travelers* decision, and returned the case to the lower court for new proceedings.

Cigna hasn't announced whether it will appeal this decision to the US Supreme Court.

But Norbeck lauded the state high court's action. "It's extremely important to the physicians, other providers, and patients in this state that [self-insured managed care] plans be held to the few regulations that we have."

Cuts both ways

But narrower ERISA preemptions aren't necessarily good news for all doctors.

"ERISA is ideology-neutral," says Richard Raskin, partner with the Chicago law office of Sidley & Austin. "It can be a very friendly device when you have state laws that are oppressive. And it can be a fairly unfavorable problem when you want to see state laws enforced."

For example, many state medical societies may applaud *Travelers* for enabling wider enforcement of managed care laws that they support.

But some doctors have used ERISA successfully to dismiss medical liability cases, a defense that could soon disappear, experts say. *Travelers* also could hurt doctor ventures that have adopted global capitation and now wish to side-step heavy new regulation of provider risk-sharing set by states like Pennsylvania.

"I think we'll see litigation soon on whether ERISA preempts state law that would force capitated providers to seek [HMO] licensure," Jacobson predicts.

Interestingly, the capitation issue could prove harmful for employer-sponsored ventures, too, he notes. In fact, employers who share global capitation directly with

E

physicians may risk losing all federal immunity from state law.

ERISA law currently establishes a three-step analysis to determine whether plans are preempted from state law.

First, state laws are superseded if they "relate to" an ERISA plan and have more than an indirect economic effect upon the plan. Any preemption found under the first clause is dropped if the laws also regulate the business of insurance.

If there's still any question, the courts look at whether the plan is self-funded. If so, it is preempted from state oversight. This analysis, known as the "deemer clause," is "the ultimate," Jacobson says. "It trumps everything else."

To date, few legal cases have explored the deemer clause, he adds. That's because before *Travelers*, most contested laws were either found to be applicable insurance regulations or were nullified because they related to self-insured plans.

"But now we get into the question of whether an employer plan is self-funded or not," Jacobson says. "The deemer clause itself doesn't offer any guidance as to what fundamentally is a self-funded plan. You have to look to state or federal law."

This could be problematic for employers, because some states consider entities to be subject to insurance regulation—and thus not covered by ERISA—if they purchase stop-loss coverage or reinsurance, or if they share risk with provider networks that aren't licensed as HMOs.

Such findings likely would squelch cutting-edge employer initiatives. "This is going to be the wave of the future, because increasingly employers want control over quality and benefits," he adds. "But they want to manage their group's experience through capitation or carve-outs."

Jacobson predicts that ultimately the courts will make a distinction under ERISA between employers and the HMOs or provider groups they subcontract with to provide health care.

"I really think we're headed to a doctrine where we preempt state laws if they affect plan choices by benefit plan managers or employers," he adds. "But if the laws are primarily directed at physician groups, provider networks or HMOs, they're not going to be preempted."

Travelers blues—for health plans

Since the seminal 1994 U.S. Supreme Court decision in *Travelers*, other courts increasingly have lowered the shield from state oversight that managed care plans can claim under ERISA. Some recent court cases:

1996

Napoletano v. Cigna Healthcare of Connecticut

Action: State Supreme Court ruled that Cigna can't use ERISA to duck a state law requiring health plans to report all physician deselections and the basis for those decisions.

BPS Clinical Laboratories v. Blue Cross and Blue Shield of Michigan

Action: State appellate court held that the Blues aren't preempted from state laws on provider selection, breach of contract, and antitrust.

1995

Pacificare of Oklahoma v. Burrage

Action: Tenth circuit federal appeals court found no ERISA shield against claims that an HMO was vicariously liable for the acts of its physicians.

Dukes v. U.S. Healthcare and *Rice v. Panchal*

Action: Third and Seventh circuits respectively established principle of "conflict preemption" under ERISA: Health plans aren't automatically immune from state oversight if ERISA provides the only federal defense to an otherwise cognizable state claim.

Resources
Contact your state medical society, state insurance office, or state department of labor for further information.

Ethics

Principles of Medical Ethics

Preamble:
The medical profession has long subscribed to a body of ethical statements developed primarily for the benefit of the patient. As a member of this profession, a physician must recognize responsibility not only to patients, but also to society, to other health professionals, and to self. The following principles adopted by the American Medical Association are not laws, but standards of conduct which define the essentials of honorable behavior for the physician.

I. A physician shall be dedicated to providing competent medical service with compassion and respect.

II. A physician shall deal honestly with patients and colleagues, and strive to expose those physicians deficient in character or competence, or who engage in fraud or deception.

III. A physician shall respect the law and also recognize a responsibility to seek changes in those requirements which are contrary to the best interests of the patients.

IV. A physician shall respect the rights of patients, of colleagues, and of other health professionals, and shall safeguard patient confidences within the constraints of the law.

V. A physician shall continue to study, apply and advance scientific knowledge, make relevant information available to patients, colleagues, and the public, obtain consultation, and use the talents of other health professionals when indicated.

VI. A physician shall, in the provision of appropriate patient care, except in emergencies, be free to choose whom to serve, with whom to associate, and the environment in which to provide medical services.

VII. A physician shall recognize a responsibility to participate in activities contributing to an improved community.

Code of Medical Ethics, Current Opinions with Annotations: including the Principles of Medical Ethics and the Rules of the Council for Ethical and Judicial Affairs. Chicago, Ill: American Medical Association; 1996:191pp. ISBN 0-89970-859-5 OP632396

Resources

Hastings Center
255 Elm Rd, Briarcliff Manor, NY 10510
914 762-8500   Fax 914 762-2124

Institute for Ethics
American Medical Association
515 N State St, Chicago, IL 60610
312 464-5619

Joseph and Rose Kennedy Institute of Ethics
National Reference Center for Bioethics Literature
Georgetown University, Washington, DC 20057
800 MED-ETHX (800-633-3849)

Ethnic Physicians Associations

National Medical Association **(African-American)**
1012 Tenth St NW, Washington, DC 20001
202 347-1895   Fax 202 842-3293

Association of **American Indian** Physicians
1235 Sovereign Row, Ste C-7
Oklahoma City, OK 73108
405 946-7072   Fax 405 946-7651

Asian-American Medical Society (Only for Indiana)
8695 Connecticut, Ste D, Merrillville, IN 46410
219 769-1124

Chinese American Medical Society
c/o Dr H. H. Wang
281 Edgewood Ave, Teaneck, NJ 07666
201 833-1506   Fax 201 833-8252

Colombian Medical Association
PO Box 857, Northbrook, IL 60065-0857

California Hispanic-American Medical Association
1020 S Arroyo Pkwy, Ste 200, Pasadena, CA 91066
818 799-5456

American Association of Physicians of **India**
PO 4370, Flint, MI 48504
313 767-4946

Islamic Medical Association
4121 S Fairview Ave, Ste 203
Downers Grove, IL 60515-2236
630 852-2122   630 852-7622   Fax 630 852-2151
E-mail: imana@aol.com

Italian American Medical Association
1127 Wilshire Blvd, Los Angeles, CA 90017
213 481-0896

Association of **Pakistani** Physicians
6414 S Cast Ave, Ste L-2, Westmont, IL 60559
630 968-8585   Fax 630 968-8677

Association of **Philippine** Physicians in America
2717 W Olive Ave, Ste 200, Burbank, CA 91505
818 843-8616   Fax 818 845-2119

Association of **Philippine** Surgeons in America
2147 Old Greenbrier Rd, Chesapeake, VA 23320
804 424-5485

National Medical and Dental Association **(Polish)**
72-41 Grand Ave, Maspleth, NY 11378
607 733-7503

American **Russian** Medical and Dental Society
6221 Wilshire Blvd, #607, Los Angeles, CA 90048
213 933-0711

Turkish American Physicians Association
c/o Dr Cemil Bikmen
222 Middle County Rd, Smithtown, NY 11787
516 724-0777

Executives (Medical)

Director, Dental Services. Administers dental program in hospital and directs departmental activities in accordance with accepted national standards and administrative policies: Confers with hospital administrators to formulate policies and recommend procedural changes. Establishes training program to advance knowledge and clinical skill levels of resident dentists studying for dental specializations. Implements procedures for hiring of professional staff and approves hiring and promotion of staff members. Establishes work schedules and assigns staff members to duty stations to maximize efficient use of staff. Observes and assists staff members at work to ensure safe and ethical practices and to solve problems and demonstrate techniques. Confers with hospital administrator to submit budget and statistical reports used to justify expenditures for equipment, supplies, and personnel. (DOT-1991)

Adminstrator, Health Care Facility. Directs adminstration of hospital, nursing home, or other health care facility within authority of governing board: Administers fiscal operations, such as budget planning, accounting, and establishing rates for health care services. Directs hiring and training of personnel. Negotiates for improvement of and additions to buildings and equipment. Directs and coordinates activities of medical, nursing, and administrative staffs and services. Develops policies and procedures for various establishment activities. May represent establishment at community meetings and promote programs through various news media. May develop or expand programs or services for scientific research, preventive medicine, medical and vocational rehabilitation, and community health and welfare promotion. May be designated according to type of health care facility as Hospital Administrator (medical service) or Nursing Home Adminstrator (medical service). (DOT-1991)

Director, Pharmacy Services. Directs and coordinates, through subordinate supervisory personnel, activities and functions of hospital pharmacy. Plans and implements procedures in hospital pharmacy according to hospital policies, and legal requirements. Directs pharmacy personnel programs, such as hiring, training, and intern programs. Confers with computer personnel to develop computer programs for pharmacy information management systems, patient and department charge systems, and inventory control. Analyzes records to indicate prescribing trends and excessive usage. Prepares pharmacy budget and department reports required by hospital administrators. Attends staff meetings to advise and inform hospital medical staff of drug applications and characteristics. Observes pharmacy personnel at work and develops quality assurance techniques to ensure safe, legal, and ethical practices. Oversees preparation and dispensation of experimental drugs. (DOT-1991)

Resources

American Association of Medical Society Executives
515 N State St, Chicago, IL 60610
312 464-2555   Fax 312 646-2467

American College of Healthcare Executives
1 N Franklin, Ste 1700, Chicago, IL 60606-3491
312 424-2800   Fax 312 424-0023
E-mail: webmaster@ache.org
Web address: http://www.ache.org

American College of Physician Executives
4890 W Kennedy Blvd, Ste 200, Tampa, FL 33609
800 562-8088   813 287-2000   Fax 813 287-8993

American Medical Directors Association
10480 Little Patuxent Pkwy, Ste 760
Columbia, MD 21044
800 876-AMDA   410 740-9743   301 596-5774
Fax 410 740-4527

Medical Group Management Association
104 Inverness Terrace E, Englewood, CO 80112
303 799-1111   Fax 303 643-4427

National Association of Health Services Executives
10320 Little Patuxent Pkwy, Ste 1106
Columbia, MD 21044
202 628-3953

Exercise

Tell patients: get physical

AM News July 26, 1996 pp 2

The first ever Surgeon General's report on physical activity and health, released July 11, 1996, found that more than 60% of American adults do not achieve recommended levels of physical activity, and that 25% do not exercise at all. Physical activity declines sharply during adolescence—nearly half of Americans between ages 12 and 21 are not vigorously active. Experts recommend that people of all ages engage in at least 30 minutes of moderate activity, such as walking briskly, on most or all days of the week.

JAMA Article of Note: Physical activity and public Health: a recommendation from the Centers of Disease Control and Prevention and the American College of Sports Medicine.

JAMA 1995 Feb 1: 273(5): 402-7.

Resources
Aerobics and Fitness Association of America
15250 Ventura Blvd, Ste 310, Sherman Oaks, CA 91403
800 446-AFAA   818 905-0040   Fax 818 990-5468

Aquatic Exercise Association
PO Box 1609, Nokomu, FL 34274-1609
941 486-8600   Fax 941 786-8820

National Health Club Association
12596 W Bayaud, 1st Fl, Denver, CO 80228
800 765-6422   303 753-6422   Fax 303 986-6813

President's Council on Physical Fitness and Sports
701 Pennsylvania Ave NW, Ste 250
Washington, DC 20004
202 272-3421
Web address: http:// www.hoptechno.com/book II.htm

Exercise Physiology

Exercise Physiologist. Develops, implements, and coordinates exercise programs and administers medical tests, under physician's supervision, to program participants to promote physical fitness. Explains program and test procedures to participant. Interviews participant to obtain vital statistics and medical history and records information. Records heart activity, using electrocardiograph (EKG) machine, while participant undergoes stress test on treadmill, under physician's supervision. Measures oxygen consumption and lung functioning, using spirometer. Measures amount of fat in body, using such equipment as hydrostatic scale, skinfold calipers, and tape measure, to assess body composition. Performs routine laboratory test of blood samples for cholesterol level and glucose tolerance, or interprets test results. Schedules other examinations and tests, such as a physical examination, chest x-ray, and urinalysis.

Records test data in patient's chart or enters data into computer. Writes initial and follow-up exercise prescriptions for participants, following physician's recommendation, specifying equipment, such as treadmill, track, or bike. Demonstrates correct use of exercise equipment and exercise routines. Conducts individual and group aerobic, strength, and flexibility exercises. Observes participants during exercise for signs of stress. Teaches behavior modification classes, such as stress management, weight control, and related subjects. Orders material and supplies and calibrates equipment. May supervise work activities of other staff members. (DOT-1991)

Resources
American Physiological Society
9650 Rockville Pike, Bethesda, MD 20014-3991
301 530-7164   Fax 301 571-8305
Web address: http://www.faseb.org/aps

National Dance Association
1900 Association Dr, Reston, VA 22091
800 321-0789   703 476-3436   703 476-3421
Fax 703 476-9527
E-mail: nda@aahpend.org
Web address: http://www.aahpend.org/cgi-bin/
counter.pl/nada.htm

Exhibits, Health Care

Healthcare Convention and Exhibitors Association
5775 Peachtree-Dunwoody Rd, Ste 500-G
Atlanta, GA 30342
404 252-3663   Fax 404 252-0774

Eyes

Eye Bank Association of America
1001 Connecticut Ave NW, Ste 601
Washington, DC 20036-5504
202 775-4999   Fax 202 429-6036

National Eye Institute
Office of Scientific Reporting, Bldg 31, Rm 6A32
Bethesda, MD 20892 (free brochures)

National Eye Care Project (for needy)
PO Box 429098, San Francisco, CA 94142
800 222-EYES   415 561-8520   Fax 415 561-8567

National Eye Research Foundation
c/o Andrew Kim, 910 Skokie Blvd, Ste 207A
Northbrook, IL 60062
800 621-2258   847 564-4652   Fax 847 564-0807

Familial Polyposis

Familial Polyposis Registry
Department of Colorectal Surgery
Cleveland Clinic Foundation
9500 Euclid Ave, Cleveland, OH 44195-5044
216 444-6470

Family Practice

Family Practitioner. Alternate title: family physician. Provides comprehensive medical services for members of family, regardless of age or sex, on continuing basis. Examines patients, using medical instruments and equipment. Elicits and records information about patient's medical history. Orders or executes various tests, analyses, and diagnostic images to provide information on patient's condition. Analyzes reports and findings of tests and examination, and diagnoses condition of patient. Administers or prescribes treatments and medications. Promotes health by advising patients concerning diet, hygiene, and methods for prevention of disease. Inoculates and vaccinates patients to immunize them from communicable diseases. Provides prenatal care to pregnant women, delivers babies, and provides postnatal care to mothers and infants. Performs surgical procedures commensurate with surgical competency. Refers patients to medical specialists for consultant services when necessary for patient's well-being. (DOT-1991)

Resources

American Board of Family Practice
2228 Young Dr, Lexington, KY 40505
606 269-5626   Fax 606 266-9699

American Academy of Family Physicians
8880 Ward Pkwy, Kansas City, MO 64114
800 274-2237   816 333-9700   Fax 816 822-0580

Federal Trade Commission

The objective of the Federal Trade Commission is to maintain competitive enterprise as the keystone of the American economic system, and to prevent the free enterprise system from being fettered by monopoly or restraints on trade or corrupted by unfair or deceptive trade practices. The Commission is charged with keeping competition both free and fair.

The purpose of the Federal Trade Commission (FTC) is expressed in the Federal Trade Commission Act (15 USC 41-58) and the Clayton Act (15 USC 12), both passed in 1914 and both successively amended in the years since. The Federal Trade Commission Act prohibits the use in or affecting commerce of "unfair methods of competi-

tion" and "unfair or deceptive acts or practices." The Clayton Act outlaws specific practices recognized as instruments of monopoly. As an administrative agency, acting quasi-judicially and quasi-legislatively, the Commission was established to deal with trade practices on a continuing and corrective basis. It has no authority to punish; its function is to "prevent," through cease-and-desist orders and other means, those practices condemned by the law of federal trade regulation; however, court-ordered civil penalties of up to $10,000 may be obtained for each violation of a Commission order or trade regulation rule. (USG-1996)

Federal Trade Commission
Pennsylvania Ave at Sixth St NW
Washington, DC 20580
202 326-2222
E-mail: antitrust@ftc.gov
Web address: http://www.ftc.gov

Fertility

Poetry and Medicine

Infertility Clinic

Joan I. Siegel
JAMA 1995 Jan 18; 273(3): 176d

I call you from darkness
where you have waited all my life
like a thought before the words
that name it.
I name you daughter.
I want to plant you
like a ripe grain
in the earth of me.
I want you born in the spring
so your eyes open to a green world
where moths flower beside dandelions
and everywhere songbirds
back from the rain forests
festoon pale trees like party lights
celebrating you.
I will name the world for you:
stones
the moon
the sound geese make leaving
the sky.
Someday you
will name the world
for me.

Resources

American Society for Reproductive Medicine
1209 Montgomery Hwy, Birmingham, AL 35216-2809
205 978-5000   Fax 205 978-5005

Fertility Research Foundation
877 Park Ave, New York, NY 10021
212 744-5500   Fax 212 744-6536

Resolve, Inc
1310 Broadway, Somerville, MA 02144-1731
617 623-1156   617 623-0744   Fax 617 623-0252

Fetal Tissue

JAMA Article of Note: Medical application of fetal tissue transplantation. Council on Scientific Affairs and Council on Ethical and Judicial Affairs.

JAMA 1990 Jan 26; 263(4): 565-70

Abstract: Fetal tissue transplantation has been attempted for a limited number of clinical disorders, including Parkinson disease, diabetes, immunodeficiency disorders, and several metabolic disorders. Fetal tissue has intrinsic properties—the ability to differentiate into multiple cell types, growth and proliferative ability, growth factor production, and reduced antigenicity—that make it attractive for transplantation research. At this time the results from fetal tissue grafts for Parkinson disease and diabetes have not demonstrated significant long-term clinical benefit to patients with these disorders. Further research will be necessary to determine the potential value of fetal tissue transplantation. For these clinical investigations to proceed, specific ethical guidelines are needed to ensure that fetal tissue derived from elective abortions is used in a morally acceptable manner. These guidelines should separate, to the greatest extent possible, the decision by a woman to have an abortion from her consent to donate the postmortem tissue for transplantation purposes. Such ethical guidelines are offered in this report.

Fifth Pathway

AMA Policy

Fifth Pathway (255.997) CME Rep D, A-81; reaffirment: CLRPD Rep F, I-91

(1) The AMA believes that the Fifth Pathway is fulfilling its purpose of improving the education of US FMGs who have completed the program and has served to help maintain standards for licensure in those jurisdictions that would have been politically pressed to lower them to accommodate these students without additional education. (2) To reaffirm the intent of the Fifth Pathway policy, namely to provide an alternative route of entry to graduate medical education for qualified students studying abroad who are not eligible through the ECFMG route, the policy should be revised to ask the sponsoring medical schools to establish more stringent requirements for admission to and successful completion of a Fifth Pathway program. (3) The AMA supports the principle that any existing or proposed alternative programs conducted by US medical schools to facilitate entry of US citizens studying in foreign medical schools into US

programs should assure that those who complete such programs are reasonably comparable to the school's regularly enrolled and graduated students.

Firearms

A Piece of My Mind

Frozen in time

Robert Burns, MD
JAMA 1994 Apr 6; 271(13): 965

I should not be here. I feel guilty, out of place. Much like a teenager getting ready to buy liquor with a forged ID card, I look around the room and make sure I don't know anyone. The shop is busy, the customers look like me, my friends. Everyone else looks out of place too.

"I've got it. This is the one for you."

The owner places it on a velvet-lined tray and slides it toward me. I think about the merchants of Paris, refusing to exchange money with customers because it reduces the transaction to a business deal. This merchant is no different. I am no longer just a potential buyer. I am a friend. I am welcomed into the family. I hesitate just a second, then pick up the piece of hardened steel and hold it in my right hand. The Browning 9-mm is heavy, heavier than I thought. It is cold. I rub my fingers along the smooth barrel. I wrap both hands around the handle and draw it toward me, pointing the barrel toward the ceiling. The smell of the steel enters my nostrils, and a sudden rush of warmth penetrates my hands.

I do not want to be surprised. 'What've ya got?' I ask as I walk down the hall and out the door of the emergency room. I pause. The cold night air enters my lungs, stings my nostrils, and revives me if only for a few minutes. It is Saturday night, and the ER is busier than usual. The checks are late this month, and people had to make a choice between food and medicines. It is my first break in eight hours and the next six already look worse. A few stars show through the clear sky. I take another breath, savoring its crisp freshness before dealing with the task at hand.

The paramedic has not answered my question. We have gone through this ritual before. Each of us has our refuge from the insanity of everyday work, of the world, and he knows mine. I will pay for these few moments of tranquillity when I enter the ambulance. He allows me my time, alone. Free. I walk toward the ambulance.

"Gunshot," he finally says, timing the words to the instant my foot touches the rear step of the ambulance. "Lovers' spat. Close range." There is no emotion in his voice.

He reaches in and turns on the light and I climb into the van. Medical supplies dangle from the cabinets and encroach into the already-too-small space. The overhead light flickers, plunging the cabin into intermittent darkness. A black body bag is strapped on the stretcher. I put down my paperwork. I hold onto the leather strap and pull the zipper.

The last remaining heat from the lifeless body escapes into the frigid March night. I open the bag, stretching a strand of thick, dark blood from the inside cover. The blood smells damp, metallic. I touch his neck, feeling for the pulse that his vacant eyes tell me has long since stopped. I usually check for five seconds, a perfunctory examination that matches the bureaucratic formality, not wanting it to last longer than necessary. Tonight, I search for the extinguished beat for 20, 30 seconds, staring into his still, brown eyes. His face appears pained. A crease across his brow, the muscles of his jaw tight, a grimace to his lips, frozen in time, at least until the mortician eases his suffering for eternity. He becomes my patient, and I want to know his history. What happened, or more importantly, why did it happen? What were his last thoughts? Did it hurt? Was his last vision of this life his lover at close range? I move my hand across his eyes and close them, trying to bring peace to us both.

"Remember, it's just the two of you. You never aim a gun unless your intention is to kill."

My instructor slaps my shoulder and steps aside, and I extend my arms above my head. The glasses are in place. The sweet, slightly acrid smell of gunpowder fills the air. Ear plugs are in place. I hear the melodic muted exploding of shells in the distance. I lower my arms. Elbows locked. The gun is level with my eyes. Twenty-five feet beyond the sight is a paper torso. Concentric circles radiate from the chest, the heart, an imaginary vortex ready to pull the missiles to their target.

He was wrong. There is no other rational explanation for it. He was at the wrong place at the wrong time. I had been with him minutes earlier. It was his turn to drive to the hockey game, and he had left me in my driveway. He flashed his headlights at me as I entered the house, and his car disappeared into the cloud of exhaust left in the cold winter night as the tires crunched the gravel. I remember when I was a child that sound gave me comfort. It meant my father was finally home. We were all home. Safe.

He was wrong. Why did he stop for money on the way home? It could have waited until morning. The bank of floodlights, in place for safety, illuminated his every step. As if he were an actor on stage, his audience watched from the shadows as he filled his wallet with the money and moved to his car. And then they followed him home.

He was wrong. He should have left his porch light on when he left the house. It would have protected him. When he pulled into his driveway he would have been home. Safe.

He was wrong. All he had to do was hand them the wallet. It was probably all they wanted. Give them what they want, the police always say. It was just paper, plastic, and leather. Nothing more. No heirlooms. No memories. Disposable, like a life. He must have punched and struggled with them. It is the only rational explanation. Why else was he pushed to the ground, the barrel of the handgun placed at his temple, and the trigger pulled?

I grip the handle. The muscles in my arms tense. My finger pulls against the trigger, but stops.

"Squeeze the trigger," he says.

Sweat drips into my eyes. The target, just paper, plastic, and metal, blurs beyond my sight. Squeeze the trigger. My finger cramps. I feel the blood pulse in my fingers. I close my eyes. The rhythmic beating of my heart in-

creases, my pulse pounds in my neck, in my temples, and finally in my skull. I see the torso. My palms sweat and I loosen my grip. I open my eyes, the torso is closer. It's moving, no longer just a target but a body, rushing toward me to challenge. My arms tense; I grip the pistol, lowering the site to the center of the chest. I pull the trigger and a deafening shot explodes. The gun pushes back against me; I step back to maintain my balance. A curl of smoke escapes from the barrel as shredded paper gently floats to the ground. The target sways from its hanger, a hole ripped through the center.

My arms drop to my sides; the gun feels heavier. My pulse slows; I wipe the sweat from my eyes. A chill rushes through my body, and I need to vomit.

"Again," the instructor says. "Do it again. The second one is always easier."

Rates of homicide, suicide, and firearm-related death among children—26 industrialized countries

CDC's *Morbidity and Mortality Weekly Report*

Div of Violence Prevention, National Center for Injury Prevention and Control, CDC.
Feb 7, 1997. p101

During 1950-1993, the overall annual death rate for US children aged less than 15 years declined substantially,[1] primarily reflecting decreases in deaths associated with unintentional injuries, pneumonia, influenza, cancer, and congenital anomalies. However, during the same period, childhood homicide rates tripled, and suicide rates quadrupled.[2] In 1994, among children aged 1–4 years, homicide was the fourth leading cause of death; among children aged 5–14 years, homicide was the third leading cause of death, and suicide was the sixth.[3] To compare patterns and the impact of violent deaths among children in the United States and other industrialized countries, CDC analyzed data on childhood homicide, suicide, and firearm-related death in the United States and 25 other industrialized countries for the most recent year for which data were available in each country.[4]

This report presents the findings of this analysis, which indicate that the United States has the highest rates of childhood homicide, suicide, and firearm-related death among industrialized countries.

In the 1994 *World Development Report*,[5] 208 nations were classified by gross national product; from that list, the United States and all 25 of the other countries in the high-income group and with populations of greater than or equal to 1 million were selected because of their economic comparability and the likelihood that those countries maintained vital records most accurately. In January and February 1996, the ministry of health or the national statistics institute in each of the 26 countries was asked to provide denominator data and counts by sex and by five-year age groups for the most recent year data were available for the number of suicides (International Classification of Diseases, Ninth Revision [ICD-9], codes E950.0-E959), homicides (E960.0-E969), suicides by firearm (E955.0-E955.4), homicides by firearm (E965.0-E965.4), unintentional deaths caused by firearm (E922.0-E922.9), and firearm-related deaths for which intention was undetermined (E985.0-E985.4); 26 (96%)

F countries, including the United States, provided complete data.* Twenty (77%) countries provided data for 1993 or 1994; the remaining countries provided data for 1990, 1991, 1992, or 1995. Cause-specific rates per 100,000 population were calculated for three groups (children aged 0-4 years, 5-14 years, and 0-14 years). The rates for homicide and suicide by means other than firearms were calculated by subtracting the firearm-related homicide and firearm-related suicide rates from the overall homicide and suicide rates. Rates for the United States were compared with rates based on pooled data for the other 25 countries. Of the 161 million children aged less than 15 years during the one year for which data were provided, 57 million (35%) were in the United States and 104 million (65%) were in the other 25 countries.

Overall, the data provided by the 26 countries included a total of 2,872 deaths among children aged less than 15 years for a period of one year. Homicides accounted for 1,995 deaths, including 1,177 (59%) in boys and 818 (41%) in girls. Of the homicides, 1,464 (73%) occurred among US children. The homicide rate for children in the United States was five times higher than that for children in the other 25 countries combined (2.57 per 100,000 compared with 0.51).

Suicide accounted for the deaths of 599 children, including 431 (72%) in boys and 168 (28%) in girls. Of the suicides, 321 (54%) occurred among US children. The suicide rate for children in the United States was two times higher than that in the other 25 countries combined (0.55 compared with 0.27). No suicides were reported among children aged less than five years.

A firearm was reported to have been involved in the deaths of 1,107 children; 957 (86%) of those occurred in the United States. Of all firearm-related deaths, 55% were reported as homicides; 20%, as suicides; 22%, as unintentional; and 3%, as intention undetermined. The overall firearm-related death rate among US children aged less than 15 years was nearly 12 times higher than among children in the other 25 countries combined (1.66 compared with 0.14). The firearm-related homicide rate in the United States was nearly 16 times higher than that in all of the other countries combined (0.94 compared with 0.06); the firearm-related suicide rate was nearly 11 times higher (0.32 compared with 0.03); and the unintentional firearm-related death rate was nine times higher (0.36 compared with 0.04). For all countries, males accounted for most of the firearm-related homicides (67%), firearm-related suicides (77%), and unintentional firearm-related deaths (89%). The nonfirearm-related homicide rate in the United States was nearly four times the rate in all of the other countries (1.63 compared with 0.45), and nonfirearm-related suicide rates were similar in the United States and in all of the other countries combined (0.23 compared with 0.24).

The rate for firearm-related deaths among children in the United States (1.66) was 2.7-fold greater than that in the country with the next highest rate (Finland, 0.62). Except for rates for firearm-related suicide in Northern Ireland and firearm-related fatalities of unknown intent in Austria, Belgium, and Israel, rates for all types of firearm-related deaths were higher in the United States than in the other countries. However, among all other countries, the impact of firearm-related deaths varied substantially. For example, five countries, including three of the four countries in Asia, reported no firearm-related deaths among children. In comparison, firearms were the primary cause of homicide in Finland, Israel, Australia, Italy, Germany, and England and Wales. Five countries (Denmark, Ireland, New Zealand, Scotland, and Taiwan) reported only unintentional firearm-related deaths.

Editorial Note: The findings in this report document a high rate of death among US children associated with violence and unintentional firearm-related injuries, particularly in comparison with other industrialized countries. Even though rates in all other countries were lower than those in the United States, rates among other countries varied substantially and were particularly low in some countries. Although specific reasons for the differences in rates among countries are unknown, previous studies have reported on the associations between rates of violent childhood death and low funding for social programs,[6] economic stress related to participation of women in the labor force,[7,8] divorce, ethnic-linguistic heterogeneity, and social acceptability of violence.[9]

The findings of the analysis in this report are subject to at least three limitations. First, although the data were obtained from official sources and were based on ICD-9 codes, the sensitivity and specificity of the vital records and reporting systems may have varied by country. Second, because 21 (81%) countries each reported less than 10 firearm-related deaths among children aged 0-14 years, the firearm-related death rates for those countries, when not pooled, are unstable and may vary substantially for different years. Finally, only one half of the countries (including the United States) reported all four digits of the ICD-9 codes for firearm-related deaths; the fourth digit distinguishes whether deaths were caused by injuries from firearms or by other explosives. For countries in which this distinction could not be made, the firearm-related death rates may be overestimated slightly.

In May 1996, the 49th World Health Assembly adopted a resolution that declared violence a leading worldwide public health problem and urged all member states to assess the problem of violence and to communicate their findings to the World Health Organization.[10] Cross-cultural comparisons may identify key factors (eg, attitudinal, behavioral, educational, socioeconomic, or regulatory) not evident from intranational studies that could assist in the development of new country-specific strategies for preventing such deaths.

References

1. Singh GK, Yu SM. US childhood mortality, 1950 through 1993: trends and socioeconomic differentials. *Am J Public Health* 1996;86:505-12.

2. National Center for Health Statistics. *Health, United States, 1994.* Hyattsville, Maryland: US Department of Health and Human Services, Public Health Service, CDC, 1995.

3. Singh GK, Kochanek KD, MacDorman MF. *Advance report of final mortality statistics, 1994.* Hyattsville, Maryland: US Department of Health and Human Services, Public Health Service, CDC, National Center for Health Statistics, 1996. (Monthly vital statistics report; vol 45, no. 3, suppl).

4. Krug EG, Dahlberg LL, Powell KE. Childhood homicide, suicide, and firearm deaths: an international comparison. *World Health Stat Q* 1996;49(4) (in press).

5. World Bank. *World development report.* New York, New York: Oxford University Press, 1994:251-2.

6. Garnter R. Family structure, welfare spending, and child homicide in developed democracies. *J Marriage Fam* 1991;53:231-40.

7. Fiala R, LaFree G. Cross-national determinants of child homicide. *Am Sociol Rev* 1988;53:432-45.

8. Gartner R. The victims of homicide: a temporal and cross-national comparison. *Am Sociol Rev* 1990;55:92-106.

9. Briggs CM, Cutright P. Structural and cultural determinants of child homicide: a cross-national analysis. *Violence Vict* 1994;9:3-16.

10. World Health Assembly. Prevention of violence: public health priority. Geneva, Switzerland: World Health Organization, 1996. (Resolution no. WHA49.25).

* Complete data were provided by Australia, Austria, Belgium, Canada, Denmark, England and Wales, Finland, France, Germany, Hong Kong, Ireland, Israel, Italy, Japan, Kuwait, Netherlands, New Zealand, Northern Ireland, Norway, Scotland, Singapore, Sweden, Spain, Switzerland, Taiwan, and the United States. In this analysis, Hong Kong, Northern Ireland, and Taiwan are considered as countries.

JAMA Theme Issue: Guns and violence

JAMA 1996, June 12: 272 (22)

This feature issue paints its picture through the use of statistics. Articles included present numbers on gun acquisition and use by adolescents, population estimates of household firearm storage practices in Oregon, and hospitalizations related to firearm injuries.

Food and Drug Administration

The name Food and Drug Administration (FDA) was first provided by the Agriculture Appropriation Act of 1931 (46 Stat 392), although similar law enforcement functions had been in existence under different organizational titles since January 1, 1907, when the Food and Drug Act of 1906 (21 USC 1-15) became effective.

The FDA's activities are directed toward protecting the health of the nation against impure and unsafe foods, drugs and cosmetics, and other potential hazards. (USG-1996)

Resource
Office of Consumer Affairs, Public Inquiries
Food and Drug Administration
5600 Fishers Ln, Rockville, MD 20857
301 443-3170
Web address: http://www.fda.gov
Breast Implant Hotline 800 532-4440

Foreign Medical Schools

World Directory of Medical Schools, 6th ed. Geneva, Switzerland: World Health Organization; 1988. 311pp.
ISBN 9-24150-008-5
Available from:
WHO Publications USA
49 Sheridan Ave, Albany, NY 12210
518 436-9686

Educational Commission for Foreign Medical Graduates
3624 Market St, Philadelphia, PA 19104
215 386-5900   Fax 215 387-9963

Forensic Medicine

Poetry and Medicine

Forensics

Paula Tatarunis, MD
JAMA 1996 November 27; 276(20): 1619

Exfoliations in the slits between the floorboards,
Catamenial sloughs behind the stove,
Stick a meat thermometer into her liver
While the old LP stammers love, love, love.

From waxy pallor to dependent purple,
the silver bullet's ricochet occults,
spattering the ontological profile,
and the fudged lab result.

Dust for double helices, uncoil the prints,
segregate the doctor from the spinster—
the missing piano wire is high C#,
the prime suspect is the minister.

Now call the chief detective's daughter—
she's playing with her Barbie on the walk.
She got an A in Art this past semester
so she's the one who always brings the chalk.

And when the house is empty as a motive,
yellow tape festooning every sill and door,
I'll slip out to pay my final homage
to your pallid outline sprawling on the floor.

Resources
American Board of Forensic Psychiatry
2100 E Broadway, Ste 313, Columbia, MO 65201
800 255-7792   573 875-1267   Fax 573 443-1199

International Reference Organization in Forensic
Medicine and Sciences
c/o Dr William G. Eckert
PO Box 16286, Panama City, FL 32406-6286
316 685-7612

Milton Helpern Institute of Forensic Medicine
520 First Ave, New York, NY 10016
212 447-2030   Fax 212 447-2716

National Association of Medical Examiners
1402 S Grand Blvd, St Louis, MO 63104
314 577-8298   Fax 314 268-5124

Foster Care

Childreach, United States Member of Plan International
155 Plan Way, Warwick, RI 02886
800 556-7918   401 738-5600   Fax 401 738-5608
TX 671 6565 PLANUSA

Contact state office of Children and Family Services.

G

Gag Clause

Gag clauses are provisions in physicians' contracts that prevent them, explicitly or implicitly, from giving patients information about treatment options that may not be covered by their health plans, even if these treatments are safe, effective, and necessary. Gag clauses also may prevent physicians from referring very sick patients outside their health plans to physicians with rare expertise in the types of care needed.

Contact the state medical association, state departments of insurance or health for questions regarding gag clauses.

Gastroenterology

American College of Gastroenterology
4900-B S 31st St, Arlington, VA 22206
703 820-7400   Fax 703 931-4520

American Gastroenterological Association
7910 Woodmont Ave, Ste 914
Bethesda, MD 20814
301 654-2055   Fax 301 654-5920
Web address: http://www.gastro.org

American Society for Gastrointestinal Endoscopy
13 Elm St, Manchester, MA 01944
508 526-8330   Fax 508 526-4018

Society of American Gastrointestinal Endoscopic Surgeons
2716 Ocean Park Blvd, Ste 3000
Santa Monica, CA 90405
310 314-2404   Fax 310 314-2585
E-mail: SAGESmail@aol.com
(For information and standards on laparoscopic cholecystectomy)

Gaucher Disease

National Gaucher Foundation
11140 Rockville Pike, Ste 350
Rockville, MD 20852-1516
301 816-1515   Fax 301 816-1516

General Practice

General practitioner. Alternate title: physician, general practice. Diagnoses and treats variety of diseases and injuries in general practice. Examines patients, using medical instruments and equipment. Orders or executes various tests, analyses, and diagnostic images to provide information on patient's condition. Analyzes reports and findings of tests and of examination, and diagnoses condition. Administers or prescribes treatments and drugs.

Inoculates and vaccinates patients to immunize patients from communicable diseases. Advises patients concerning diet, hygiene, and methods for prevention of disease. Provides prenatal care to mother and infant. Reports births, deaths, and outbreak of contagious diseases to governmental authorities. Refers patients to medical specialist or other practitioner for specialized treatment. Performs minor surgery. May make house and emergency calls to attend to patients unable to visit office or clinic. May conduct physical examinations to provide information needed for admission to school, consideration for jobs, or eligibility for insurance coverage. May provide care for passengers and crew aboard ship and be designated Ship's Doctor. (DOT-1991)

Genetic Research

Scientists flock to hear cloner Wilmut at the NIH

Charles Marwick
JAMA. 1997 April 9;277:1102-1103

Every so often the spotlight focuses on some major scientific advance that raises fears in the popular mind of implications for the future of humanity.

The announcement in February 1997 that scientists in Scotland had succeeded in cloning a sheep has raised concerns that they are only a short step from doing the same thing in humans.

"Scottish Institute under Fire after Breakthrough in Sheep Reproduction" was a headline in one Scottish newspaper, which proceeded to quote an individual, described as an authority on genetics, charging the sheep cloners with "monstrous conduct." In the following weeks this theme occupied major newspapers and magazines around the world.

Phrases such as "good and evil" and "playing God" and considerations of the moral significance of the development filled editorial and opinion pages, not to mention television screens. In the United States, President Clinton banned the funding of research on human cloning and charged the National Bioethics Advisory Commission with examining the implications of such work (*JAMA* 1997;277:1023-1026). Hearings on mammalian cloning were held in Congress. It was all very stirring, but it had little to do with the facts.

Wilmut visits United States
The leader of the sheep cloning team, Ian Wilmut, PhD, of the Roslin Institute, near Edinburgh, came to the National Institutes of Health (NIH) in Bethesda, Md, to talk about the work three weeks after the research report was published in *Nature* (1997;385:810-813). He also

G spoke in Baltimore, Md, at a meeting sponsored by the Cambridge Healthtech Institute and at the US Department of Agriculture research center in Beltsville, Md.

In 45 minutes, he quietly summarized before a packed auditorium at the NIH the 10 years of painstaking scientific work involved in nuclear transfer that led to the birth of Dolly, a Finn Dorset lamb, and to two lambs before her, Megan and Morag.

"The first thing to point out is that this sort of research is a team game. It's not something that any one of us can do on our own," Wilmut said, noting the contributions of 10 associates. "It's also important to understand that these projects are long term. We started about 10 years ago, and we have only just begun to understand the importance and implications."

What became clear as Wilmut described the Roslin results was that this work, headline news though it may be, is only another step along a road that humans have been traveling for millennia—domestic animal husbandry. Wilmut reminded his audience that he worked for an institute concerned with improving agricultural science. His use of the modern tools of biotechnology and gene manipulation, he implied, is a means to that end.

The Roslin Institute, named for the village in which it is located, has a long history. Situated at the foot of the Pentland Hills a few miles south of Edinburgh, the organization had its beginnings shortly after World War I as an animal breeding research station. It later became the Institute for Animal Genetics and was affiliated with Edinburgh University. In 1993 it became the Roslin Institute, sponsored by the Biotechnology and Biological Sciences Research Council of the United Kingdom with support from other government agencies, the European Union, and industry. Over the years the facility has become internationally recognized as a research center for the welfare, reproduction, development, and nutrition of farm animals.

Possible applications
During his talk at the NIH, Wilmut pointed out that one obvious application of the successful cloning experiment was the possibility of producing genetically identical embryos. "There must be many dairy farmers who have looked at a cow and thought, 'I wish we had more like her. She gives a lot of milk, it's of good quality, she gets pregnant easily, she stays healthy, there's no mastitis.' In the end it may be possible to use this technology to provide such animals. But with an efficiency of 1 in 300, [cloning] clearly lies in the future," Wilmut said. It took 277 embryos to get one live birth: Dolly. Right now the procedure is inefficient, Wilmut said.

He said the procedure that produced Dolly appears to involve an increase in the clone's birth weight and a prolongation of gestation. At birth, Dolly weighed 6.6 kg (the range in weight of Finn Dorset lambs born to their own breed is 1.2-5.0 kg), and the pregnancy of the Scottish Blackface ewe that carried her lasted 148 days (while the mean duration of pregnancy for Finn Dorsets is 143 days).

"Quite often parturition is sluggish [in the attempts to produce cloned lambs], Wilmut said, "and there is an increase in perinatal mortality, often not associated with any obvious abnormality. It's clear that one could not consider using this technique on a large scale, for instance, in animal breeding, until these problems have been understood and eliminated."

However, Wilmut maintained that the results do show that the nuclear transfer technique is "very robust" and that "it has been possible, in this one case at least, to reprogram development from a cell which has been in an adult animal and to obtain a normal lamb." He added, "I'm pleased to say that Dolly is still healthy and well and, like me, struggling to cope with the TV cameras."

Essentially, the procedure involves transferring the nucleus of a cell (in Dolly's case, the nucleus was taken from a cell from a mammary gland of a six-year-old ewe) into an oocyte from which the nucleus had been removed. A key element that enabled the Roslin group to perform this feat with a nonembryonic cell was inducing the donor mammary gland cells to enter a quiescent phase by reducing the nutrient-laden serum normally used to support their growth in culture—a process that evidently makes it easier to reprogram the differentiated mammary gland cells.

It is this innovation that may prove to be the most important aspect of the accomplishment, by helping researchers understand the mechanisms that control the process of differentiation that leads to specialized cells and tissues, Wilmut said.

One potential outgrowth of such work is that it may someday permit scientists to add a corrective gene or genes to cultured cells provided by a patient with an inherited disorder, using cloning as a means of producing undifferentiated "stem cells" that will then be redifferentiated into the appropriate cells, tissues, or organs with normal function to be reintroduced into the patient.

Study of the aging process is another possibility arising out of this work, Wilmut said. The donor of the mammary cells used to create Dolly was six years old. Dolly was born last July. "Is she [several] months old? Or is she really six years old?" he asked.

Wilmut also pointed out that cloned animals are apt to be less alike than genetically identical twins, because only the chromosomal genes are transferred in nuclear transfer; the donor oocyte is the source of the mitochondrial genes.

"Remember, when I describe these animals as being genetically identical, this is really shorthand," he said. "They share the same chromosomes but they may well have different cytoplasms." Also, identical twins share the same uterine environment and its influences during pregnancy, which is not the case for the cloned animal and its source.

Precise genetic changes
The immediate applications of the Roslin group's work will come from the ability to introduce precise genetic changes into livestock, said Wilmut, noting that there are now well-established techniques for such genetic manipulation in cultured cells. Cloning provides an opportunity for changing a cell's existing genetic makeup and having these changes reproduced in a cloned embryo.

Wilmut predicted that within two or three years, clones of animals that have been genetically modified to produce therapeutic human proteins in their milk will be born. He cited clotting factors for the management of hemophilia as one example of such proteins.

Wilmut noted that experience "tells us we are bad at predicting the benefits to come from new scientific opportunities." In this case, however, he is quite sure that there are going to be many.

National Center for Human Genome Research

The Center provides leadership for and formulates research goals and long-range plans to accomplish the mission of the Human Genome Project, including the study of ethical, legal, and social implications of human genome research. Through grants, contracts, cooperative agreements, and individual and institutional research training awards, the Center supports and administers research and research training programs in human genome research and the systematic, targeted effort to create detailed maps of the genomes or organisms. It provides coordination of genome research, both nationally and internationally; serves as a focal point within National Institutes of Health and the Department of Health and Human Services of federal interagency coordination and collaboration with industry and academia; and sponsors scientific meetings and symposia to promote progress through information sharing. Through its Division of Intramural Research (DIR), the Center plans and conducts a program of laboratory and clinical research related to the application of genome research to the understanding of human genetic disease and the development of DNA diagnostics and gene therapies. (USG-1996)

Resources

Association of Genetic Technologists (AGT)
PO Box 15945-288, Lenexa, KS 66285
913 541-9077

Genetics Society of America
9650 Rockville Pike, Bethesda, MD 20814-3998
301 571-1825   Fax 301 530-7079
E-mail: society@genetics.faseb.org

National Human Genome Research Institute
31 Cedar Dr, MSC 2152, Bldg 31, Rm 4B09
Bethesda, MD 20892-2152
301 496-0844
Web address: http://www.nhgri.nih.gov

Genetic Syndromes

Charcot-Marie-Tooth International
One Springbank Dr
St Catharines, Ontario, Canada L25 2K1
905 687-3670   Fax 905 687-8753
E-mail: cmtint@vaxxine.com
(Charcot-Marie Tooth is also known as peroneal muscular atrophy heredity motor and sensory neuropathy)

Cornelia De Lange Syndrome Foundation
c/o Julie Mairano, 60 Dyer Ave
Collinsville, CT 06022-1273
800 223-8355   203 693-0159   Fax 203 693-6819

Cri Du Chat Syndrome Society
11609 Oakmont, Overland Park, KS 66210
913 469-8900

National Down's Syndrome Society
666 Broadway, New York, NY 10012
212 460-9330 800 221-4602 (Hotline)
Fax 212 979-2873

National Fragile X Foundation
1441 York St, Ste 215, Denver, CO 80206
800 688-8765   303 333-6155   Fax 303 333-4369
The **fragile X syndrome** is an inherited defect of the X chromosome that causes mental retardation. Fragile X syndrome is the most common cause of mental retardation in males after Down syndrome.

The disorder occurs within families according to an X-linked recessive pattern of inheritance. Although males are mainly affected, women are able to carry the genetic defect responsible for the disorder and pass it on to some of their daughters, who in turn become carriers of the defect.

Approximately one in 1500 men is affected by the condition; one in 1000 women is a carrier. In addition to being mentally retarded, affected males are generally tall, are physically strong, have a prominent nose and jaw, increased ear length, and large testicles, and are prone to epileptic seizures. About one third of female carriers show some degree of intellectual impairment.

There is no treatment for the condition. If a woman has a history of the syndrome in her family, it is useful to seek genetic counseling regarding the risk of a child being affected. (ENC-1989)

Friedreich's Ataxia Group in America
PO Box 11116, Oakland CA 94611
415 655-0833
Friedreich's ataxia is a very rare inherited disease in which degeneration of nerve fibers in the spinal cord causes ataxia (loss of coordinated movement and balance). The disease is the result of a genetic defect, usually of the autosomal recessive type. It affects about two people per 100,000.

Symptoms first appear in late childhood or adolescence. The main symptoms are unsteadiness when walking, clumsy hand movements, slurred speech, and rapid, involuntary eye movements. In many cases there are also abnormalities of bone structure and alignment.

There is as yet no cure for the disease. Once it has developed, it becomes progressively more severe, and, within 10 years of onset, more than half the sufferers are confined to wheelchairs. If cardiomyopathy (heart muscle disease) develops, it may contribute to an early death. People who have blood relatives with Friedreich's ataxia should seek genetic counseling before starting a family. (ENC-1989)

National Marfan Foundation
382 Main St, Port Washington, NY 11050
800 862-7326   516 883-8712   Fax 516 883-8712
E-mail: staff@marfan.org

Meniere's Disease
EAR Foundation
200 Church St, Box 111, Nashville, TN 37236
800 545-HEAR   615 329-7809   Fax 615 329-7935

Spina Bifida Association of America
4590 MacArthur Blvd NW, Ste 250
Washington, DC 20007-4226
800 621-3141   202 944-3285   Fax 202 944-3295
Spina bifida is a congenital defect in which part of one (or more) vertebra fails to develop completely, leaving a portion of the spinal cord exposed. Spina bifida can occur anywhere on the spine but is most common in the lower back. The severity of the condition depends on how much nerve tissue is exposed. (ENC-1989)

National Tay-Sachs and Allied Diseases Association
2001 Beacon St, Brookline, MA 02146
800 906-8723   617 277-4463   Fax 617 277-0134
Tay-sachs disease is a serious inherited brain disorder that results in very early death. Tay-Sachs disease was formerly known as amaurotic family idiocy.

Tay-Sachs disease is caused by a deficiency of hexosamini-dase, a certain enzyme (a protein essential for regulating chemical reactions in the body). Deficiency results in a buildup of a harmful substance in the brain. The disease is most common among Ashkenazi Jews. The incidence in this group is around one in 2500, which is 100 times higher than in any other ethnic group. The gene for Tay-Sachs disease is recessive and an Ashkenazi Jew has a one in 25 chance of carrying it. If two carriers marry, there is a one in four chance that they will have an affected child.

Signs of the illness, which appear during the first six months of life, are blindness, dementia, deafness, seizures, and paralysis. An exaggerated startle response to sound is an early sign. Symptoms progress rapidly and the affected child usually dies before age 3. (ENC-1989)

Genetic Testing

AMA Policy

Insurance Companies and Genetic Information (E-2.135)

Physicians should not participate in genetic testing by health insurance companies to predict a person's predisposition for disease. As a corollary, it may be necessary for physicians to maintain separate files for genetic testing results to ensure that the results are not sent to health insurance companies when requests for copies of patient medical records are fulfilled. Physicians who withhold testing results should inform insurance companies that, when medical records are sent, genetic testing results are not included. This disclosure should occur with all patients, not just those who have undergone genetic testing. Issued June 1994 based on the report "Physician Participation in Genetic Testing by Health Insurance Companies," issued June 1993; updated June 1996.

AMA Policy

Genetic Information and Insurance Coverage
(H-185.972) BOT Rep 15, I-96

AMA believes:

1. Health insurance providers should be prohibited from using genetic information, or an individual's request for genetic services, to deny or limit any health benefit coverage or establish eligibility, continuation, enrollment, or contribution requirements.

2. Health insurance providers should be prohibited from establishing differential rates or premium payments based on genetic information or an individual's request for genetic services.

3. Health insurance providers should be prohibited from requesting or requiring collection or disclosure of genetic information.

4. Health insurance providers and other holders of genetic information should be prohibited from releasing genetic information without express prior written authorization of the individual. Written authorization should be required for each disclosure and include to whom the disclosure would be made.

Geriatrics

A Piece of My Mind

Aging and caring

Paul E. Ruskin, MD
JAMA 1983 Nov 11; 250(18): 2440

I was invited to present a lecture to a class of graduate nurses who were studying the "Psychosocial Aspects of Aging." I started my lecture with the following case presentation:

The patient is a white female who appears her reported age. She neither speaks nor comprehends the spoken word. Sometimes she babbles incoherently hours on end. She is disoriented about person, place, and time. She does, however, seem to recognize her own name. I have worked with her for the past six months, but she still does not recognize me.

She shows complete disregard for her physical appearance and makes no effort whatsoever to assist in her own care. She must be fed, bathed, and clothed by others. Because she is edentulous, her food must be pureed, and because she is incontinent of both urine and stool, she must be changed and bathed often. Her shirt is generally soiled from incessant drooling. She does not walk. Her sleep pattern is erratic. Often she wakens in the middle of the night, and her screaming awakens others.

Most of the time she is very friendly and happy. However, several times a day she gets quite agitated without apparent cause. Then she screams loudly until someone comes to comfort her.

After the case presentation, I asked the nurses how they would feel about taking care of a patient such as the one described. They used words such as "frustrated," "hopeless," "depressed," and "annoyed" to describe how they would feel.

When I stated that I enjoyed taking care of her and that I thought they would too, the class looked at me in disbelief. I then passed around a picture of the patient: my six-month-old daughter.

After the laughter had subsided, I asked why it was so much more difficult to care for a 90-year-old than a six-month-old with identical symptoms. We all agreed that it is physically easier to take care of a helpless baby weighing 15 pounds than a helpless adult weighing 100, but the answer seemed to go deeper than this.

The infant, we all agreed, represents new life, hope, and almost infinite potential. The demented senior citizen, on the other hand, represents the end of life, with little potential for growth.

We need to change our perspective. The aged patient is just as lovable as the child. Those who are ending their lives in the helplessness of old age deserve the same attention as those who are beginning their lives in the helplessness of infancy.

Resources

American Geriatrics Society
770 Lexington, Ste 300, New York, NY 10021
800 247-4779   212 308-1414   Fax 212 832-8646
E-mail: agsnyc@sono.los.com

Gerontological Society of America

1275 K St NW, Ste 350, Washington, DC 20005
202 842-1275   Fax 202 842-1150

Board Certification
American Board of Family Practice
2228 Young Dr, Lexington, KY 40505
606 269-5626   Fax 606 266-9699

American Board of Internal Medicine
3624 Market St, Philadelphia, PA 19104
800 441-ABIM (800 441-2246) 215 243-1500
Fax 215 382-4702

Gifts to Physicians From Industry

Annotated guidelines of gifts to physicians from industry

Council on Ethical and Judicial Affairs, American Medical Association, Chicago, Ill
Final Version: Issued October 9, 1991

On December 3, 1990, the Council on Ethical and Judicial Affairs issued its guidelines on gifts to physicians from industry. Since then, the Council has received numerous requests for interpretations of the guidelines. In order to facilitate application of the guidelines, the Council has developed the following annotated version that includes representative questions about the guidelines:

General question
When do the interpretations take effect?

The guidelines and interpretations are in full force. However, the interpretations do not apply retroactively to programs that have been planned in a good faith that they complied with the guidelines.

Do the guidelines apply only to pharmaceutical, device, and equipment manufacturers?

"Industry" includes all "proprietary health-related entities that might create a conflict of interest," as recommended by the American Academy of Family Physicians.

Guideline One. Any gifts accepted by physicians individually should primarily entail a benefit to patients and should not be of substantial value. Accordingly, textbooks, modest meals and other gifts are appropriate if they serve a genuine educational function. Cash payments should not be accepted.

a. *May physicians accept gram stain test kits, stethoscopes, or other diagnostic equipment?*

Diagnostic equipment primarily benefits the patient. Hence, such gifts are permissible as long as they are not of substantial value. In considering the value of the gift, the relevant measure is not the cost to the company of providing the gift. Rather, the relevant measure is the cost to the physician if he purchased the gift on the open market.

b. *May companies invite physicians to a dinner with a speaker and donate $100 to a charity or medical school on behalf of the physician?*

There are positive aspects to the proposal. The donations would be used for a worthy cause, and the physicians would receive important information about patient care. There is a direct personal benefit to the physician as well, however. An organization that is important to the physician—and one that the physician might have ordinarily felt obligated to make a contribution to—receives financial support as a result of the physician's decision to attend the meeting. On balance, physicians should make their own judgment about these inducements. If the charity is predetermined without the physician's input, there would seem to be little problem with the arrangement.

c. *May contributions to a professional society's general fund be accepted from industry?*

The guidelines are designed to deal with gifts from industry which affect, or could appear to affect, the judgment of individual practicing physicians. In general, a professional society should make its own judgment about gifts from industry to the society itself.

d. *When companies invite physicians to a dinner with a speaker, what are the relevant guidelines?*

First, the dinner must be a modest meal. Second, the guideline does allow gifts that primarily benefit patients and that are not of substantial value. Accordingly, textbooks and other gifts that primarily benefit patient care and that have a value to the physician in the general range of $100 are permissible.

e. *May physicians accept vouchers that reimburse them for uncompensated care they have provided?*

No. Such a voucher would result directly in increased income for the physician.

f. *May physicians accumulate "points" by attending several educational or promotional meetings and then choose a gift from a catalogue of educational options?*

This guideline permits gifts only if they are not of substantial value. If accumulation of points would result in physicians receiving a substantial gift by combining insubstantial gifts over a relatively short period of time, it would be inappropriate.

g. *May physicians accept gift certificates for educational materials when attending promotional or educational events?*

The Council views gift certificates as a gray area which is not per se prohibited by the guidelines. Medical textbooks are explicitly approved as gifts under the guidelines. A gift certificate for educational materials, ie, for the selection by the physician from an exclusively medical textbook catalogue, would not seem to be materially different. The issue is whether the gift certificate gives the recipient such control as to make the certificate similar to cash. As with charitable donations, preselection by the sponsor removes any question. It is up to the individual physician to make the final judgment.

Guideline Two. Individual gifts of minimal value are permissible as long as the gifts are related to the physician's work (eg, pens and notepads).

Guideline Three. Subsidies to underwrite the costs of continuing medical education conferences or professional meetings can contribute to the improvement of patient care and therefore are permissible. Since the giving of a subsidy directly to a physician by a company's sales representative may create a relationship which could influence the use of the company's products, any subsidy should be accepted by the conference's sponsor who in turn can use the money to reduce the conference's registration fee. Payments to defray the costs of a conference should not be accepted directly from the company by the physicians attending the conference.

a. *Are conference subsidies from the educational division of a company covered by the guidelines?*

Yes. When the Council says "any subsidy," it would not matter whether the subsidy comes from the sales division, the educational division, or some other section of the company.

b. *May a company or its intermediary send physicians a check or voucher to offset the registration fee at a specific conference or a conference of the physician's choice?*

Physicians should not directly accept checks or certificates that would be used to offset registration fees. The gift of a reduced registration should be made across the board and through the accredited sponsor.

Guideline Four. Subsidies from industry should not be accepted directly or indirectly to pay for the costs of travel, lodging, or other personal expenses of physicians attending conferences or meetings, nor should subsidies be accepted to compensate for the physicians' time. Subsidies for hospitality should not be accepted outside of modest meals or social events held as a part of a conference or meeting. It is appropriate for faculty at conferences or meetings to accept reasonable honoraria and to accept reimbursement for reasonable travel, lodging, and meal expenses. It is also appropriate for consultants who provide genuine services to receive reasonable compensation and to accept reimbursement for reasonable travel, lodging, and meal expenses. Token consulting or advisory arrangements cannot be used to justify compensating physicians for their time or their travel, lodging, and other out-of-pocket expenses.

a. *If a company invites physicians to visit its facilities for a tour, or to become educated about one of its products, may the company pay travel expenses and honoraria?*

This question has come up in the context of a rehabilitation facility that wants physicians to know of its existence so that they may refer their patients to the facility. It has also come up in the context of surgical device or equipment manufacturers who want physicians to become familiar with their products.

In general, travel expenses should not be reimbursed, nor should honoraria be paid for the visiting physician's time since the presentations are analogous to a pharmaceutical company's educational or promotional meetings. The Council recognizes that medical devices, equipment, and other technologies may require, in some circumstances, special evaluation or training in proper usage that cannot practically be provided except on site. Medical specialties are in a better position to advise physicians regarding the appropriateness of reimbursement with regard to these trips. In cases where the company insists on such visits as a means of protection from liability for improper usage, physicians and their specialties should make the judgment. In no case would honoraria be appropriate and any travel expenses should be only those strictly necessary.

b. *If the company invites physicians to visit its facilities for review and comment on a product, to discuss its independent research projects, or to explore the potential for collaborative research, may the company pay travel expenses and honoraria?*

If the physician is providing genuine services, reasonable compensation for time and travel expenses can be given. However, token advisory or consulting arrangements cannot be used to justify compensation.

c. *May a company hold a sweepstakes for physicians in which five entrants receive a trip to the Virgin Islands or airfare to the medical meeting of their choice?*

No. The use of a sweepstakes or raffle to deliver a gift does not affect the permissibility of the gift. Since the sweepstakes is not open to the public, the guidelines apply in full force.

d. *If a company convenes a group of physicians to recruit clinical investigators or convenes a group of clinical investigators for a meeting to discuss their results, may the company pay for their travel expenses?*

Expenses may be paid if the meetings serve a genuine research purpose. One guide to their propriety would be whether the NIH conducts similar meetings when it sponsors multicenter clinical trials. When travel subsidies are acceptable, the guidelines emphasize that they be used to pay only for "reasonable" expenses. The reasonableness of expenses would depend on a number of considerations. For example, meetings are likely to be problematic if overseas locations are used for exclusively domestic investigators. It would be inappropriate to pay for recreation or entertainment beyond the kind of modest hospitality described in this guideline.

e. *How can a physician tell whether there is a "genuine research purpose?"*

A number of factors can be considered. Signs that a genuine research purpose exists include the facts that there are (1) a valid study protocol, (2) recruitment of physicians with appropriate qualifications or expertise, and (3) recruitment of an appropriate number of physicians in light of the number of study participants needed for statistical evaluation.

f. *May a company compensate physicians for their time and travel expenses when they participate in focus groups?*

G

Yes. As long as the focus groups serve a genuine and exclusive research purpose and are not used for promotional purposes, physicians may be compensated for time and travel expenses. The number of physicians used in a particular focus group or in multiple focus groups should be an appropriate size to accomplish the research purpose, but no larger.

g. *Do the restrictions on travel, lodging, and meals apply to educational programs run by medical schools, professional societies, or other accredited organizations that are funded by industry, or do they apply only to programs developed and run by industry?*

The restrictions apply to all conferences or meetings which are funded by industry. The Council drew no distinction on the basis of the organizer of the conference or meeting. The Council felt that the gift of travel expenses is too substantial even when the conference is run by a non-industry sponsor. (Industry includes all "proprietary health-related entities that might create a conflict of interest" as recommended by the American Academy of Family Physicians.)

h. *May company funds be used for travel expenses and honoraria of bona fide faculty at educational meetings?*

This guideline draws a distinction between attendees and faculty. As was stated, "[i]t is appropriate for faculty at conferences or meetings to accept reasonable honoraria and to accept reimbursement for reasonable travel, lodging, and meal expenses."

Companies need to be mindful of the guidelines of the Accreditation Council on Continuing Medical Education. According to those guidelines, "[f]unds from a commercial source should be in the form of an educational grant made payable to the CME sponsor for the support of programming."

i. *May travel expenses be reimbursed for physicians presenting a poster or a "free paper" at a scientific conference?*

Reimbursement may be accepted only by a bona fide faculty. The presentation of a poster or a free paper does not by itself qualify a person as a member of the conference faculty for purposes of these guidelines.

j. *When a professional association schedules a long-range planning meeting, is it appropriate for industry to subsidize the travel expenses of the meeting participants?*

The guidelines are designed to deal with gifts from industry which affect, or could appear to affect, the judgment of individual practicing physicians. In general, a professional society should make its own judgment about gifts from industry to the society itself.

k. *May continuing medical education conferences be held in the Bahamas, Europe, or South America?*

There are no restrictions on the location of conferences as long as the attendees are paying their own travel expenses.

l. *May travel expenses be accepted by physicians who are being trained as speakers or faculty for educational conferences and meetings?*

In general, no. If a physician is presenting as an independent expert at a CME event, both the training and its reimbursement raise questions about independence. In

addition, the training is a gift because the physician's role is generally more analogous to that of an attendee than a participant. Speaker training sessions can be distinguished from meetings (see 4b) with leading researchers, sponsored by a company, designed primarily for an exchange of information about important developments or treatments, including the sponsor's own research, for which reimbursement for travel may be appropriate.

m. *What kinds of social events during conferences and meetings may be subsidized by industry?*

Social events should satisfy three criteria. First, the value of the event to the physician should be modest. Second, the event should facilitate discussion among attendees and/or discussion between attendees and faculty. Third, the educational part of the conference should account for a substantial majority of the total time accounted for by the educational activities and social events together. Events that would be viewed (as in the succeeding question) as lavish or expensive should be avoided. But modest social activities that are not elaborate or unusual are permissible, eg, inexpensive boat rides, barbecues, entertainment that draws on the local performers. In general, any such events that are a part of the conference program should be open to all registrants.

n. *May a company rent an expensive entertainment complex for an evening during a medical conference and invite the physicians attending the conference?*

No. The guidelines permit only modest hospitality.

o. *If physicians attending a conference engage in interactive exchange, may their travel expenses be paid by industry?*

No. Mere interactive exchange would not constitute genuine consulting services.

p. *If a company schedules a conference and provides meals for the attendees that fall within the guidelines, may the company also pay the costs of the meals for spouses?*

If a meal falls within the guidelines, then the physician's spouse may be included.

q. *May companies donate funds to sponsor a professional society's charity golf tournament?*

Yes. But it is sensible if physicians who play in the tournament make some contribution themselves to the event.

r. *If a company invites a group of consultants to a meeting and a consultant brings a spouse, may the company pay the costs of lodging or meals of the spouse? Does it matter if the meal is part of the program for the consultants?*

Since the costs of having a spouse share a hotel room or join a modest meal are nominal, it is permissible for the company to subsidize those costs. However, if the total subsidies become substantial, then they become unacceptable.

Guideline Five. Scholarship or other special funds to permit medical students, residents, and fellows to attend carefully selected educational conferences may be permissible as long as the selection of students, residents, or fellows who will receive the funds is made by the academic or training institution.

a. *When a company subsidizes the travel expenses of residents to an appropriately selected conference, may the residents receive the subsidy directly from the company?*

Funds for scholarships or other special funds should be given to the academic departments or the accredited sponsor of the conference. The disbursement of funds can then be made by the departments or the conference sponsor.

Guideline Six. No gifts should be accepted if there are strings attached. For example, physicians should not accept gifts which are given in relation to the physician's prescribing practices. In addition, when companies underwrite medical conferences or lectures other than their own, responsibility for and control over the selection of content, faculty, educational methods, and materials should belong to the organizers of the conferences or lectures.

a. *May companies send their top prescribers, purchasers, or referrers on cruises?*

No. There can be no link between prescribing or referring patterns and gifts. In addition, travel expenses, including cruises, are not permissible.

b. *May the funding company itself develop the complete educational program that is sponsored by an accredited continuing medical education sponsor?*

No. The funding company may finance the development of the program through its grant to the sponsor, but the accredited sponsor must have responsibility and control over the content and faculty of conferences, meetings, or lectures. Neither the funding company nor an independent consulting firm should develop the complete educational program for approval by the accredited sponsor.

c. *How much input may a funding company have in the development of a conference, meeting, or lectures?*

The guidelines of the Accreditation Council on Continuing Medical Education on commercial support of continuing medical education address this question.

Government Printing Office

The Government Printing Office (GPO) began operations in accordance with Congressional Joint Resolution 25 of June 23, 1860. The activities of the GPO are outlined and defined in the public printing and documents chapters of Title 44 of the US code. It produces and procures printed and electronic publications for Congress and the departments and establishments of the federal government. (USG-1996)

Government Printing Office
North Capitol and H Streets NW
Washington, DC 20401
202 512-1991

Publication orders and inquiries
202 512-1800

Information
202 275-3648
E-mail: gpo5@access.digex.net
Web address: http://www.gao.gov

Bookstores
US Government Printing Office Bookstore
710 N Capitol St NW, Washington, DC 20401
202 512-0132
1510 H St NW, Washington, DC 20005
202 653-5075

Alabama
US Government Bookstore
O'Neill Bldg
2021 Third Ave N, Birmingham, AL 35203
205 731-1056

California
US Government Bookstore
ARCO Plaza, C-Level
505 S Flower St, Los Angeles, CA 90071
213 239-9844

US Government Bookstore
Marathon Plaza, Rm 141-S
303 Second St, San Francisco, CA 94107
415 512-2770

Colorado
US Government Bookstore
Room 117, Federal Bldg
1961 Stout St, Denver, CO 80294
303 844-3964

US Government Bookstore
Norwest Banks Bldg
201 W 8th St, Pueblo, CO 81003
719 544-3142

Florida
US Government Bookstore
100 W Bay St, Ste 100, Jacksonville, FL 32202
904 353-0569

Georgia
US Government Bookstore
First Union Plaza
999 Peachtree St NE, Ste 120
Atlanta, GA 30309-3964
404 347-1900

Illinois
US Government Bookstore
1 Congress Center
401 S State St, Ste 124, Chicago, IL 60605
312 353-5133

Maryland
US Government Printing Office
Warehouse Sales Outlet
8660 Cherry Ln, Laurel, MD 20707
301 953-7974   301 792-0262

Massachusetts
US Government Bookstore
Thomas P. O'Neill Bldg
Rm 169, 10 Causeway St, Boston, MA 02222
617 720-4180

Michigan
US Government Bookstore
Ste 160, Federal Bldg
477 Michigan Ave, Detroit, MI 48226
313 226-7816

Missouri
US Government Bookstore
120 Bannister Mall
5600 E Bannister Rd, Kansas City, MO 64137
816 767-8225

New York
US Government Bookstore
Rm 110, Federal Bldg
26 Federal Plaza, New York, NY 10278
212 264-3825

Ohio
US Government Bookstore
Rm 1653, Federal Bldg
1240 E 9th St, Cleveland, OH 44199
216 522-4922

US Government Bookstore, Room 207, Federal Bldg
200 N High St, Columbus, OH 43215
614 469-6956

Oregon
US Government Bookstore
1305 SW First Ave, Portland, OR 97201-5801
503 221-6217

Pennsylvania
US Government Bookstore
Robert Morris Bldg
100 N 17th St, Philadelphia, PA 19103
215 636-1900

US Government Bookstore
Rm 118, Federal Bldg
1000 Liberty Ave, Pittsburgh, PA 15222
412 644-2721

Texas
US Government Bookstore
Rm IC50, Federal Bldg
1100 Commerce St, Dallas, TX 75242
214 767-0076

US Government Bookstore
Texas Crude Bldg
801 Travis St, Ste 120, Houston, TX 77002
713 228-1187

Washington
US Government Bookstore
Rm 194, Federal Bldg
915 Second Ave, Seattle, WA 98174
206 553-4271

Wisconsin
US Government Bookstore
Ste 150, Reuss Federal Plaza
310 W Wisconsin Ave, Milwaukee, WI 53203
414 297-1304

Graduate Medical Education

Graduate Medical Education Directory. Chicago, Ill:
American Medical Association. Annual. 1995/96 ed,
1133 pp. ISBN 0-89970-675-4 OP416795

*Fellowship & Residency Electronic Interactive Database
Access* 1995 (FREIDA)
(3 1/2" Disk) OP411695
(5 1/4" Disk) OP411795

AMA-FREIDA Database Hotline
800 464-4936

Resources
Accreditation Council on Graduate Medical Education
515 N State St, Ste 2000, Chicago, IL 60610
312 464-4920   Fax 312 464-4098

Council on Graduate Medical Education (COGME)
Bureau of Health Professions
Department of Health and Human Services
5600 Fishers Ln, Rockville, MD 20857
301 443-5794

Fellowships:
FREIDA Hotline
312 464-4936
Certification of subspecialty programs
Internal Medicine, Pathology, and Pediatrics will be listed
in the *Graduate Medical Education Directory,* also part of
the FREIDA program.

For Internal Medicine:
National Study for Internal Medicine Manpower
Center for Health Administration
University of Chicago
1101 E 58th St, Chicago, IL 60637
312 702-7753

*Contact the specialty societies for certification
information on subspecialty programs. No formal list of
them exists.*

Grammar Hotline

Grammar Hotline, Eastern Illinois University
217 581-5929

Grammar Hotline, Illinois State University
309 438-2345

Grammarline, Illinois Valley Community College
815 224-2720

Grammarphone, Triton College
708 456-0300

Purdue University
765 494-3723

Grief

The Compassionate Friends
PO Box 3696, Oak Brook, IL 60522-3696
630 990-0010   Fax 630 990-0246

Grief Education Institute
2422 S Downing St, Denver, CO 80210
303 759-6048

G

Group Practice

The acceleration of medical costs during the 1980s, coupled with the explosion of managed care options, has increased the focus on medical group practices and their relationships to health care delivery systems. Nearly three fourths of respondents in a 1991 Health Care Benefits Survey (Foster Higgins, 1992) offered at least one type of managed care plan: 60% an HMO, 31% a PPO, and 11% a point-of-service option. As corporations and other health care purchasers focus increasingly on ways to reduce employee health care costs, managed care entities continue to boost market share.[1] Recognizing the diversity of health care delivery systems and the need for high-quality, low-cost care, medical groups have formed a variety of relationships with these providers.

Reference

1. Johnsson T. HMOs dominate, shape the market. *Am Med News* Jan 22/29, 1996; 39:27. (MDG-1996)

Table G-1

Percentage[a] of Groups Related to HMOs and PPOs

Type of Relationship	%	Total N
Staff model HMO	1.0	13,193[b]
Organized to provide services to HMO	11.9	13,193[b]
One or more HMO contracts	94.9	13,193[b]
HMO referrals	16.3	13,193[b]
PPO contracts	83.9	15,521[c]

a. Percentages do not total 100 because groups could check more than one response. For example, groups that contract with HMOs may also contract with PPOs.

b. Total Ns for relationships of groups to HMOs do not differ because all options in question 7 on the Census of Medical Groups were treated as a single question; for example, if the respondent indicated staff model HMO, and left other HMO relationship options blank, it was assumed that a "no" response was meant for these options (see Appendix A Survey Instruments). Excludes 4374 long-form respondents for whom HMO relationship is unknown.

c. Excludes 2046 long-form respondents for whom PPO contract is unknown.

Table G-2

Distribution of Groups by Group Size and Specialty Composition

Group Size	Single Specialty %	N	Multi-specialty %	N	Family/General Practice %	N	Total %	N
3	27.1	3659	13.8	597	31.5	493	24.5	4749
4	23.1	3122	13.3	576	29.3	458	21.4	4156
5-6	24.5	3312	18.2	789	21.6	337	22.9	4438
7-9	12.7	1716	13.6	588	9.0	140	12.6	2444
10-15	7.6	1027	14.3	618	4.0	63	8.8	1708
16-25	3.3	443	10.3	446	3.0	48	4.8	937
26-49	1.3	173	7.8	339	1.0	15	2.7	527
50-75	0.2	26	2.9	124	0.5	7	0.8	157
76-99	0.1	9	1.4	59	0.0	0	0.4	68
100 or more	0.1	17	4.6	198	0.1	2	1.1	217
Total	**100.0**	**13,504**	**100.2***	**4334**	**100.0**	**1563**	**100.0**	**19,401**

*Percentages do not sum to 100 due to rounding.

Multispecialty groups tend to be larger than single specialty or family/general practice groups. Although 50.2% of all single specialty groups and 60.8% of all family/ general practice groups have three or four physicians, only 27.1% of multispecialty groups do. (MDG-1996)

Resources

American Medial Group Association
1422 Duke St, Alexandria, VA 22314-3430
703 838-0033   Fax 703 548-1890
Web address: http://www.amga.org

Medical Group Management Association
104 Inverness Terrace E, Englewood, CO 80112
303 799-1111   303 643-4427

Growth

Human Growth Foundation
7777 Leesburg Pike, Falls Church, VA 22043
800 451-6434   703 883-1773   Fax 703 883-1776
E-mail: hgfound@erol.com

G

Gynecology

Gynecologist. Diagnoses and treats diseases and disorders of female genital, urinary, and rectal organs. Examines patient to determine medical problem, utilizing physical findings, diagnostic images, laboratory test results, and patient's statements as diagnostic aids. Discusses problem with patient, and prescribes medication and exercise or hygiene regimen, or performs surgery as needed to correct malfunctions or remove diseased organ. May care for throughout pregnancy and deliver babies. (DOT-1991)

Resources

American Board of Obstetrics and Gynecology
2915 Vine St, Dallas, TX 78504
214 871-1619   Fax 214 871-1943

American College of Obstetricians and Gynecologists
409 12th St SW, Washington, DC 20024-2188
202 638-5577   Fax 202 484-8107

American Association of Gynecologic Laparoscopists
13021 E Florence Ave
Santa Fe Springs, CA 90670
800 554-2245   310 946-8774   Fax 310 946-0073
E-mail: 102254.3033@compuserve.com
Web address: http://pages.prodigy.com/CA/jmp/jmp.html

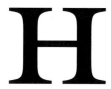

H

Hair Loss

American Hair Loss Council
401 N Michigan Ave, 22nd Fl, Chicago, IL 60611-4212
800 274-8717   Fax 312 245-1080

National Alopecia Areata Foundation
PO Box 150760, San Rafael, CA 94915-0760
415 456-4644   Fax 415 456-4274

Hand Surgery

American Association for Hand Surgery
444 E Algonguin Rd, Arlington Heights, IL 60005
847 228-9758   Fax 847 228-6509

American Society for Surgery of the Hand
6060 Greenwood Plaza Blvd, Ste 100
Englewood, CO 80111-4801
303 771-9236   Fax 303 771-9269

Board Certification:
American Board of Orthopaedic Surgery
400 Silver Cedar Ct, Chapel Hill, NC 27514
919 929-7103   Fax 919 942-8988

American Board of Plastic Surgery
7 Penn Center, Ste 400
1635 Market St, Philadelphia, PA 19103
215 587-9322

American Board of Surgery
1617 John F. Kennedy Blvd, Ste 860
Philadelphia, PA 19103
215 568-4000   Fax 215 563-5718

Head Injury

Brain Injury Association
1776 Massachusetts Ave NW, Ste 100
Washington, DC 20036
800 444-6443   202 296-6443   Fax 202 296-8850

Headaches

American Association for the Study of the Headache
875 Kings Hwy, Ste 200, Woodbury, NJ 08096
609 845-0322   Fax 609 384-5811

National Headache Foundation
(formerly National Migraine Foundation)
428 W Saint James Pl, 2nd fl, Chicago, IL 60614-2750
800 843-2256   800 523-8858 (IL only)
Fax 773 525-7357

Health Administration

Association of University Programs in
Health Administration
1911 N Fort Myer Dr, Ste 503
Arlington, VA 22209
703 524-5500

Health and Human Services, Department of

The US Department of Health and Human Services (HHS) is the Cabinet-level department of the federal executive branch most concerned with people and most involved with the nation's human concerns. In one way or another, whether it is mailing out Social Security checks or making health services more widely available, HHS touches the lives of more Americans than any other federal agency. It is literally a department of people serving people, from newborn infants to our most elderly citizens. The Department of Health and Human Services was created as the Department of Health, Education and Welfare on April 11, 1953 (USC app), and redesignated, effective May 4, 1980, by the Department of Education Organization Act (20 USC 3508).
(USG-1996)

Resource

Department of Health and Human Services
200 Independence Ave SW
Washington, DC 20201
202 245-6296
Web address: http://www.os.dhhs.gov

Health Associations

American Council on Science and Health
1995 Broadway, New York, NY 10023-5860
212 362-7044   Fax 212 362-4919

Catholic Health Association of the US
4455 Woodson Rd, St Louis, MO 63134-3797
314 427-2500   Fax 314 427-0029

Group Health Association of America
1129 20th St NW, 2nd Fl, #600
Washington, DC 20036
202 778-3200   Fax 202 331-7487

National Health Council
1730 M St NW, Ste 500
Washington, DC 20036
202 785-3910   Fax 202 785-5923
Web address: http://www.social.com

Healthcare Financial Management Association
2 Westbrook Corp, Ste 700
Westchester, IL 60154
800 252-HFMA   708 531-9600

Health Care Financing Administration

The Health Care Financing Administration (HCFA) was created as a principal operating component of the US Department of Health and Human Services (HHS) by the Secretary of HHS in 1977, to combine under one administration the oversight of the Medicare program, the federal portion of the Medicaid program, and related quality assurance activities. Today, HCFA serves 68 million people, or one in four elderly, disabled, and poor Americans through Medicare and Medicaid.

The Medicare and Medicaid programs include a quality assurance focal point to carry out the quality assurance provisions of the Medicare and Medicaid programs; the development and implementation of health and safety standards for providers of care in federal health programs; and the implementation of the End-Stage Renal Disease Program and the Professional Review provisions.

For further information, contact the Administrator, Health Care Financing Administration, Department of Health and Human Services, 200 Independence Ave SW, Washington, DC 20201. Phone, 410 786-3151. (USG-1996)

(For the Health Care Financing Administration statement of organization, see the *Federal Register* of March 29, 1994, 59 FR 14628)

Regional HCFA Offices

Region I—Boston
(Connecticut, Maine, Massachusetts, New Hampshire, Rhode Island, and Vermont.)
Associate Regional Administrator, HCFA Program Operations
John F. Kennedy Federal Bldg, Government Center, Rm 2325, Boston, MA 02203-0033
617 565-1273

Region II—New York
(New Jersey, New York, Puerto Rico, and Virgin Islands.)
Associate Regional Administrator, HCFA Program Operations
Jacob K. Javits Federal Bldg, 26 Federal Plaza, Rm 3811, New York, NY 10278-0063
212 264-8517

Region III—Philadelphia
(Delaware, District of Columbia, Maryland, Pennsylvania, Virginia, and West Virginia.)
Associate Regional Administrator
HCFA Program Operations
3535 Market St, PO Box 7760
Philadelphia, PA 19101-3363
215 596-6828

Region IV—Atlanta
(Alabama, Florida, Georgia, Kentucky, Mississippi, North Carolina, South Carolina, and Tennessee.)
Associate Regional Administrator
HCFA Program Operations
101 Marietta Tower, Ste 701, Atlanta, GA 30323-2711
404 331-2548

Region V—Chicago
(Indiana, Illinois, Michigan, Minnesota, Ohio, and Wisconsin.)
Associate Regional Administrator, HCFA Program Operations
105 W Adams St, 15th Fl, Chicago, IL 60603-6201
312 353-9840

Region VI—Dallas
(Arkansas, Louisiana, Oklahoma, New Mexico, and Texas.)
Associate Regional Administrator
HCFA Program Operations
1200 Main Tower Bldg, Ste 2000
Dallas, TX 75202-4305
214 767-6418

Region VII—Kansas City
(Iowa, Kansas, Missouri, and Nebraska.)
Associate Regional Administrator
HCFA Program Operations
601 East 12th St, Rm 235
Kansas City, MO 64106-2808
816 426-3539

Region VIII—Denver
(Colorado, Montana, North Dakota, South Dakota, Wyoming, and Utah.)
Associate Regional Administrator
HCFA Program Operations
1961 Stout St, Rm 1185, Denver, CO 80294-3538
303 844-6149 ext 233

Region IX—San Francisco
(Arizona, California, Nevada, Guam, Hawaii, and American Samoa.)
Associate Regional Administrator
HCFA Program Operations
75 Hawthorne St, 4th and 5th Fl
San Francisco, CA 94105-3903
415 744-3628

Region X—Seattle
(Alaska, Idaho, Oregon, and Washington.)
Associate Regional Administrator
HCFA Program Operations
2201 Sixth Ave, DPO-RX40
Seattle, WA 98121-2500
206 553-0440

Health Fraud

Guide to the American Medical Association Historical Health Fraud and Alternative Medicine Collection. Chicago, Ill: American Medical Association; 1992. 215 pp. ISBN 0-89907-044-17 OP310492

National Council Against Health Fraud
PO Box 1276, Loma Linda, CA 92354-1276
909 824-4690   Fax 909 824-4838

Health Information Management

Definition of the profession
Health information management is the profession that focuses on health care data and the management of health care information resources. The profession addresses the nature, structure, and translation of data into usable forms of information for the advancement of health and health care of individuals and populations.

Health information management professionals collect, integrate, and analyze primary and secondary health care data; disseminate information; and manage information resources related to the research, planning, provision, and evaluation of health care services.

History
Standards for educational programs for medical record administrators (formerly librarians) were established in 1935 by the American Medical Record Association (now the American Health Information Management Association [AHIMA]) through its committee on training. The first four programs for medical record administrators were accredited in that year, three of which were hospital based and one of which was a college-based program. In 1942, the AHIMA invited the American Medical Association (AMA) to serve as the official accrediting agency for educational programs for medical record administrators. This responsibility was accepted by the AMA House of Delegates. *Standards (Essentials)* for educational programs for medical record administrators were initially developed and adopted in 1943, and were subsequently revised in 1952, 1960, 1967, 1974, 1981, 1988, and 1994.

In 1953, the first *Standards* for educational programs for medical record technicians were established and approved by both the AHIMA and the AMA. The first educational programs for medical record technicians were hospital based. Over the years there has been a gradual transition from hospital-based educational programs for medical record administrators and medical record technicians to college- and university-based programs. In 1965, 1976, 1983, 1988, and 1994, the AHIMA, in collaboration with the AMA Council on Medical Education (CME), revised and adopted the *Standards and Guidelines for Accredited Programs for the Health Information Technician and the Health Information Administrator.* Today, the *Standards* are adopted by the Commission on Accreditation of Allied Health Education Programs (CAAHEP) in collaboration with AHIMA.

Health Information Administrator

Occupational description
Health information administrators manage health information systems consistent with the medical, administrative, ethical, and legal requirements of the health care delivery system. Although these administrators are not often directly involved in patient contact, their work with the medical and hospital administrative staff is of critical importance to patient care. Because they deal with patient records and information, they should not be confused with medical librarians, who work chiefly with books, periodicals, and other medical publications.

Job description
The health information administrator is the professional responsible for the management of health information systems consistent with professional standards and the medical, administrative, ethical, and legal requirements of the health care delivery system. The administrator possesses the administrative knowledge and skills necessary to plan and develop health information systems that meet standards of accrediting and regulating agencies; to design health information systems appropriate for various sizes and types of health care facilities; to manage the human, financial, and physical resources of a health information service; to participate in medical staff and institutional activities, including utilization management, risk management, and quality assessment; to collect and analyze patient and facility data for reimbursement, facility planning, marketing, risk management, utilization management, quality assessment, and research; to serve as an advocate for privacy and confidentiality of health information; and to plan and offer in-service educational programs for health care personnel.

Employment characteristics
The demand for health information administrators is greatest in hospitals. Other growing areas of employment are ambulatory and long-term care facilities, state health departments, peer review organizations, government agencies, and private industry. Health information administrators interested in teaching may accept faculty appointments in academic programs for health information administration.

According to the AHIMA, entry-level salaries average between $25,000 and $30,000. (AHRP-1997)

Health Information Technician

Occupational description
The medical record is a permanent document prepared for each person treated in a health care facility. It contains the "who, what, why, where, when, and how" details of patient care during diagnosis and treatment, as well as information of medical, scientific, and legal value. Health information technicians are important members of the health care team. Traditionally, health information technicians have been employed in the medical records department of hospitals. With the increasing expansion of health care needs, opportunities for employment are also available in ambulatory health care facilities, industrial clinics, state and federal health agencies, long-term care facilities, and a number of other areas.

Job description

The health information technician is the professional responsible for maintaining components of health information systems in a manner consistent with the medical, administrative, ethical, legal, accreditation, and regulatory requirements of the health care delivery system. In all types of facilities, and in various locations within a facility, the technician possesses the technical knowledge and skills necessary to process, maintain, compile, and report patient data for reimbursement, facility planning, marketing, risk management, utilization management, quality assessment, and research; to abstract and code clinical data using appropriate classification systems; and to analyze health records according to standards. The health information technician may be responsible for functional supervision of the various components of the health information system.

Employment characteristics

Although the demand for health information technicians is greatest in hospitals, other growing areas of employment may include long-term care facilities, ambulatory care centers, rehabilitation centers, state and local health departments, and large group medical practices. According to the AHIMA, entry-level salaries average $22,000. (AHRP-1997)

Resources

AMA Allied Health Department
312 553-9355

American Health Information Management Association
919 N Michigan Ave, Ste 1400
Chicago, IL 60611-1683
312 787-2672   Fax 312 787-9793
Web address: http://www.ahima.org/

Health Maintenance Organizations

Poetry and Medicine

With HMOs—Well, Who Really Knows?

Deborah Smith Parker
JAMA 1996 Oct 2; 276(13):1006u

Employers got nervous with just fee for service,
     their medical bills were too high
So they gave up their voice and physician choice
     to give HMOs a try.
But how we now cringe that this rationing binge
     has sidetracked good care and health
Which today is replaced by a shiny new face,
     the accumulation of wealth.
What we hope now prevails is a lifting of veils
     to reveal the HMOs' greed,
To see through the sell and pull out of hell
     subscribers who are truly in need.

With HMOs—well, who really knows,
     since data collection's not done;
Now they are aware the data are there,
     it's just a function they shun.
It's hard to take looks at their open books,
     there's little they must disclose;
So what really occurred is oddly obscured
     and lines pockets for their CEOs.

They limit access while alleging success
     and to customers they state
How much has been saved by excesses they've shaved
     and then they raise the rate.

But God save your soul if you've a bad mole
     or are losing your body hair,
Or a cyst pilonidal or you're suicidal
     and need a specialist's care
If you've a strange rash, then you'd better have cash
     for a skin doc you'll never see;
You'll first be deterred from being referred
     for medical necessity.
It takes a magician to get past that physician,
     your primary care designee,
Who must be a whiz to manage the biz
     and is called a PCP.

On them you depend, but they must defend
     the profit; on them is the onus
To keep the costs low (as to treatment you go)
     so executives share in a bonus.
Now physicians who care feel great despair
     that they must so closely ration,
But if they want work, they should act like clerks
     and try to stifle all passions.
If they want to be good, then like Robin Hood
     they steal from the lords of risk pools.
It's not treating disease or suffering to ease,
     it's the almighty dollar that rules.

Health maintenance organizations (HMOs) are responsible for both financing and providing an agreed-upon set of comprehensive health maintenance and treatment services to a specifically defined and voluntarily enrolled population for a prepaid, fixed sum. Thus, an HMO serves as both an insurer and a provider (or an arranger) of health care services. In contrast to traditional indemnity health insurance, which simply reimburses covered individuals or those who provide health care services to them, the close relationship between insuring and providing services requires HMOs and their providers to carefully monitor and manage both the quantity and the quality of care.

HMOs are typically separated into five types: the staff model, the group practice model, the individual practice association model, the direct contract model, and the network model. It is significant to note, like so many distinctions in managed care, that the lines between these catagories appear to be blurring. (DRS 1-1993)

How HMOs evolved

In his 1971 health message to Congress, President Richard Nixon focused on prepaid medical practices, which had become known as HMOs, as the centerpiece of national health policy. Two years elapsed before passage of the Health Maintenance Act of 1973 (PL93-222). Federal funds in the form of loans and grants were used by individual HMOs for 2 or 3 years of initial study and development.

An integral part of the Health Maintenance Act of 1973 concerned federal HMO qualification. For an HMO to qualify for federal financial support it must have been deemed financially viable and able to supply certain health services to its members. These included diagnostic and therapeutic services, inpatient hospital services, short-term rehabilitation services, emergency services, mental health care services for alcohol or drug abuse, home health care, family planning, and preventive health care. No HMO could offer lower-priced contracts with benefits less than those specified and obtain federal qualification. An additional provision in the law that gave added impetus to the growth of HMOs was the stipulation that all employers with more than 25 workers must offer their employees the opportunity to enroll in a federally qualified HMO if one was available in their geographic area. This was the "dual choice option" provision.

Continued federal commitment to the HMO concept included 1976 and 1978 legislation that eased existing regulations to encourage HMO growth. The 1976 amendment waived the 1973 requirement in which physicians were to devote at least one half of their practice to the HMO for 3 years. The legislation also repealed the 30-day open enrollment periods for smaller, newly developed HMOs and allowed the HMOs to deny enrollment or delay coverage to persons institutionalized with chronic illness or permanent injury. Mandatory dual-choice option regulation was also reiterated in the new legislation. These changes removed many of the barriers that had limited HMO growth.

In 1978, the federal government passed legislation to provide further financial assistance to HMOs. The amendment extended HMO program authorization for 3 years, increased the maximum dollar limit for initial development grants, and raised loan guarantees from 1 to 2 million dollars. Although the 1978 amendment increased federal financing for HMOs, the legislation also established strict financial reporting guidelines and enrollment practices.

A new era of HMO development began with the Reagan Administration, which viewed the HMO approach as a way to encourage competition in the health care marketplace while reducing federal government involvement. In the 1980s, the Reagan Administration slowly removed federal assistance from HMOs. Thus, an increasing number of new and existing HMOs became for-profit entities. Growing national concern with health care costs, the increased role of for-profit health care, and wider public acceptance of prepaid health care delivery are among the factors that have accelerated recent HMO growth. (HDS-1988)

Resources

Health Resources and Services Administration
Bureau of Health Maintenance
Organizations and Resources
5600 Fishers Ln, Rm 903, Rockville, MD 20857
301 966-0474

Complaints:
Contact state department of insurance.

HMOs that accept Medicare recipients:
Contact regional Health Care Financing Administration office.

Health Maintenance Organizations, State Associations of

Alabama HMO Guaranty Association
600 Beacon Pky W, Ste 280
Birmingham, AL 35209-3140

California Association of HMOs (CAHMO)
910 K Str, Ste 350, Sacramento, CA 95814-3512
916 552-2910   Fax 916 443-1037

District of Columbia Association of HMOs
1901 Pennsylvania Ave NW, Ste 600
Washington DC 20006-3405

Association of HMOs in Michigan
327 Seymore, PO Box 19333, Lansing, MI 48901
517 371-3181

Minnesota Council of HMOs
2550 University Ave W, Ste 330N
St Paul, MN 55114-1052

New York State HMO Conference
Carriage House
21 Elk St, Albany, NY 12207-1008
518 462-2293   Fax 518 462-2150

HMO Association of Ohio
65 E State St, Ste 1000, Columbus, OH 43215
614 460-3503

Tennessee Association of HMOs
611 Commerce St, Ste 2900, Nashville, TN 37203-3742

Texas HMO Association
1400 Lavaca, Ste 101, Austin, TX 78701-3283
512 476-2091   Fax 512 476-2870

Health Officials

Association of State and Territorial Health Officials
415 2nd St NE, Ste 315, Washington, DC 20001
202 624-5828   Fax 202 624-7875

Health Policy

National Governor's Association Health Policy Group—
Hall of States
444 N Capitol St, Ste 267
Washington, DC 20001
202 624-5300   Fax 202 624-5313

Health Professional Shortage Areas

Financial assistance and education programs to encourage care to the underserved

JAMA 1992 Sept 2; 268(9): 1089

Concerns about the adequacy of physician supply in certain areas of the US have been raised,[1] and there are data to support the existence of shortages.[2,3] For more than two decades, attempts have been made at the federal and state levels to correct the geographic imbalance in physician supply. In general, corrective actions tied to medical education have been of two kinds: financial support to educational programs or the sites where educational experiences are offered, and direct financial assistance to medical students in return for service to defined populations. Most often, the goal of both kinds of programs is to increase the number of primary care providers practicing in areas of need.

Financial support to educational programs or sites

The federal government, in 1971, began supporting primary care physician training through Title VII of the Public Health Service Act. At about the same time, Congress passed legislation to support the creation of Area Health Education Centers (AHECs). AHECs function to enhance the level of care to underserved populations and to provide sites of training for physicians and other health professionals.[4] In fiscal year 1989, the AHEC program was modified to add Health Education and Training Centers, which support regions and populations with acute and longstanding shortages of health personnel.[5]

With the passage of the Health Professions Education Assistance Act of 1963 (Pub L No. 88-129), medical schools began to receive federal aid to support expansion of their class sizes. In 1976, an amendment to this legislation (Pub L No. 94-484) tied this support, in part, to expanding primary care residency positions.[6] While capitation was successful in its primary objective—increasing the total number of physicians graduated—less clear was the specific impact on the supply of primary care physicians and the availability of care to the underserved.[1]

States also participated in the expansion of medical education during the 1960s and 1970s. Of the 39 medical schools organized between 1960 and 1979, 30 were publicly supported and nine were private.[7] Many of these schools were founded with a mission of serving their regions and producing practitioners for the state (Politzer et al[1] and Liaison Committee on Medical Education Annual Medical Questionnaire, Part II, 1992, data kept at American Medical Association, Chicago, Ill).

Financial assistance programs

The federal mechanism for providing financial support to physicians-in-training has been through the National Health Service Corps and the Indian Health Service, both of which currently have scholarship and loan repayment programs tied to eventual service in areas of need. The level of support for all these programs has varied over the years. For example, the National Health Service Corps program decreased sharply from 2339 new scholarships to medical students in 1978-1979 to 25 in 1986-1987.[8] The availability of scholarships has increased in recent years, to a total of 400 for all health professions in 1992-1993.

Sixteen states have one or more types of financial assistance programs tied to service in rural shortage areas for set periods of time. These include direct scholarship or loan programs and loan repayment programs.[9] The programs often are managed through state rural health offices. For more information about federal or state financial assistance programs tied to service in shortage areas, contact the American Medical Association Division of Undergraduate Medical Education.

References

1. Politzer R, Harris D, Gaston M, Mullan F. Primary care physician supply and the medically underserved. *JAMA.* 1991;266:104-109.

2. Kindig D, Movassaghi H. The adequacy of physician supply in small rural counties. *Health Aff.* 1989;8:63-76.

3. Kindig D, Movassaghi H, Dunham N, Zwick D, Taylor C. Trends in physician availability in 10 urban areas from 1963 to 1980. *Inquiry.* 1987;24:136-146.

4. Cranford C. Linking medical education and training to rural America: the rural Arkansas AHEC program (1991) (testimony before the Special Senate Committee on Aging).

5. *The Health Education and Training Centers (HECT) of the National AHEC Program.* San Francisco: The California AHEC System; 1991.

6. Scofield J. *New and Expanded Medical Schools, Mid-Century to the 1980s.* San Francisco, Calif: Jossey-Bass Inc; 1984.

7. Medical schools in the United States. *JAMA.* 1991;266: 1007-1011. Appendix II.

8. *AAMC Data Book (January 1992).* Washington, DC: Association of American Medical Colleges; 1992.

9. McCloskey A, Luehrs J. *State Initiatives to Improve Rural Health Care.* Washington, DC: National Governors' Association; 1990.

List of primary health manpower shortage areas

Federal Register. 1990 June 29, 55(126): 27010-85 (published periodically in the *Federal Register*)

Summary

This notice provides two lists. The first is a list of all areas, population groups, or facilities designated as primary medical care health manpower shortage areas (HMSAs) as of December 31, 1989. Second is a list of previously designated primary medical care HMSAs that have been found to no longer meet the HMSA criteria and are therefore being withdrawn from the HMSA list. HMSAs are designated or withdrawn by the Secretary of Health and Human Services under the authority of section 332 of the Public Health Service Act.

Background information

Section 332 of the Public Health Service Act provides that the Secretary of Health and Human Services shall designate health manpower shortage areas based on criteria established by regulation. Health manpower shortage areas (HMSAs) are defined in section 332 to include (1) urban and rural geographic areas, (2) population groups, and (3) facilities with shortages of health manpower. Section 332 further requires that the Secretary publish a list of the designated geographic areas, population groups, and facilities. The list of areas is to be reviewed at least annually and revised as necessary. The Health Resources and Services Administration's Bureau of Health Care Delivery and Assistance has the responsibility for designating and updating these HMSAs.

Public or nonprofit entities in (or with a demonstrated interest in) these HMSAs are eligible to apply for assignment of National Health Service Corps (NHSC) personnel to provide health services in, or to, the areas or populations involved. These HMSAs are also eligible obligated-service areas for certain Public Health Service scholarship, loan repayment, and traineeship programs; entities located therein are eligible to apply for (or receive preference for) certain Public Health Service grant programs; physicians delivering services in nonmetropolitan HMSAs may be eligible for increased Medicare reimbursement; and nurse practitioners and physician's assistants serving Rural Health Clinics in HMSAs are eligible for Medicaid or Medicare reimbursement.

Resources

Marder WD. *Physician Supply and Utilization by Specialty: Trends and Projections.* Chicago, Ill: American Medical Association; 1988; 135 pp.
ISBN 0-89970-315-1   OP193788

Bureau of Health Care Delivery and Assistance
Office of Shortage Design
Parklawn Bldg, Rm 8-47
5600 Fishers Ln, Rockville, MD 20857
301 443-6932

Health Professions

Accredited by 13 agencies, 5000 educational programs for 41 professions are overseen. The organizations and the professions involved in this effort are the following:

Accreditation Council for Occupational Therapy Education (ACOTE)

American Art Therapy Association (AATA)

Commission on Accreditation of Allied Health Education Programs (CAAHEP)

Commission on Accreditation/Approval for Dietetics Education of the American Dietetic Association (CAADE)

Commission on Dental Accreditation of the American Dental Association (CDA)

Commission on Opticianry Accreditation (COA)

Council on Academic Accreditation in Audiology and Speech-Language Pathology (CAA)

Council on Accreditation of the National Recreation and Park Association (NRPA)

Council on Rehabilitation Education (CORE)

Joint Review Committee on Educational Programs in Nuclear Medicine Technology (JRCNMT)

Joint Review Committee on Education in Radiologic Technology (JRCERT)

National Accrediting Agency for Clinical Laboratory Sciences (NAACLS)

National Association for Schools of Music (NASM)

Includes the following fields:

Anesthesiologist Assistant

Art Therapist

Athletic Trainer

Audiologist

Cardiovascular Technologist

Clinical Laboratory Scientist/Medical Technologist

Clinical Lab Technician/Medical Lab Technician

Cytotechnologist

Dental Assistant

Dental Hygienist

Dental Laboratory Technician

Diagnostic Medical Sonographer

Dietetic Technician

Dietition/Nutritionist

Electroneurodiagnostic Technologist

Emergency Medical Technician—Paramedic

Health Information Administrator

Health Information Technician/Technologist

Histologic Technician/Technologist

Medical Assistant

Medical Illustrator

Music Therapist

Nuclear Medicine Technologist

Occupational Therapist

Occupational Therapy Assistant

Ophthalmic Dispensing Technician

Ophthalmic Laboratory Technician

Ophthalmic Medical Technician/Technologist

Orthotist/Prosthetist

Pathologists' Assistant

Perfusionist

Physician Assistant

Radiation Therapist

Radiographer

Rehabilitation Counselor

Respiratory Therapist

Respiratory Therapy Technician

Specialist in Blood Bank Technology

Speech-Language Pathologist

Surgical Technologist (AHRP-1997)

Resources

Health Professions Education Directory 1997-1998. 25th ed. Chicago, Ill: American Medical Association; 1997; 459 pp. ISBN 0-89970-834-X   OP417597

American Society of Allied Health Professions
1101 Connecticut Ave NW, Ste 700
Washington, DC 20036
202 857-1150

Health Services

Accrediting Commission on Education for Health Services Administration
1911 N Fort Myer Dr, Ste 503, Arlington, VA 22209
703 524-0511   Fax 703 525-4791
E-mail: accredcom@aol.com

US National Center for Health Services Research
5600 Fisher Ln, Rm 1812, Rockville, MD 20857
301 443-4100

Health System Agencies

Federation of American Health Systems
1405 N Pierce, #311, Little Rock, AR 72217-8708
501 661-9555   Fax 501 663-4903

Administrative Offices:
1405 N Pierce, #311, Little Rock, AR 72207
501 661-9555

Hearing Impaired

American Deafness and Rehabilitation Association
PO Box 251554, Little Rock, AR 72225
501 868-8850   Fax 501 868-8812
E-mail: adarahuie@aol.com

American Hearing Research Foundation
55 E Washington, Ste 2022, Chicago, IL 60602
312 726-9670   Fax 312 726-9695

American Speech-Language-Hearing Association
10801 Rockville Pike, Rockville, MD 20852
800 638-8255 (800 638-TALK) 301 897-5700
Fax 301 879-7348
E-mail: irc@asha.org

Captioned Films for the Deaf
800 237-6213

Deafness Research Foundation
9 E 38th St, 7th Fl, New York, NY 10016
800 535-3323   212 684-6556   Fax 212 779-2125

Gallaudet College (Deaf education)
800 Florida Ave NE, Washington, DC 20002
800 672-6720   202 651-5206   Fax 202 651-5458

International Hearing Dog Inc
5901 E 89th Ave, Henderson, CO 80640
303 287-3277   Fax 303 287-3425

National Captioning Institute
1900 Gallows Rd, Ste 3000, Vienna, VA 22182
703 917-7600   Fax 703 917-9878

International Hearing Society
20361 Middlebelt Rd, Livonia, MI 48152
800 521-5247   810 478-2610   Fax 810 478-4520

Occupational Hearing Service
PO Box 1880, Media, PA 19063
800 222-3277

SHHH (Self-Help for Hard of Hearing People, Inc)
c/o Carla Beyer,7910 Woodmont Ave, Ste 1200,
Bethesda, MD 20814
301 657-2248   Fax 301 913-9413
TDD (Telecommunication Device for the Deaf)
800 325-0778

TRIPOD (Information for families with deaf children)
c/o Barbara Lincoln, 2901 N Keystone St
Burbank, CA 91504
800 2-TRIPOD   818 972-2080   Fax 818 972-2090
E-mail: tripodla@aol.com

Heart Associations, Statewide

American Heart Association Alabama Affiliate
1449 Medical Park Dr, Birmingham, AL 35213
205 592-7100   Fax 205 592-0727

American Heart Association Alaska Affiliate
2330 E 42nd Ave, Anchorage, AK 99508
907 563-3111   Fax 907 563-5321

American Heart Association Arizona Affiliate
2929 S 48th St, Tempe, AZ 85282
602 414-5353   Fax 602 414-5355

American Heart Association Arkansas Affiliate
909 W 2nd St, Little Rock, AR 72201
501 375-9148   Fax 501 375-9066

American Heart Association
Greater Los Angeles Affiliate
3550 Wilshire Blvd, 5th Fl, Los Angeles, CA 90010
213 385-4231   Fax 213 386-4057

American Heart Association California Affiliate
1710 Gilbreth Rd, Burlingame, CA 94010
415 259-6700   Fax 415 259-6891

American Heart Association of Colorado
1280 S Parker Rd, Denver, CO 80231
303 369-5433   Fax 303 369-8087

American Heart Association Connecticut Affiliate
5 Brookside Dr, Wallingford, CT 06492
203 294-0088   Fax 203 297-3329

American Heart Association of Delaware
1096 Old Churchman's Rd, Newark, DE 19713
302 633-0200   Fax 302 633-3964

American Heart Association
Nation's Capitol Affiliate
5335 Wisconsin Ave NW, Ste 940
Washington, DC 20015
202 686-6888   Fax 202 686-6162

American Heart Association Florida Affiliate
1213 16th St N, St Petersburg, FL 33705-1092
813 894-7400   Fax 813 894-8561

American Heart Association Georgia Affiliate
1685 Terrell Mill Road, Marietta, GA 30067
404 952-1316   Fax 404 952-2208

American Heart Association Hawaii Affiliate
245 N Kukui St, Ste 204, Honolulu, HI 96817
808 538-7021   Fax 808 538-3443

American Heart Association Idaho/Montana Affiliate
270 S Orchard, Ste B, Boise, ID 83705
208 384-5066   Fax 208 336-5867

American Heart Association of Metropolitan Chicago
208 S LaSalle St, Ste 900
Chicago, IL 60604-1197
312 346-4675   312 346-7375

American Heart Association Illinois Affiliate
1181 N Dirksen Pkwy, Springfield, IL 62708
217 525-1350   Fax 217 525-6970

American Heart Association Indiana Affiliate
PO Box 681550, 8645 Guion Rd, Ste H
Indianapolis, IN 46268
317 876-4850   Fax 317 876-4859

American Heart Association Iowa Affiliate
1111 9th St, Ste 280, Des Moines, IA 50314
515 224-3278   Fax 515 244-5164

American Heart Association Kansas Affiliate
5375 SW 7th St, Topeka, KS 66606
913 272-7056   Fax 913 272-2425

American Heart Association Kentucky Affiliate
333 Guthrie St, Ste 207, Louisville, KY 40202
502 587-8641   Fax 502 585-7001

American Heart Association of Louisiana
105 Campus Dr E, Destrehan, LA 70047
504 764-8711   Fax 504 764-8712

American Heart Association Maine Affiliate
20 Winter St, Augusta, ME 04330
207 623-8432   Fax 207 626-3213

American Heart Association Maryland Affiliate
415 N Charles St, Baltimore, MD 21201-4441
410 685-7074   Fax 410 539-5049

American Heart Association Massachusetts Affiliate
20 Speen St, Framingham, MA 02194
508 620-1700   Fax 508 620-6137

American Heart Association of Michigan
16310 W 12 Mile Rd, Lathrup Village, MI 48076
810 557-9500   Fax 810 569-3353

American Heart Association Minnesota Affiliate
4701 W 77th St, Minneapolis, MN 55435
612 835-3300   Fax 612 835-5828

American Heart Association Mississippi Affiliate
4830 E McWillie Circle, Jackson, MS 39204
601 981-4721   Fax 601 981-7536

American Heart Association Missouri Affiliate
4643 Lindell Blvd, St Louis, MO 63108
314 367-3383   Fax 314 367-8605

American Heart Association Idaho/Montana Affiliate
270 S Orchard, Ste B, Boise, ID 83705
208 384-5066   Fax 208 336-5867

American Heart Association Nebraska Affiliate
3624 Farnam, Omaha, NE 68131
402 346-0771   Fax 402 346-1717

American Heart Association Nevada Affiliate
6370 W Flamingo, Ste 1, Las Vegas, NV 89103
702 367-1366   Fax 702 367-1975

American Heart Association New Hampshire Affiliate
309 Pine St, Manchester, NH 03103
603 669-5833   Fax 603 669-6745

American Heart Association New Jersey Affiliate
2550 Route 1, North Brunswick, NJ 08902
908 821-2610   Fax 908 821-2736

American Heart Association New Mexico Affiliate
1330 San Pedro NE, Ste 105
Albuquerque, NM 87110
505 268-3711   Fax 505 268-7680

American Heart Association New York City Affiliate
122 E 42nd St, 18th Fl, New York, NY 10168
212 661-5335   Fax 212 697-7232

American Heart Association New York State Affiliate
100 N Concourse, North Syracuse, NY 13212
315 454-8166   Fax 315 454-8778

American Heart Association North Carolina Affiliate
300 Silver Cedar Ct, Chapel Hill, NC 27515
919 968-4453   Fax 919 968-7229

American Heart Association Dakota Affiliate
1005 12th Ave SE, Jamestown, ND 58401-1287
701 252-5122   Fax 701 251-2092

American Heart Association Northeast Ohio Affiliate
1689 E 115th St, Cleveland, OH 44106
216 791-7500   Fax 216 791-5202

American Heart Association Ohio Affiliate
5455 N High St, Columbus, OH 43216
614 848-6676   Fax 614 848-4227

American Heart Association Oklahoma Affiliate
3545 NW 58th St, Ste 400C
Oklahoma City, OK 73112
405 942-2444   Fax 405 942-6616

American Heart Association Oregon Affiliate
1425 NE Irving, #100, Portland, OR 97232-4201
503 233-0100   Fax 503 233-4464

American Heart Association
Southeastern Pennsylvania Affiliate
625 W Ridge Pike Bldg A, Ste 100
Conshohocken, PA 19428
610 940-9540   Fax 610 940-9541

American Heart Association Pennsylvania Affiliate
Pennsboro Center, 1019 Mumma Rd
PO Box 8835, Camp Hill, PA 17011-8835
717 975-4800   Fax 717 975-5597

Puerto Rico Heart Association
Cabo Alverio 554, Hato Rey, PR 00918
809 751-6569   Fax 809 250-0281

American Heart Association Rhode Island Affiliate
40 Broad St, Pawtucket, RI 02860
401 728-5300   Fax 401 728-5376

American Heart Association South Carolina Affiliate
400 Percival Rd, Columbia, SC 29206
803 738-9540   Fax 803 787-0804

American Heart Association Tennessee Affiliate
1200 Division St, Ste 201
Nashville, TN 37203-4012
615 726-0108   Fax 615 242-9727

American Heart Association Texas Affiliate
1700 Rutherford Ln, Austin, TX 78754
512 836-7220   Fax 512 832-5880

American Heart Association Utah Affiliate
645 E 400 South, Salt Lake City, UT 84102
801 322-5601   Fax 801 364-6732

American Heart Association Vermont Affiliate
PO Box 485, 12 Hurricane Ln, Williston, VT 05495
802 878-7700   Fax 802 878-7850

American Heart Association Virginia Affiliate
4217 Park Place Ct, Glen Allen, VA 23060
804 747-8334   Fax 804 346-8567

American Heart Association Washington Affiliate
4414 Woodland Park Ave N, Seattle, WA 98103
206 632-6881   Fax 206 632-8478

American Heart Association West Virginia Affiliate
211 35th St SE, Charleston, WV 25304
304 346-5381   Fax 304 346-5560

American Heart Association Wisconsin Affiliate
795 N Van Buren St, Milwaukee, WI 53202
414 271-9999   Fax 414 271-3299

American Heart Association of Wyoming
200 W 17th St, Ste 10, Cheyenne, WY 82001
307 632-1746   Fax 307 634-7292

Heart Disease

American Heart Association
7320 Greenville Ave, Dallas, TX 75231
800 242-1793   214 373-6300   Fax 214 706-1341
Web address: http://www.amhrt.org

American College of Angiology
1044 Northern Blvd, Ste 103, Roslyn, NY 11576
516 484-6880   Fax 516 625-1174

American College of Cardiology
9111 Old Georgetown Rd
Bethesda, MD 20814-1699
800 253-4636   301 897-5400   Fax 301 897-9745

National Heart, Lung and Blood Institute
9000 Rockville Pike, Bethesda, MD 20892
301 496-4236
Web address: http://gopher.nhlbi.nih.gov

Board Certification in Cardiovascular Disease:
American Board of Internal Medicine
3624 Market St, Philadelphia, PA 19104
800 441-2246   215 243-1500   Fax 215 382-4702

Height-Weight Tables

For adults:
Metropolitan Life Insurance Co.
Attn: Health and Safety Education Dept—16W
1 Madison Ave, New York, NY 10010
212 578-2211

Heimlich Maneuver Poster

Card chart single copies free
Employers Insurance of Wausau
Wausau, WI 54402-8017
715 845-5211

Hematology

American Society of Hematology
1200 19th St NW, Ste 300
Washington, DC 20036-2412
202 857-1118   Fax 202 857-1164

Board Certification:
American Board of Internal Medicine
3624 Market St, Philadelphia, PA 19104
800 441-ABIM (800 441-2246)
215 243-1500   Fax 215 382-4702

American Board of Pathology
5401 W Kennedy Blvd, PO Box 25915
Tampa, FL 33622
813 286-2444   Fax 813 289-5279

Hemochromatosis

Hemochromatosis Foundation
PO Box 8569, Albany, NY 12208
518 489-0972   Fax 518 489-0227

Hemophilia

National Hemophilia Foundation
110 Green St, Ste 303, New York, NY 10012
212 219-8180   Fax 212 431-0906

Hippocrates (460?-377? BC)

The oath

I swear by Apollo the Physician, and Aesculapius, and health, and all-heal, and all the Gods and Goddesses, that, according to my ability and judgment, I will keep this oath and stipulation:

To reckon him who taught me this art equally dear to me as my parents, to share my substance with him, and relieve his necessities if required; to regard his offspring as on the same footing with my own brothers, and teach them this art, if they shall wish to learn it, without fee or stipulation; and that by precept, lecture, and every other mode of instruction, I will impart a knowledge of the Art to my own sons, and those of my teachers, and to disciples bound by a stipulation and oath according to the law of medicine, but to none others.

I will follow that method of treatment which, according to my ability and judgment, I consider for the benefit of my patients, and abstain from whatever is deleterious and mischievous. I will give no deadly medicine to any one if asked, nor suggest any such counsel; furthermore, I will not give to a woman an instrument to produce abortion.

With Purity and with Holiness I will pass my life and practice my Art. I will not cut a person who is suffering with a stone, but will leave this to be done by men who are practitioners of this work. Into whatever houses I enter I will go into them for the benefit of the sick and will abstain from every voluntary act of mischief and corruption; and further from the seduction of females or males, bond or free.

Whatever, in connexion with my professional practice, or not in connexion with it, I may see or hear in the lives of men which ought not to be spoken abroad I will not divulge, as reckoning that all such should be kept secret.

While I continue to keep this oath unviolated, may it be granted to me to enjoy life and the practice of the art, respected by all men at all times but should I trespass and violate this oath, may the reverse be my lot.

Histologic Technology

Occupational description

Physicians (usually pathologists) and other scientists specializing in biological sciences or related clinical areas such as chemistry work in partnership with medical laboratory workers to analyze blood, tissues, and fluids from humans (and sometimes animals), using a variety of precision instruments. The results of these tests are used to detect and diagnose disease and other abnormalities.

The main responsibility of the histologic technician/histotechnologist in the clinical laboratory is preparing sections of body tissue for examination by a pathologist. This includes the preparation of tissue specimens of human and animal origin for diagnostic, research, or teaching purposes. Tissue sections prepared by the histologic technician/technologist for a variety of disease entities enable the pathologist to diagnose body dysfunction and malignancy.

Job description

Histologic technicians process sections of body tissue by fixation, dehydration, embedding, sectioning, decalcification, microincineration, mounting, and routine and special staining. Histotechnologists perform all functions of the histotechnician, as well as the more complex procedures for processing tissues. They identify tissue structures, cell components, and their staining characteristics, and relate them to physiological functions; implement and test new techniques and procedures; make judgments concerning the results of quality control measures; and institute proper procedures to maintain accuracy and precision. Histotechnologists apply the principles of management and supervision when they function as section supervisors and of educational methodology when they teach students.

Employment characteristics

Most histologic technicians/histotechnologists work in hospital laboratories, averaging a 40-hour week.

Based upon a 1994 survey by the American Society of Clinical Pathologists' Board of Registry, the median entry-level salary for histologic technicians was $20,800, the median entry-level salary for histotechnologists was $24,752, and the supervisor entry-level salary was $29,099. (AHRP-1997)

Resource

AMA Department of Allied Health
312 553-9355

National Society for Histotechnology
4201 Northview Dr, Ste 502
Bowie, MD 20716-9188
301 262-6221   301 262-9188
Web address: http://www.mwrn.com/nsh

History of Medicine

Bibliography of the History of Medicine. Bethesda, Md: National Library of Medicine. Annual: series begun 1965. ISSN 0067-7280 For sale by the GPO.

The *Bibliography of the History of Medicine* focuses on the history of medicine and its related sciences, professional associations, and institutions. The general history and philosophy of science have been admitted only sparingly. All chronological periods and geographic areas are covered. Journal articles, monographs, and analytical entries for symposia, congresses, and similar composite publications, as well as historical chapters in general monographs, are included. (BIB-1992)

Resource

American Association for the History of Medicine
Arthur J. Viseltear, PhD, Yale School of Medicine
333 Cedar St, New Haven, CT 06510
203 785-4338

HIV

AMA Policy

AMA HIV Policy Update H-20.966 (BOT Rep X, I-89; Reaffirmed: BOT Rep I-93-34)

The AMA: National Policy (1) supports continuing its recommendation for, and pledges its support to, a national commission on HIV. Such a Commission, modeled after the commission which made recommendations on the problems of Social Security financing in the early 1980s, should be constituted with representatives from the Executive Branch of the federal government, the Congress, state and local governments, and the private sector and directed to develop a consensus position for consideration by the Congress, the Executive Branch, state and local governments, and private associations and institutions;

Media (2a) supports being a catalyst to bring the communications industry together. Government officials and the health care communities should design and direct efforts for more effective and better targeted messages, especially for those persons at increased risk of infection; (2b) continues to encourage public service announcements on abstinence, condom usage, and safer sex, and encourages specifically targeted messages. Among the audiences that should receive focused messages in an appropriate language and style are intravenous drug users and their sexual partners and minority groups such as blacks and Hispanics; (2c) continues to encourage federal, state, and local governments to allocate funds for HIV education programs presented through the various public media;

Prevalence and Incidence Study (3a) encourages and advocates for an anonymous, representative, cross-sectional study to determine the degree of HIV infection in the US population as a whole, as well as in groups of special interest such as adolescents and minorities. The study should be repeated at appropriate intervals; (3b) supports offering to assist the CDC in the design and implementation of these studies; (3c) encourages public and private sector prevention and care efforts that are proportionate to the best available statistics on HIV incidence and prevalence rates; (3d) continues support for a national health survey which should incorporate a representative sample of the US population of all ages (including adolescents) and should include questions on sexual orientation and sexual behavior (CSA Rep. 8 - I-94);

Financing Care (4) supports incorporating into CMS's continuing study consideration of the estimated cost of care in each stage of HIV infection, and on the estimated number of persons in each stage of HIV disease now and through the next five years;

Funding (5a) continues to support adequate public and private funding for all aspects of this epidemic, including research, education, and patient care for the full spectrum of the disease; (5b) supports increased funding for reimbursement and other incentives to encourage expanded availability of alternatives to inpatient care of persons with HIV disease, including intermediate care facilities, skilled nursing facilities, home care, residential hospice, home hospice, and other support systems;

Education for Health Care Professionals (6a) supports continued efforts to work with other physician organizations, public health officials, universities, and others to assure (1) an easily accessible method of receiving the most current authoritative information on HIV; (2) readily available training in HIV counseling and education; (3) identification of effective ways to change those behaviors that place a person at risk of HIV infection; (4) a review of methods other than education and counseling that might be effective in preventing the spread of HIV; and (5) special attention to reducing the spread of HIV among intravenous drug users; (6b) recognizing that it is unlikely that the care of HIV-infected persons will be provided entirely by specialists and referral centers, supports publishing information and offering training to encourage large numbers of physicians and other health care workers to become involved in the care of HIV-infected patients; (6c) encourages and assists physicians to provide HIV prevention information to their patients and, when the opportunity arises, to the public and supports providing educational efforts targeted to persons at increased risk of HIV infection; (6d) continues to emphasize the importance of providing information and training to physicians, medical societies, and auxiliaries so that they can create and implement programs of prevention and treatment; (6e) encourages physicians to provide accurate, current information to the public and to help determine local and national policy on HIV. Public statements on HIV disease, including efficacy of experimental therapies, should be based only on current scientific and medical studies;

Medical Student and Residency Training (7a) supports collaborating in a survey of medical schools and residency programs to review and report on HIV programs and policies; (7b) strongly supports indemnification of medical students and resident physicians infected with HIV as a result of contact with assigned patients. The AMA supports examining the possible mechanisms to achieve the intent of this recommendation, realizing that the issues for medical students and resident physicians differ.

Collaboration, Research, Education (8a) supports continued collaboration with other concerned professional groups to provide prevention and treatment information to physicians and other health professionals and to encourage physicians and other health care professionals to educate the public on methods of prevention; (8b) continues to encourage that research on HIV be prioritized, funded, and implemented in the speediest fashion consistent with appropriate scientific rigor, and that the results of research form the basis for future programs of prevention and treatment; (8c) continues to review risk factors for hospitals, medical staffs, and health workers who care for HIV-infected patients; (8d) in coordination with appropriate medical specialty societies, supports addressing the special issues of heterosexual HIV infection, the role of intravenous drugs and HIV infection in women, and initiatives to prevent the spread of HIV infection through prostitutes; (8e) supports reviewing and reporting on progress in the use of AZT and other drugs to inhibit HIV infection generally, to prevent HIV infection from a mother to her newborn infant, and to reduce symptom expression in HIV-infected persons; (8f) supports consulting with appropriate federal agencies and

drug manufacturers to encourage the expansion of the availability of drugs with demonstrated effectiveness for any stage of HIV disease;

Physician Ethical Responsibilities (9) believes that a physician may not ethically refuse to treat a patient whose condition is within the physician's current realm of competence solely because the patient is HIV seropositive. Persons who are seropositive should not be subjected to discrimination based on fear or prejudice. Physicians who are unable to provide the services required by HIV-infected patients should make referrals to those physicians or facilities equipped to provide such services. It is in the best interest of the patient for the physician to focus on treatment of the disease, rather than on making value judgments about how the disease was contracted (CEJA);

Sexual and Drug History (10a) encourages physicians to take a sexual and substance abuse history, sufficient to identify the usual modes of HIV transmission, on every adolescent and adult patient, with a more comprehensive history taken when warranted; (10b) encourages and provides continuing physician education and training on techniques related to nonjudgmental history taking of sexual practices and drug use;

Blood Donations and Transfusions (11a) supports working with blood banking organizations to educate prospective donors about the safety of blood donation and blood transfusion; (11b) supports providing educational information to physicians on alternatives to transfusion; (11c) continues to encourage physicians to inform high-risk patients of the value of self-deferral from blood and blood product donations;

Health Care Settings (12a) supports regularly reviewing and publishing commentary on infection control guidelines for medical settings; (12b) continues to endorse and recommend adherence to the CDC guidelines for infection control; (12c) encourages institutions to develop recommendations to suit specific procedures and situations which may not be covered by currently published guidelines; (12d) supports addressing home care and the training of nonprofessional home care givers, with special attention to infection control; (12e) encourages immediate publication of peer-reviewed reports of any case of HIV transmission from skin or mucous membrane exposure, and any case of a health care worker with occupation-related HIV infection; (12f) encourages employers of health care workers to provide, at the employer's expense, serologic testing for HIV infection to all health care workers who have documented occupational exposure to HIV; (12g) supports helping provide physicians with an awareness of the role that can be played in patient care by self-help and support groups for those who are HIV positive; (12h) supports using its resources in cooperation with other health organizations and agencies to facilitate the distribution of information on drug therapies available for HIV disease;

HIV-Infected health care workers (13a) encourages health care workers who perform invasive procedures to voluntarily determine their serostatus and/or to act as if their serostatus were positive; (13b) encourages an infected health care worker who performs invasive medical procedures as part of his/her duties to request that an ad hoc committee be constituted to consider which activities can continue to be engaged in without an identifiable risk of infection to patients. Membership of this committee may be composed of, but not necessarily limited to, an infectious disease specialist familiar with HIV transmission risks, the pertinent hospital department chairperson, a hospital administrator, the infected health care worker's personal physician, and the infected health care worker; (13c) encourages that a confidential review system be established by the ad hoc committee to monitor the health care worker's fitness to engage in invasive health care activities. Any restrictions or modifications to health care activities for patient safety should be determined by the ad hoc committee based on current medical and scientific information; (13d) encourages that knowledge of the health care worker's status be restricted to those few professionals who have a medical need to know the status. Except for those with a need to know, all information on the serostatus of the health care worker must be held in the strictest confidence; (13e) encourages that, as a general rule and consistent with current scientific information, the infected health care worker be permitted to provide services as long as there is no identifiable risk of patient infection and no compromise in the physical or mental ability of the worker to perform the required health care procedures; (13f) encourages that, where restrictions, limitations, or changes in health care activities are recommended, the ad hoc committee do its utmost to assist the health care worker to obtain financial and social support for these changes. Consideration should be given to adapting programs for impaired health care workers to serve those who are HIV infected; (13g) encourages that, if intra-institutional confidentiality cannot be assured, health care facilities make arrangements with other organizations, such as local or state medical societies, to serve the functions of the ad hoc committee. Health care workers not affiliated with a hospital may also use this procedure to form an ad hoc committee; (13h) believes that, since there are a variety of disability insurance coverages available and a diversity of practice modes among health care workers, each health professional should individually assess his or her risk of infection and that of his or her employees and select disability coverage accordingly.

Encouraging School HIV Education (14a) commends school administrations, boards of education, teachers, health educators, and all others who have helped implement HIV curricula in school systems. This effort needs to continue. Appropriate means must be found to provide HIV education for those who are not currently receiving such education through the school system, including individualized educational materials; (14b) endorses and supports the education of elementary, secondary, and college students regarding the modes of HIV transmission and prevention; (14c) supports efforts to obtain adequate funding from local, state, and national sources for the immediate development and implementation of HIV educational programs as part of comprehensive health education in the schools; (14d) encourages the development of language- and culture-specific HIV educational materials to inform minorities of risk behaviors associated with HIV infection; (14e) encourages religious organizations and social service organizations to implement HIV education programs for those they serve;

School Children with AIDS (15a) supports day-care, preschool, and school attendance of HIV-infected children; (15b) encourages the physician responsible for care of an infected child in a day-care, preschool, or school setting to receive information from the school on other infectious diseases in the environment and temporarily remove the HIV-infected child from a setting that might pose a threat to his/her health; (15c) encourages that HIV-infected children who are adopted or placed in a foster-care setting have access to special health care benefits to encourage adoption or foster-care;

Education about Condoms (16a) continues to endorse the use of condoms as one useful measure to help contain the spread of HIV; (16b) supports cooperating with the public health community, government agencies, and the media to develop standards for public service announcements on condoms related to sexually transmitted diseases including HIV; (16c) encourages the production of condom education materials that meet standards of accuracy, completeness, social appropriateness, clarity, and simplicity; (16d) in cooperation with state, county, and specialty medical societies, encourages physicians to educate their patients about the role of condom use in reducing the risk of sexually transmitted diseases, including HIV disease. While such counseling may not be appropriate for all patients, physicians should be encouraged to provide this information to any patient who may benefit from being more aware of the risks of sexually transmitted diseases; (16e) in collaboration with appropriate specialty medical societies, supports exploring with condom manufacturers the development of a condom-education kit to train physicians to educate patients on condom use (Reaffirmed by CSA Rep. 3, A-95);

HIV Testing Availability (17a) continues to recommend that HIV testing be readily available to all who wish to be tested, including having available sites for confidential testing; (17b) encourages persons who suspect that they have been exposed to HIV to be tested so that appropriate treatment and counseling can begin for those who are seropositive; (17c) encourages physicians and laboratories to review their procedures to assure that HIV testing conforms to standards that will produce the highest level of accuracy; (17d) supports considering an award recognition program for physicians who donate a portion of their professional time to testing and counseling those patients who could not otherwise afford services;

Testing Procedures (18a) recommends that appropriate medical organizations establish rigorous proficiency testing and quality control procedures for testing laboratories on a frequent and regular basis; (18b) recommends that appropriate medical organizations establish a standard that a second blood sample be taken and tested on all persons found to be positive or indeterminate for HIV antibodies on the first blood sample. This practice is also advised for any unexpected negative result; (18c) recommends that appropriate medical organizations establish a policy that results from a single unconfirmed positive ELISA test never be reported to the patient as a valid indication of infection; (18d) recommends that appropriate medical organizations establish a policy that laboratories specify the tests performed and the criteria used for positive, negative, and indeterminate Western blots or other confirmatory procedures; (18e) recommends that

H training for HIV blood test counselors encourage patients with an indeterminate Western blot to be advised that three- to six-month follow-up specimens may be needed to resolve their status. Because of the uncertain status of their contagiousness, it is prudent to counsel such patients as though they were seropositive until such time as the findings can be resolved;

Mandatory HIV Testing (19a) supports mandatory HIV testing of donors of blood and blood fractions, and breast milk; organs and other tissues intended for transplantation; semen or ova for artificial conception; immigrants to the United States; and military personnel; (19b) supports reviewing its policy on mandatory testing periodically to incorporate information from studies of the unintended consequences or unexpected benefits of HIV testing in special settings;

Mandatory Testing of Prisoners (20a) continues to recommend that testing be mandatory for inmates in federal and state prisons; (20b) continues to encourage the inclusion of HIV-prevention information as a regular part of correctional staff and inmate education; (20c) continues to encourage physicians who practice in correctional institutions to evaluate all tuberculin-positive inmates for HIV infection and all HIV-positive patients for tuberculosis, since HIV status may affect subsequent management of tuberculosis infection or disease and tuberculosis may accompany HIV infection;

Voluntary Testing (21a) continues to strongly support the provision of voluntary HIV testing with informed consent for individuals who may have come into contact with the blood, semen, or vaginal secretions of an infected person in a manner that has been shown to transmit HIV infection; (21b) continues to support voluntary HIV testing with counseling for patients whose care may benefit from this information. Voluntary testing should be encouraged for patients, especially those requiring surgical or other invasive procedures, for whom the physician's knowledge of the patient's serostatus would improve treatment. The prevalence of HIV infection in the community should be considered in determining the likelihood of infection. If voluntary HIV testing is not sufficiently accepted, the hospital and medical staff may consider requiring HIV testing;

Neonates (22a) continues to urge the U.S. Public Health Service to develop confirmatory tests and procedures for HIV infection in newborns; (22b) continues to support voluntary, routine HIV antibody testing of the newborn in areas with a high prevalence of HIV infection, and that confidentiality of test results be strictly observed; (22c) supports mandatory HIV testing of all newborns in high prevalence areas when treatment modalities with proven benefits for infected neonates are available; (22d) continues to recommend that, where safe and alternative nutrition is widely available, HIV seropositive women should be counseled not to breast feed and not to donate breast milk. HIV testing of all human milk donors should be mandatory, and milk from HIV-infected donors should not be used for human consumption;

Counseling Considerations (23) supports promoting the standards that (a) appropriate pretest and posttest voluntary counseling be considered an integral and essential component of HIV testing and (b) appropriate posttest counseling be an integral component of diagnostic HIV testing;

HIV Test Consent (24a) supports the standard that individuals should knowingly and willingly give consent before a voluntary test is conducted, in a manner that is the least burdensome to the individual and to those administering the test; (24b) supports the development of hospital medical staff guidelines to allow HIV testing of a patient at the physician's discretion without prior consent in cases of puncture injury or mucosal contact of health caregivers by potentially infected fluids;

Discrimination Laws (25a) condemns any act, and opposes any legislation of categorical discrimination based on someone's actual or imagined disease, including HIV infection; this includes Congressional mandates calling for the discharge of otherwise qualified individuals from the armed services solely because of their HIV seropositivity (Modified by Sub. Res. 401, I-96); (25b) encourages vigorous enforcement of existing antidiscrimination statutes; incorporation of HIV in future federal legislation that addresses discrimination; and enactment and enforcement of state and local laws, ordinances, and regulations to penalize those who illegally discriminate against persons based on disease; (25c) encourages medical staff to work closely with hospital administration and governing bodies to establish appropriate policies regarding HIV-positive patients;

Confidentiality Laws (26a) supports uniform protection, at all levels of government, of the identity of those with HIV disease, except where the public health requires otherwise. The AMA has drafted model state legislation on confidentiality; (26b) encourages that patients receive general information on the limits of confidentiality of medical records on the initial physician visit. Specific information on the limits of confidentiality of HIV testing and results should be given when the disclosure of HIV results to the physician is imminent or when the physician counsels patients about taking the HIV test; (26c) endorses policy to enable physicians to confidentially discuss a patient's serostatus with other health care providers involved in the patient's care without fear of legal sanctions. Medical societies should be encouraged to support changes in laws that interfere with such an exchange;

Contact Tracing and Partner Notification (27a) strongly recommends that a system for contact-tracing and partner notification for unsuspecting sexual or needle-sharing partners who might have been HIV-infected should be established in each community; (27b) requests that states make provisions in any contact-tracing and notification program for adequate safeguards to protect the confidentiality of seropositive persons and their contacts, for counseling of the parties involved, and for the provision of information on counseling, testing, and treatment resources for partners who might be infected; (27c) in collaboration with state medical societies, supports legislation on the physician's right to exercise ethical and clinical judgment regarding whether or not to warn unsuspecting and endangered sexual or needle-sharing partners; (27d) promulgates the standard that a physician attempt to persuade an HIV-infected patient to cease all activities which endanger unsuspecting others and to inform those whom he/she might have infected. If such persuasion fails, the physician should pursue notification through means other than by reliance on the patient, such as by the Public Health Department or by the physician directly; (27e) strongly recommends the reportability of HIV seropositive patients to the Departments of Health of the 50 states for the purposes of contact-tracing and partner notification;

Sanctions for Willfully Infecting Others (28) requests that states provide sanctions for an infected individual who knowingly and willingly risks infecting an unsuspecting person when that person subsequently discovers his/her risk and makes a complaint to the authorities. Preemptive sanctions are not being endorsed by this recommendation;

Drug Abuse (29a) encourages federal and state agencies to determine the number and demographic characteristics of intravenous drug users, and the characteristics and conditions under which intravenous drug equipment is shared; (29b) urges federal, state, and local governments to increase funding for research and treatment of intravenous drug users; (29c) calls for removal of any federal and state regulations which are based on incomplete or inaccurate scientific and medical data that restrict or inhibit methadone maintenance treatment; (29d) encourages the availability of methadone maintenance for persons addicted to opioids; (29e) encourages the development of health education outreach programs for sexual partners of intravenous drug users; (29f) advocates continued attention to HIV risk reduction for adolescent drug users, including those with special needs such as the homeless, runaways, and detained adolescents;

FDA (30a) encourages continued FDA review of ways to improve drug trials and the associated drug approval processing; (30b) encourages the FDA to continue to expedite evaluations of available drugs used in the treatment of HIV disease;

Research Animals (31) supports exploring ways to bring to the attention of the public the positive contributions of animal studies on advances in HIV disease;

State and Local Cooperation (32a) encourages each state health department to involve local health departments in planning the delivery of HIV testing, counseling, and prevention campaigns. State and local health department systems, in cooperation with all other concerned organizations, are the appropriate mechanisms for determining whether HIV infection will be designated a sexually transmitted or communicable disease in that state; (32b) encourages each state health department to involve state and local medical societies in the planning and delivery of all aspects of the state's HIV prevention and service efforts;

International (33a) supports joining with other international medical, professional, and health organizations to develop worldwide strategies for cooperation in prevention and care of HIV disease; and (33b) encourages worldwide projection of the number of HIV cases expected in the next 5 to 10 years.

What is the distinction between AIDS and HIV?

AIDS, the acquired immunodeficiency syndrome, was originally defined by the US Centers for Disease Control and Prevention (CDC) as a disease, at least moderately predictive of a defect in cell-mediated immunity, occurring in a person with no known cause for diminished resistance to that disease. Kaposi sarcoma (KS) and *Pneumocystis carinii* pneumonia (PCP) were the most frequently recognized clinical manifestations of the immunodeficiency syndrome.

It is now known that the syndrome AIDS is simply the end-stage manifestation of a prolonged, chronic erosion of the immune system caused by the human immunodeficiency virus (HIV). The clinical manifestations of disease in any given individual are largely due to a reactivation and/or uncontrolled proliferation of microorganisms or neoplasms that are normally held in check by the intact human immune system.

Two related but distinct types of HIV have been isolated and characterized, HIV-1 and HIV-2. All but a few of the HIV infections in the United States are HIV-1. At present HIV-2 is largely confined to Western Africa. The clinical disease associated with HIV-1 is well recognized. However, the clinical spectrum of disease associated with HIV-2 remains to be clarified.

The original syndrome-defined categorization of AIDS was a brilliantly effective epidemiological tool: by 1985 the major modes of transmission had been elucidated and the etiologic retrovirus HIV had been isolated and characterized. Over the ensuing years the relationship between HIV infection and AIDS has become clear. In 1987, the CDC published a revised definition of AIDS and the current definition is evolving. AIDS is an aggregate of preterminal manifestations of a predictable, progressive loss of immune competence caused by HIV. In the remainder of this essay the outdated syndrome-defined term AIDS will not be used; the omission is intentional. Instead, the term "late-stage HIV infection" will be used to emphasize the concept that HIV causes a spectrum of disease.

Optimal medical management of HIV infection, as with all medical conditions, requires two fundamental steps. First, an accurate diagnosis must be established, and second, the extent of target organ damage must be precisely measured. Armed with this information, the knowledgeable physician can offer improvements in the quality and duration of life to his or her HIV-infected patient. Although HIV disease is not (at present) curable, it is most certainly treatable. (HIV-1989)

HIV prevention in primary care: overcoming the obstacles

Physicians are an important source of information about medical and health issues. Studies further show that patients want to talk about their sexual concerns with their physicians. As well, parents frequently mention concerns about how to discuss HIV with their children and adolescents, and may ask physicians for information about what to teach them. Since most people see a physician about three times a year, primary care physicians are uniquely positioned to help patients identify risks and to support them in changing their behavior to reduce or eliminate risk of HIV infection.

It can be difficult for physicians to know when a prevention intervention is appropriate. While some physicians offer routine HIV prevention services to their patients, most do not. HIV prevention opportunities are more obvious when patients present for treatment of sexually transmissible diseases, or for family planning, or with other sex-related health concerns. Other prevention opportunities may be missed because physicians assume their patients are not at high risk for HIV infection or that patients would raise concerns about personal risks if they had concerns. Identifying patients at risk can often only be accomplished by *asking* patients about their sexual and injecting drug use behaviors.

Discussions about sex can cause discomfort for patients and physicians. Developing ease of communication about sexual issues and about concerns of gay men and of people who inject or otherwise use drugs can facilitate effective communication. Ease of communication is important, because without evincing a particular moral, philosophical, or religious position, physicians' verbal and nonverbal messages can have a chilling effect on patients' willingness to share information about personal experiences. By expressing acceptance of patients while challenging unaddressed risk taking, physicians can show an appreciation for the complexity of decision making in behavior change.

Interventions related to sexual behavior and injecting drug use can be time consuming. Considering today's demands on physicians, prevention efforts must be intentional and systematic, if they are to occur. Prevention should be ongoing, because repeated prevention efforts tend to have a cumulative effect. Ultimately, individuals are responsible for their own behavior, and physicians, like anyone else, can only assist them to a point. Developing synergies with public and community-based organizations can help physicians confidently refer patients who need further education or counseling. Referral can also help patients maximize their chances for successful risk reduction while creating more time for primary care physicians to focus on other health concerns.

Patients at risk . . .
Incidence of AIDS is six times higher among *African-Americans* and three times higher among *Latinos* than among *whites.*

More than 50% of all AIDS cases in the United States have occurred among *gay men* and among other *men who have sex with men.*

Eighteen percent of all AIDS cases reported in the United States during 1994 and 1995 occurred among *women.*

References

1. Centers for Disease Control and Prevention. U.S. HIV and AIDS cases reported through December 1995. *HIV/AIDS Surveillance Report.* 1995;7 [inclusive page numbers].

2. Rabin DL, Boekeloo BO, Marx ES, Bowman MA, Russell NK, Willis AG. Improving office-based physicians' practices for sexually transmitted diseases. *Ann Intern Med.* 1994;121:513-519.

3. Gabel LL, Crane R, Ostrow DG. HIV-related disease: family physicians' multiple opportunities for preventive intervention. *J Am Board Fam Pract.* 1994;7:218-224.

4. Makadon HJ, Silin JG. Prevention of HIV infection in primary care: current practices, future possibilities. *Ann Intern Med.* 1995;123:715-719.

5. Gerbert B, MaGuire BT, Coates TJ. Are patients talking to their physicians about AIDS? *Am J Publ Health.* 1990;80:467-468.

6. Rawitscher LA, Saitz R, Friedman LS. Adolescents' preferences regarding human immunodeficiency virus (HIV)-related physician counseling and HIV testing. *Pediatrics.* 1995;96:52-58.

7. The Henry J. Kaiser Family Foundation. *The Kaiser Survey on Americans and AIDS/HIV: Questionnaire and National Toplines.* March 1996.

8. Adams PF, Benson V. Current estimates from the National Health Interview Survey, 1990. *Vital Health Stat.* 1991;10:1-212.

9. Cohen SJ, Halvorson HW, Gosselink CA. Changing physician behavior to improve disease prevention. *Prev Med.* 1994;23:284-291.

10. Gemson DH, Colombotos J, Elinson J, Fordyce EJ, Hynes M, Stoneburner R. Acquired immunodeficiency syndrome prevention: knowledge, attitudes, and practices of primary care physicians. *Arch Intern Med.* 1991;151:1102-1108.

11. Fredman L, Rabin DL, Bowman M, et al. Primary care physicians' assessment and prevention of HIV infection. *Am J Prev Med.* 1989;5:188-195.

12. Patton C. *Fatal Advice: How Safe-Sex Education Went Wrong.* Durham, NC: Duke University Press; 1996.

13. Council on Scientific Affairs, American Medical Association. Health care needs of gay men and lesbians in the United States. *JAMA.*1996;275:1354-1359.

14. Thompson RS, Taplin SH, McAfee TA, Mandelson MT, Smith AE. Primary and secondary prevention services in clinical practice. *JAMA.* 1995;273:1130-1135.

15. Kottke TE, Brekke ML, Solberg LI. Making "time" for preventive services. *Mayo Clin Proc.* 1993;68:785-791.

16. Centers for Disease Control and Prevention. *HIV Counseling, Testing and Referral: Standards and Guidelines.* May 1994. (PHIV-1996)

Holistic Medicine

A form of therapy aimed at treating the whole person—body and mind—not just the part or parts in which symptoms occur. A holistic approach is claimed to be emphasized by practitioners of alternative medicine, such as homeopathists, acupuncturists, and herbalists. (ENC-1989)

Resource
American Holistic Medical Association
4101 Lake Boone Trail, Ste 201
Raleigh, NC 27607
919 787-5146   Fax 919 787-4916
Web address: http://www.doubleclicked.com/about_ahma.html

Home Births
Informed Homebirth/Informed Birth and Parenting
PO Box 3675, Ann Arbor, MI 48106
313 662-6857

Position on Homebirth:
American College of Obstetricians and Gynecologists
409 12th St SW, Washington, DC 20024
202 638-5577   Fax 202 484-8107

Home Health Care

AMA Policy

On-Site Physician Home Health Care (H-210.981) CSA Rep 9, I-96

The AMA:

(1) recognizes that timely access to physician care for the frail, chronically ill, or disabled patient is a goal that can only be met by an increase in physician house calls to this vulnerable, underserved population.

(2) strongly supports the role of interdisciplinary teams in providing direct care in the patient's own home, but recognizes that physician oversight of that care from a distance must sometimes be supplemented by on-site physician care through house calls.

(3) recognizes the value of the house call in establishing and enhancing the physician-patient and physician-family relationship and rapport, in assessing the effects of the social, functional, and physical environment on the patient's illness, and in incorporating the knowledge gained into subsequent health care decisions.

(4) believes that physician on-site care through house calls is important when there is a change in condition that cannot be diagnosed over the telephone with the assistance of allied health personnel in the home and assisted transportation to the physician's office is costly, difficult to arrange, or excessively tiring and painful for the patient.

(5) recognizes the importance of improving communication systems to integrate the activities of the disparate health professionals delivering home care to the same patient. Frequent and comprehensive communication between all team members is crucial to quality care, must be part of every care plan, and can occur via telephone, FAX, e-mail, videotelemedicine, and in person.

(6) recognizes the importance of removing economic, institutional, and regulatory barriers to physician house calls.

(7) supports the requirement for a medical director for all home health agencies, comparable to the statutory requirements for medical directors for nursing homes and hospice.

(8) recommends that all specialty societies address the effect of dehospitalization on the patients that they care for and examine how their specialty is preparing its residents in-training to provide quality care in the home.

(9) encourages appropriate specialty societies to continue to develop educational programs for practicing physicians interested in expanding their involvement in home care.

A Piece of My Mind

House calls

Ronald F. Galloway
JAMA 1991 Aug 14; 266(6): 786

The first time I saw him, Mr. Henry was standing in front of a mirror, his back to the door of his hospital room, tinkering with his electric razor and fixing to shave. I called his name; he turned, put down his razor, smiled, and reached out to grasp my hand. He was tall, skinny as a rail, a bit stoop-shouldered, but he moved about pretty spryly.

As a thoracic surgeon, I had been asked to see Mr. Henry regarding a possible resection for a lemon-sized tumor in his left lung. He was 80 years old at the time. I had already seen his chest film and reviewed his chart and was, I admit, trying to think of a gentle way to explain to him that, at his age, he would not likely do well after major chest surgery. My preconceived notion was reinforced by the fact that he had been admitted with a proved diagnosis of carcinoma of the prostate. However, his smile and his firm handshake cut through that preconception, so I explained to him all the ifs, ands, and buts of a pulmonary lobectomy and informed him that his attending urologist planned a total orchiectomy at the same sitting. At the end of my detailed talk I paused and asked for questions. He had only one: "When do we do this?" I told him. He smiled again and said, "I'm ready."

Mr. Henry tolerated both surgical procedures well, had no complications, and soon went home. At his follow-up visit at my office a few weeks later, I learned that his wife's health was poor, that he didn't drive a car especially well, and that his coming to my office for checkups was difficult at best. So, I told him that on occasion I drive to the South Carolina coast and that his town was on the way. I offered to stop by to visit him from time to time. He seemed surprised but obviously appreciative that I would volunteer to do this.

Some weeks later I drove through that small town, followed his directions to its outskirts, and found the house trailer on concrete blocks that Mr. and Mrs. Henry called home. The yard was well kept, a small, neat garden decorated one corner. I hadn't called for an "appointment" but had presumed that his wife's poor health kept Mr. Henry close to home. I knocked on the door and was greeted by Mr. Henry with a smile as big as all outdoors and his special warm handshake. I examined him, noted that he was doing quite well, and spent a while just visiting with them both. As I left, felt absolutely wonderful.

I've returned to the Henrys' several times since that first encounter. They seemed to enjoy my visits, and each trip has been an unqualified blessing for me.

It has occurred to me that I could, if I wished, file a claim with Medicare for reimbursement for these 72-mile (144 miles round-trip) "house calls." But, the thought of the hassle the Medicare people would give me and the probability that they wouldn't believe I made the 72-mile house calls in the first place have deterred me. Then, too, the frozen boiled peanuts Mr. Henry gave me on one trip, the tomatoes he promised me this summer, the pride he takes in showing me his garden, the look in his eyes when I appear at his door, and my personal "hands-on" knowledge that he continues to do well are worth far more than any amount I might be able to argue out of Medicare.

And there's no deductible to meet.

Article of Note: Guidelines for the medical management of the home-care patient

Arch Fam Med 1993 Feb; 1993(2): 194-206

Abstract: Increasing numbers of patients of all ages are receiving needed health care services in noninstitutional settings. Acute, subacute, rehabilitative, preventive, long-term, and hospice services are provided in the home under the physician's supervision. The safe and appropriate treatment of these patients involves the physician in a team effort as most home care is provided by nurses, other allied health professionals, and family members. The guidelines cover such areas as the role of the physician; the physician-patient relationship; the elements of medical management in home care, including the evaluation assessment process, the selection of the interdisciplinary team, and the development of the care plan; patient's rights and responsibilities; the coordination of care; and the use of community resources.

JAMA Article of Note: Educating physicians in home health care. Council on Scientific Affairs and Council on Medical Education. [corrected] [published erratum appears in *JAMA* 1991 May 8;265(18):2340]

JAMA. 1991 Feb 13; 265(6): 769-71

Abstract: A growing proportion of health care, especially long-term care, should best and most appropriately be provided in the home setting. Physicians have largely remained on the periphery of this reemerging area of health care. Yet if home health care is to reach its full potential, physicians must fulfill their essential role as members of the home health team. Direct physician input and participation are needed to ensure that home health care is safe and medically appropriate. Physician involvement will enhance the supervision of medical care in the home, and physicians' expertise is also much needed for home health care quality assurance and clinical research. Role models and training experiences must be developed for new physicians so that they can integrate home health care skills and values into their future practices. Although most of the usual physician objections to home health care involvement can be addressed by education, the problem of inadequate reimbursement is substantive and must be addressed by policy change.

Resources

American Federation of Home Health Agencies
1320 Fenwick Lane, Ste 100, Silver Spring, MD 20910
301 588-1454   Fax 301 588-4732

Joint Commission on Accreditation of
Healthcare Organizations, Home Care Project
1 Renaissance Blvd, Oakbrook Terrace, IL 60181
630 792-5000   Fax 630 792-5001
Web address: http://www.jcaho.org

National Association for Home Care
519 C St NE, Stanton Park, Washington, DC 20002
202 547-7424   Fax 202 547-3540

National Association of Professional
Geriatric Care Managers
1604 N Country Club Rd, Tucson, AZ 85716
520 881-8008   Fax 520 325-7925

Contact local medical society for referrals to physicians who make house calls.

Homeless

National Coalition for the Homeless
1612 K St NW, Ste 1004, Washington, DC 20006
202 775-1322   Fax 202 775-1316
E-mail: ncn@ari.net

Contact local Travelers and Immigrants Aid.

Homeopathic Medicine

A system of alternative medicine that seeks to treat patients by administering small doses of medicines that would bring on symptoms similar to those of the patient in a healthy person. For example, the homeopathic treatment for diarrhea would be a minuscule amount of a laxative. (ENC-1989)

Resource

National Center for Homeopathy
801 N Fairfax St, Ste 306, Alexandria, VA 22314
703 548-7790   Fax 703 548-7792

Hormone

National Hormone and Pituitary Program
685 Lofstrand Dr, Rockville, MD 20850
301 309-3667   Fax 301 340-9245

Hospice

Celebrating its 20th anniversary in the United States this year, hospice care is an increasingly popular option for people at the end of life. In 1992, some 246,000 terminally ill people entered a US hospice program, 56% more than in 1985, when the first hospice census was conducted. Hospice has won the support of many organizations and individuals, including the AMA. Routinely, people in medicine say that hospice provides good care for patients and useful services for physicians.

Hospice bill could improve end-of-life care—experts

Diane M. Gianelli
AM News Feb 24, 1997, p15

A new hospice bill before Congress "reflects some necessary changes" that will allow physicians to provide "even better care at the bedside," said Carlos Gomez, MD, director of the University of Virginia's Palliative Care Service. The bill, a series of technical amendments to the Medicare hospice benefit, restructures the benefit periods, allowing patients to opt back into the hospice system after leaving it during times of remission.

Patients currently have four opportunities to receive hospice benefits. They enter the hospice program when they have been determined to have six months or less to live. The first two periods last 90 days, the third lasts 30 days, and the fourth is of unlimited duration.

If beneficiaries revoke their hospice benefits during the fourth period, however—usually because their disease has gone into remission—they are unable to receive hospice benefits when their condition worsens.

The bill—called the Medicare Hospice Benefit Amendments of 1997—would alter the status quo by creating multiple benefit periods: two initial 90-day periods, followed by an unlimited number of 60-day periods, resulting in more frequent evaluations of patients who outlive their initial prognoses.

Care improves outcome
"What sometimes happens is that the patients get into the fourth benefit period while they have a prognosis of six months, but during that unlimited period it becomes more apparent that they may not die within a six-month period of time," said Jay Mahoney, president of the National Hospice Organization.

"Good hospice care can change prognosis," he added.

The new proposal, Mahoney said, will allow patients to feel more comfortable about being discharged, knowing they have the option of coming back into the program when they need it. "It allows closer scrutiny without any negative impact on the patient," he said.

Covered services clarified
The bill also clarifies a point of confusion for many physicians caring for terminally ill patients. It specifies that the program will pay for services that some think are not normally associated with the hospice benefit, such as diagnostic tests and radiation therapy. Such services would be viewed appropriate when they are considered part of the patient's plan of care and are necessary for palliative purposes, Mahoney said.

"I often will approve radiation therapy or diagnostic testing in the interest of palliating a patient's symptoms," said Dr. Gomez, senior consultant to the AMA's end-of-life educational campaign. "Radiation can shrink a tumor, particularly when it has metastasized to the bone or the brain."

This can decrease the pain, he said, even if it doesn't lengthen a person's life. The new language "just clarifies for physicians or for hospice programs who may have thought otherwise that, indeed, these services can be offered appropriately in a hospice setting," Mahoney said.

The bill also amends the "core services" requirement to allow hospices to contract for physician services with independent contractor doctors as well as with physician groups. Under Medicare rules, physicians must be considered "employees" of the hospice.

In 1982, when the hospice benefit was initiated, most physicians were solo practitioners, said Mahoney, so establishing a W-2 employer/employee relationship was relatively easy. In recent years, however, more and more physicians have moved into group practices, making it much more difficult to establish a traditional "employee relationship" between an individual doctor and a hospice. The new language would make it easier for a hospice to contract with a group for an individual doctor's services.

The bill would allow rural hospices waivers for certain staffing requirements, and it would amend the "waiver of liability" provisions to protect beneficiaries if hospice claims are denied by Medicare because the terminal illness eligibility requirement was not met. It also would give physicians more leeway in meeting deadlines for completing paperwork certifying a patient's terminal illness.

When patients sign up for hospice, they waive all other Medicare benefits except those unrelated to the care of the terminal disease. The majority of all hospice care is provided in the patient's own home. Hospice pays for all services for the patient, including their nursing and physician care as well as other necessary services. It also provides counseling services, paying for bereavement care for families. Except for some nominal copayments on drugs and inpatient respite care, there is very little cost to the beneficiary, Mahoney said.

The hospice benefit is paid under four different levels. Ninety percent of it is paid under the routine home rate, averaging roughly $95 per day. Regardless of what services are provided, the hospice program gets paid at the same rate. Other types of hospice care—inpatient, respite and continuous care—are all paid at different rates.

Hospice payments surging
In 1994, hospice care was elected by roughly one of every three people who died from AIDS or cancer. The Medicare program spent $1.85 billion for hospice care in fiscal 1995, a 36% increase from the previous year.

The bill, introduced by Reps. Benjamin L. Cardin (D, Md.) and Rob Portman (R, Ohio), "streamlines the process for physicians," Mahoney said.

"I think this will give physicians greater ability to make sure that appropriate patients are referred to hospice programs at a time when they can provide the best care," he said. "Hospice can't do its best work when it's getting patients with three or four days to live."

Dr. Gomez added an additional perspective.

A smoother-running hospice program provides a credible response to the assisted-suicide movement, he said.

"The goal of hospice is to make the dying process as comfortable as it possibly can be for patients and families, with as many choices as they possibly can have. People are afraid of being bankrupt at the end of life, due to medical costs. They're afraid of suffering needlessly. They're afraid of losing control," Dr. Gomez said.

"One of the beauties of the hospice program is that the financial concerns get taken out of the equation immediately, because the government pays for almost everything."

Resources
The American Academy of Hospice Physicians
PO Box 14288, Gainesville, FL 32604-2288
904 377-8900

Children's Hospice International
1850 M St N, Ste 900
Washington, DC 20036
800 24-CHILD 703 684-0330 Fax 703 684-0226

Hospice Association of America
228 7th SE, Washington, DC 20003
202 546 4759 202 547-7424 Fax 202 547-3540
E-mail: jen@nanc.org

Hospice Education Institute
190 Westbrook Rd, Essex, CT 06426-1511
800 331-1620 203 767-1620 Fax 203 767-2746

National Hospice Organization
1901 N Moore St, Ste 901, Arlington, VA 22209
800 658-8898 703 243-5900 Fax 703 525-5762

Accreditation:
Joint Commission on Accreditation
of Healthcare Organizations
1 Renaissance Blvd, Oakbrook Terrace, IL 60181
630 792-5000   Fax 630 792-5001
Web address: http://www.jcaho.org

Hospitals

American Hospital Association
1 N Franklin St, Chicago, IL 60606-3421
312 422-3000   Fax 312 422-4796

Health Statistics Group: 312 422-3990
Library: 312 422-2000 Fax 312 422-4700
E-mail: rc@aha.org
Order Dept: 800 242-2626

Accreditation Manual for Hospitals, Joint Commission on Accreditation of Healthcare Organizations, Oakbrook, Ill. Annual.

For questions regarding

Accreditation:
Joint Commission on Accreditation of Healthcare Organizations
(to check on hospital's accreditation standing)

Charges:
Contact state/local cost containment council.

Hospital Management Companies:
Federation of American Health Systems
1405 N Pierce, #311, Little Rock, AR 72217-8708
501 661-9555   Fax 501 663-4903

Hospital Medical Staff:
National Association of Medical Staff Services
PO Box 23350, Knoxville, TN 37933-1350
615 531-3571   Fax 615 531-9939

Public:
Tips on Choosing a Hospital
Send $.25 and stamped self-addressed envelope to:
Council of Better Business Bureaus
4200 Wilson Blvd, Ste 800, Arlington, VA 22203
703 276-0100   Fax 703 525-8277

Complaints

In general:
Contact local state health care council or department of public health.

About fees:
American Hospital Association: 312 422-3000

Booklet on how to catch problems in hospital bills is available from:
National Emergency Medicine Alliance
800 553-0735

Hospital Associations, Statewide

Alabama Hospital Association
500 N East Blvd, Montgomery, AL 36117
205 272-8781   Fax 205 272-9527

Alaska State Hospital & Nursing Home Association
319 Seward St, Ste 11, Juneau, AK 99801
907 586-1790   Fax 907 463-3573

Arizona Hospital Association
1501 W Fountainhead Pkwy, Ste 650
Tempe, AZ 85281-6943
602 968-1083   Fax 602 967-2029

Arkansas Hospital Association
419 Natural Resources Drive
Little Rock, AR 72205-1539
501 224-7878   Fax 501 224-0519

California Association of Hospitals and Health Systems
1201 K St, Ste 800, Sacramento, CA 95812-1100
916 443-7401   Fax 916 552-7596

Colorado Hospital Association
2140 S Holly St, Denver, CO 80222-5607
303 758-1630   Fax 303 758-0047

Connecticut Hospital Association
110 Barnes Rd, PO Box 90
Wallingford, CT 06492-0090
203 265-7611   Fax 203 284-9318

Association of Delaware Hospitals
1280 S Governors Ave, PO Box 471
Dover, DE 19901-4802
302 674-2853   Fax 302 734-2731

District of Columbia Hospital Association
1250 I St NW, Ste 700, Washington, DC 20005-3922
202 682-1581   Fax 202 371-8151

Florida Hospital Association
307 Park Lake Circle, PO Box 531107
Orlando, FL 32853-1107
407 841-6230   Fax 407 422-5948

Georgia Hospital Association
1675 Terrell Mill Rd, Marietta, GA 30067
404 955-0324   Fax 404 955-5801

Healthcare Association of Hawaii
932 Ward Ave, Ste 430, Honolulu, HI 96814-2126
808 521-8961   Fax 808 599-2879

Idaho Hospital Association
802 W Bannock St, Ste 500, PO Box 1278
Boise, ID 83702
208 338-5100   Fax 208 338-7800

Illinois Hospital Association
1151 E Warrenville Rd, PO Box 3015
Naperville, IL 60566-7015
630 505-7777   Fax 630 505-9457

Indiana Hospital Association
1 American Square, PO Box 82063
Indianapolis, IN 46282
317 633-4870   Fax 317 633-4875

Iowa Hospital Association
100 E Grand Ave, Ste 100, Des Moines, IA 50309
515 288-1955   Fax 515 283-9366

Kansas Hospital Association
1263 Topeka Ave, PO Box 2308, Topeka, KS 66601
913 233-7436   Fax 913 233-6955

Kentucky Hospital Association
1302 Clear Spring Trace, PO Box 24163
Louisville, KY 40224
502 426-6220   Fax 502 426-6226

Louisiana Hospital Association
9521 Brookline Ave, PO Box 80720
Baton Rouge, LA 70898-0720
504 928-0026   Fax 504 923-1004

Maine Hospital Association
150 Capitol St, Augusta, ME 04330
207 622-4794   Fax 207 622-3073

Maryland Hospital Association
1301 York Rd, Ste 800
Lutherville, MD 21093-6087
410 321-6200   Fax 410 321-6268

Massachusetts Hospital Association
5 New England Executive Park
Burlington, MA 01803
617 272-8000   Fax 617 272-0466

Michigan Hospital Association
6215 W Saint Joseph Hwy, Lansing, MI 48917
517 323-3443   Fax 517 323-0946

Minnesota Hospital Association
2221 University Office Plaza, Ste 425
Minneapolis, MN 55414-3085
612 331-5571   Fax 612 331-1001

Mississippi Hospital Association
6425 Lakeover Rd, PO Box 16444
Jackson, MS 39213-6444
601 982-3251   Fax 601 982-2992

Missouri Hospital Association
4712 Country Club Dr, PO Box 60
Jefferson City, MO 65102-0060
314 893-3700   Fax 314 893-2809

Montana Hospital Association
1720 Ninth Ave, PO Box 5119, Helena, MT 59604
406 442-1911   Fax 406 443-3894

Nebraska Hospital Association
1640 L St, Ste D, Lincoln, NE 68508-2509
402 476-0141   Fax 402 475-4091

Nevada Hospital Association
4600 Kietzke Ln, Ste A-108, Reno, NV 89502
702 827-0184   Fax 702 827-0190

New Hampshire Hospital Association
125 Airport Rd, Concord, NH 03301-5388
603 225-0900   Fax 630 225-4346

New Jersey Hospital Association
746-760 Alexander Rd, CN-1
Princeton, NJ 08543-0001
609 275-4000   Fax 609 275-4100

New Mexico Hospital and Health System Association
2121 Osuna Rd NE, Albuquerque, NM 87113
505 343-0010   Fax 505 343-0012

Healthcare Association of New York State
74 N Pearl St, Albany, NY 12207
518 434-7600   Fax 518 431-7915

North Carolina Hospital Association
PO Box 80428, Raleigh, NC 27623-0428
919 677-2400   Fax 919 677-4200

North Dakota Hospital Association
1120 College Dr, PO Box 7340
Bismark, ND 58507-7340
701 224-9732   Fax 701 224-9529

Ohio Hospital Association
155 E Broad St, Columbus, OH 43215
614 221-7614   Fax 614 221-4771

Oklahoma Hospital Association
4000 Lincoln Blvd, Oklahoma City, OK 73105
405 427-9537   Fax 405 424-4507

Oregon Association of Hospitals
4000 Kruse Way Pl, Bldg 2, Ste 100
Lake Oswego, OR 97035-2543
503 636-2204   Fax 503 636-8310

Pennsylvania Hospital Association
4750 Lindle Rd, PO Box 8600
Harrisburg, PA 17105-8600
717 564-9200   Fax 717 561-5333

Puerto Rico Hospital Association
Villa Nevarez Professional Ctr, Stes 101-103
Rio Piedras, PR 00927
809 764-0290   Fax 809 753-9748

Rhode Island Hospital Association
Weld Building, 345 Blackstone Blvd, 2nd Fl
Providence, RI 02906
401 453-8400   Fax 401 453-8411

South Carolina Hospital Association
101 Medical Circle, PO Box 6009
West Columbia, SC 29171-6009
803 796-3080   Fax 803 796-2938

South Dakota Hospital Association
3708 Brooks Place, Ste 1, Sioux Falls, SD 57106
605 361-2281   Fax 605 361-5175

Tennessee Hospital Association
500 Interstate Blvd S, Nashville, TN 37210
615 256-8240   Fax 615 242-4803

Texas Hospital Association
6225 US Highway 290 E, PO Box 15587
Austin, TX 78761-5587
512 465-1000   Fax 512 465-1090

Utah Hospital Association
127 S 500 East, Ste 625
Salt Lake City, UT 84102
801 364-1515   Fax 801 532-4806

Vermont Hospital Association
148 Main St, Montpelier, VT 05602
802 223-3461   Fax 802 223-0364

Virginia Hospital Association
PO Box 31394, Richmond, VA 23294
804 747-8600   Fax 804 965-0475

Washington State Hospital Association
300 Elliott Ave W, Ste 300
Seattle, WA 98119-4118
206 281-7211   Fax 206 283-6122

West Virginia Hospital Association
600 D St, 2nd Level
South Charleston, WV 25303-3112
304 744-9842   Fax 304 744-9889

Wisconsin Hospital Association
5721 Odana Rd, Madison, WI 53719-1289
608 274-1820   Fax 608 274-8554

Wyoming Hospital Association
2005 Warren Ave, PO Box 5539
Cheyenne, WY 82003
307 632-9344   Fax 307 632-9347

Huntington's Disease

Huntington's Disease Society of America
140 W 22nd St, 6th Fl
New York, NY 10011-2420
800 345-4372   212 242-1968   Fax 212 243-2443

Hypertension

Citizens for Public Action on Blood Pressure
and Cholesterol
PO Box 30374, Bethesda, MD 20824
301 770-1711   Fax 301 770-1113

National High Blood Pressure Education Program
National Institutes of Health, Bethesda, MD 20014
301 496-1051

Free publication:
High Blood Pressure 120/80
National Institutes of Health, Bethesda, MD 20014

Hypnosis

Hypnotherapist. Induces hypnotic state in client to increase motivation or alter behavior patterns. Consults with client to determine nature of problem. Prepares client to enter hypnotic state by explaining how hypnosis works and what client will experience. Tests subject to determine degree of physical and emotional suggestibility. Induces hypnotic state in client, using individualized methods and techniques of hypnosis based on interpretation of test results and analysis of client's problem. May train client in self-hypnosis conditioning. (DOT-1991)

Resource

American Society of Clinical Hypnosis
22050 E Devon Ave, Ste 291
Des Plaines, IL 60018-4534
847 297-3317   Fax 847 297-7309

Hypoglycemia

National Hypoglycemia Association
PO Box 120, Ridgewood, NJ 07451
201 670-1189

Identification Cards (Emergency)

Medic Alert Foundation International
1735 N Lynn St, Ste 950, Arlington, VA 22209-2022
703 524-7710

National Safety Council
1121 Spring Lake Dr, Itasca, IL 60143-3201
630 285-1121   Fax 630 285-1315
Web address: http://www.nsc.org
(medical information on microfilm)

Immunization

Vaccines for children program

AM News Nov 14, 1994 p54
- Created by Omnibus Budget Reconciliation Act of 1993
- Physicians file simple form with state health department
- Administrative fee caps from $13 to $17
- Vaccine shipped to doctors or distributed by health departments
- Physicians agree to do simple eligibility screen, not charge for shots, comply with immunization schedule and rules for patient education and record-keeping
- Eligible groups: uninsured, Native American or Alaskan Eskimo, Medicaid recipients. Underinsured are eligible at federally qualified health centers
- To learn more, call state health department immunization program

Contact state/local public health department for guidelines.

Resources
Children
American Academy of Pediatrics
141 Northwest Point Blvd, PO Box 927
Elk Grove Village, IL 60009-0927
800 433-9016 847 228-5005   Fax 847 228-5097
E-mail: kidsdocs@aap.org
Web address: http://www.aap.org

International travel
Vaccination Requirements and Health Advice for International Travel (World Health Organization — Geneva)—available from:
WHO Publications Center USA
49 Sheridan Ave, Albany, NY 12210
518 436-9686

Blair F ed. *Countries of the World and Their Leaders Yearbook*. Detroit, Mich: Gale Research Inc. Annual. ISSN 0196-2809. Vol 2 section entitled "Foreign Travel: Health Information."
(May be available in many public libraries.)

Immunology

Immunologists share Nobel

AM News Oct 21, 1996 p2

The 1996 Nobel Prize for Medicine went to two researchers who discovered how white blood cells identify virus-infected cells. Sharing the award are Peter Doherty, PhD, chair of the department of immunology at St. Jude's Medical Center in Memphis, and Rolf Zinkernagel, MD, head of the Institute of Experimental Immunology at the University of Zurich in Switzerland.

Poetry and Medicine

Toccata

Paula Tatarunis, MD
JAMA 1996 February 28; 275(8): 578j

Louis Pasteur
What begins, begins with a knock on the door.
He looks up from his notebook long enough
to see the doomed boy's eyes,
the fresh gauze, the eyes
of the mother and the father.
They have pled their case with him—
the dog dead in the usual fury,
Negri bodies fairly leaping off the slide.
Behind him, the rabbits rustle in their cages,
even the ones who should have died.
With a knock on the door,
Paris has entered his laboratory.
His heart quivers and fills its narrow flask.
He knows the boy will live, and once again
he's frightened and humbled by his power.

Josef Meister
What ends, ends with a knock on the door,
on the door of le Musée Louis Pasteur,
where he's tended his savior's lab
into the dark years beyond his death.
In the morning they'll return to claim the key,
for the glorious *Reich and Fuhrer*.
Tonight Paris is black as oil; as their bootheels blink away
in the light of the swung blunt torches, he thinks,

The world, o père Louis, is strangling between
its dumb and furious rages. The little
housepainter froths, howls, bites and will not die.
I drift alone through our cold, brown rooms
for one last time, past the quiet cages,
the empty flasks, the straight spines
of your notebooks, still as upright and unbroken
as a fresh regiment. History must tend them now,
if it can, mon Père, for there is no other way
for me to end my song of gratitude than this,

I

just short of the coda of betrayal
(oh, somewhere, somewhere here
I know there's a rope
a rope to close this throat of mine,
the throat that rabies didn't.)

Footnote: In 1885 Louis Pasteur used his experimental rabies vaccination on a small boy, Joseph Meister, who'd been bitten by a rabid dog; he survived and went on to serve Pasteur, even tending the Pasteur museum after his death. Meister hanged himself rather than turn over the laboratory to the occupying German army during World War II.

Resources

American Association of Immunologists
9650 Rockville Pike, Bethesda, MD 20814
301 530-7178   Fax 301 571-1816
E-mail: infaai@aai.faseb.org
Web address: http://glamdring.ucsd.edu/others/aai

American Board of Allergy and Immunology
University City Science Center
510 Walnut St, Ste 1701, Philadelphia, PA 19106-3699
215 592-9466   Fax 215 592-9411

Impaired Physician

AMA Policy

Reporting Impaired, Incompetent or Unethical Colleages (H-275.952) Amended CEJA Rep A, I-91

1. Impairment: (*a*) Impairment should be reported to the hospital's in-house impairment program, if available, or if the type of impairment is not normally addressed by an impairment program, eg, extreme fatigue and emotional distress, then the chief of an appropriate clinical service, the chief of staff of the hospital, or other appropriate supervisor (eg, the chief resident) should be alerted. (*b*) If a report cannot be made through the usual hospital channels, then a report should be made to an external impaired physician program. Such programs typically would be operated by the local medical societies or state licensing boards. (*c*) Physicians in office-based practices who do not have the clinical privileges at an area hospital should be reportedly directly to an impaired physician program. (*d*) If reporting to an individual or program which would facilitate the entrance of the impaired physician into an impaired physician program cannot be accomplished, then the impaired physician should be reportedly directly to the state licensing board.

What is impairment?

In general terms, impairment exists when physical or mental illness and/or drug or alcohol abuse interfere with family, social, or work life.

The American Medical Association has operationally defined the impaired physician as one who is unable to practice medicine with reasonable skill and safety because of mental illness or excessive use or abuse of drugs, including alcohol.

Actual diagnosis of impairment must be made by professionals because the problem can exist in many different forms. For example, in some cases, mental illness may be the underlying cause of substance abuse. Alcoholism is the most common cause of impairment, though many people become addicted to other drugs. Some people may combine the use of alcohol with other drugs.

The following are some of the most commonly used substances that can cause impairment.

Alcohol. The use of alcohol is the number one drug problem. Alcohol is considered a drug because it dramatically affects the central nervous system, producing slowed reflexes and drowsiness. It is the major psychoactive chemical ingredient in wines, beers, and distilled beverages such as scotch, gin, and vodka.

Depressants. As prescription drugs, depressants are used for the relief of anxiety, irritability, and tension, and for the treatment of insomnia. In excessive amounts, they produce a state of intoxication similar to alcohol, including impaired judgment, slurred speech, and loss of motor coordination. Among the more commonly used depressants are antianxiety drugs such as the benzodiazepines (which include Valium and Librium) and barbiturates (such as Nembutal, Seconal, and Amytal). Barbiturates can be highly addictive and especially dangerous when mixed with alcohol, a practice that sometimes can cause accidental death.

Narcotics. As prescription drugs, narcotics are the most effective agents known for the relief of intense pain. Narcotics tend to induce pinpoint pupils and reduced vision, drowsiness, decreased physical activity, and constipation. Larger doses may induce sleep, but there is an increased possibility of nausea, vomiting, and respiratory depression, the major toxic effect of these drugs. Except in cases of acute intoxication, there is no loss of motor coordination or slurred speech, as in the case of depressants. Narcotics include opium, morphine, codeine, heroin, and meperidine (Demerol).

Stimulants. These drugs stimulate the central nervous system, causing the user to feel stronger and more decisive, and to experience a rush of exhilaration, wakefulness, and loss of appetite. Stimulants include amphetamines, such as Dexedrine and Benzedrine, which have been prescribed for the treatment of obesity and narcolepsy. One of the more commonly abused stimulants is methamphetamine or "speed." Cocaine, also considered a stimulant, is commonly regarded as a "status" recreational drug and produces intense euphoria. Early signs of stimulant use include repetitive grinding of the teeth, performing a task repeatedly, suspiciousness, and paranoia. (SPI-1986)

The impaired physician

Physicians are no different from other people in experiencing the difficulties in life that can lead to impairment. And, in fact, the characteristics physicians often develop to adapt to the extremes stresses involved in the training and practice of medicine may put them at special risk for the problem.

Risks for impairment

The process of training physicians can be like an endurance test. The demands of the profession are so great that trainees may feel overworked and overstressed. To succeed, medical students and residents may become obsessed with work, self-sacrificing, highly competitive, and outwardly unemotional.

Medical school and residency often create an environment with intense competition for grades, excessive workloads, pressure to learn "everything," a continual pursuit of perfection, and fear of failure, which is a particularly pervasive problem. Medical students and residents may be afraid of flunking out, not keeping up with the workload, failing board exams, or making an incorrect diagnosis.

Sleep deprivation is one of the most debilitating aspects of medical school. Medical students may stay up all night to study, and residents can be up all night treating patients while on call. Residents may be overwhelmed by the stress of making their own decisions about patients during the middle of the night. Yet they are afraid to ask for help from peers, because it will appear that they are unable to handle the pressure. Residents may also feel further debilitation from the pressure to perform competently without having had any sleep the night before.

These intense pressures on medical students and residents leave them with little time or energy for personal relationships or other life-enriching experiences, a factor that alienates them from society.

Once physicians begin to practice, stresses and behavior patterns tend to stay much the same. Excessive time demands still exist or may increase, with pressures to keep up with patient care and with new technology and medical advances. Physicians feel required to suppress emotions toward their patients and to distance themselves from death. They also continue to feel pressure over whether they have provided the proper treatment for difficult cases.

In addition to these continual stresses, other frustrations occur for physicians after they begin practice. During the training years, physicians may have dreamed about the independence they would have. Yet once in practice, many become disillusioned when they find that the independence does not really exist, particularly today with constraints from the government and third-party payers.

As in the training years, the marriages and family lives of physicians may be adversely affected by the demands of the medical profession. Too little time at home may make it difficult for them to maintain successful relationships with family members. This may be especially true for those physicians who are compelled to use time at home to do paperwork or catch up on their reading of medical journals. The promises of what can be bought with the money that results from the physician's hard work will not replace the love and involvement family members want and need.

When physicians bring home the autocratic sense of authority that is often used in the office, family members may resent being treated like patients and being told what to do. Physicians may also strain marital relations in other ways. They may postpone or cancel family outings and vacations due to work demands or expect spouses to handle all household problems because of their concerns with the medical practice.

A lack of fulfillment may develop in physicians who have been in practice for some time. Physicians go into practice with the ideals of saving lives and making great contributions to the community and sometimes it is difficult for them to accept the everyday, routine work that is a part of a medical practice. These physicians may start to question whether all of the hard work has been worth it and may feel a sense of emptiness and failure.

The demands of medical practice cause physicians to experience numerous pressures throughout their careers and to deny many of the human needs for social and family interaction. These pressures and deprivations can cause anger, anxiety, fear, and stress—factors that may lead to mental illness and/or drug and alcohol abuse in some physicians.

The psychiatric disorders that lead to impairment most often involve depressive illnesses. While depression alone can cause impairment in physicians, it can often lead to further impairment through alcohol and/or drug abuse.

Alcohol or drug abuse may have begun as early as the training years as a way to cope with the stress. Physicians are especially at risk for drug abuse—and not just because of their easy access to drugs. As medical students, they are trained to use medication to solve patients' problems and they may come to view drugs as an easy and appropriate way to solve their own problems as well. Also, because of their medical training, physicians may feel that they are knowledgeable enough to control drug use without becoming addicted. (SPI-1986)

Coping mechanisms

Obviously, all physicians suffer from stressors that can potentially lead to impairment. Yet not all physicians become impaired. It depends on how the stressors affect them. If physicians are aware of the inherent risks of impairment in the medical profession and employ certain coping mechanisms, the pressures are less likely to result in impairment.

Due to an increased awareness of the risks for impairment, many medical schools and residency training programs are offering workshops, seminars, and support groups to help trainees learn to cope with stress, improve and maintain their personal communication skills, and manage their practices. By learning these skills in the training years, students and residents can avoid developing the counterproductive coping mechanism (such as alcohol or drugs) that may lead to impairment.

Some of the coping mechanisms recommended for all physicians include:
- establishing good communications and intimacy with spouses, children, and friends so that a solid support system can be established for coping with life's pressures;
- leaving medical concerns at the office or hospital so that physicians can experience quality time with family and friends;
- ensuring successful family interactions by taking 30 minutes to decompress from office pressure before getting involved in situations at home;
- learning to manage time and define goals so that physicians can be involved with one activity without worrying about other responsibilities;
- cultivating outside interests or hobbies that are fun, not work, so that medicine does not become so all-consuming;
- taking care of personal health by getting plenty of exercise, eating properly, and avoiding excessive use of alcohol, tobacco, and caffeine. (SPI-1986)

I

Resources
Impaired Physician Program
c/o Georgia Impaired Health Professional
5448 Yorktown Dr, College Park, GA 30349
800 445-4232   404 994-0185   Fax 404 994-2024

*Contact state medical societies for local support
mechanisms for impaired physicians.*

Incorporating a Medical Practice
Making the decision to incorporate

Should a professional corporation[1] for a medical practice
be formed? Unfortunately, there is no simple answer to
that question. First, the choice depends on personal and
professional circumstances and interests—so much so
that incorporation might be ideal for one practitioner, yet
unwise for another. Second, the choice involves some
very complex questions, and it will take careful analysis
and planning to reach an appropriate decision. Since the
benefits and drawbacks of that decision will be borne by
the physician, it is important to learn as much about the
subject as possible in order to make an informed
decision.

Many physicians avoid investigating the possibility of
forming a professional corporation because they believe it
will take too much time, or it will be too complicated to
figure out, or that it doesn't matter one way or the other.
As a result, some of these practitioners may be paying
more than they should in taxes, or exposing themselves
to unnecessary legal and financial risks. A decision against
incorporation should never be made by default.

A corporation is nothing more than a particular form of
legal organization for a business enterprise, and it is only
one form out of many. Whatever current situation a
practice is in, that practice has a specific legal status,
whether run by a sole proprietor, a salaried employee, a
partnership, a shareholder in a professional corporation,
or some other status. Each kind of legal status has a
different impact on financial operations, the taxes paid,
and the potential legal and business risks faced. Contrary
to what some people say, no one form of legal organization is perfect for all physicians, or even for any particular
physician; each kind involves both benefits and drawbacks. For example, some of the more complex forms of
legal organization may involve a good deal more paperwork, administrative detail, and start-up costs than the
simpler forms. But the trade-off might be a good one for
many physicians in terms of tax savings. Carefully investigate both the good points and bad points of incorporation as compared with other forms of organization, to
determine which is the optimum choice. The following
definitions should provide a starting point.

A corporation is an artificial form of business organization created by state laws, and recognized by the federal
government's tax and other laws. A professional service
corporation is a specific kind of corporation that has
some things in common with every other corporation, no
matter how large, but also has other aspects that are
specific to professional service corporations and no other
kind. Every state has laws governing the formation and
operation of corporations of all kinds, and though the
laws are generally similar, any one state may have certain
peculiarities in its law that could affect a practice. By all
means, consult experts before making any final decisions.

The professional corporation is not a new concept. The
Federal Revenue Act of 1918, enacted only 5 years after
the first income taxes were authorized, contained a definition of a professional service corporation as one that
receives income primarily from the rendering of professional services, as opposed to the manufacturing of goods
or providing of nonprofessional services. That definition
is still a good starting point today. However, until recently professional corporations were quite rare, due
primarily to the lack of state professional service incorporation statutes and the refusal of the Internal Revenue
Service to acquiesce to the idea that professional corporations were entitled to the same federal tax advantages
that other kinds of corporations enjoyed. However, the
courts rejected the IRS position in the late 1960s, and
the professional corporation approach has since been
widely adopted, particularly in the medical profession.

Perhaps the professional corporation's most important
feature is that it separates a person from a practice, in a
legal sense. The corporation has a separate existence from
the physician, even if that physician is the only stock-
holder, only officer, only director, and only employee.
That can be an advantage compared with a sole propri-
etorship (the form a practice normally takes if a professional practices independently and takes no legal steps to
form any other sort of organization). For example, if a
sole proprietor owes a business debt, that debt can be
collected from the sole proprietor's personal assets as well
as his or her business assets. For federal tax purposes, all
of the practice income and expenses are reported on the
personal 1040 return.

Partners in partnerships fare the same in some states,
where the practice is recognized as being separate from
the personal affairs of the individual partners, but their
tax status is generally no different from that of the solo
practitioner. The partnership may have a legal status as a
separate and distinct business, but the taxes that each
partner pays are basically the same as if each partner were
practicing independently and splitting all income and
expense. Here it should be noted that while physicians
may share office space or expenses, that does not necessarily mean those involved are or are not partners: partnership is a specific legal form that involves a sharing of
income, costs, and business and legal risks within the
scope of the partnership.

But if a practice incorporates, the corporation becomes
an independent taxpaying entity completely separate
from the physicians who are its shareholders. The way
the group actually practices medicine won't change in
any way, of course, but for accounting purposes the
income and expenses of the corporation are kept absolutely and completely separate from the personal finances
of the physician-shareholders. Once a corporation is
created, it must obey a completely different set of state
and federal laws with regard to legal rights and obligations, including tax obligations. These laws can be rather
rigid; that is, the legal and financial advantages of some
of these laws cannot be claimed unless all are obeyed
quite strictly. For example, a corporation may not simply
be formed on paper and then forgotten about, while
conducting financial affairs prior to restructuring. Both
the IRS and the courts may regard the corporation as

nonexistent, and, therefore, it is possible to lose all the tax and legal advantages.

Note: 1. Professional corporation and professional service corporation, as used in this essay, mean essentially the same thing. Each state has its own terminology to describe corporations that may be used by physicians and other professionals. In describing the applicable tax rules, the Internal Revenue Code generally uses the term professional service corporations, but the rules are applicable to all such entities regardless of the terminology used in the applicable state law. (PRO-1989, adaptation)

Independent Practice Association (IPA)

An IPA is a corporation formed by physicians who maintain their independent practices but participate in the IPA to secure managed care business. IPAs accept financial risk for their members through capitation or discounted fees. The group is spread out geographically and is less formal than a group or staff model HMO. The only association between IPA providers is an individual contract between the physicians and the insurance company.

IPAs were originally formed to allow independent, community-based physicians a vehicle to compete with staff and group model HMOs. IPAs typically have a core of primary care physicians responsible for acting as gatekeepers (providing basic primary care) by managing all medical services and authorizing all referrals to specialists. Experts disagree about the long-term success of an IPA to compete effectively against staff and group model providers due to the inherent efficiencies in these other models. (MMCMP-1996)

The Independent Practice Association of America
333 Hegenderger Rd, Ste 305
Oakland, CA 94621
510 569-6561

Indigent Health Care

Contact county/state board of health

Industrial Health

American Industrial Health Council
2001 Pennsylvania Ave NW, Ste 760
Washington, DC 20006
202 833-2131   Fax 202 833-2201
E-mail: membershipservices@ainc.com

American Industrial Hygiene Association
2700 Prosperity Ave, Ste 250, Fairfax VA 22031
703 849-8888   Fax 703 207-3561

Industry, Health

Health Industry Distributors Association
225 Reinekers Ln, #650
Alexandria, VA 22314-2875
703 549-4432   Fax 703 549-6495

Health Industry Manufacturers Association
1200 G St NW, Ste 400, Washington, DC 20005
202 783-8700   Fax 202 783-8750

Infectious Diseases

JAMA Theme Issue: Emerging and reemerging microbial threats

JAMA 1996 Jan 17; 275(3)

This theme issue looks at trends in infectious disease. It also looks at the impact they have on society and how society has changed the way they can affect the human species. Specific topics include malaria, antimicrobial tuberculosis, and measles.

Resources

National Foundation for Infectious Diseases
4733 Bethesda Ave, Ste 750, Bethesda, MD 20814
301 656-0003   Fax 301 907-0878
E-mail: NFID@aol.com
Web address: http://www.scp.com/NFID

Board Certification:
American Board of Internal Medicine
3624 Market St, Philadelphia, PA 19104
800 441-ABIM (800 441-2246)   215 243-1500
Fax 215 382-4702

Board Certification in Pediatric Infectious Disease:
American Board of Pediatrics
111 Silver Cedar Ct, Chapel Hill, NC 27514
919 929-0461   Fax 919 929-9255

Informed Consent

AMA Policy

Informed Consent and Decision Making in Health Care (H-140.989) BOT Rep NN, A87

(1) Health care professionals should inform patients or their surrogates of their clinical impression or diagnosis; alternative treatments and consequences of treatments, including the consequence of no treatment; and recommendations for treatment. Full disclosure is appropriate in all cases, except in rare situations in which such information would, in the opinion of the health care professional, cause serious harm to the patient.

(2) Individuals should, at their own option, provide instructions regarding their wishes in the event of their incapacity. Individuals may also wish to designate a surrogate decisionmaker. When a patient is incapable of making health care decisions, such decisions should be made by a surrogate acting pursuant to the previously expressed wishes of the patient, and when such wishes are not known or ascertainable, the surrogate should act in the best interests of the patient.

(3) A patient's health record should include sufficient information for another health care professional to assess previous treatment, to ensure continuity of care, and to avoid unnecessary or inappropriate tests or therapy.

(4) Conflicts between a patient's right to privacy and a third party's need to know should be resolved in favor of patient privacy, except where that would result in serious health hazard or harm to the patient or others.

(5) Holders of health-record information should be held responsible for reasonable security measures through respective licensing laws. Third parties that are granted access to patient health care information should be held

I

responsible for reasonable security measures and should be subject to sanctions when confidentiality is breached.

(6) A patient should have access to the information in his or her health record, except for that information which, in the opinion of the health care professional, would cause harm to the patient or to other people.

(7) Disclosures of health information about a patient to a third party may only be made upon consent by the patient or the patient's lawfully authorized nominee, except in those cases in which the third party has a legal or predetermined right to gain access to such information.

Injury

National Injury Information Clearinghouse
5401 Westbard Ave, Rm 625, Bethesda, MD 20207
301 492-6424

Insurance, Health

JAMA Theme Issue: Caring for the uninsured and underinsured

(Beginning in May of 1991, the goal of the series is to keep in the minds of the medical community the work that still needs to be done to make the American health care system effective and available to all Americans.)

Caring for the uninsured and underinsured

JAMA Series. *JAMA* addresses the issues involved with this distinct population via a yearly theme issue each May, and an article series that appears at various times throughout each volume (see bibliography below).

JAMA Volume 277, Jan-June 1997

Extending health maintenance organization insurance to the uninsured: a controlled measure of health care utilization [Bograd], p 1067

JAMA Volume 276, July-Dec 1996

Characteristics and needs of sheltered homeless and low-income housed mothers [Bassuk], p 640

Uncompensated hospital care: will it be there if we need it? [Weissman], p 823

JAMA Volume 274, July-Dec 1995

New estimates of the underinsured younger than 65 years [Short], p 1302

Protecting children with chronic illness in a competitive marketplace [Neff], p 1866

Tenn-Care—health system reform for Tennessee [Mirvis], p 1235

JAMA Volume 273, Jan-June 1995

Health care mess: a bit of history [Richmond], p 69

JAMA Volume 272, July-Dec 1994

Better-quality alternative: single-payer national health system reform, p 803

Community-academic health center partnerships for underserved minority populations: one solution to a national crisis, p 309

Job loss due to health insurance mandates, p 552

Where is the health in health system reform? p 1292

JAMA Volume 271, Jan-June 1994

Dynamics of people without health insurance: don't let the numbers fool you, p 64

Evaluating health system reform: the case for a single-payer approach, p 782

Financing long-term care: a proposal by the American College of Physicians and the American Geriatrics Society, p 1525

Health system reform in the Czech Republic: policy lessons from the initial experience of the general health insurance company, p 1870

How will changes in health insurance tax policy and employer health plan contributions affect access to health care and health care costs? p 939

Improving health care for the poor: lessons from the 1980s, p 464

Policy options for public long-term care insurance, p 1520

JAMA Volume 270, July-Dec 1993

Health care unreform: the New Jersey approach, p 2968

Holes in the Jackson Hole approach to health care reform, p 1357

Lessons from a clinic for the homeless: the Camillus Health Concern, p 2721

Lessons from France 'vive la difference': the French health care system and US health system reform, p 748

United States needs a health system like other countries, p 980

JAMA Volume 269, Jan-June 1993

Access to prenatal care following major Medicaid eligibility expansions, p 1285

Community-oriented primary care: the cornerstone of health care reform, p 2544

Hawaii's employer mandate and its contribution to universal access, p 2538

MinnesotaCare (HealthRight): myths and miracles, p 511

Physician utilization disparities between the uninsured and insured: comparisons of the chronically ill, acutely ill, and well nonelderly populations, p 787

Socioeconomic inequalities in health: no easy solution, p 3140

JAMA Volume 268, July-Dec 1992

Can states take the lead in health care reform? p 1588

Physician supply policies and health reform, p 3115

Problem of discrimination in health care priority setting, p 1454

Single-source financing systems: a solution for the United States? p 774

What are we teaching about indigent patients? p 2561

JAMA Volume 267, Jan-June 1992

Balancing incentives: how should physicians be reimbursed? p 403

Consumer competence and the reform of American health care, p 1511

Health USA: a national health program for the United States, p 552

Making the critical choices, p 2509

Patient care and professional staffing patterns in McKinney Act clinics providing primary care to the homeless, p 698

Practice and ethics of risk-rated health insurance, p 2503

Uninsured and the debate over the repeal of the Massachusetts universal health care law, p 1113

JAMA Volume 266, July-Dec 1991

Another pound of cure, p 1692

Free clinics: a solution that can work...now! p 838

Maryland experience and a practical proposal to expand existing models in ambulatory primary care, p 1118

Medical apartheid: an American perspective, p 2746

Model for primary care delivery to a widely dispersed medically indigent population, p 563

National long-term care program for the United States: a caring vision, p 3023

Primary care and health: a cross-national comparison, p 2268

Primary care physician supply and the medically underserved: a status report and recommendations, p 104

JAMA Volume 265, Jan-June 1991

Access to health care for the uninsured: the perspective of the American Academy of Family Physicians, p 2856

American approach to health system reform, p 2537

Beyond universal health insurance to effective health care, p 2559

Call for action: the Pepper Commission's blueprint for health care reform, p 2507

Caring for the uninsured: choices for reform, p 2563

Expanding Medicare and employer plans to achieve universal health insurance, p 2525

Expansion of health care to the uninsured and underinsured has to be cost neutral, p 2388

Framework for reform of the US health care financing and provision system [Kansas Employer Coalition on Health, Task Force on Long-term Solutions], p 2529

Health Access America—strengthening the US health care system, p 2503

Health care financing for all Americans: an attainable goal, p 3296

Health care in crisis: a proposed role for the individual physician as advocate, p 1991

Health care insurance values and implementation in the Netherlands and the Federal Republic of Germany: an alternative path to universal coverage, p 2496

Health security partnership: a federal-state universal insurance and cost-containment program, p 2555

Health, health insurance, and the uninsured, p 2998

Is the Oregon rationing plan fair? p 2232

Let's provide primary care to all uninsured Americans—now! p 2108

Liberal benefits, conservative spending: the Physicians for a National Health Program proposal, p 2549

National health care reform: an aura of inevitability is upon us, p 2566

Physicians Who Care Plan: preserving quality and equitability in American medicine, p 2511

Restructuring health care in the United States: a proposal for the 1990s, p 2516

Tax Reform strategy to deal with the uninsured, p 2541

Uninsured: from dilemma to crisis, p 2491

Universal health insurance through incentives reform, p 2532

US Health Act: comprehensive reform for a caring America, p 2545

Resources

Alliance of American Insurers
1501 Woodfield Rd, Ste 400W
Schaumburg, IL 60173-4980
847 330-8500   Fax 847 330-8602

American Association of Health Plans (AAHP)
1129 20th St NW, Ste 600, Washington, DC 20036
202 778 3200
Web address: http://www.aahp.org

American Insurance Association
1130 Connecticut Ave NW, Ste 1000
Washington, DC 20036
202 828-7100   202 828-7183   Fax 202 293-1219

Understanding and Choosing Your Health Insurance
American Society of Internal Medicine
2011 Pennsylvania Ave NW, Ste 100
Washington, DC 20006-1808
202 835-2746   Fax 202 835-0443

Insurance Information Institute
110 William St, New York, NY 10038
212 669-9200   Fax 212 732-1916

National Insurance Consumer Hotline
(Sponsored by the insurance industry; can answer questions about life, health, home, or auto insurance)
800 942-4242

National Healthcare Anti-Fraud Association
1255 23rd St NW, Ste 850, Washington, DC 20037
202 659-5955   Fax 202 833-3636

Complaints: Contact state department of insurance.

I Insurance Departments, Statewide

Alabama Insurance Department
135 S Union St, Montgomery, AL 36130
205 269-3550

Alaska Division of Insurance
Commerce & Economic Development Department
PO Box D, Juneau, AK 99811
907 465-2515

Arizona Department of Insurance
3030 N Third St, Rm 1100, Phoenix, AZ 85012
602 255-5400

Arkansas Insurance Department
400 University Tower Bldg, Little Rock, AR 72204
501 686-2900

California Department of Insurance
770 L St, Ste 1120, Sacramento, CA 95814
916 445-5544

Colorado Division of Insurance
Department of Regulatory Agencies
303 W Colfax Ave, 5th Fl, Denver, CO 80204
303 866-3201

Connecticut Department of Insurance
PO Box 816, Hartford, CT 06142
203 297-3802

District of Columbia
Insurance Administration
Consumer & Regulatory Affairs
613 C St NW, Rm 600, Washington, DC 20001
202 727-8000

Delaware Department of Insurance
The Green, Dover, DE 19901
302 739-4251

Florida Department of Insurance
State Capitol, PL 11, Tallahassee, FL 32399
904 922-3100

Georgia Office of the Insurance Commissioner
704 W Tower, 2 Martin Luther King Jr Dr
Atlanta, GA 30334
404 656-2056

Hawaii Division of Insurance
Commerce & Consumer Affairs Department
1010 Richards St, Honolulu, HI 96813
808 586-2790

Idaho Department of Insurance
500 S 10th, Boise, ID 83720
208 334-2250

Illinois Department of Insurance
320 W Washington St, 4th Fl, Springfield, IL 62767
217 782-4515

Indiana Department of Insurance
311 W Washington St, Ste 300, Indianapolis, IN 46204
317 232-2406

Iowa Insurance Division
Department of Commerce
Lucas State Office Bldg, Des Moines, IA 50319
515 281-5705

Kansas Insurance Department
420 SW Ninth St, Topeka, KS 66612
913 296-3071

Kentucky Department of Insurance
Public Protection & Regulation Cabinet
229 W Main St, Frankfort, KY 40601
502 564-6027

Louisiana Department of Insurance
PO Box 94214, Baton Rouge, LA 70804
504 342-5900

Maine Bureau of Insurance
Professional & Financial Regulations
State House Station #34, Augusta, ME 04333
207 582-8707

Maryland Division of Insurance
Licensing & Regulation Department
501 St Paul St, Baltimore, MD 21202
410 333-2520

Massachusetts Division of Insurance
Executive Office of Consumer Affairs
280 Friend St, Boston, MA 02114
617 727-7189

Michigan Commissioner of Insurance
Licensing & Regulation Department
611 W Ottawa, PO Box 30220, Lansing, MI 48909
517 373-9273

Minnesota Department of Commerce
133 E Seventh St, St Paul, MN 55101
612 296-4026

Missouri Division of Insurance
Department of Economic Development
Truman Bldg, Box 690, Jefferson City, MO 65102
314 751-4126

Mississippi Department of Insurance
1804 Sillers Bldg, Jackson, MS 39201
601 359-3569

Montana Insurance Division
Office of the State Auditor
Mitchell Bldg, Helena, MT 59620
406 444-2040

Nebraska Department of Insurance
The Terminal Bldg, 941 O St, Ste 400
Lincoln, NE 68508
402 471-2201

Nevada Insurance Division
Department of Commerce
1665 Hot Springs Rd, Carson City, NV 89710
702 687-4270

New Hampshire Insurance Department
169 Manchester St, Concord, NH 03301
603 271-2261

New Jersey Department of Insurance
20 W State St, CN 325, Trenton, NJ 08625
609 633-7667

New Mexico Department of Insurance
PERA Bldg, Rm 428, Santa Fe, NM 87503
505 827-4297

New York Insurance Department
Empire State Plaza, Agency Bldg #1
Albany, NY 12257
518 474-4550

North Carolina Department of Insurance
430 N Salisbury St, Raleigh, NC 27603
919 733-7343

North Dakota Insurance Department
State Capitol, 5th Fl
600 East Blvd, Bismarck, ND 58505
701 224-2440

Ohio Department of Insurance
2100 Stella Ct, Columbus, OH 43266
614 644-2651

Oklahoma Insurance Department
408 Will Rogers Bldg, Oklahoma City, OK 73105
405 521-2828

Oregon Department of Insurance and Finance
21 Labor & Industries Bldg, Salem, OR 97310
503 378-4120

Pennsylvania Insurance Department
Strawberry Square, 13th Fl, Harrisburg, PA 17120
717 787-6835

Rhode Island Department of Business Regulation
233 Richmond St, Ste 233, Providence, RI 02903
401 277-2223

South Carolina Department of Insurance
1612 Marion St, Columbia, SC 29201
803 737-6117

South Dakota Division of Insurance
Commerce & Regulations Department
910 Sioux, State Capitol, Pierre, SD 57501
605 773-3563

Tennessee Department of Commerce and Insurance
500 James Robertson Pkwy, Nashville, TN 37243
615 741-2241

Texas Board of Insurance
1110 San Jacinto Blvd, Austin, TX 78701
512 463-6464

Utah State Insurance Department
3110 State Office Bldg, Salt Lake City, UT 84114
801 538-3800

Vermont Department of Banking and Insurance
120 State St, Montpelier, VT 05602
802 828-3301

Virginia State Corporation Commission
1220 Bank St, 13th Fl, Richmond, VA 23219
804 786-3603

Washington Office of the Insurance Commissioner
Insurance Bldg, M/S: AQ-21, Olympia, WA 98504
206 753-7301

West Virginia Division of Insurance
2100 Washington St E, Charleston, WV 25305
304 348-3394

Wisconsin Office of the Commissioner of Insurance
123 W Washington Ave, PO Box 7873
Madison, WI 53707
608 266-3585

Wyoming Insurance Department
Herschler Bldg, Cheyenne, WY 82002
307 777-7401

American Samoa Insurance Commissioner
Office of the Governor, Pago Pago, AS 96799
684 633-4116

Guam Department of Revenue and Taxation
855 W Marine Drive, Agana, GU 96910
671 477-5144

Northern Mariana Islands Commerce and Labor
Department
Office of the Governor, Saipan, MP 96950
670 322-8711

Puerto Rico Insurance Commission
PO Box 8330, Santurce, PR 00910
809 722-8686

US Virgin Islands
Lieutenant Governor
7 & 8 King St, Kongens Gade, St Thomas, VI 00802
809 774-2991

Internal Medicine

Internist. Alternate title: internal medicine specialist. Diagnoses and treats diseases and injuries of human internal organ systems. Examines patient for symptoms or congenital disorders and determines nature and extent of injury or disorder, referring to diagnostic images and tests, and using medical instruments and equipment. Prescribes medication and recommends dietary and activity program, as indicated by diagnosis. Refers patient to medical specialist when indicated. (DOT-1991)

Resources

American Board of Internal Medicine
3624 Market St, Philadelphia, PA 19104
800 441-ABIM (800 441-2246)   215 243-1500
Fax 215 382-4702

American Society of Internal Medicine
2011 Pennsylvania Ave NW, Ste 800
Washington DC 20006-1808
202 835-2746   Fax 202 835-0443

International Classification of Diseases (ICD-9-CM)

The International Classification of Diseases, 9th Revision, Clinical Modification (ICD-9-CM) is based on the official version of the World Health Organization's 9th Revision, *International Classification of Diseases (ICD-9)*. *ICD-9* is designed for the classification of morbidity and mortality information for statistical purposes, and for the indexing of hospital records by disease and operations, for data storage and retrieval. The historical background of the *International Classification of Diseases* may be found in the Introduction to ICD-9*(see below).

The concept of extending the *International Classification of Diseases* for use in hospital indexing was originally developed in response to a need for a more efficient basis for storage and retrieval of diagnostic data. In 1950, the US Public Health Service and the Veterans Administration began independent tests of the *International Classification of Diseases* for hospital indexing purposes. In the following year, the Columbia Presbyterian Medical Center in New York City adopted the *International Classifi-*

---

*Manual of the International Classification of Diseases, Injuries, and Causes of Death, World Health Organization, Geneva, Switzerland, 1977.

I *cation of Diseases*, 6th Revision, with some modifications for use in its medical record department. A few years later, the Commission on Professional and Hospital Activities adopted the *International Classification of Diseases* for use in hospitals participating in the Professional Activity Study.

The problem of adapting *ICD* for indexing hospital records was taken up by the US National Committee on Vital and Health Statistics through its subcommittee on hospital statistics. The subcommittee reviewed the modifications made by the various users of *ICD* and proposed that uniform changes be made. This was done by a small working party.

In view of the growing interest in the use of the *International Classification of Diseases* for hospital indexing, a study was undertaken in 1956 by the American Hospital Association and the American Medical Record Association (the American Association of Medical Record Librarians) of the relative efficiencies of coding systems for diagnostic indexing. This study indicated that the *International Classification of Diseases* provided a suitable and efficient framework for indexing hospital records. The major users of the *International Classifications of Diseases* for hospital indexing purposes then consolidated their experiences and an adaptation was first published in December 1959. A revision was issued in 1962 and the first "Classification of Operations and Treatments" was included.

In 1966, the international conference for the revision of the *International Classification of Diseases* noted that the 8th revision of *ICD* had been constructed with hospital indexing in mind and considered that the revised classification would be suitable, in itself, for hospital use in some countries. However, it was recognized that the basic classification might provide inadequate detail for diagnostic indexing in other countries. A group of consultants was asked to study the 8th revision of *ICD* (*ICD-8*) for applicability to various users in the United States. This group recommended that further detail be provided for coding of hospital and morbidity data. The American Hospital Association was requested to develop the needed adaptation proposals. This was done by advisory committee (the Advisory Committee to the Central Office on ICDA). In 1968 the US Public Health Service published the product, *Eighth Revision International Classification of Diseases, Adapted for Use in the United States* (PHS publication 1693). This became commonly known as *ICDA-8*, and beginning in 1968 it served as the basis for coding diagnostic data for both official morbidity and mortality statistics in the United States.

Other adaptations
In 1968, the Commission on Professional and Hospital Activities (CPHA) of Ann Arbor, Michigan, published the *Hospital Adaptation of ICDA (H-ICDA)* based on both the original *ICD-8* and *ICDA-8*. In 1973, CPHA published a revision of *H-ICDA*, referred to as *H-ICDA-2*. Hospitals throughout the United States were divided in their usage of these classifications. Effective January 1979, *ICD-9-CM* provided a single classification intended primarily for use in the United States, replacing these earlier related but somewhat dissimilar classifications.

ICD-9-CM background
In 1977, a steering committee was convened by the National Center for Health Statistics to provide advice and counsel to the development of a clinical modification of the *ICD-9*.

The organizations represented on the steering committee included:

American Association of Health Data Systems

American Hospital Association

American Medical Record Association

Association for Health Records

Council on Clinical Classifications

Health Care Financing Administration, Department of Health and Human Services

WHO Center for Classification of Diseases for North America, sponsored by the National Center for Health Statistics, Department of Health and Human Services

The Council on Clinical Classifications was sponsored by:

American Academy of Pediatrics

American College of Obstetricians and Gynecologists

American College of Physicians

American College of Surgeons

American Psychiatric Association

Commission on Professional and Hospital Activities

The steering committee met periodically in 1977. Clinical guidance and technical output were provided by Task Forces on Classification from the Council on Clinical Classification's sponsoring organizations.

ICD-9-CM is a clinical modification of the World Health Organizations's *International Classification of Diseases, 9th Revision (ICD-9)*. The term "clinical" is used to emphasize the modification's intent: to serve as a useful tool in the area of classification of morbidity data for indexing of medical records, medical care review, and ambulatory and other medical care programs, as well as for basic health statistics. To describe the clinical picture of the patient, the codes must be more precise than those needed only for statistical groupings and trend analysis.

The procedure classification
An important new development occurred with the publication of *ICD-9*: a Classification of Procedures in Medicine. Heretofore, procedure classifications had not been a part of *ICD*, but were published with the adaptations to it produced in the United States.

The *ICD-9* Classification of Procedures in Medicine is published separately from the disease classification in a series of supplementary documents called fascicles. Each fascicle contains a classification of modes of therapy, surgery, radiology, laboratory, and other diagnostic procedures. The decision to publish each fascicle as a unique document was made in order to permit its revision on a separate schedule from the disease classification. Primary input to Fascicle V, "Surgical Procedures," came from the United States, whose adaptations of *ICD* had contained a procedure classification since 1962. This experience was invaluable in constructing a classification to permit analysis of health care services in hospitals and primary care settings.

The *ICD-9-CM* Procedure Classification is a modification of WHO's Fascicle V, "Surgical Procedures," and is published as Volume 3 of *ICD-9-CM*. It contains both a Tabular List and an Alphabetic Index. Greater detail has been added to the *ICD-9-CM* Procedure Classification, necessitating expansion of the codes from three to four digits. Approximately 90% of the rubrics refer to surgical procedures, with the remaining 10% accounting for other investigative and therapeutic procedures.

Specifications for the procedure classification

1. The *ICD-9-CM* Procedure Classification is published in its own volume containing both a Tabular List and an Alphabetic Index.

2. The classification is a modification of Fascicle V, "Surgical Procedures," of the *ICD-9* Classification of Procedures in Medicine, working from the draft dated Geneva, 30 September-6 October 1975, and labeled WHO *ICD-9* Rev. Conf. 75.4.

3. All three-digit rubrics in the range 01-86 are maintained as they appear in Fascicle V, whenever feasible.

4. Nonsurgical procedures are aggregated from the surgical procedures and confined to the rubrics 87-99, whenever feasible.

5. Selected detail contained in the remaining fascicles of the *ICD-9* Classification of Procedures in Medicine is accommodated where possible.

6. The structure of the classification is based on anatomy rather than surgical specialty.

7. The *ICD-9-CM* Procedure Classification is numeric only, ie, no alphabetic characters are used.

8. The classification is based on a two-digit structure with two decimal digits where necessary.

9. Compatibility with the *ICD-9* Classification of Procedures in Medicine was not maintained when a different axis was deemed more clinically appropriate.

Guidance in the use of *ICD-9-CM*

To code accurately, it is necessary to have a working knowledge of medical terminology and to understand the characteristics, terminology, and conventions of the *ICD-9-CM*. Transforming verbal descriptions of diseases, injuries, conditions, and procedures into numerical designations (coding) is a complex activity and should not be undertaken without proper training.

Originally coding was accomplished to provide access to medical records by diagnoses and operations through retrieval for medical research, education, and administration. Medical codes today are used to facilitate payment of health services, to evaluate utilization patterns, and to study the appropriateness of health care costs. Coding provides the bases for epidemiological studies and research into the quality of health care.

Coding must be performed correctly and consistently to produced meaningful statistics to aid in the planning for the health needs of the nation.

Questions regarding the use and interpretation of the *International Classification of Diseases, 9th Revision, Clinical Modification,* can be directed to any of the organizations listed below. (ICD-1989)

International Classification of Diseases, 9th Revision, Clinical Modification (ICD-9-CM), Vols 1 and 2. National Center for Health Statistics; 1989. ISBN 0-68540-119-7

Resources

American Hospital Association Center for ICD-9
1 North Franklin St, Chicago, IL 60606
312 422-3000

National Center for Health Statistics
6525 Belcrest Rd, Hyattsville, MD 20782
301 436-7016
Web address: http://www.cdc.gov/nchswww/nchshome.htm

Office of Research, Demonstrations, and Statistics
Health Care Financing Administration
Department of Health and Human Services
330 Independence Ave SW, HHS Bldg
Washington, DC 20201
Web address: http://www.hcfa.gov

International Health

American College of International Physicians
711 2nd St NE, Ste 200, Washington, DC 20002
202 544-7498   Fax 202 546-7105

National Council for International Health
1701 K St NW, Ste 600, Washington, DC 20006
202 833-5900   Fax 202 833-0075

Project Hope, People-to-People Health Foundation
Project Hope Health Sciences
Education Center, Carter Hall, Millwood, VA 22646
800 544-4673   703 837-2100   Fax 703 837-1813

International Medical Graduates, Physicians, and Schools

AMA Policy

Foreign Medical Graduates (H-255.988) CME Rep F, A-81; Reaffirmed: CLRPD Rep F, I-91.

The AMA supports the following principles, based on recommendations of the Ad Hoc Committee on Foreign Medical Graduates (FMGs):

1. The AMA encourages American specialty boards to adjust certification procedures to FMGs returning to their home countries. This does not suggest that FMGs should be awarded certificates on the basis of lower standards, but that requisites such as post-qualifying practice in the US should be adapted to FMG diplomates returning home.

2. The AMA supports the practice of US teaching hospitals and foreign medical educational institutions entering into appropriate relationships directed toward providing clinical educational experiences for advanced medical students who have completed the equivalent of US core clinical clerkships. Policies governing the accreditation of US medical education programs specify that core clinical training be provided by the parent medical school; consequently, the AMA strongly objects to the practice of substituting clinical experiences provided by US institutions for core clinical curriculum of foreign medical

Ischools. Moreover, it strongly disapproves of the placement of any medical school undergraduate students in hospitals and other medical care delivery facilities which lack educational resources and experience for supervised teaching of clinical medicine.

3. The AMA urges the ECFMG to evaluate current standards for determining the proficiency of alien FMGs in the use of English.

4. The AMA recognizes that certain state and local medical societies have provided English language training programs to FMGs and encourages other medical societies, in areas where there are concentrations of FMGs needing such training, to consider providing it. Medical societies in areas where there are a few FMGs are encouraged to recommend appropriate language programs to FMGs in need of them.

A Piece of My Mind

Training too many, training too few

Samer Jabbour, MD
JAMA 1996 September 4; 276(9): 729

September 4
It was a Friday morning in June 1995, and my final day at the hospital where I had virtually lived for four years. I arrived there at 6 am, and by 10 I had visited my patients, joined in a meeting for quality improvement, and listened to the residents complain about coverage the previous night. As one of the departing chief medical residents, I was to deliver a graduation speech in the hospital's main auditorium. The ceremony was beginning in an hour, and I still had not translated all my ideas into words.

There was much to say. I was among the first few exchange visitor international medical graduates (EVIMGs) to join the program and the first to have become a chief resident. I wanted my speech to capture the experiences that other EVIMGs and I had lived through during training. Despite our different backgrounds, we had confronted similar challenges and shared related aspirations.

My fellow chief residents gave their speeches first. They each talked about what had made the past four years so exciting: the family-oriented structure of the residency program, the reward of watching a very ill patient improve, the joy of learning, the shared frustration of work and call schedules, and the friendships that developed from these experiences. Finally it was my turn; I decided to let my memories speak:

"Dear friends," I began, "when I first came to this country a few years ago, I had one dream: to return to my home city as a well-trained cardiologist; everything else was secondary. Looking back now, I know there was a lot more to it. I learned the pivotal role of the primary care physician in patient management, and the high-quality care the internist can provide. I came to understand and appreciate values such as patient autonomy and the right to self-determination, nonpaternalistic patient-physician relationships, patient advocacy, and principles of ethical practice. Like all of you, I struggled with the changes in the health care system, the pressure of defensive medicine and overutilization of modern technology, the culture of

documentation, and the deteriorating public image of the physician.

"Graduate medical education for EVIMGs in the United States is publicly funded. We try to pay back with hard work and gratitude. The road we've traveled has not been easy, but it has been worthwhile. On many occasions we had to walk the extra mile. The medical community needed to appreciate our potential, and our patients needed to see us as capable doctors. We had to be recognized beyond our strange names and funny accents. While some of us minded this, most did not; we were all eager to demonstrate our abilities. The support that I had from most people helped to overcome the prejudice and discrimination of a few.

"Like many foreigners who enter the United States every day, I had many prejudices about your culture. Ridding myself of many misconceptions was a slow but rewarding process. Living here for a few years has revealed many treasured aspects of your lives that have become a part of mine: the strong work ethic, the appreciation of diversity and multiethnicity, the community activities of the holiday seasons, the celebration of family through Thanksgiving, and the world of jazz. I have shared your fears and uncertainties regarding violence, family integrity, and the future of the economy. In turn, many of you have learned about the values and challenges that concern my culture. Our respect for each other enabled us to communicate. I hope we will continue this model of dialogue in our future community experiences.

Thank you all."

Later that day, I read an article that described the escalating costs of graduate medical education and outlined commonly discussed options for its refinancing. In most current proposals, training funds are reduced for international medical graduates, including exchange visitors, affecting both the number of slots and per-resident allocations. With these forthcoming changes, I am concerned that future international physicians will miss the opportunities that other EVs and I had for higher education and cultural exchange.

Developed societies have trained medical graduates from developing countries for many years. Many of these graduates have elected, or have been encouraged if they possess special talents, to stay in the countries where they trained, unfortunately for their compatriots. Those who return home, however, are vital to the countries they serve. Because of their privileged education, they can become model clinicians, health care policymakers, and teachers of future generations of physicians. For example, a colleague of mine, Saundy, is a physician from Africa. Despite many odds (his home country did not have the resources to train him), he found the means to pursue training in pediatrics and infectious diseases in the United States. Saundy now codirects a new infectious disease control center in his native city.

In the United States, increasing numbers of IMGs entering the workforce, a physician surplus, personnel maldistribution, and budget constraints have instigated the implementation of tighter regulations for training IMGs, including exchange visitors. Along with limiting the number of EVIMGs who find the means to stay in the States after training, these regulations will also restrict the training opportunities for those committed to returning home, and their home countries, in turn, will be deprived of the new skills and ideas generated in graduate training programs. This will threaten the progress made in international medical education in developing nations. Our countries have already lost many physicians and other professionals—the so-called brain drain—to industrialized nations in the past few decades. Can we afford to lose these training opportunities as well?

Cross-cultural education of health professionals worldwide is a prerequisite for providing better global health. All societies benefit from these shared educational responsibilities. It is time for these issues to be addressed in a global context; the policies that follow will, ideally, promote international education and health.

During my first month as an intern in medicine, I quickly learned that the key to survival was working together with others, hand in hand. Through our commitment to teamwork and to the exchange of ideas, we realized our common goals. This lesson certainly applies to how we can achieve the goal of better health and education for everyone.

In less than two years, I finish my training in cardiovascular medicine. What am I expected to bring back to my country? Quality patient care, problem solving–oriented knowledge, and the ability to establish and maintain channels of communication across our cultures. These are the skills that EVIMGs acquire in graduate medical education programs in the United States. To ensure continued dissemination of these skills, training opportunities for exchange visitors who are committed to returning to their communities need to be preserved.

Resources

American College of International Physicians
711 Second St NE, Ste 200
Washington, DC 20002
202 544-7498   Fax 202 546-7105

Educational Commission for Foreign Medical Graduates
3624 Market St, Philadelphia, PA 19104
215 386-5900   Fax 215 387-9963

Internet

Traveling the new information highway

Editorial

Thomas L. Lincoln, MD
JAMA 1994 June 22/29; 271(24): 1955-6

Editorials represent the opinions of the authors and *The Journal* and not those of the American Medical Association.

Every new technical advance in communication, as it becomes practical, has been adopted by medicine. As a consequence, the article on the Internet by Glowniak and Bushway,[1] excerpted above, is worthy of the reader's attention, even if the subject of personal and direct information retrieval and message exchange by networked computers is not a part of his or her practice or present mode of continuing medical education. At many levels, interactive long-distance computing is becoming a phenomenon that is difficult to ignore. Like the physical highways before it, the electronic information highway is stretching itself across the nation and around the world,

this time by glass fiber networks and satellite, thereby changing how work will be done and, ultimately, how professions will be organized. Clearly, information and communication technologies are converging, so that information exchange is different today than it has ever been in the past and will be different again tomorrow.

Through the National Library of Medicine, the United States has been an innovative leader in the electronic organization of medical information for scientific and professional use. Now the National Library of Medicine is at work on the wider organization of scientific medical information, for example, on genome information by supporting GenBank, the National Institutes of Health international database of genetic sequence information.[2]

Such efforts have led scientists and medical researchers into a broader computerized world that is increasingly dependent on shared information.

However, practicing medical professionals remain conservative in the means they use day to day to acquire medical knowledge. This may result from a prudent regard for the predictability of established ways of doing things (and the fact that they work), but also there is often a lack of time to directly investigate the ins and outs of some new technological approach that may impose many demands. Some of those who venture out on the Internet data highway may report results that vary from the greatest enthusiasm to the deepest frustration and despair. There are few personal chauffeurs to help. Thus, the user must drive (or navigate) the system alone or use automated aids that are sometimes as hard to decipher as the task itself, all with an uncertain payoff. And for some, interactive information retrieval by computer represents just one more of those not yet mature "halfway technologies"[3] that require more effort than will be returned over the near term. Fortunately, the instructions provided for accessing and using the Internet in the article by Glowniak and Bushway improve the odds of success.

For medicine, the long-term potential of interactive information exchange and retrieval is truly open-ended. In other fields of interest, extremely active collegial groups have come together through electronic bulletin boards on the Internet and other services to exchange information and opinion, giving rise to the description "global villages."[4] Similar electronic discussions have also started in some specialized areas of medicine, but particularly in research and among students.

In the future, the same set of computing technologies will provide us with a fully electronic clinical chart—a radically new medical record in which digitized images and sound will augment encounter documents and patient data sets. As such clinical records come into existence, the information highway will become an evident means of exchanging information among responsible parties. As an extension of teleconferencing, collaborative software applications already allow all sorts of electronic data to be examined, discussed, and modified at multiple sites at the same time as if all parties were in the same room. Thus, for example, physicians can hold a working tumor conference that extends across wide geographic boundaries, allowing, in addition to joint discussion, an on-line review of the literature and the results of clinical trials, an interactive comparison of radiation strategies,

I

and pharmacokinetic simulations of chemotherapy. Here we have the makings of a global university without walls.

It is now well understood that technologies are double-edged swords, often enhancing problems as well as solutions. Networked communication vastly facilitates access to computer databases, where information is power. In the shadow of everyday health care use, significant new policy issues arise concerning the confidentiality of patient information.[5] In the highly automated future era, patient data will be available to an increasingly large number of people who are not bound by the traditions and ethics of the medical profession. At the margins, there are those who seek to profit from the data they can extract from any service database. On the other side, those in authority can rationalize "a need to know" that violates individual privacy. Already there have been lawsuits that demand access to the exchange of informal electronic messages as if they were formal documents, not private mail or conversations.

All new technologies require that proper rules be established for their use, including how these rules should be followed. How will electronic health care data be used? Who will make these decisions? Would we accept laissez-faire usage, as with mailing lists? Or limits by law, as with copying rented videotapes? Would we rely on regulation? Or on societal acceptance, as with junk mail? Or on medical ethics and tradition, as with present clinical records? If we do accept a set of rules, how will they be policed? What constraints and remedies will be provided? How are confidential data to be protected? How are transmissions between distant sites to be safeguarded?

Quite clearly, encryption is one way to protect messages so that they cannot be monitored by others. There are excellent ways to do this that depend on "public keys" in which the encoding is too complex for easy decoding.[6] Privacy is primarily an issue of information use. Direct security controls of information systems to limit access to personal data offer an incomplete answer. The dominant problem, little different today from earlier times but magnified by the technology, remains the unauthorized actions of authorized users.

However, to police the highway, some in government may want access to what is said or transmitted in any communication. In Congress today, on the general issue of privacy and confidentiality of electronic message traffic, there is an emerging debate between those who take the formal view that all such messages, like first-class mail, are only the concern of the parties involved, and the pragmatists (largely government agencies) who feel a need to examine the traffic in order to find and control illegal uses of it. Thus, if messages are encrypted for privacy, authorities want "trapdoors" so that, under suitable legal constraints, they can monitor, decode, and read them. At the extreme, there are proposals that these constraints should not require a court order, but only a "finding" of some sort by the agency itself.[7] Although the debate about what should be free of government control and what should be regulated is at least as old as the Constitution, the outcome of the current debate will have many implications for the medical use of the information highway or its avoidance.

Beyond the everyday exercise of electronic resources to exchange and retrieve information, the issues of privacy, confidentiality, and security on the new information highway serve to highlight a much broader range of information policy questions. These will surely impinge on the health care professions in the coming years. In order to consider such problems both as citizens and as professionals, it behooves us to first gather experience with these technologies by traveling the Internet under less-pressured circumstances.

References

1. Glowniak JV, Bushway MK. Computer networks as a medical resource: accessing and using the Internet. *JAMA.* 1994;271:1934-1939.

2. Benson DA, Lipman DJ, Ostell J. GenBank. *Nucleic Acids Res.* 1993;21:2963-2965.

3. Thomas L. *The Youngest Science: Notes of a Medicine-Watcher.* New York, NY: Viking Press; 1983.

4. Gore A. Infrastructure for the global village. *Sci Am.* 1991;265:150-153.

5. Gostin LO, Turek-Brezina J, Powers M, Kozloff R, Faden R, Steinhower DD. Privacy and security of personal information in a new health care system. *JAMA* 1993;270:2487-2494.

6. Helman ME. The mathematics of public-key cryptography. *Sci Am.* 1979;241:146-157.

7. US General Accounting Office. *FBI Advanced Communications Technologies Pose Wiretapping Challenges.* Washington, DC: Briefing Report to the Chairman, Subcommittee on Telecommunications and Finance, Committee on Energy and Commerce, House of Representatives; July 1992. US General Accounting Office publication GAO IMTEC-92-68BR. Obtainable by: **ftp ftp.cpsr.org** login: **anonymous** password: **you\@your.internet.address, cd cpsr, cd privacy, cd wiretap, get gao-report-digital-telephony.txt**

Iron Overload

Iron Overload Diseases Association
433 Westwind Dr, North Palm Beach, FL 33408
407 840-8512   407 840-8513   Fax 407 842-9881
E-mail: LADYIRON@aol.com

J K

J

Journalism

JAMA 100 Years Ago

JAMA 1994 Aug 17; 272(7): 496b

'Scare-head' journalism

JAMA 1894 July 14; 23: 88

The temptation to sensationalizing in matters affecting the public health, is so generally yielded to by the average newspaper that the *Journal* hastens to recognize the value of such an exceptionally level-headed editorial as that in a recent issue of the *Washington Post* under the caption, "Beware of Scare-Heads," in which it advises its readers not to be alarmed because of the plague in China, or the cholera in Europe, or the yellow fever in Cuba. It summarizes the situation substantially as it has been given in this department from time to time and says, as to cholera: "The interests of the United States in this matter were never so vigilantly represented abroad as they are now and our Eastern seaboard was never so well fortified against the introduction of cholera from Europe." As to the plague in China: "It is gratifying to know that all along the Western coast, from British Columbia down, the authorities both of the Dominion and of the United States have taken every precaution that medical skill could suggest to prevent the introduction of plague germs by shipboard." And, finally: "The symptoms of an epidemic visitation of any sort from any country are too slight to warrant anxiety, still less anything like a panicky sensation. They are just enough pronounced to remind the sanitary authorities all along the line that they have their duty to perform, which admits of no relaxation, and this, we entertain no doubt, they fully realize. The people have also a duty to discharge on their own account in exercising all possible precautions as to their own immediate conditions and the importance of carefully regulating their habits of life and maintaining the cleanliness of their surroundings." Such timely advice, so intelligently given, is in sharp contrast to the startling head-lines, sensational exaggerations, denunciation of quarantine regulations and vilification of sanitary authorities which would follow the advent of the first case of Asiatic cholera or bubonic plague upon our shores.

More newspaper medicine

JAMA 1894 Aug 11; 23: 211

A London, England, dispatch speaks of an American found dead recently in the slums of Glasgow, at whose post-mortem examination it was found that "the body showed that he had died of fright." Whereupon our esteemed contemporary, the *New York Medical Journal,* expresses a desire to learn what the post-mortem signs of fright are, and adds that newspaper medicine is almost always amusing, but generally without intention. An entertaining example of intentional humor in connection with medical matters was given in an editorial article recently published in the *New York Times,* in which the writer evolved a theory of the American tendency to use middle names. He says: "The middle letter made its appearance in America immediately after the first great epidemic of influenza. We may therefore feel reasonably certain that it was one of the innumerable sequelae of that exasperating disease. It attacked nearly every boy and girl in the country, and in most cases assumed a chronic form. The recent epidemic of influenza, which has for the last five years devastated the noses and throats of America, has been followed by the development of the middle name in full, and this in its turn will become chronic. The fact that the middle letter appeared in England before the influenza merely shows that so far as Englishmen are concerned, the two have no relation to each other. When, on the other hand, we find that immediately after a severe attack of influenza Mr. W. D. Howells becomes 'William Dean Howells,' and Mr. James W. Riley becomes 'James Whitcomb Riley,' it is impossible that we should fail to see that these facts stand to each other in the relation of cause and effect."

K

Kidney Disease

Disorders of the kidney

The kidneys are susceptible to a wide range of disorders. However, only one normal kidney is needed for good health, so disease is rarely life-threatening unless it affects both kidneys and has reached an advanced stage.

Hypertension

High blood pressure, or hypertension, can be both a cause and effect of kidney damage. Other effects of serious disease or damage include the nephrotic syndrome (in which large amounts of protein are lost in the urine and fluid collects in body tissues) and acute or chronic renal failure.

Congenital and genetic disorders
Congenital abnormalities of the kidneys are fairly common. In horseshoe kidney, the two kidneys are joined at their base. Some people are born with one kidney missing, both kidneys on one side, or a kidney that is partially duplicated and gives rise to two ureters (duplex kidney). These conditions seldom cause problems. In rare cases, a baby is born with kidneys that are so underdeveloped that they are barely functional.

Polycystic disease of the kidneys is a serious inherited disorder in which multiple cysts develop on both kidneys. In Fanconi syndrome and renal tubular acidosis (which are rare), there are subtle abnormalities in the functioning of the kidney tubules, so that certain substances are inappropriately lost in the urine.

Impaired blood supply
Various diseases may cause damage to, or lead to obstruction of, the small blood vessels within the kidneys, impairing blood flow. Diabetes mellitus and hemolytic-uremic syndrome are examples. In physiological shock, blood pressure and flow through the kidneys are seriously reduced; this can cause a type of damage known as acute tubular necrosis. The larger blood vessels in the kidney may be affected by periarteritis nodosa and systemic lupus erythematosus. In rare cases, there is a defect of the renal artery supplying a kidney, which may lead to hypertension and tissue damage.

Autoimmune disorders
Glomerulonephritis refers to an important group of autoimmune disorders in which the glomerular filtering units of the kidneys become inflamed. It sometimes develops after infection with streptococcal bacteria.

Tumors
Benign kidney tumors are rare. They may cause hematuria (blood in the urine), although most cause no symptoms. Malignant tumors are also rare. Renal cell carcinoma, the most common type, occurs mostly in adults over 40; nephroblastoma (Wilms tumor) affects mainly children under 4.

Metabolic disorders
Kidney stones are common in middle age. They are usually caused by excessive concentrations of various substances (such as calcium) or lack of inhibitors of crystallization in the urine. In hyperuricemia, there is a tendency for uric acid stones to form.

Infection
Infection of a kidney is called pyelonephritis. An important predisposing factor is obstruction of the flow of urine through the urinary tract, leading to stagnation and subsequent infection spreading up from the bladder. The cause of the obstruction may be a congenital defect of the kidney or ureter, a kidney or ureteral stone, a bladder tumor, or, in a man, enlargement of the prostate gland.

Drugs
Allergic reactions to certain drugs can cause an acute kidney disease, with most of the damage affecting the kidney tubules. Other drugs may directly damage the kidneys if taken in large amounts for prolonged periods. For example, renal failure can develop after many years of taking excessive amounts of analgesics. Some potent antibiotics can damage the kidney tubules, producing acute tubular necrosis.

Other disorders
Hydronephrosis refers to a kidney swollen with urine as a result of obstruction further down the urinary tract. In the crush syndrome, kidney function is disrupted by proteins (released into the blood from severely damaged muscles) that block the filtering mechanisms.

Investigation
Kidney disorders are investigated by kidney imaging techniques such as ultrasound scanning, intravenous or retrograde pyelography, angiography, and CT scanning; by renal biopsy (removal of a small amount of tissue for analysis); by blood tests; and by kidney function tests, such as urinalysis. (ENC-1989)

Resources
American Association of Kidney Patients
100 S Ashley Dr, Ste 280, Tampa, FL 33602-5346
800 749-2257   Fax 813 223-0001

American Kidney Fund
6110 Executive Blvd, Ste 1010
Rockville, MD 20852
800 638-8299   301 881-3052   Fax 301 881-0898
(in Maryland 800 492-8361; in DC 301 881-3052)

American Society of Nephrology
1200 19th St NW, Ste 300, Washington, DC 20036
202 857-1190   Fax 202 223-4579
E-mail: asn@sba.com

National Institute of Diabetes, Digestive and Kidney Disease
9000 Rockville Pike, Bethesda, MD 20892
301 496-3583
Web address: http://www.niddk.nih.gov

National Kidney Foundation
30 E 33rd St, Ste 1100, New York, NY 10016
800 622-9010   212 889-2210   Fax 212 689-9261
Web address: http://www.kidney.org

Renal Physicians Association
2011 Pennsylvania Ave NW
Washington, DC 20006-1808
800 RPA-7525   202 835-0436   Fax 202 835-0443

L

Language

American Speech-Language-Hearing Association
10801 Rockville Pike, Rockville, MD 20852
800 638-8255   Fax 301 897-7348
For referrals 301 897-5700
E-mail: irc@asha.org

Laryngology

American Laryngological Association
c/o Gerald B. Healy, MD
Children's Hospital, 300 Longwood Ave
Boston, MA 02115
617 355-6417   Fax 617 735-8041

American Laryngological, Rhinological and
Otological Society
(Also called the Triological Society)
10 S Broadway, Ste 1401, St Louis, MO 63102
314 621-6550   Fax 314 621-6688

Laser

American Society for Laser Medicine and Surgery
2404 Stewart Square, Wausau, WI 54401
715 845-9283   Fax 715 848-2493

Laser argon photocoagulation:
American Academy of Ophthalmology
655 Beach St, San Francisco, CA 94109
415 561-8500   Fax 415 561-8533

Legal Affairs

American Bar Association
750 N Lake Shore Dr, Chicago, IL 60611
800 285-2221   312 988-5000   Fax 312 988-6281
Web address: http://www.abanet.org

American College of Legal Medicine
(persons with both law and medical degrees)
611 E Wells St, Milwaukee, WI 53202
800 433-9137 414 276-1881   Fax 414 276-3349
Web address: http://execp.com/~aclm

American Society of Law, Medicine and Ethics
765 Commonwealth Ave, 16th Fl
Boston, MA 02215
617 262-4990   Fax 617 437-7596
E-mail: aslme@bu.edu

National Health Lawyers Association
1120 Connecticut Ave NW, Ste 950
Washington, DC 20036
202 833-1100   Fax 202 833-1105
E-mail: healthlaw@nhla.org
Web address: http://www.nhla.org

Legal Affairs, Statewide

Alabama State Bar
415 Dexter Ave, PO Box 671, Montgomery, AL 36101
334 269-1515   Fax 334 261-6310

Alaska Bar Association
510 L St, Ste 602, PO Box 100279
Anchorage, AK 99510
907 272-7469   Fax 907 272-2932

State Bar of Arizona
111 W Monroe St, Phoenix, AZ 85003-1742
602 252-4804   Fax 602 271-4930

Arkansas Bar Association
Arkansas Bar Center
400 W Markham St, Little Rock, AR 72201
800 482-9406   501 375-4605   Fax 501 375-4930

California
The State Bar of California—Los Angeles
1230 W Third St, Los Angeles, CA 90017
213 482-8220

The State Bar of California—Sacramento
1100 11th St, Ste 315, Sacramento, CA 95814
916 444-2762

The State Bar of California—San Francisco
555 Franklin St, San Francisco, CA 94102-4498
415 561-8200   Fax 415 561-8305

The Colorado Bar Association
1900 Grant St, Ste 950, Denver, CO 80203-4309
800 332-6736   303 860-1115   Fax 303 894-0821

Connecticut Bar Association
101 Corporate Pl, Rocky Hill, CT 06067
203 721-0025   Fax 203 257-4125

Delaware State Bar Association
1201 Orange St, Ste 1100, Wilmington, DE 19801
302 658-5279   Fax 302 658-5212

Bar Association of DC
1819 H St NW, 12th Fl, Washington, DC 20036-4202
202 223-6600   Fax 202 293-3388

The Florida Bar
650 Apalachee Pkwy, Tallahassee, FL 32399-2300
904 561-5600   Fax 904 561-5827

State Bar of Georgia
800 The Hurt Bldg, 50 Hurt Plaza, Atlanta, GA 30303
404 527-8700   Fax 404 527-8717

Hawaii State Bar Association
Penthouse One, 1136 Union Mall, Honolulu, HI 96813
808 537-1868   Fax 808 521-7936

Idaho State Bar
204 W State St, PO Box 895, Boise, ID 83701-0895
208 334-4500   Fax 208 334-4515

L

Illinois

Illinois State Bar Association
Illinois Bar Center, 424 S 2nd St
Springfield, IL 62701
800 252-8908   217 525-1760   Fax 217 525-0712

Illinois State Bar Association—Chicago Regional Office
20 S Clark St, Ste 900, Chicago, IL 60603-1802
312 726-8775

Indiana State Bar Association
Indiana Bar Center, 230 E Ohio St
Indianapolis, IN 46204
317 639-5465   Fax 317 266-2588

Iowa State Bar Association
521 E Locust St, Des Moines, IA 50309-1939
515 243-3179   Fax 515 243-2511

Kansas Bar Association
1200 Harrison St, PO Box 1037
Topeka, KS 66601-1037
913 234-5696   Fax 913 234-3813

Kentucky Bar Association
Kentucky Bar Center
514 W Main St, Frankfort, KY 40601-1883
502 564-3795   Fax 502 564-3225

Louisiana State Bar Association
601 St Charles Ave, New Orleans, LA 70130
504 566-1600   Fax 504 566-1600

Maine State Bar Association
124 State St, PO Box 788, Augusta, ME 04332-0788
207 622-7523   Fax 207 623-0083

Maryland State Bar Association, Inc
520 W Fayette St, Baltimore, MD 21201
410 685-7878   Fax 410 837-0518

Massachusetts Bar Association
20 West St, Boston, MA 02111-1218
617 542-3602   Fax 617 426-4344

State Bar of Michigan
306 Townsend St, Lansing, MI 48933-2083
517 372-9030, ext 3027   Fax 517 482-6248

Minnesota State Bar Association
514 Miollet Mall, Minneapolis, MN 55402
612 333-1183   Fax 612 333-4927

Mississippi State Bar
643 N State St, PO Box 2168, Jackson, MS 39202
601 948-4471   Fax 601 355-8635

The Missouri Bar
The Missouri Bar Center
326 Monroe St, PO Box 119, Jefferson City, MO 65102
314 635-4128   Fax 314 635-2811

State Bar of Montana
46 N Last Chance Gulch, Ste 2A
PO Box 577, Helena, MT 59624-0577
406 442-7660   Fax 406 442-7763

Nebraska State Bar Association
635 S 14th St, 2nd Fl, Lincoln, NE 68508
402 475-7091   Fax 402 475-7098

State Bar of Nevada
600 E Charleston Blvd
Las Vegas, NV 89104
702 382-2200   Fax 702 385-2878

New Hampshire Bar Association
112 Pleasant St, Concord, NH 03301
603 224-6942   Fax 603 224-2910

The New Jersey State Bar Association
New Jersey Law Center
One Constitution Square
New Brunswick, NJ 08901-1500
908 249-5000   Fax 908 249-2815

State Bar of New Mexico
121 Tijeras NE, Springer Square
PO Box 25883, Albuquerque, NM 87102
505 842-6132   800 876-6227   Fax 505 843-8765

New York State Bar Association
1 Elk St, Albany, NY 12207
518 463-3200   Fax 518 463-4276

The North Carolina State Bar
North Carolina State Bar Bldg
208 Fayetteville Street Mall, PO Box 25908
Raleigh, NC 27611
919 828-4620   Fax 919 821-9168

State Bar Association of North Dakota
515 1/2 E Broadway, Ste 101, Bismarck, ND 58502
800 472-2685   701 255-1404   Fax 701 224-1621

Ohio State Bar Association
1700 Lake Shore Dr, Columbus, OH 43216-1008
614 487-2050   Fax 614 487-1008

Oklahoma Bar Association
1901 N Lincoln Blvd, PO Box 53036
State Capitol Station, Oklahoma City, OK 73105
800 522-8065   405 524-2365   Fax 405 524-1115

Oregon State Bar Association
5200 SW Meadows Rd
PO Box 1689, Lake Oswego, OR 97035-0889
503 620-0222   Fax 503 684-1366

Pennsylvania Bar Association
100 South St, PO Box 186, Harrisburg, PA 17108
717 238-6715   Fax 717 238-1204

Rhode Island Bar Association
115 Cedar St, Providence, RI 02903
401 421-5740

South Carolina Bar
950 Taylor St, PO Box 608, Columbia, SC 29202-0608
803 799-6653   Fax 803 799-4118

State Bar of South Dakota
222 E Capitol, Pierre, SD 57501
605 224-7554   Fax 605 224-0282

Tennessee Bar Association
3622 West End Ave, Nashville, TN 37205
615 383-7421   Fax 615 297-8058

State Bar of Texas
1414 Colorado, PO Box 12487
Capitol Station, Austin, TX 78711
512 463-1400

Utah State Bar
Utah Law & Justice Center
645 S 200 E, Ste 310, Salt Lake City, UT 84111
801 531-9077   Fax 801 531-0660

Vermont Bar Association
PO Box 100, Montpelier, VT 05601
802 223-2020   Fax 802 223-1573

Virginia State Bar
707 E Main St, Ste 1500
Richmond, VA 23219-2803
804 775-0500   Fax 804 775-0501

Washington State Bar Association
500 Westin Bldg, 2001 6th Ave
Seattle, WA 98121-2599
206 727-8200   Fax 206 727-8320

The West Virginia State Bar
2006 Kanawha Blvd E, Charleston, WV 25311
304 558-2456   Fax 304 558-2467

State Bar of Wisconsin
402 W Wilson St, PO Box 7158
Madison, WI 53707-7158
608 257-3838   Fax 608 257-5502

Wyoming State Bar
500 Randall Ave, PO Box 109, Cheyenne, WY 82001
307 632-9061   Fax 307 632-3737

Leprosy

American Leprosy Foundation (Leonard Wood Memorial)
11600 Nebel St, Ste 210, Rockville, MD 20852
301 984-1336   Fax 301 770-0580

American Leprosy Missions
1 ALM Way, Greenville, SC 29601-7407
800 543-3131   803 271-7040   Fax 803 271-7062

Leukemia

Leukemia Society of America, Inc
600 Third Ave, New York, NY 10016
800 955-4LSA   212 573-8484   Fax 212 856-9686
Web address: http://www.leukemia.org/infopage.htm

National Leukemia Association
585 Stewart Ave, Ste 536, Garden City, NY 11530
516 222-1944

Libraries, Medical Regional

National Network of Libraries of Medicine

The purpose of the National Network of Libraries of Medicine (NNLM) is to provide health science practitioners, investigators, educators, and administrators in the United States with timely, convenient access to biomedical and health care information resources.

The Network is administered by the National Library of Medicine. It consists of eight regional medical libraries (major institutions under contract with the National Library of Medicine), 140 resource libraries (primarily at medical schools), and some 4500 primary access libraries (primarily at hospitals). The regional medical libraries administer and coordinate services in the Network's eight geographic regions.

New programs focus on reaching health professionals in rural, inner city, and other areas who do not have access to medical library resources. The goal is to make them aware of the services that Network libraries can provide. Other important Network programs include the interlibrary lending of more than 2 million journal articles, books and other published materials each year; reference services; training and consultation; and online access to MEDLINE and other databases made available by the National Library of Medicine.

Three of the regional medical libraries have been designated online centers, to conduct National Library of Medicine online training classes and coordinate online services in several regions.

For general Network information, contact the National Library of Medicine.

For more information about specific network programs in a region, call the appropriate Regional Medical Library at 800 338-7657.

Resource Libraries by Region

The following is a list of Regional Medical Libraries and the areas served by each.

Middle Atlantic Region—Region 1
New York Academy of Medicine
1216 Fifth Ave, New York, NY 10029
212 822-7300   Fax 212 534-7042
E-mail: RML1@nyam.org
Wbe address: http://www.nnlm.nlm.nih.gov/mar
States served: DE, NJ, NY, PA
Online Center for all regions

Southeastern Atlantic Region—Region 2
University of Maryland at Baltimore
Health Sciences Library
111 S Greene St
Baltimore, MD 21201-1583
410 706-2855   Fax 410 706-0099
Web address: http://www.nnlm.nlm.nih.gov/sar
States served: AL, FL, GA, MD, MS, NC, SC, TN, VA, WV, District of Columbia, Puerto Rico, and the US Virgin Islands

Greater Midwest Region—Region 3
University of Illinois at Chicago
Library of the Health Sciences
1750 W Polk St, Chicago, IL 60612-7223
312 996-2464   Fax 312 996-2226
Web address: http://www.nnlm.nlm.nih.gov/gmr
States served: IA, IL, IN, KY, MI, MN, ND, OH, SD, WI

Midcontinental Region—Region 4
University of Nebraska Medical Center
Leon S. McGoogan Library of Medicine
600 S 42nd St, Omaha, NE 68198-6706
402 559-4326   Fax 402 559-5482
Web address: http://www.nnlm.nlm.nih.gov/mr
States served: CO, KS, MO, NE, UT, WY
Online Center for Regions 3, 4, and 5

South Central Region—Region 5
Houston Academy of Medicine—Texas Medical Center Library
1133 M. D. Anderson Blvd, Houston, TX 77030-2809
713 790-7053   Fax 713 790-7030
E-mail: #nnlm@library.tmc.edu
Web address: http://www.nnlm.nlm.nih.gov/scr
States served: AR, LA, NM, OK, TX

Pacific Northwest Region—Region 6
University of Washington
Health Sciences Center Library, Box 357155
Seattle, WA 98195-7155
206 543-8262   Fax 206 543-2469
E-mail: nnlm@u.washington.edu
Web address: http://www.nnlm.nlm.nih.gov/pnr
States served: AK, ID, MT, OR, WA

L

Pacific Southwest Region—Region 7
University of California, Los Angeles
Louise M. Darling Biomedical Library
12-077 Center for the Health Sciences, Box 951798
Los Angeles, CA 90095-1798
310 825-1200   Fax 310 825-5389
Web address: http://www.nnlm.nlm.nih.gov/psr
States served: AZ, CA, HI, NV, and US Territories in the Pacific Basin
(Online Center for Regions 6 and 7)

New England Region—Region 8
University of Connecticut Health Center
Lyman Maynard Stowe Library
263 Farmington Ave, Farmington, CT 06030-5370
860 679-4500   Fax 860 679-1305
States served: CT, MA, ME, NH, RI, VT

Following is a partial list of Regional Medical Libraries. To locate additional libraries, contact the National Network of Libraries of Medicine, 800 338-7657.

Region 1

New Jersey
University of Medicine and Dentistry of New Jersey
George F. Smith Library of the Health Sciences
30 12th Ave, Newark, NJ 07103-2706
201 982-4580   Fax 201 982-7474

New York
Columbia University Libraries
Butler Library, Rm 313
535 W 114th St, New York, NY 10027
212 305-3692

State University of New York at Buffalo
University Libraries
433 Capen Hall, Buffalo, NY 14260
716 831-3900

SUNY Health Science Center at Syracuse
Health Science Library
766 Irving Ave, Syracuse, NY 13210
315 464-4582   Fax 315 464-7199

New York Academy of Medicine Library
1216 5th St, New York, NY 10029-5293
212 876-0375 (for librarians)
212 876-8200 ext 321 (for general)   Fax 212 432-0276

Pennsylvania
University of Pennsylvania
Biomedical Library Johnson Pavilion
36th and Hamilton Walk, Philadelphia, PA 19104-6060
215 898-5817

University of Pittsburgh
Maurice and Laura Falk Library of the Health Sciences
Scaife Hall, 2nd Fl, Pittsburg, PA 15261
412 648-8824   Fax 412 648-9020

Region 2

Alabama
University of Alabama at Birmingham
Lister Hill Library of the Health Sciences
1700 University Blvd, Birmingham, AL 35294-0013
250 934-5460   Fax 250 934-3545

University of South Alabama Biomedical Library
Library 312
Mobile, AL 36688-0002
205 460-7043   Fax 205 460-7638

District of Columbia
George Washington University Medical Center
Himmelfarb Health Sciences Library
2300 Eye St NW, Washington, DC 20037
202 994-3528   Fax 202 223-3691

Howard University, Health Sciences Library
600 W St NW, Washington, DC 20059
202 806-6433   Fax 202 806-4567

Georgetown University Medical Center
Dahlgren Memorial Library
3900 Reservoir Rd NW, Washington, DC 20007
202 687-1187   Fax 202 687-1862

Florida
University of South Florida
Health Sciences Center Library
12901 Bruce B. Downs Blvd
Tampa, FL 33612-4799
813 974-2399   Fax 813 974-4930

University of Florida, Health Sciences Center Library
Box J-206, JHMHC, Gainesville, FL 32611
904 392-4016   Fax 904 392-6803

University of Miami School Library
Louis Calder Memorial Library
PO Box 016950, Miami, FL 33101
305 547-6441   Fax 305 325-8853

Georgia
Emory University, Health Sciences Center Library
1462 Clifton Rd NE, Atlanta, GA 30322
404 727-5820   Fax 404 727-8469

Medical College of Georgia
Robert B. Greenblatt, MD, Library
Augusta, GA 30912-4400
706 721-3441   Fax 706 721-6006

Morehouse School of Medicine Multi-Media Center
720 Westview Dr SW, Atlanta, GA 30310-1495
404 752-1531   Fax 404 755-7318

Mercer University School of Medicine
Medical Library, Macon, GA 31207
912 752-2515   Fax 912 752-2051

Maryland
University of Maryland at Baltimore Health Sciences Library
111 S Greene St, Baltimore, MD 21201
410 706-7545   Fax 410 706-3101

William H. Welch Medical Library
1900 E Monument St, Baltimore, MD 21205-2113
410 955-3411   Fax 410 955-0985

Mississippi
University of Mississippi Medical Center Rowland Medical Library
2500 N State St, Jackson, MS 39216-4505
601 984-1290   Fax 601 984-1251

North Carolina
Bowman Gray School of Medicine
Wake Forest University, Coy C. Carpenter Library
Medical Center Blvd, Winston-Salem, NC 27157-1069
919 716-4691   Fax 919 716-2186

Duke University Medical Center Library
S. G. Mudd Building
Box 3702 Medical Center, Durham, NC 27710-3702
919 684-2092   Fax 919 684-5906

University of North Carolina at Chapel Hill
Health Sciences Library, CB# 7585
Chapel Hill, NC 27599-7585
919 966-2111   Fax 919 966-1029

East Carolina University Health Sciences Library
Brody Medical Sciences Building
Greenville, NC 27858-4354
919 816-2212   Fax 919 816-2224

Puerto Rico
University of Puerto Rico
Medical Sciences Campus Library
PO Box 365067, San Juan, PR 00936-5067
809 758-2525   Fax 809 759-6713

South Carolina
Medical University of South Carolina Library
171 Ashley Ave, CSB912, Charleston, SC 29425-3001
803 792-2000   Fax 803 792-7121

University of South Carolina School of Medicine Library
Columbia, SC 29208
803 733-3344   Fax 803 733-1509

Tennessee
East Tennessee State University
Department of Learning Resources Medical Library
PO Box 701693, Johnson City, TN 37614-0693
615 929-6252   Fax 615 461-7025

Meharry Medical College Library
1005 D. B. Todd Blvd, Nashville, TN 37208-3599
615 327-6728   Fax 615 327-6448

University of Tennessee, Memphis
Health Sciences Library
877 Madison Ave, Memphis, TN 38163
901 448-5638   Fax 901 448-7235

Vanderbilt University Medical Center Library
Nashville, TN 37232-8340
800 288-0110   615 936-4029   Fax 615 936-1384

Virginia
Eastern Virginia Medical School
Moorman Memorial Library
700 W Olney Rd, PO Box 1980, Norfolk, VA 23501
804 446-5841   Fax 804 446-5134

Virginia Commonwealth University
Tomkins-McCaw Library
Box 980582, 509 N 12th St
Richmond, VA 23298-0582
804 428-0633   Fax 804 828-6089

University of Virginia
Claude Moore Health Sciences Library
Box 234, UVA Health Sciences Center
Charlottesville, VA 22908
804 924-5464   Fax 804 924-0379

West Virginia
West Virginia University Health Sciences Library
Basic Sciences Building
Morgantown, WV 26506-6306
304 293-2113   Fax 304 293-7319

Region 3
Note: Interlibrary loan (InterLibrary Loan) number is a library contact *only.*

Illinois
American Dental Association Bureau of Library Services
211 E Chicago Ave, Chicago, IL 60611
312 440-2642   Fax 312 440-2774
312 440-2653 (InterLibrary Loan)

Chicago College of Osteopathic Medicine
Alumni Memorial Library
555 W 31st St, Downers Grove, IL 60515
630 515-6185   Fax 630 515-6195
630 515-6176 (InterLibrary Loan)

John Crerar Library of the University of Chicago
5730 S Ellis, Chicago, IL 60637
312 702-7715 Fax 312 702-3022
312 702-7031 (InterLibrary Loan)

Loyola University of Chicago
Loyola Medical Center Library
2160 S First Ave, Maywood, IL 60153
708 216-9192 (InterLibrary Loan)   Fax 708 216-8115

Northwestern University
Galter Health Sciences Library
303 E Chicago Ave, Chicago, IL 60611
312 503-8133   Fax 312 908-8028
312 503-1908 (InterLibrary Loan)

Southern Illinois University
School of Medicine Library
801 N Rutledge St
PO Box 19231, Springfield, IL 62794
217 782-2658   Fax 217-782-0988
217 785-2124 (InterLibrary Loan)

Chicago Medical School
University of the Health Sciences Library
3333 Green Bay Rd, North Chicago, IL 60064
847 578-3242   Fax 847 578-3401
847 578-3000 ex 648 (InterLibrary Loan)

University of Illinois at Chicago
Library of the Health Sciences
1750 W Polk St, Chicago, IL 60612
312 996-8974   Fax 312 996-1899
312 996-8991 (InterLibrary Loan)

Indiana
Indiana University, Ruth Lilly Library
975 W Walnut St, Indianapolis, IN 46202-5121
317 274-7182   Fax 317 274-2088
317 274-7184 (InterLibrary Loan)

Iowa
University of Iowa
Hardin Library for the Health Sciences
Iowa City, IA 52242
319 335-9871   Fax 319 335-9897
319 335-9874 (InterLibrary Loan)

Kentucky
University of Kentucky, Medical Center Library
800 Rose St, Lexington, KY 40536-0084
606 323-1040   Fax 606 223-6514
606 323-5726 (InterLibrary Loan)

University of Louisville
Kornhauser Health Sciences Library
Lexington, KY 40292
502 588-5771   Fax 502 852-8300
502 588-5769 (InterLibrary Loan)

Michigan
Michigan State University Science Library
East Lansing, MI 48824-1048
517 355-2347   Fax 517 432-3693
517 355-7641 (InterLibrary Loan)

University of Michigan
Alfred Taubman Medical Library
1135 E Catherine St, Ann Arbor, MI 48109-0726
313 764-1210   Fax 313 763-1473
313 763-6407 (InterLibrary Loan)

Wayne State University, Shiffman Medical Library
4325 Brush St, Detroit, MI 48201
313 577-1088   Fax 313 577-0706
313 577-1100 (InterLibrary Loan)

Minnesota
Mayo Foundation Medical Center Libraries
200 First St SW, Rochester, MN 55905
507 284-2061   Fax 507 284-1038
507 284-2042 (InterLibrary Loan)

University of Minnesota, Bio-Medical Library
450 Diehl Hall, 505 Essex St SE
Minneapolis, MN 55455
612 626-3260   Fax 612 626-3824
612 626-2969 (InterLibrary Loan)

University of Minnesota, Duluth
Health Sciences Library
215 Health Science Library
10 University Dr, Duluth, MN 55812
218 726-8587   Fax 218 726-6205
218 726-8585; 218 726-8589 (InterLibrary Loan)

North Dakota
University of North Dakota
Harley E. French Library of the Health Sciences
Grand Forks, ND 58202-9002
701 777-3993   Fax 701 772-4790
701 777-2606 (InterLibrary Loan)

Ohio
Cleveland Health Sciences Library
2119 Abington Rd, Cleveland, OH 44106
216 368-3647   Fax 216 368-3008

Medical College of Ohio at Toledo
Raymond H. Mulford Library
3000 Arlington Ave, Toledo, OH 43614
419 381-4225   Fax 419 382-8842
419 381-4215, ext 3406 (InterLibrary Loan)

Northeastern Ohio University College of Medicine
Oliver Ocasek Regional Medical Information Center
4209 SR 44, PO Box 95
Rootstown, OH 44272-0095
216 325-2511   Fax 216 325-0522
216 325-2511, ext 530 (InterLibrary Loan)

Ohio State University
John A. Prior Health Sciences Library
376 W 10th Ave, Columbus, OH 43210-1240
614 292-4861   Fax 614-292-5717
614 292-4894 (InterLibrary Loan)

Ohio University Alden Health Science Library
Athens, OH 45701-2978
614 593-2680   Fax 614 593-4693
614 593-2690, ext 2691 (LL)

State Library of Ohio
65 S Front St, Columbus, OH 43215-4163
614 644-7061   Fax 614 466-3584
614 644-6956 (InterLibrary Loan)

University of Cincinnati, Health Sciences Library
231 Bethesda Ave, PO Box 670574
Cincinnati, OH 45267-0574
513 558-5627   Fax 513 558-2682
513 558-4637 (InterLibrary Loan)

Wright State University
Fordham Health Sciences Library
3640 Colonel Glenn Hwy, Dayton, OH 45435
513 873-2266   Fax 513 879-2675
513 873-4110 (InterLibrary Loan)

South Dakota
University of South Dakota
Lommen Health Sciences Library, School of Medicine
414 E Clark, Vermillion, SD 57069-2390
605 677-5347   Fax 605 677-5124

Wisconsin
Medical College of Wisconsin Libraries
8701 Watertown Plank Rd, Milwaukee, WI 53226
414 456-8323   Fax 414 266-8681
414 257-8460 (InterLibrary Loan)

University of Wisconsin
Center for Health Science Libraries
1305 Linden Dr, Madison, WI 53706-1593
608 262-6594   Fax 608 262-4732
608 262-6524 (InterLibrary Loan)

Region 4
Colorado
University of Colorado Health Science Center
Denison Memorial Library
4200 E Ninth Ave, Denver, CO 80262
303 270-5125   Fax 303 270-6255

Kansas
The Archie R. Dykes Library of the Health Sciences
University of Kansas Medical Center
2100 W 39th St, Kansas City, KS 66160-7180
913 588-7166 800 332-4193 (KS only)
Fax 913 588-7304

Missouri
University of Missouri-Columbia
J. Otto Lottes Health Sciences Library
Health Sciences Center, Columbia, MO 65212
314 882-7033   Fax 314 882-5574

Washington University School of Medicine Library
660 S Euclid Ave, Campus Box 8132
St Louis, MO 63110
314 362-7080   Fax 314 362-0190

St Louis University Health Science Center Library
1401 S Grand Blvd, St Louis, MO 63104
314 577-8605   Fax 314 772-1307

Nebraska
Creighton University Health Sciences Library
2500 California Ave, Omaha, NE 68178
402 280-5108   Fax 402 280-5134

McGoogan Library of Medicine
University of Nebraska Medical Center
600 S 42nd St, PO Box 986705
Omaha, NE 68198-6705
402 559-4006   Fax 402 559-5498

Utah
Spenser S. Eccles Health Sciences Library
Building 589, 10 N Medical Drive
University of Utah, Salt Lake City, UT 84112
801 581-8771   Fax 801 581-3632

Wyoming
University of Wyoming
Science and Technology Library
University Station Box 3262, Laramie, WY 82071
307 766-6203   Fax 307 766-3611

Region 5
Arkansas
University of Arkansas for Medical Sciences Library
Slot 586, 4301 W Markham Ave
Little Rock, AR 77205-7186
501 686-5980   Fax 501 686-6745

Louisiana
Louisiana State University—Medical Center Library
433 Bolivar St, New Orleans, LA 70112-2882
504 568-6105   Fax 504 568-7720

Louisiana State University—Medical Center Library
PO Box 33932, Shreveport, LA 71130-3932
318 674-5445   Fax 318 675-5442

Tulane Medical Center
Rudolph Matas Medical Library
1430 Tulane Ave, PO Box SL86
New Orleans, LA 70112-2699
504 588-5155   Fax 504 587-7417

New Mexico
University of New Mexico Health Science Center Library
North Campus, Albuquerque, NM 87131
505 277-2548 Fax 505 277-5350

Oklahoma
Oklahoma College of Osetopathic Medicine and
Surgery—Medical Library
1111 W 17th St, Tulsa, OK 74107-1898
918 561-8449   Fax 918 561-8412

University of Oklahoma Health Sciences Center
2808 S Sheridan, Tulsa, OK 74129
918 838-4616   Fax 918 838-4624

University of Oklahoma Health Science Center
Robert M. Bird Health Sciences Library
100 Stanton L. Young Blvd, PO Box 26901
Oklahoma City, OK 73190-3046
405 271-2285   Fax 405 271-3297

Texas
Texas A&M University
Medical Sciences Library
College Station, TX 77843-4462
409 845-7427   Fax 409 845-7493

University of Texas Health Sciences Center at
San Antonio
Dolph Brisco Library
7703 Floyd Curl Dr, San Antonio, TX 78284-7940
210 567-2400   Fax 210 567-2490

Texas College of Osteopathic Medicine Health
Sciences Library
3500 Camp Bowie, Fort Worth, TX 76107
817 735-2380   Fax 817 735-2283

University of Texas Medical Branch
Moody Medical Library
301 University Blvd, Galveston, TX 77555-1035
409 772-1971   Fax 409 765-9852

Houston Academy of Medicine
Texas Medical Center Library
1133 M. D. Anderson Blvd, Houston, TX 77030
713 795-4200   Fax 713 790-7052

University of Texas
Southwestern Medical Center at Dallas Library
5323 Harry Hines Blvd, Dallas, TX 75235-9049
214 648-2001   Fax 214 648-2826

Texas Tech University Health Sciences Center
Library of the Health Sciences
3601 Fourth St, Lubbock, TX 79430-0001
806 743-2203   Fax 806 743-2218

Region 6
Oregon Health Science University Library
3181 SW Sam Jackson Park Rd
PO Box 573, Portland, OR 97207-0573
503 494-8026   Fax 503 494-5241

Region 7
Arizona
University of Arizona, Arizona Health
Sciences Center Library
1501 N Campbell Ave, Tucson, AZ 85724
602 626-6121   Fax 602 626-2922

California
University of California, Davis
Carlson Health Sciences Library
Davis, CA 95616
916 752-1214 Fax 916 752-4718

University of California, Irvine, Biomedical Library
PO Box 19556, Irvine, CA 92712
714 856-5212   Fax 714 856-8095

University of California, San Diego
Biomedical Library, 9500 Gilman Dr 0175B
La Jolla, CA 92093-0175
619 534-3253   Fax 619 534-6609

Loma Linda University
Del E. Webb Memorial Library
Anderson and University Streets, Loma Linda, CA 92350
909 824-4585   Fax 909 824-4188

University of Southern California
Norris Medical Library
2003 Zonal Ave, Los Angeles, CA 90033-4582
213 342-1116   Fax 213 221-1235

University of Southern California, Dental Library
DEN 201, University Park-MC 0641
Los Angeles, CA 90089-0641
213 740-6476   Fax 213 748-8565

University of California, Irvine
Medical Center Library
101 City Drive S, Rt 82, Bldg 22A, Orange, CA 92668
714 456-5585

L

University of California, Davis
Medical Center Library
4301 X St, Rm 1005, Sacramento, CA 95817
916 734-3529   Fax 916 734-7418

University of California, San Diego
Medical Center Library
200 W Arbor Dr, San Diego, CA 92103
619 543-6520   Fax 619 543-3289

University of California, San Francisco, Library
513 Parnassus Ave, Ste 257
San Francisco, CA 94143-0840
415 476-8293   Fax 415 476-4653

Stanford University Medical Center
Lane Medical Library
Stanford, CA 94305-5323
415 723-6831   Fax 415 725-7471

Hawaii
Hawaii Medical Library
1221 Punchbowl St, Honolulu, HI 96813
808 536-9302   Fax 808 524-6956

Nevada
University of Nevada-Reno
Savitt Medical Library Building 306
School of Medicine, Reno, NV 89557-0046
702 784-4625   Fax 702 784-4489

Region 8
Connecticut
University of Connecticut Health Center
Lyman Maynard Stowe Library
PO Box 4003, Farmington, CT 06034-4003
206 679-2839   Fax 203 679-4046

Yale University
Harvey Cushing John Hay Whitney Medical Library
333 Cedar St, PO Box 208014
New Haven, CT 06520-8014
203 785-5352   Fax 203 785-4369

Maine
Veteran's Administration Medical Center Learning
Resource Service
Togus, ME 04330
207 623-5773   Fax 207 623-5766

Massachusetts
Boston College O'Neill Library
O'Neill 410, Chestnut Hill, MA 02167
617 552-4489 Fax 617 552-2600

Boston University School of Medicine Alumni
Medical Library
80 E Concord St, L-12, Boston, MA 02118-2394
617 638-4230   Fax 617 638-4233

Harvard University Schools of Medicine, Dental Medicine
and Public Health
Boston Medical Library
10 Shattuck St, Boston, MA 02115
617 432-2142   Fax 617 432-0693

Massachusetts College of Pharmacy and Allied
Health Sciences
Sheppard Library
179 Longwood Ave, Boston, MA 02115
617 732-2813   Fax 617 278-1566

Tufts University Health Sciences Library
145 Harrison Ave, Boston, MA 02111
617 956-7481 Fax 617 350-8039

University of Massachusetts Medical Center
Lamar Soutter Medical School Library
55 Lake Ave N, Worcester, MA 01655
508 856-2511   Fax 508 856-5899

New Hampshire
Dartmouth College Dana Biomedical Library
Hanover, NH 03755
603 650-1658 Fax 603 650-1354

Rhode Island
Brown University Sciences Library
Box I, Providence, RI 02912
401 863-2405   Fax 401 863-2753

Vermont
University of Vermont
Charles A. Dana Medical Library
Given Building, Burlington, VT 05405
802 656-2200   Fax 802 656-0762

Libraries, National

National Library of Medicine
The Library, which serves as the nation's chief medical information source, is authorized to provide medical library services and online bibliographic searching capabilities, such as MEDLINE, TOXLINE, and others, to public and private agencies and organizations, institutions, and individuals. It is responsible for the development and management of a biomedical communications network, applying advanced technology to the improvement of biomedical communications, and operates a computer-based toxicology information system for the scientific community, industry, and other federal agencies. Through its National Center for Biotechnology Information, the Library has a leadership role in development of new information technologies to aid in the understanding of the molecular processes that control health and disease. In addition, the Library acquires and makes available for distribution audiovisual instruction material, and develops prototype audiovisual communication programs for the health educational community. Through grants and contracts, the Library administers programs of assistance to the nation's medical libraries that include support of a regional medical library network, research in the field of medical library science, establishment and improvement of the basic library resources, and supporting biomedical scientific publications of a nonprofit nature. (USG-1996)

Resources
National Library of Medicine
8600 Rockville Pike, Bethesda, MD 20894
General Information 301 496-6095
MEDLINE 800 638-8480
Web address: http://www.nlm.nih.gov/top_level.dir/
nlm_online_info.html

National Agricultural Library
Agriculture Department
10301 Baltimore Blvd, Beltsville, MD 20705
301 504-5719

United States Library of Congress
101 Independence Ave SE, Washington, DC 20540
202 287-5000
For information on tours or exhibits, 800 334-4465.

Library Associations

Obituary

Billings, John Shaw (1840?-1913)
JAMA 1913 Mar 15; 60(11): 846

John Shaw Billings, MD, lieutenant-colonel US Army, retired. Curator of the Army Medical Museum and Library for many years, the Index Catalogue of which will stand as a lasting monument to his industry and genius; died in the New York Hospital, March 11, from pneumonia, aged 73.

He was born in Switzerland County, Ind, and was graduated from the Medical College of Ohio, Cincinnati, in 1860. He also has had conferred on him the honorary degree of LLD by the University of Munich in 1889 and by Dublin University in 1892 and the degree of DCL by the University of Oxford in 1889.

After serving for a year as demonstrator in anatomy in his alma mater, he entered the United States Army as assistant surgeon, April 16, 1862; was made captain and assistant surgeon four years later; after 10 years was promoted to major and surgeon, and June 6, 1894, was made lieutenant-colonel and deputy surgeon-general and was retired from the Army at his own request, after more than thirty years service, Oct. 1, 1895. In 1869 he was ordered to the Surgeon-General's office, Washington, where he had charge of the organization of the Veteran Reserve Corps; of matters pertaining to contract surgeons and of all property and disbursing accounts until 1885, when he was placed in charge of the Library of the Surgeon-General's office, serving in this capacity until 1893, when he was appointed curator of the Army Medical Museum and Library. He was placed in charge of the division of vital and social statistics of the tenth and eleventh censuses. In 1870 Dr. Billings was engaged in the reorganization of the United States Marine Hospital Service and from 1879 to 1882 served as vice-president of the National Board of Health.

His contributions to the medical literature were numerous and varied, the best known being the *Index Catalogue of the Library of the Surgeon General's Office* and the *National Medical Dictionary*. He was professor of hygiene in the University of Pennsylvania and director of its laboratory of hygiene from 1893 to 1896, when he accepted the directorship of the New York Public Library, Astor, Lenox and Tilden Foundations, holding this position until his death.

Dr. Billings survived his coworker, Dr. Robert Fletcher, by only 4 months. His work as an administrative officer and as a bibliographer is unique in the history of American medicine.

Resources

American Library Association
Public Library Association (c/o)
50 E Huron St, Chicago, IL 60611
800 545-2433   312 944-6780   Fax 312 280-3255

Medical Library Association
6 N Michigan Ave, Ste 300, Chicago, IL 60602
312 419-9094   Fax 312 419-8950
Web address: http://www.kumc.edu/MLA

Special Libraries Association
1700 18th St NW, Washington, DC 20009
202 234-4700   Fax 202 265-9317
E-mail: SLA@CADON.NET
Web address: http://www.sla.org

Licensure

Licensing: what doctors should know

An increasing public awareness and demand for protection, coupled with the growth in the number and sophistication of fraudulent practitioners over the past 14 years, has resulted in stronger and more complex state licensing boards and licensing statutes throughout the country. As might be expected, the rate of change differs widely among the states' licensing boards, depending on each state's resources and Medical Practice Acts as well as on legislative, media, and public expectations. All states, however, have improved dramatically over the decade and will continue to improve, although at different rates.

Within this context, a physician seeking licensure for the first time or in another state should anticipate the possibility of necessary delays for investigation of credentials and past practice, as well as the need to comply with increasingly stringent licensing standards. To assist a physician in the quest for licensure, a rough set of ground rules is provided below. These suggestions obviously will not apply in all cases but generally will help most physicians applying for licensure, as well as benefit the licensing board of the state in which the physician wishes to practice. The ground rules are as follows:

1. When contacting a licensing board for the first time, ask how long it takes to process applications and for a copy of its current licensing requirements. This will provide the physician with a solid idea of when to close an existing practice and/or plan a move, as well as with information about the potential problem areas to be addressed in completing an application.

2. At the initial contact in writing, the physician should provide the licensing board with a resume or curriculum vitae. This will allow a licensing board to evaluate potential problem areas early in the process. In short, the initial contact should be used to develop a set of reasonable expectations about the duration and complexity of the licensing process in a state. A physician who fails to develop appropriate expectations will likely end up frustrated with the licensing process. More important, unreasonable expectations can result in financial jeopardy due to the premature closing of a practice or failure to meet a starting date with an employer in the new state.

3. A physician should never try to hide derogatory information from a licensing board. It is much better to come forward with the information, assist the board in obtaining records and other necessary data, and present the reasons the situation should not result in the denial of the license. Full and frank disclosure of all information requested is by far the best approach to being successfully licensed. A physician should remember that in most states, making a false statement on a license application is grounds for denial or future restriction.

4. A physician who is actively involved in the licensing process often can shorten the length of time it takes to

L get licensed. Personally contacting the medical schools, training programs, and appropriate hospitals and then following up will motivate these institutions to more expeditiously verify credentials. Following up with the licensing boards in other states where the physician holds or has held a license also may assist in shortening the time for licensure. It is important to note that there is a difference between follow-up and overutilization of phone contact, which often delays the processing of requested verification materials, since the physician's application or request may need to be pulled from the "stack" to answer an inquiry. A short note to the organization processing the request for information 30 days after the initial letter or form was mailed may be a better course to follow than frequent phone contact.

5. A physician should not confuse reciprocity with endorsement. In medical licensing, reciprocity has largely become a thing of the past, as most states' legislatures wish to establish their own eligibility criteria and require licensure from a credentialing process based on original documents or direct contact with educational training or licensing boards. Endorsement of the licensing examination scores of another state is really the only form of reciprocity left in medical licensing, and even it has mutated to the point that it can hardly be called endorsement. A physician should be prepared to engage in the gathering and submission of original documents.

6. A wise physician will exercise patience and courtesy in the licensing process. State licensing boards, in most cases, do the best job possible with the resources provided them. The staffs of licensing boards are there to do the best possible job of protecting the public. This requires taking the time necessary to fairly evaluate each application for licensure. (LIC–1996)

Licensure, Examinations

The Federation of State Medical Boards (FSMB) and the National Board of Medical Examiners (NBME) have established a single, three-step examination for licensure in the United States. The United States Medical Licensing Examination (USMLE) provides a commmon evaluation system for applicants for medical licensure. The USMLE has replaced the Federation Licensing Examinations (FLEX) and the NBME Parts I, II, and III.

The USMLE is designed to assess a physician's ability to apply knowledge, concepts, and principles that are important in health and disease and that constitute the basis of safe and effective patient care. The USMLE is a single examination with three steps. Each step is complementary to the others; no step can stand alone in the assessment of readiness for medical licensure. Each USMLE step is composed of multiple choice questions and requires 2 days of testing. Each step is administered twice annually.

Since this article was originally written for the 1989 Edition of *US Medical Licensure Statistics and Current Licensure Requirements,* many innovative changes have occurred to increase cooperation among national and state agencies to expedite the processing of licensure applications. Organizations such as the Federation of State Medical Boards of the United States, the American Medical Association, the National Board of Medical

Examiners, the Educational Commission for Foreign Medical Graduates, and the state medical boards are taking steps toward technological advances with data transmission in order to expedite the sharing of data. Ultimately, this will further reduce delays in processing credentials.

Each of these organizations will allow the quick and necessary exchange of information needed to determine whether physicians meet licensing standards for licensure in participating states.

Both physicians and state licensing boards will soon be able to benefit from a less restrictive flow of data that, in the past, relied on completing similar forms each time a new license or a change in hospital privileges was pursued.

Although a physician may have a perfect and clean track record, those intending to apply should plan for a delay in obtaining a medical license, just to be safe. A 60-day leeway period from the anticipated date of licensure is suggested. For example, if applying for a medical license in State X in April, after talking to everyone in State X, estimate that a license will be granted in July. Starting practice should not even be considered until after September. Just about everyone wants to be licensed between the months of June and August of each year. Physicians with families want to relocate before the academic school year starts for their children; residents want and need licensure to begin practicing in order to pay off loans; contracts with HMOs, IPAs, and PPOs generally start during the summer months, and state employees with school-age children often take their earned vacation time during this period. It is easy to see that state licensing boards experience the highest workload demand from April to September of each year, which also contributes to the increased potential for the delay in processing a license application. It is never too early to begin the process of applying for a state medical license. Don't forget that hospital credentialing and obtaining medical malpractice insurance are based on being fully licensed and that the process may add additional time before a physician can actually practice.

Finally, physicians willing to inform themselves and work cooperatively with a licensing board need not find licensing an unpleasant experience. Members of the medical profession should never forget that the business of licensing boards is to protect the public from unprofessional and incompetent physicians. However, licensing boards also strive to ensure a process that protects the legal rights and privileges of physicians. While maintaining this balance often appears bureaucratic and cumbersome, the end result is improved health care for the people of our country. (LIC–1997)

US Medical Licensure Statistics and Current Licensure Requirements. Chicago, Ill: American Medical Association; 1997; 96 pp
ISBN 0-89970-771-8 OP3999097

Resources

Council on Licensure, Enforcement and Regulation
404 Lafayette Ave, Lexington, KY 40502
606 231-1892 Fax 606 231-1943
E-mail: clear@ukcc.uky.edu

Council of State Government
c/o Phyllis Santos
3560 Iron Works Pike, PO Box 11910
Lexington, KY 40578-1910
800 800-1910   606 244-8000
606 244-8111   Fax 606 244-8001

Federation of State Medical Boards of the
United States, Inc
400 Fuller Wise Rd, Ste 300, Euless, TX 76039-3855
817 868-4000   Fax 817 868-4099
Web address: http://www.fsmb.org

National Board of Medical Examiners
3930 Chestnut St, Philadelphia, PA 19104
215 590-9500   Fax 215 590-9555

Licensure, State

Alabama State Board of Medical Examiners
848 Washington Ave, Montgomery, AL 36102-0946
205 242-4116

Alaska State Medical Board
3601 C St, #722, Anchorage, AK 99503
907 561-2878

Arizona Board of Medical Examiners
2001 W Camelback Rd, Ste 300, Phoenix, AZ 85015
602 255-3751

Arkansas State Medical Board
2100 Riverfront Dr, Ste 200, Harrisburg, AR 72202
501 324-9410

California Medical Board
1426 Howe Ave, Sacramento, CA 95825
916 263-2499

Canal Zone:
Previous holders of a Canal Zone license may obtain
information concerning their license from:
Office of Health and Safety
Panama Canal Commission
APO Miami, FL 34011

Colorado State Board of Medical Examiners
1560 Sherman St, Ste 1300, Denver, CO 80203-1750
303 866-2468

Connecticut Division of Medical Quality Assurance
150 Washington St, Hartford, CT 06106
203 566-7398

Delaware Board of Medical Practice
O'Neil Bldg, 2nd Fl, PO Box 1401, Dover, DE 19903
302 736-4522

District of Columbia Board of Medicine
605 G St NW, Rm 202-Lower Level, PO Box 37200
Washington, DC 20013-7200
202 727-9794

Florida Board of Medicine, Northwood Centre, #60
1940 N Monroe St, Tallahassee, FL 32399-0750
904 488-0595

Georgia Composite State Board of Medical Examiners
166 Pryor St SW, Atlanta, GA 30303
404 656-3913

Guam Board of Medical Examiners
Department of Public Health and Social Services
PO Box 2810, Agana, GU 96910
671 734-7296

Board of Medical Examiners
PO Box 3469, Honolulu, HI 96801
808 586-2708

Idaho State Board of Medicine
State House, 280 N 8th St, Ste 202, Boise, ID 83720
208 334-2822

Illinois Department of Professional Regulation
100 W Randolph, Ste 9-300, Chicago, IL 60601
312 785-0820

Indiana Medical Licensing Board
402 W Washington, Ste 041, Indianapolis, IN 46204
317 232-2960

Iowa State Board of Medical Examiners
State Capitol Complex, Executive Hills West
1209 E Court Ave, Des Moines, IA 50319-0075
515 281-5171

Kansas State Board of Healing Arts
235 SW Topeka Blvd, Topeka, KS 66603-3068
913 296-7413

Kentucky Board of Medical Licensure
310 Whittington Pkwy, Ste 1B, Louisville, KY 40222
502 429-8046

Louisiana State Board of Medical Examiners
830 Union St, Ste 100, New Orleans, LA 70112-1499
504 524-6763

Maine Board of Registration and Medicine
State House Station #137, 2 Bangor St
Augusta, ME 04333
207 287-3601

Maryland State Board of Physician Quality Assurance
4201 Patterson Ave, 3rd Fl, Baltimore, MD 21215
410 764-4777

Massachusetts Board of Registration in Medicine
10 West St, 3rd Fl, Boston, MA 02111
617 727-3086   617 727-3087

Michigan Board of Medicine
611 W Ottawa St, 4th Fl, PO Box 30192
Lansing, MI 48909
517 373-9102

Minnesota Board of Medical Examiners
University Park Plaza
2829 University Ave SE, Ste 400
Minneapolis, MN 55414-3246
612 617-2130   Fax 612 617-2166

Mississippi State Board of Medical Licensure
2688-D Insurance Center Dr, Jackson, MS 39216
601 354-6645

Missouri State Board of Registration of the Healing Arts
3605 Missouri Blvd, PO Box 4
Jefferson City, MO 65102
314 751-0171

Montana Board of Medical Examiners
111 N Jackson, PO Box 200513
Helena, MT 59620-0513
406 444-4284

Nebraska State Board of Examiners in Medicine
& Surgery
301 Centennial Mall S, PO Box 95007
Lincoln, NE 68509-5007
402 471-2115

L

Nevada State Board of Medical Examiners
1105 Terminal Way, Ste 301, PO Box 7238
Reno, NV 89510
702 688-2559

New Hampshire Board of Registration in Medicine
Health and Welfare Bldg, 6 Hazen Dr
Concord, NH 03301
603 271-1203

New Jersey State Board of Medical Examiners
28 W State St, Rm 602, Trenton, NJ 08608
609 292-4843

New Mexico State Board of Medical Examiners
491 Old Santa Fe Trail, Rm 129, PO Box 20001
Santa Fe, NM 87504
505 827-7317

New York State Board for Medicine
Cultural Education Center, Rm 3013
Empire State Plaza, Albany, NY 12230
518 474-3841

North Carolina Board of Medical Examiners
1203 Front St, PO Box 26808
Raleigh, NC 27611-6808
919 828-1212

North Dakota State Board of Medical Examiners
418 E Broadway Ave, Ste 12, Bismarck, ND 58501
701 223-9485

Ohio State Medical Board
77 S High St, 17th Fl, Columbus, OH 43266-0315
614 466-3934

Oklahoma State Board of Medical Licensure and
Supervision
5104 N Francis, Ste C, PO Box 18256
Oklahoma City, OK 73154-0256
405 848-2189

Oregon Board of Medical Examiners
Crown Plaza, 1500 1st Ave, Ste 620
Portland, OR 97201-5826
503 229-5770

Pennsylvania State Board of Medicine
Transportation & Safety Bldg, Ste 612
Harrisburg, PA 17105-2649
717 787-1400

Puerto Rico Board of Medical Examiners
Call Box 13969, Santurce, PR 00908
809 782-8989

Rhode Island Board of Licensure and Discipline
205 Cannon Bldg, 3 Capitol Hill
Providence, RI 02908-5097
401 277-3855

South Carolina State Board of Medical Examiners
1220 Pickens St, PO Box 12245, Columbia, SC 29211
803 731-1650

South Dakota State Board of Medical and
Osteopathic Examiners
1323 S Minnesota Ave, Sioux Falls, SD 57105
605 336-1965

Tennessee Board of Medical Examiners
283 Plus Park Blvd, Nashville, TN 37247-1010
615 367-6231

Texas State Board of Medical Examiners
1812 Centre Creek, Ste 300, Austin, TX 78714-9134
512 834-7728

Utah Physicians Licensing Board
160 E 300 S, PO Box 45802
Salt Lake City, UT 84145-0805
801 530-6511

Vermont Board of Medical Practice
Pavillion Office Bldg, 109 State St
Montpelier, VT 05609-1106
802 828-2673

Virginia Board of Medicine
6606 W Broad St, 4th Fl, Richmond, VA 23230-1717
804 662-9908

Virgin Islands Board of Medical Examiners
48 Sugar Estate, St Thomas, VI 00802
809 776-8311

Washington Board of Medical Examiners
1300 S Quince St, PO Box 47866
Olympia, WA 98504-7866
206 753-2205

West Virginia Board of Medicine
101 Dee Dr, Charleston, WV 25311
304 558-2921

Wisconsin Medical Examining Board
1400 E Washington Ave, PO Box 8935
Madison, WI 53708
608 266-2811

Wyoming Board of Medicine
2301 Central Ave, Ste 208, Barrett Bldg
Cheyenne, WY 82002
307 777-6463

Life Insurance

American Council on Life Insurance
Strategic Research Department
1001 Pennsylvania Ave NW
Washington, DC 20004-2599
800 942-4242   202 624-2000   Fax 202 624-2319

American Academy of Insurance Medicine
c/o Paul R. Bell, MD
2211 Congress St, Portland, ME 04122
207 770-2946

Lipid Diseases

National Lipid Diseases Foundation
1201 Corbin St, Elizabeth, NJ 07201
201 527-8000

Liposuction

American Society of Lipo-Suction Surgery
401 N Michigan Ave, Chicago, IL 60611-4212
312 527-6713   Fax 312 344-1815

American Society of Plastic and
Reconstructive Surgeons
444 E Algonquin Rd, Arlington Heights, IL 60005
847 228-9900   Fax 847 228-9131
Referral Line: 800 635-0635

Literacy

Barbara Bush Foundation for Family Literacy
1002 Wisconsin Ave NW, Washington, DC 20007
202 338-2006   Fax 202 337-6754

Literacy Volunteers of America
5795 Widewaters Pkwy, Syracuse, NY 13214
315 445-8000   Fax 315 445-8006
E-mail: lvanat@aol.com

Literature, Medical

A Piece of My Mind

Keeping up with the literature

Howard Bennett, MD
JAMA 1992 Feb 19; 267(7): 920

When I began my medical education almost 20 years ago, I had no idea what a medical article was. In those days I was a textbook man—a rather plodding fellow who liked his information organized, summarized, and neatly packaged between the covers of a book. The first time I actually saw an article I was sitting in pathology lab looking at a slide of my own blood. In between glances at neutrophils and lymphocytes, my lab partner handed me a copy of an article from a pediatric journal. "What's this?" I asked, glad for the chance to talk to a multicellular organism. "It's an article on CBCs," he said. "Did you know there's a shift to the right with viral infections?" "No," I said rather sheepishly. The only shifting I knew about was shifting dullness, and I had only learned about that the week before. Nevertheless, since ignorance is something medical students learn to live with, I leaned forward with my best "I'm really interested in this" face. "What else does it say?" I queried. "A lot," he said. "I'll copy it for you after class." At which point we went back to looking at doughnut-shaped RBCs, platelets, and the like.

I still remember how excited I was after class. Wow! I thought. So this is what the medical literature is all about. Copying articles and reading stuff that's so new it hasn't made it into the textbooks yet. When we got to the library, I actually felt taller, as though I had traversed some major evolutionary step in an instant. Little did I know, however, that one day I would look back on this afternoon with a somewhat different perspective.

The problem, I learned, is that it is impossible to keep up with the medical literature. This is not the fault of the medical literature itself, but rather of those individuals who keep adding to it as though it were an endangered species. Unfortunately, while most of us cannot keep up with our reading, we all know people who say they can. But is this really true? Are there people out there who do not need to eat or sleep? People who never need to change diapers, attend ballet recitals, or plant azaleas? People who take their journals with them wherever they go?

To settle this issue, I spent the last few years examining the reading habits of all the physicians I know. What I found out is that few physicians actually go to bed with their journals at night (this was a comforting observation). I also discovered that physicians go through stages in their reading just like other areas of development.

And, as we all know, the important thing about developmental stages is finding out whether you are reaching your milestones. Therefore, I have compiled the information I collected into a table for your review. If your reading habits are in sync with the listed categories, you can relax and should no longer feel guilty when you pick up a beer instead of a medical journal. (Remember, older golfers don't hit in the 70s anymore, so why should you?) On the other hand, if you don't "fit" anywhere on the table, perhaps now is the time to take a sabbatical and open up that restaurant you've been talking about all these years.

Bennett's Classification for Reading Medical Articles

Medical Student:	Reads entire article but does not understand what any of it means.
Intern:	Uses journal as a pillow during nights on call.
Resident:	Would like to read entire article but eats dinner instead.
Chief resident:	Skips article entirely and reads the classifieds.
Junior attending:	Reads and analyzes entire article in order to pimp medical students.
Senior attending:	Reads abstracts and quotes the literature liberally.
Research attending:	Reads entire article, reanalyzes statistics, and looks up all references, usually in lieu of sex.
Chief of service:	Reads references to see if he was cited anywhere.
Private attending:	Doesn't buy journals in the first place but keeps an eye open for medical articles that make it into *Time* or *Newsweek*.
Emeritus attending:	Reads entire article but doesn't understand what any of it means.

JAMA Series of Note: Users' guide to the medical literature

I: How to get started. *JAMA* 1993 Nov 3; 270(17): 2093-5

II: How to use an article about therapy or prevention. What were the results and will they help me in caring for my patients? *JAMA* 1994 Jan 5; 271(1): 59-63

III: How to use an article about a diagnostic test. What were the results and will they help me in caring for my patients? *JAMA* 1994 Mar 2; 271(9): 703-7

IV: How to use an article about harm. *JAMA* 1994 May 25; 271(20): 1615-9

V: How to use an article about prognosis. *JAMA* 1994 July 20; 272(3): 234-7

VI: How to use an overview. *JAMA* 1994 Nov 2; 272(17): 1367-71

VII: How to use a clinical decision analysis: (A) Are the results of the study valid? *JAMA* 1995 Apr 26; 273(16): 1292-5

L

VII: How to use a clinical decision analysis: (B) What are the results and will they help me in caring for my patients? *JAMA* 1995 May 24/31; 273(20): 1610-3

VIII: How to use clinical practice guidelines: (A) Are the recommendations valid? *JAMA* 1995 Aug 16; 274(7): 570-574

VIII: How to use clinical practice guidelines: (B) What are the recommendations and will they help you in caring for your patients? *JAMA* 1995 Nov 22/29; 274(20): 1630-1632

IX: A method for grading health care recommendations. *JAMA* 1995 Dec 13; 274 (22): 1800-1804

X: How to use an article reporting variations in the outcomes of health services. *JAMA* 1996 Feb 21; 275 (7): 554-558

XI: How to use an article about clinical utilization review. *JAMA* 1996 May 8; 275(18): 1435-1439

XII: How to use articles about health-related quality of life. *JAMA* 1997 Apr 16; 277(15): 1232 -1237

XIII: How to use an article on economic analysis of clinical practice: (A) Are the results of the study valid? *JAMA* 1997 May 21; 277(19): 1552-1557

XIII: How to use an article on economic analysis of clinical practice: (B) What are the results and will they help me in caring for my patients? *JAMA* 1997 June 11; 277(22): 1802-1806

Editorial

The Second International Congress on Peer Review in Biomedical Publication

JAMA 1994 July 13; 272(2): 91
Drummond Rennie, MD, Annette Flanagin, RN, MA

Editorials represent the opinions of the authors and *The Journal* and not those of the American Medical Association.

In this issue of the *Journal* (272[2]), we publish 26 of the papers presented at the Second International Congress on Peer Review in Biomedical Publication, held in Chicago, Ill, September 9-11, 1993. Of these 26 papers, two, those by Kassirer and Campion[1] and Judson,[2] were invited. The others were submitted in response to a concerted effort we have made during the past eight years to stimulate research into editorial peer review.[3,4]

Given the subject, it is appropriate to comment on the review process used to help select these papers. We received 110 abstracts describing work to be presented at the congress. These were sent to seven independent reviewers (from the United States, Canada, and the United Kingdom) who allotted scores to each abstract; selection was made according to these scores. Thirty-three abstracts (30%) were selected for oral presentation, and 21 abstracts (19%) were presented as posters. Subsequently, the presentations were thoroughly revised for consideration for inclusion in this issue. Thirty-four manuscripts were submitted. Each was sent for review to a wide variety of reviewers (overall, 63 reviewers contributed to this effort, several of whom had not attended the congress). Eight of these papers were rejected after review, and the others were again revised into their current form.

We at *JAMA* have already commented on the vigorous debates that followed each presentation during the congress,[5,6] and others have written about it in the scientific press.[7,8] Our purpose, then, is to tell the readers something about who attended and what they thought of this initiative.

Two hundred seventy-five editors, researchers, and others interested in biomedical publication from 20 countries attended the congress, which was similar to the 283 from 22 countries who attended the first congress in 1989. We have heard from some of our more vocal colleagues that we have been preaching to the choir, and that a self-appointed clique has conducted, presented, and discussed all the research and generated all the controversies that have come out of these two congresses. Irked and intrigued by this possibility, we reviewed the attendance records for each congress. If any such groups had in fact formed, they could only have been drawn from at most a quarter of those who attended the second congress; only 26% of the 1993 participants had attended the first congress.

As we did during the first congress,[9] we asked the participants of the second congress to give us their opinions on a number of subjects related to peer review and the integrity of the publication process by completing precongress and postcongress attitude surveys. Since we did not count the heads of those specifically attending the first and last days of the meeting, we do not know how many registrants actually participated in the congress on each day of the survey. However, from the total number of registrants (275), we calculated minimum response rates of 85% for the initial survey and 68 percent for the final survey. Despite the limitations of this approach, we can still glean a few trends from the replies to the congress surveys. For example, the vast majority of respondents (95% precongress and 92% postcongress) agreed that peer review improves the quality of manuscripts for publication. No other question, except the one asking whether or not to hold another congress, received such high accord.

Two additional questions generated agreement among the respondents before the meeting that became stronger afterward. From the precongress survey, 68% thought journals should adopt more uniform standards for peer review. After the congress, this number increased to 81%. Similarly, the majority of respondents concurred that editors should assist in or encourage research to establish baseline data on the prevalence of scientific fraud (75% precongress and 85% postcongress). While reflecting only moderate agreement, responses to two other questions changed during the meeting. Before the congress, 49% of respondents reported that journals should publish retractions if the research institution, but not the authors, requested it; this number increased to 58% after the congress. Demonstrating a change in the opposite direction, 56% of respondents initially agreed that journals should establish a section for speculative and unconventional work; after the congress, this number decreased to 48%.

As alluded to earlier, 95% of postcongress survey respondents said that we should hold future, regular conferences on editorial peer review. In order to hold another congress, say in four years, we need prospective participants to begin thinking of innovative ways to assess peer review and to set up study protocols, since the whole point of this initiative is to stimulate and present research.

References

1. Kassirer JP, Campion EW. Peer review: crude and understudied, but indispensable. *JAMA*.1994;272:96-97.

2. Judson HF. Structural transformation of the sciences and the end of peer review. *JAMA* 1994;272:92-94.

3. Rennie D. Guarding the guardians: a conference on editorial peer review. *JAMA*.1986;256:2391-2392.

4. Rennie D. Editorial peer review in biomedical publication: the first international congress. *JAMA*.1990;263:1317.

5. Rennie D. More peering into peer review. *JAMA*. 1993;270:2856-2858.

6. Cotton P. Flaws documented, reforms debated at congress on journal peer review. *JAMA*.1993;270:2775-2778.

7. Taubes G. Peer review goes under the microscope. *Science*. 1993;262:25-26.

8. Vanchieri C. Peer review out to the test: credibility at stake. *J Natl Cancer Inst.* 1993;85:1632-1633.

9. Flanagin A, Rennie D, Lundberg G. Attitudes of Peer Review Congress attendees. In: *Peer Review in Scientific Publishing*. Chicago, Ill: Council of Biology Editors; 1991:260-263.

A third congress on international peer review took place in fall 1997.

JAMA Article of Note: Uniform Requirements for Manuscripts Submitted to Biomedical Journals. International Committee of Medical Journal Editors

JAMA 1993 May 5; 269(17): 2282-6

A small group of editors of general medical journals met informally in Vancouver, British Columbia, in January 1978 to establish guidelines for the format of manuscripts submitted to their journals. The group, now expanded and known as the International Committee of Medical Journal Editors (also known as the Vancouver Group), has met annually since then and its concerns have broadened. The committee has produced four editions of the *Uniform Requirements for Manuscripts Submitted to Biomedical Journals;* this fourth edition was revised slightly in January 1993. During discussions of manuscript requirements, questions have been raised about other issues surrounding publication, especially ethics. Some of these concerns are now covered in the *Uniform Requirements;* others are addressed in separate statements issued by the committee. The total content of this communication may be reproduced for educational, not-for-profit purposes without regard for copyright; the committee encourages distribution of the material, which we hope will be useful. Journals that agree to use the *Uniform Requirements* are asked to cite the document in their instructions to authors.

Inquiries and comments should be sent to Secretariat Office, *Annals of Internal Medicine,* Independence Mall West, Sixth St at Race, Philadelphia, PA 19106-1572.

Single copies of *Uniform Requirements for Manuscripts Submitted to Biomedical Journals* are available free of charge from the Secretariat Office. The telephone number is 800 523-1546, ext 2631. Prices for purchases of

10 or more copies are available from the Secretariat Office.

L

Liver Diseases

Poetry and Medicine

44

Richard Donze
JAMA 1997 Mar 26; 277(12): 943

44
and gone after only
one year of the
colon-to-liver
usual yellow alacrity

husband and daughters
stand straight, serene, and smiling
in the receiving line
without pharmacy brain buzz
they welcome other addled 44's to
"the celebration of her rebirth"
saying, "she's an angel now"
and soberly mean every word
as clear-eyed and radiant as
she ever was

looking so all right they
give us space
to indulge self
they comfort our red
swollen eyes not
quite ready to see her or us
with wings and harps at
44

we scramble for meaning and
pretend to find some as
we hiccup around the wake
promising to grab gusto since
life is short when
what we really want are
answers
data

unwilling to accept
random circumstance
we strain to see
something different about her
in genes
or diet
or swallowed stress

something we don't have
or don't do
or won't ever do again

something that will let us
sleep tonight and
work tomorrow
feeling safe at
44

L

Resources

American Association for the Study of Liver Disease
6900 Grove Rd, Thorofare, NJ 08086
609 848-1000   Fax 609 848-5274
E-mail: aasid@siackinc.com

American Liver Foundation
1425 Pompton Ave, Cedar Grove, NJ 07009
800 GO-LIVER   800 223-0179
201 256-2550 (in NJ)   Fax 201 256-3214
Web address: http://sadieo.ucf.edu/alf/alffinal/homepagealf.html

Refer to National Institutes of Health
9000 Rockville Pike, Bethesda, MD 20892
301 496-5787
(Liver transplant status)

Living Will

AMA Policy

Living Wills, Durable Powers of Attorney and Durable Powers of Attorney for Health Care (W-140.985) BOT Rep 00, A-89

The AMA believes that (1) state medical associations should encourage the 40 legislatures that have not enacted a durable power of attorney for health care statute to enact the model state bill adopted by the AMA in 1986; and (2) physicians should encourage their patients to document their wishes regarding the use of life-prolonging medical treatments.

Resources

Advance medical directives: a guide to living wills and powers of attorney for health care. Patient and Physician brochures are available from the AMA.

Choice in Dying—The National Council for the Right to Die
200 Varick St, 10th Fl, New York, NY 10014-4810
800 989-WILL   212 366-5540   Fax 212 366-5337
E-mail: 72420.1653@compuserve.com

Medical Directive
c/o Harvard Medical School Health Letter
164 Longwood Ave, Boston, MA 02115
Medical Directive forms:
($5 for two forms with a self-addressed, stamped envelope)

Loans

The loan application process

A loan officer will request the type of information outlined in the Loan Application Checklist. In addition, some banks may require the applicant to complete the bank's loan application. Once the physician or group has submitted all requested documents, the loan officer will verify the information and evaluate the application. The approval process generally is completed within 1 to 4 weeks after all requested documents are provided.

Loan application checklist

The following checklist indicates the type of information that should be included in the physician's loan application package.

Market and service analysis
New and existing practices include:
- Type of services to be provided
- Market area to be served

New practices, programs, or market include:
- Estimated demand in market area for services to be provided
- Estimated fees for service
- Estimated collection rate
- List of competitors and estimated volume of business provided
- Identification of where patients will come from and how they will be attracted to the practice

Existing practices include:
- Historical volumes and net revenues

Financial information
New and existing practices include:
- Projected income statement for practice (for 1 to 5 years; in some cases, month-by-month projections are suggested for the first year)
- Projected cash flow statement (for 1 to 5 years)
- Projected capital expenditures
- Estimated repayment term

Existing practices include:
- Three years of audited historical financial statements or corporate and personal tax returns

General information
New and existing practices may include:
- Physicians' credentials, including places of education and training
- Credentials of business management, including education and experience
- Personal statement of net worth
- Personal tax returns
- Long-term plans for the business
- Personal and professional references

Conclusion
The requirements to obtain a loan vary from institution to institution. A well-developed business plan will provide a significant portion of the information required by lenders and also will assist the physician or group in realistically evaluating the potential of the practice. In addition, the applicant stands a better chance of getting the loan by appearing fully prepared, since loan application reviews include a subjective component. (FIN-1991)

Resources
National Association of Residents and Interns
292 Madison Ave, New York, NY 10017
800 221-2168   212 949-5900

Physicians beginning practice:
American Professional Practice Association
292 Madison Ave, New York, NY 10017
212 949-5900

Locations for Practice

Checklist for deciding where to practice

Geographic factors:
- Which areas need physicians? How many other doctors practice in the area? What are their specialties? How old are they? Check the local telephone classified directory, and the AMA's *Physician Characteristics and Distribution in the US.*
- Will the town support a physician in your specialty? Where do people go now for the type of medical service you provide? If they go outside the community, will they break existing medical ties to come to you?
- Is the town without a doctor? Why? How long has it been without one and why did the last physician leave?
- What is the trade area? Does the town have a bank, stores, or facilities that will draw people to it? Are there new or recent retail and commercial enterprises?
- Is the area gaining or losing population?
- Is the area prosperous or depressed? Compare per capita income with other areas in the state of similar size.
- What is the tax delinquency rate? Check with the local or county taxing body.
- What are the vacancy rates for apartments and commercial property? Check with the local real estate board.
- Has major industry moved into the area recently, or is it expected?
- Is the local construction industry vigorous, or in a decline?
- Are bank deposits going up or down, and how do they compare with areas of similar population? Your local bank can furnish you with data from the Federal Reserve system.
- Is the local economy subject to seasonal fluctuations or the fortunes of a single company or industry?

Professional factors:
- Can you practice your kind of medicine in this community?
- Can you obtain adequate, well-located, reasonably priced office space with ample parking and transportation facilities?
- If you are associating with another physician or a group, are office facilities well located and well equipped?
- Is there a good hospital? How far from your prospective office?
- Will you be able to obtain hospital privileges?
- Are special diagnostic and therapeutic facilities available in the area?
- Is there a good pharmacy? A good laboratory?
- Are other doctors in the community receptive to your coming?
- Are qualified practitioners in other specialties and subspecialties available for consultation?
- If you're going into solo practice, are there doctors with whom you can share coverage?
- Will allied health personnel be available when you need them?
- Will there be opportunities for continuing medical education and professional growth?
- How do physicians in the area get along together? Will you be able to develop the referral sources you need among other physicians?
- Is there hostility between local hospitals that involves the medical staffs?
- Is the county medical society active, and what level of participation will be expected of you?
- Are nursing homes or other extended care facilities available?

Economic factors:
- Can you make a good living in the area?
- Will living expenses be drastically different from those to which you've been accustomed?
- How do doctors' incomes compare with those of MDs in other similarly populated parts of the state?
- Do doctors' fees seem in line with charges for other services? Have they kept pace or lagged behind?
- Can you rent or buy office space and equip it at a reasonable price?
- Is there good housing, fairly priced?
- How about state and local taxes? Are they in line with income and living costs?
- Will banks or other institutions provide the financial backing you need to set up practice?
- What is the prevailing salary level for medical office personnel?

Personal factors:
- Can you and your spouse live the kind of life you want in the community? Will the rest of your family like living there?
- Will you fit into the community? Religion, ethnic background, and personal lifestyle might be considerations.
- Is good housing available? Are there good schools? Churches, other houses of worship?
- Are there shopping facilities within reasonable distance that offer a range of high-quality goods and services?
- Are there community organizations that interest you?
- Are there congenial people in the area with ages and interests that are similar to those of you and your marriage partner? Will the recreational and cultural outlets meet the needs of yourself and your family? (BUS-1989)

Locum Tenens

More and more medical practices are using locum tenens

"Locum tenens," the Latin term for someone holding a place, has a specific connotation in the medical field. The term has been adapted to physicians who hold temporary positions for other physicians when they must be absent from their practices.

Locum tenens physicians take temporary assignments to fill vacancies in solo practices, on hospital staffs, in group practices, and in managed care organizations. Temporary assignments are both short- and long-term, ranging from 1-week to 1-year commitments. Today, there is a growing demand for locum tenens physicians.

Locum tenens help practices balance workl.... new services in the marketplace. Duri.... patient loads, such as flu season.... practices to balance staffing.... the permanent medica.... additional service.... to test out n....

L acceptance before hiring permanent staff. When new medical centers open, locum tenens can be used to free up the time of the medical directors to concentrate on administrative activities, and to test the market before hiring staff for the demonstrated patient volume.

Checklist for locum tenens recruitment

- If possible, begin the process of recruitment 3 to 4 months in advance.
- Select the prospective candidates you wish to interview.
- Interview candidates over the telephone. Request that candidates submit the necessary documentation and recommendations.
- Verify all credentials.
- Verify that the locum tenens and the medical practice have adequate malpractice coverage.
- Check references.
- Make locum tenens offer and negotiate contract terms.
- Obtain state licensure and malpractice insurance, as needed.
- Arrange for travel and housing, as needed.
- Prepare the practice, hospital, and pharmaceutical staff for the arrival of the locum tenens. Welcome the locum tenens and provide adequate orientation to the practice, hospital, pharmacy, and community.
- Monitor the work of the locum tenens. (LOC-1992)

Lung Diseases

Disorders of the lung

The lungs are continuously exposed to airborne particles, such as bacteria, viruses, and allergens, all of which can cause lungs disorders. Most of these disorders do not interfere with oxygen supply; those that do are a major threat to health.

Infection

Infective disorders are common, especially tracheitis (inflammation of the lining of the windpipe) and croup (a viral infection of young children). Bronchitis (inflammation of the bronchi), bronchiectasis (swelling of the bronchi), and bronchiolitis (inflammation of the bronchioles) commonly follow colds or influenza. Pneumonia (inflammatio᷐ he lung) is usually caused by infection by virus᷐   a. Fungal infections of the lungs, suc᷐   ctinomycosis, histoplasmosis, and ᷐   ᷐v uncommon.

the muscles of the bronchi ᷐ passage of air, often occurs pollens, house mites, ᷐d many other agents. ᷐ the alveoli) may be as moldy hay.

᷐ of all malignant ᷐ cigarette smok- ᷐ve spread ᷐ common.

᷐hest

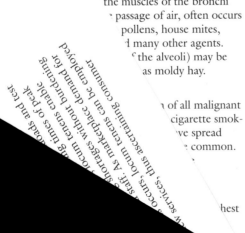

hemothorax (blood in the pleural cavity) are usually caused by a penetrating injury; either may cause collapse of the lung. Injury can also occur from the inhalation of poisonous dusts, gases, or toxic substances. Silicosis and asbestosis are caused by inhalation of silica and asbestos, respectively; they may lead to progressive fibrosis of the lung.

Impaired blood and oxygen supply

The most serious disorder is pulmonary embolism, in which a blood clot formed in one of the major veins breaks free and is carried to the lungs. The clot may block the pulmonary arteries and cause death. Heart failure may cause pulmonary edema, in which the lungs become filled with fluid. Respiratory distress syndrome, which may affect newborn babies or adults, has many causes. In this condition, leakage of fluid into the alveoli seriously interferes with oxygen supply. Emphysema, in which the walls of the alveoli break down so that the area for oxygen exchange is reduced, is frequently seen in people suffering from chronic bronchitis and asthma.

Investigation

Lung disorders are investigated by chest x-ray, bronchoscopy, pulmonary function tests, sputum analysis, blood tests, and physical examination. Sometimes a biopsy of lung tissue is taken for analysis. (ENC-1989)

Resources

American Lung Association
1740 Broadway, New York, NY 10019-4374
212 315-8700   Fax 212 265-5642
Web address: http://www.lungusa.org

LUNGLINE—National Jewish Center for Immunology and Respiratory Medicine
1400 Jackson St, Denver, CO 80206
303 388-4461   Fax 303 270-2165
Web address: http:// www.njc.org/mfhtml/ mflist_subj.html

Lung Associations, Statewide

American Lung Association of Alabama
PO Box 55209, Birmingham, AL 35255
205 933-8821

American Lung Association of Alaska
1057 W Fireweed Ln, Ste 201
Anchorage, AK 99503-1736
907 276-5864   Fax 907 263-2090

Arizona Lung Association
102 W McDowell Rd, Phoenix, AZ 85003
602 258-7505   Fax 602 258-7507

American Lung Association of Arkansas
211 Natural Resources Dr
Little Rock, AR 72205-1539
501 224-5864   Fax 501 224-5645

American Lung Association of California
424 Pendleton Way, Oakland, CA 94621-2189
510 638-5864   Fax 510 638-8984

American Lung Association of Colorado
1600 Race St, Denver, CO 80206-1198
303 388-4327   Fax 303 377-1102

American Lung Association of Connecticut
45 Ash St, East Hartford, CT 06108-3272
800 992-2263   203 289-5401   Fax 203 289-5405

American Lung Association of Delaware
1021 Gilpin Ave, Ste 202, Wilmington, DE 19806
302 655-7258   Fax 302 655-8546

American Lung Association of the District of Columbia
475 H St NW, Washington, DC 20001-2617
202 682-5864   Fax 202 682-5874

American Lung Association of Florida
5526 Arlington Rd, PO Box 8127
Jacksonville, FL 32239-0127
800 940-2933   904 743-2933   Fax 904 743-2916

American Lung Association of Georgia
2452 Spring Rd, Smyrna, GA 30080-3862
404 434-5864   Fax 404 319-0349

American Lung Association of Hawaii
245 N Kukui St, Honolulu, HI 96817
808 537-5966   Fax 808 537-5971

American Lung Association of Idaho
1111 S Orchard, Ste 245, Boise, ID 83705-1966
208 344-6567   Fax 208 345-5896

American Lung Association of Illinois
PO Box 25769, Springfield, IL 62708-2576
217 528-3441   Fax 217 528-9192

American Lung Association of Indiana
9410 Priority Way W Dr, Indianapolis, IN 46240-1470
317 573-3900   Fax 317 573-3909

American Lung Association of Iowa
1025 Ashworth Rd, Ste 410
West Des Moines, IA 50265-6600
800 362-1643   515 224-0800   Fax 515 224-0540

American Lung Association of Kansas
4300 Drury Ln, Topeka, KS 66604-2419
913 272-9290   Fax 913 272-9297

American Lung Association of Kentucky
4100 Churchman Ave, Louisville, KY 40209-0067
502 363-2652   Fax 502 363-0222

American Lung Association of Louisiana
333 St Charles Ave, Ste 500
New Orleans, LA 70130-3180
504 523-5864   Fax 504 523-5867

American Lung Association of Maine
128 Sewall St, Augusta, ME 04330
800 499-5864   207 622-6394   Fax 207 626-2919

American Lung Association of Maryland
1840 York Rd, Ste K-M, Timonium, MD 21093-5156
410 560-2120   Fax 410 560-0829

American Lung Association of Massachusetts
1505 Commonwealth Ave, Brighton, MA 02135-3605
617 787-5864   Fax 617 787-2446

American Lung Association of Michigan
18860 W 10 Mile Rd, Southfield, MI 48075-2689
810 559-5100   Fax 810 559-7434

American Lung Association of Minnesota
490 Concordia Ave, St Paul, MN 55103-2441
612 227-8014   Fax 612 227-5459

American Lung Association Mississippi
353 N Mart Plaza, PO Box 9865, Jackson, MS 39286
800 737-5453   601 362-5453   Fax 601 362-5456

American Lung Association of Eastern Missouri
1118 Hampton Ave, St Louis, MO 63139-3196
314 645-5505   Fax 314 645-7128

American Lung Association of Western Missouri
2007 Broadway, Kansas City, MO 64108-2080
816 842-5242   Fax 816 842-5470

American Lung Association of Montana
Christmas Seal Bldg, 825 Helena Ave
Helena, MT 59601-3459
406 442-6556   Fax 406 442-2346

American Lung Association of Nebraska
7101 Newport Ave, Ste 303, Omaha, NE 68152
402 572-3030   Fax 402 572-3028

American Lung Association of Nevada
619 Ridgeview Ct, Ste 100, PO Box 7056
Reno, NV 89510-7056
702 829-5864   Fax 702 829-5850

American Lung Association of New Hampshire
PO Box 1014, Manchester, NH 03105-1014
603 669-2411   Fax 603 627-9833

American Lung Association of New Jersey
1600 Route 22 E, Union, NJ 07083-3407
908 687-9340   Fax 908 851-2625

American Lung Association of New Mexico
216 Truman Ave NE, Albuquerque, NM 87108
800 221-5864   505 265-0732   Fax 505 260-1739

American Lung Association of New York State
8 Mountain View Ave, Albany, NY 12205-2899
518 459-4197   Fax 518 489-5864

American Lung Association of North Carolina
916 W Morgan St, PO Box 27985
Raleigh, NC 27611-7985
800 892-5650   919 832-8326   Fax 919 856-8530

American Lung Association of North Dakota
212 N 2nd St, PO Box 5004, Bismarck, ND 58502-5004
800 252-6325   701 223-5613   Fax 701 223-5727

American Lung Association of Ohio
1700 Arlingate Ln, Columbus, OH 43228-4102
614 279-1700   Fax 614 279-4940

American Lung Association of Oklahoma
2442 N Walnut, PO Box 53303
Oklahoma City, OK 73152-3303
800 522-8577   405 524-8471   Fax 405 525-6979

American Lung Association of Oregon
Capital Plaza Bldg, 9320 SW Barbur Blvd, Ste 140
Portland, OR 97219-5430
503 246-1997   Fax 503 246-1924

American Lung Association of Pennsylvania
6041 Linglestown Rd, Harrisburg, PA 17112-1208
717 541-5864   Fax 717 541-8828

Asociacion Puertorriquena del Pulmon
PO Box 195247, San Juan, PR 00019-5247
809 765-5664   Fax 809 765-5964

Rhode Island Lung Association
10 Abbott Park Pl, Providence, RI 02903-3700
401 421-6487   Fax 401 331-5266

American Lung Association of South Carolina
1817 Gadsden St, Columbia, SC 29201-2392
800 849-5864   803 779-5864   Fax 803 254-2711

South Dakota Lung Association
208 E 13th St, Sioux Falls, SD 57102-1099
800 873-5864   605 336-7222   Fax 605 336-7227

American Lung Association of Tennessee
1808 West End Ave, Ste 514, Nashville, TN 37203
615 329-1151   Fax 615 329-1723

American Lung Association of Texas
3520 Executive Center Dr, Ste G-100
Austin, TX 78755-0460
512 343-0502   Fax 512 343-0598

American Lung Association of Utah
1930 S 1100 E, Salt Lake City, UT 84106-2317
801 484-4456   Fax 801 484-5461

Vermont Lung Association
30 Farrell St, South Burlington, VT 05403
802 863-6817   Fax 802 863-6818

American Lung Association of the Virgin Islands
PO Box 974, St Thomas, VI 00804
809 774-8620   Fax 809 776-2320

American Lung Association of Virginia
311 South Blvd, PO Box 7065
Richmond, VA 23221-0065
804 355-3295   Fax 804 342-1063

American Lung Association of Washington
2625 Third Ave, Seattle, WA 98121-1213
206 441-5100   Fax 206 441-3277

American Lung Association of West Virginia
415 Dickinson St, PO Box 3980
Charleston, WV 25339-3980
304 342-6600   Fax 304 342-6096

American Lung Association of Wisconsin
150 S Sunny Slope Rd, Ste 105
Brookfield, WI 53005-6461
414 782-7833   Fax 414 782-7834

American Lung Association of Wyoming
c/o American Lung Association Field Services, Planning
and Marketing
1740 Broadway, New York, NY 10019-4374
800 586-4872   212 315-8716   Fax 307 772-6599

Lupus

Lupus Foundation of America, Inc
4 Research Pl, Ste 180, Rockville, MD 20850-3226
800 558-0121   301 670-9292   Fax 301 670-9486
Web address: http://www.lupus.org/lupus

Lyme Disease

Lyme Disease Foundation
1 Financial Plaza, 18th Fl, Hartford, CT 06103
800 886-LYME   203 525-2000   Fax 203 525-8425

Rush Lyme Disease Center
1653 W Congress Pkwy, Chicago, IL 60612
312 942-5963

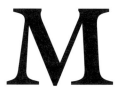

Macular Diseases

Association for Macular Diseases
210 E 64th St, New York, NY 10021
212 605-3719

Magnetic Resonance Imaging

Poetry and Medicine

MRI Scan

David Watts, MD
JAMA 1994 July 27; 272(4): 251

I arrive
in a place of strange
light, the kind
of place that takes away
intelligence.

I am dreamless.
I am made of the same stuff
the walls are made of.

I am a photograph.
The long door,
the closet, empty
in the center where I sit.

They say the magnet
draws particles
from air through the body,
energy that shakes the cells
and makes them cough up
their whereabouts.

I am a tube in a tube
with no exit sign,
a plastic cone
with sides that clack
and groan, my heart
shudders, my bones ache, I
could swear my skin rises
on a bed of crepitations
like tinfoil over Jiffy-Pop.

I can no longer tell
what is real. I imagine
the Van Allen Belt
sucked through my body,
my flesh shimmering like atmospheres
after space wind.

And I wonder
if now the soul
might leave the body
and drift as vapor

over the ordeal of tissues.
But then
the body would be alone.
So I lie still and witness
the dissection of my form.

And like Indians who feared
the photograph, knowing something
is lost there,
I wonder afterwards
if we ever are the same,
ever are,
after anything.

Mammography

Wrong focus for the mammography debate?

Stephanie Stapleton
AM News May 5, 1997 pp 3-4

Only one member of the National Cancer Advisory Board cast a vote against the panel's March 27 mammogram screening recommendations for women ages 40 to 49.

The guidelines, accepted on the same day by the National Cancer Institute, advise that women with average risk factors have screening mammograms every one to two years in their 40s. Women at higher risk should seek expert medical advice about whether to begin screenings even earlier.

But to Kay Dickersin, PhD, the board member who cast the lone dissenting vote, the process was an example of skewed priorities that were not grounded in science.

"I certainly think it is an example of spending energy and dollars in the wrong place," said Dr. Dickersin, an associate professor of epidemiology at the University of Maryland School of Medicine.

The resources, she said, could have been better spent improving preventive care for women over 50, a population for whom there is no scientific debate regarding the benefits of regular mammograms.

Her concerns are echoed by others in the public health community who worry that the national preoccupation over the 40- to 49-year-old age group—and the recent wave of conflicting screening recommendations for that group—do nothing to improve compliance rates among older women.

"I do not criticize anyone in particular regarding the ongoing debate," said Otis Brawley, director of NCI's Office of Special Populations. "I'm not against women in their 40s being screened."

High toll, low compliance

But, he noted, very few people mention the fact that if the proportion of women over 50 who get regular screenings were increased by 15% to 20%, the annual number of lives saved would be far more than those saved by a universal recommendation to begin mammograms at age 40. One third of breast cancer deaths in the over-50 population could be prevented through early detection via mammograms.

About 80% of breast cancers occur in this population, and incidence rates increase as women age past 60, according to National Cancer Information Center statistics.

More than half of these women, however, have not had a mammogram in the last two years—leading to speculation that the current debate reinforces complacency by blurring this message.

"We don't hear that [prevention message] clearly enunciated when we talk about the dispute," said American Cancer Society spokeswoman Lois Callahan, despite the organization's efforts to reiterate the importance of regular screenings for all women.

"Yes, there is a controversy about when to start," said Barbara Levine, director of governmental affairs for the American Public Health Association. "But we better get on with getting women who are 50 and older in for mammograms. There's no debate there, and we're not paying enough attention to doing it."

JAMA Article of Note: Early detection of breast cancer. Council on Scientific Affairs.

JAMA 1984 Dec 7; 252(21): 3008-11

Recommendations:
American College of Radiology
1891 Preston White Dr, Reston, VA 22091
703 648-8900

Cancer Information Service Hotline
800 4CANCER
(FDA certified mammography facilities)

Managed Care

A Piece of My Mind

Back to basics

Phillip Van Swearingen, MD
JAMA 1997 March 19; 277(11): 862

It's like a scene from a movie—one of the old ones. Think in black and white. I'm in bed, propped up a bit on my pillow. The clock downstairs has just gone through its chimes—it's 4 am. The sheer lace curtains that frame the open window hang still, the early evening breeze having gone who knows where, perhaps hushed by the approaching dawn. I can hear the coal train slowly making its way around the bend, down along the edge of the Monongahela River. The sound is carried well on the still night air. The diesel's horn blasts, then dies away into a lonely moan each time the train goes through a crossing. Cardinals let out an occasional chirping note; they are early risers.

Turning slightly to my left I see her, bathed in the moonlight, curled into a peaceful, secure world. On this warm night, her shoulders are bare. I reach out and gently touch her. Her skin is still velvety smooth. She's aged well. One might think the movie scene complete if a cigarette were glowing next to my lips, a ribbon of smoke trailing toward the ceiling. The smoke would silently weave its way through rings that undulated and expanded through moonlit shadows. Afterglow? No. I don't smoke, and I've just come back to bed.

Sighing, I lean over and kiss a soft shoulder and pull the sheet up over her. The response is only a tiny murmur and a subtle shift in position. She did not even know I had left—just before midnight. After 20 years, three or more times a week, she has become immune. I envy her. This time there was a great deal of blood. The melena was constant. The smell still lingers somewhere in my nose, even, I imagine, in my lungs. Each breath I take intensifies the odor. After 2 hours of lavage, eight units of blood, and finally an almost acceptable blood pressure, I found it. It really was not a large ulcer, but it was situated over a significant branch of the pancreaticoduodenal artery, which was erupting viciously with each heartbeat. I murmured a prayer of thanks for the technical wizards who make long slender black tubes, cautery probes, and injector needles as this volcano stopped blowing its top for a second and looked poutingly at me. We knew each other. There was almost a kinship, I thought, as it started to swell. But I was faster. I touched it, then burned it out of existence.

Stepping back, I breathed a sigh of relief. But it was only a short-lived moment, for all the monitor alarms went off, again. It seems we weren't through. The little green blips that lived in the cardiac monitor had decided to do some sort of hectic junctional dance. So—we injected a bolus of this potion and dripped some of that concoction until they were finally whipped back into line, denoting a normal cardiac rate and rhythm.

"Well, what's next?" I asked the nurse. "Murphy's law?" I should have known not to make it sound like a joke. The unit clerk brought me coffee and a lab slip. I should have been wary of her impish smile.

"Do you want sugar in your coffee, Doctor? Your patient seems to have some to spare. See here, her blood glucose level is close to 700. That's just a bit high, isn't it?"

Now, more birds are chirping. It's nearly 5 o'clock. I shouldn't drink coffee at 3 am. At least it's quiet here. But, my thoughts drift back to the bright lights. Her family now is at her bedside. At least, for now, there is good news.

I remember turning to leave as they all stepped close to speak to her. The blood had been cleaned up, everything was neat and orderly again. I stopped and looked at them. No one spoke. No one thanked me. I won't get paid either. Her husband was laid off last year, no new job, no insurance, too proud to apply for Medicaid.

I turned again to leave but glanced back one more time. A small child, perhaps 4 or 5 years old, watched me, tracking my every move. She had been crying, her eyes were puffy. A half-eaten doughnut that one of the nurses had given her was clutched in one hand. Sugar flakes stuck to her cheeks. On impulse I looked directly at her and winked. She fled instantly to her mother and buried her sticky face into the folds of her dress. One eye slowly peeked into view and as she looked to see if I had gone, I winked again. She smiled.

So, now it's 5 am. The alarm clock is unforgiving and the sun is already pinking the sky. It is time to go back. Today there will be more of the same. More contracts to read. HMO this, PPO that. Take this business course to survive. Downsize your practice. Don't you know that medicine is a business now? An insurance company rep on one telephone line tells me I can't give this medication more than once a day, and my patient on the other informs me that if he doesn't take it twice a day, his heartburn is unbearable. My insurance rates are doubling and there are four letters on my desk, each of which has four or more names in the upper left-hand corner. Damn them all.

What will I do? I will think of the little girl. Her smile will be enough for today. Will the feeling last? Probably not. What has happened to the simple satisfaction of a job well done? For saving a life? I hope, at least, that reward will still be there tomorrow. Something has to sustain me.

I'm tired.

Guidelines

For the reasons described in its 1994 report, the AMA Council on Ethical and Judicial Affairs issues the following guidelines: This report was adopted by the House of Delegates of the American Medical Association on June 14, 1994, and subsequently revised in response to comments from the peer reviewers.

1. The duty of patient advocacy is a fundamental element of the physician-patient relationship that should not be altered by the system of health care delivery in which physicians practice. Physicians must continue to place the interests of their patients first.

2. When managed care plans place restrictions on the care that physicians in the plan may provide to their patients, the following principles should be followed:
   a. Any broad allocation guidelines that restrict care and choices that go beyond the cost-benefit judgments made by physicians as a part of their normal professional responsibilities should be established at a policymaking level so that individual physicians are not asked to engage in ad hoc bedside rationing. Regardless of any allocation guidelines or gatekeeper directives, physicians must advocate for any care they believe will materially benefit their patients.
   b. Physicians should be given an active role in contributing their expertise to any allocation process and should advocate for guidelines that are sensitive to differences among patients. Managed care plans should create structures similar to hospital medical staffs that allow physicians to have meaningful input into the plan's development of allocation guidelines. Guidelines for allocating health care should be reviewed on a regular basis and updated to reflect advances in medical knowledge and changes in relative costs.
   c. Adequate appellate mechanisms for both patients and physicians should be in place to address disputes regarding medically necessary care. In some circumstances, physicians have an obligation to initiate appeals on behalf of their patients. Cases may arise in which a health plan has an allocation guideline that is generally fair but in particular circumstances results in unfair denials of care, ie, denial of care that, in the physician's judgment, would materially benefit the patient. In such cases, the physician's duty as patient advocate requires that the physician challenge the denial and argue for the provision of treatment in the specific case. Cases may also arise in which a health plan has an allocation guideline that is generally unfair in its operation. In such cases, the physician's duty as patient advocate requires not only a challenge to any denials of treatment from the guideline but also advocacy at the health plan's policymaking level to seek an elimination or modification of the guideline. Physicians should assist patients who wish to seek additional appropriate care outside the plan when the physician believes the care is in the patient's best interests.
   d. Managed care plans must adhere to the requirement of informed consent that patients be given full disclosure of material information. Full disclosure requires that managed care plans inform potential subscribers of limitations or restrictions on the benefits package when they are considering entering the plan. Physicians also should continue to promote full disclosure to patients enrolled in managed care organizations. The physician's obligation to disclose treatment alternatives to patients is not altered by any limitations in the coverage provided by the patient's managed care plan. Full disclosure includes informing patients of all their treatment options, even those that may not be covered under the terms of the managed care plan. Patients may then determine whether an appeal is appropriate or whether they wish to seek care outside the plan for treatment alternatives that are not covered.
   e. Physicians should not participate in any plan that encourages or requires care at or below minimum professional standards.

3. When physicians are employed or reimbursed by managed care plans that offer financial incentives to limit care, serious potential conflicts are created between the physicians' personal financial interests and the needs of their patients. Efforts to contain health care costs should not place patient welfare at risk. Thus, financial incentives are permissible only if they promote the cost-effective delivery of health care and not the withholding of medically necessary care.
   a. Any incentives to limit care must be disclosed fully to patients by plan administrators on enrollment and at least annually thereafter.
   b. Limits should be placed on the magnitude of fee withholds, bonuses, and other financial incentives to limit care. Calculating incentive payments according to the performance of a sizable group of physicians rather than on an individual basis should be encouraged.
   c. Health plans or other groups should develop financial incentives based on quality of care. Such incentives should complement financial incentives based on the quantity of services used.

4. Patients have an individual responsibility to be aware of the benefits and limitations of their health care coverage. Patients should exercise their autonomy by public participation in the formulation of benefits packages and by prudent selection of health care coverage that best suits their needs.

Glossary of managed care terminology

Administrative costs—Costs related to utilization review, insurance marketing, medical underwriting, agents' commissions, premium collection, claims processing, insurer profit, quality assurance programs, and risk management.

Adverse selection—Among applicants for a given group or individual program, the tendency for those with an impaired health status, or who are prone to higher than average utilization of benefits, to be enrolled in disproportionate numbers and lower deductible plans.

Agency for Health Care Policy and Research (AHCPR)—The agency of the Public Health Service responsible for enhancing the quality, appropriateness, and effectiveness of health care services.

Ambulatory care—Health care services provided on an outpatient basis. No overnight stay in a hospital is required. The services of ambulatory care centers, hospital outpatient departments, physicians' offices, and home health care services fall under this heading.

Beneficiary—Individual who is either using or eligible to use insurance benefits, including health insurance benefits, under an insurance contract.

Benefit payment schedule—List of amounts an insurance plan will pay for covered health care services.

Capitation—A payment system whereby managed care plans pay health care providers a fixed amount to care for a patient over a given period. Providers are not reimbursed for services that exceed the allotted amount. The rate may be fixed for all members or it can be adjusted for the age and gender of the member, based on actuarial projections of medical utilization.

Case management—The process by which all health-related matters of a case are managed by a physician or nurse or designated health professional. Physician case managers coordinate designated components of health care, such as appropriate referral to consultants, specialists, hospitals, ancillary providers, and services. Case management is intended to ensure continuity of services and accessibility to overcome rigidity, fragmented services, and the misutilization of facilities and resources. It also attempts to match the appropriate intensity of services with the patient's needs over time.

Claims review—The method by which an enrollee's health care service claims are reviewed prior to reimbursement. The purpose is to validate the medical necessity of the provided services and to be sure the cost of the service is not excessive.

Closed panel—Medical services are delivered in the HMO-owned health center or satellite clinic by physicians who belong to a specially formed, but legally separate, medical group that only serves the HMO. This term usually refers to group or staff HMO models.

Coinsurance—A cost-sharing requirement under a health insurance policy that provides that the insured will assume a portion or percentage of the costs of covered services. After the deductible is paid, this provision forces the subscriber to pay for a certain percentage of any remaining medical bills, usually 20%.

Community rating—Setting insurance rates based on the average cost of providing health services to all people in a geographic area, without adjusting for each individual's medical history or likelihood of using medical services.

Concurrent review—Review of a procedure or hospital admission done by a health care professional (usually a nurse) other than the one providing the care.

Coordination of benefits (COB)—Provisions and procedures used by third-party payers to determine the amount payable to each payer when a claimant is covered under two or more group health plans.

Copayment—A type of cost-sharing that requires the insured or subscriber to pay a specified flat dollar amount, usually on a per unit of service basis, with the third-party payer reimbursing some portion of remaining charges.

Cost sharing—The general set of financing arrangements whereby the consumer must pay out-of-pocket to receive care, either at the time of initiating care, or during the provision of health care services, or both. Cost sharing can also occur when an insured pays a portion of the monthly premium for health care insurance.

Cost shifting—Charging one group of patients more in order to make up for underpayment by others. Most commonly, charging some privately insured patients more in order to make up for underpayment by Medicaid or Medicare.

Credentialing—The process of reviewing a practitioner's credentials, ie, training, experience, or demonstrated ability, for the purpose of determining if criteria for clinical privileging are met.

Deductible—The out-of-pocket expenses that must be borne by an insurance subscriber before the insurer will begin reimbursing the subscriber for additional expenses.

Diagnosis-related groups (DRGs)—A system used by Medicare and other insurers to classify illnesses according to diagnosis and treatment. All Medicare inpatient hospital operating costs are determined in advance and paid on a per-case basis, according to fixed amount or weight established for each DRG.

Early and periodic screening, diagnosis, and treatment (EPSDT)—EPSDT program covers screening and diagnostic services to determine physical or mental defects in recipients under age 21, as well as health care and other measures to correct or ameliorate any defects and chronic conditions discovered.

Employee Retirement Income Security Act (ERISA)—ERISA exempts self-insured health plans from state laws governing health insurance, including contribution to risk pools, prohibitions against disease discrimination, and other state health reforms.

Exclusions—Clauses in an insurance contract that deny coverage for select individuals, groups, locations, properties, or risks.

Exclusive provider organization (EPO)—A managed care organization that is organized similarly to PPOs in that physicians do not receive capitated payments, but that only allows patients to choose medical care from network providers. If a patient elects to seek care outside of the network, then he or she will not be reimbursed for the cost of the treatment.

Exclusivity clause—A part of a contract that prohibits physicians from contracting with more than one managed care organization (HMO, PPO, IPA, etc).

Experience rating—A system where an insurance company evaluates the risk of an individual or group by looking at the applicant's health history.

Federally qualified HMOs—HMOs that meet certain federally stipulated provisions aimed at protecting consumers, eg, providing a broad range of basic health services, assuring financial solvency, and monitoring the quality of care. HMOs must apply to the federal government for qualification. The process is administered by the Health Care Financing Administration (HCFA), Department of Health and Human Services (DHHS).

Fee disclosure—Physicians and caregivers discussing their charges with patients prior to treatment.

Fee-for-service—The traditional payment method whereby patients pay doctors, hospitals, and other providers for services rendered and then bill private insurers or the government.

Fee schedule—A comprehensive listing of fees used by either a health care plan or the government to reimburse physicians and/or other providers on a fee-for-service basis.

Fiscal intermediary—The agent (eg, Blue Cross) that has contracted with providers of service to process claims for reimbursement under health care coverage. In addition to handling financial matters, it may perform other functions such as providing consultative services or serving as a center for communication with providers and making audits of providers' needs.

Formulary—A list of selected pharmaceuticals and their appropriate dosages felt to be the most useful and cost effective for patient care. Organizations often develop a formulary under the aegis of a pharmacy and therapeutics committee. In HMOs, physicians are often required to prescribe from the formulary.

Gatekeeper—A primary care physician responsible for overseeing and coordinating all aspects of a patient's medical care. In order for a patient to receive a specialty care referral or hospital admission, the gatekeeper must preauthorize the visit, unless there is an emergency.

Group insurance—Any insurance policy or health services contract by which groups of employees (and often their dependents) are covered under a single policy or contract, issued by their employer or other group entity.

Group model HMO—An HMO that contracts with a multispecialty medical group to provide care for HMO members; members are required to receive medical care from a physician within the group unless a referral is made outside the network.

Inpatient services—Inpatient hospital services are items and services furnished to an inpatient of a hospital by the hospital, including bed and board, nursing and related services, diagnostic and therapeutic services, and medical or surgical services.

Health maintenance organization (HMO)—HMOs offer prepaid, comprehensive health coverage for both hospital and physician services. An HMO contracts with health care providers, eg, physicians, hospitals, and other health professionals, and members are required to use participating providers for all health services. Members are enrolled for a specified period of time. Model types include staff, group practice, network, and IPA (for additional information, see staff, group, network, and IPA model definitions).

Health plan employer data and information set (HEDIS)—A set of performance measures designed to standardize the way health plans report data to employers. HEDIS currently measures five major areas of health plan performance: quality, access and patient satisfaction, membership and utilization, finance, and descriptive information on health plan management.

Hold harmless clause—A clause frequently found in managed care contracts whereby the HMO and the physician hold each other not liable for malpractice or corporate malfeasance if either of the parties is found to be liable. Many insurance carriers exclude this type of liability from coverage. It may also refer to language that prohibits the provider from billing patients if their managed care company becomes insolvent. State and federal regulations may require this language.

Indemnify—To make good a loss.

Independent practice association (IPA)—A health maintenance organization delivery model in which the HMO contracts with a physician organization, which, in turn, contracts with individual physicians. The IPA physicians practice in their own offices and continue to see fee-for-service patients. The HMO reimburses the IPA on a capitated basis; however, the IPA usually reimburses the physicians on a fee-for-service basis. This type of system combines prepayment with the traditional means of delivering health care.

Managed care—A general term for organizing doctors, hospitals, and other providers into groups in order to enhance the quality and cost-effectiveness of health care. Managed care organizations include HMOs, PPOs, POSs, EPOs, etc.

Market share—That part of the market potential that a managed care company has captured; usually market share is expressed as a percentage of the market potential.

Medical group practice—The American Group Practice Association, the American Medical Association, and the Medical Group Management Association define medical group practice as: "provision of health care services by a group of at least three licensed physicians engaged in a formally organized and legally recognized entity sharing equipment, facilities, common records, and personnel involved in both patient care and business management."

Medically necessary—Those covered services required to preserve and maintain the health status of a member or eligible person in accordance with the area standards of medical practice.

Multispecialty group—A group of doctors who represent various medical specialties and who work together in a group practice.

National Committee for Quality Assurance (NCQA)—A nonprofit organization created to improve patient care quality and health plan performance in partnership with managed care plans, purchasers, consumers, and the public sector.

Network model HMO—An HMO that contracts with two or more independent group practices to provide health services. This type may include a few solo practices but is primarily organized around groups.

Open enrollment—A period of time in which eligible subscribers may elect to enroll in, or transfer between, available programs providing health care coverage.

Outcomes management—A clinical outcome is the result of medical or surgical intervention or nonintervention. It is thought that through a database of outcomes experience, caregivers will know better which treatment modalities result in consistently better outcomes for patients. Outcomes management may lead to the development of clinical protocols.

Outlier—One who does not fall within the norm; term typically used in utilization review. A provider who uses either too many or too few services (eg, anyone whose utilization differs two standard deviations from the mean on a bell curve is termed an "outlier").

Out-of-area benefits—The coverage allowed to HMO members for emergency situations outside of the prescribed geographic area of the HMO.

Outpatient services—Medical and other services provided by a hospital or other qualified facility, such as a mental health clinic, rural health clinic, mobile X-ray unit, or freestanding dialysis unit. Such services include outpatient physical therapy services, diagnostic X-ray, and laboratory tests.

Participating provider—A health care provider who participates through a contractual arrangement with a health care service contractor, HMO, PPO, IPA, or other managed care organization.

Peer review—A review by members of the profession ("peers") regarding the quality of care provided a patient, including documentation of care (medical audit), diagnostic steps used, conclusions reached, therapy given, appropriateness of utilization (utilization review), and reasonableness of charges/claims.

Performance standards—Standards an individual provider is expected to meet, especially with respect to quality of care. The standards may define volume of care delivered per time period. Thus, performance standards for obstetrician/gynecologist may specify some or all of the following: office hours and office visits per week or month, on-call days, deliveries per year, gynecological operations per year, etc.

Point-of-service plan (POS)—Also known as an open-ended HMO, POS plans encourage, but do not require, members to choose a primary care physician. As in traditional HMOs, the primary care physician acts as a "gatekeeper" when making referrals; plan members may, however, opt to visit non-network providers at their discretion. Subscribers choosing not to use the primary care physician must pay higher deductibles and copays than those using network physicians.

Practice parameters—Defined by the American Medical Association as strategies for patient management, developed to assist physicians in clinical decision making. Practice parameters may also be referred to as practice options, practice guidelines, practice policies, or practice standards.

Preadmission review—The practice of reviewing claims for inpatient admission prior to the patient's entering the hospital to ensure that the admission is medically necessary.

Preferred provider organization (PPO)—Health care arrangement between purchasers of care (eg, employers, insurance companies) and providers that provides benefits at a reasonable cost by providing members incentives (such as lower deductibles and copays) to use providers within the network. Members who prefer to use nonpreferred physicians may do so, but only at a higher cost. Preferred providers must agree to specified fee schedules in exchange for a preferred status and are required to comply with certain utilization review guidelines.

Preauthorization—A method of monitoring and controlling utilization by evaluating the need for medical service prior to its being performed.

Quality assurance (QA)—Activities and programs intended to ensure the quality of care in a defined medical setting. Such programs include peer or utilization review components to identify and remedy deficiencies in quality. The program must have a mechanism for assessing its effectiveness and may measure care against preestablished standards.

Risk—The chance or possibility of loss. For example, physicians may be held at risk if hospitalization rates exceed agreed-upon thresholds. The sharing of risk is often employed as a utilization control mechanism within the HMO setting. Risk is also defined in insurance terms as the possibility of loss associated with a given population.

Risk pool—A pool of money that is to be used for defined expenses. Commonly, if the money that is put at risk is not expended by the end of the year, some or all of it is returned to those managing the risk.

Staff model HMO—An HMO that delivers health services through a physician group that is controlled by the HMO unit; most physicians are salaried employees who deal exclusively with HMO members.

Self-insurance—The practice of an employer or organization assuming responsibility for health care losses of its employees. This usually includes setting up a fund against which claim payments are drawn and claims processing is often handled through an administrative services contract with an independent organization.

Stop loss—That point at which a third party has reinsurance to protect against the overly large single claim or the excessively high aggregate claim during a given period of time. Large employers, who are self-insured, may also purchase "reinsurance" for stop-loss purposes.

Tertiary care—Subspecialty care usually requiring the facilities of a university-affiliated or teaching hospital that has extensive diagnostic and treatment capabilities.

Third-party—Administrator or individual or company that contracts with employers who want to self-insure the health of their employees. They develop and coordinate self-insurance programs, process and pay the claims and may help locate stop-loss insurance for the employer. They also can analyze the effectiveness of the program and trace the patterns of those using the benefits.

Usual, customary and reasonable (UCR)—Health insurance plans that pay a physician's full charge if it is reasonable and does not exceed his or her usual charges and the amount customarily charged for the service by other physicians in the area.

Utilization review (UR)—Also known as utilization management or utilization control, utilization review is a systematic means for reviewing and controlling patients' use of medical care services as well as the appropriateness and quality of that care. Usually involves data collection, review, and/or authorization, especially for services such as specialist referrals, emergency room use, and hospitalization.

Utilization—The patterns of use of a service or type of service within a specified time. Utilization is usually expressed in rate per unit of population-at-risk for a given period (eg, the number of hospital admissions per year per 1000 persons enrolled in an HMO).

Withhold—That portion of the monthly capitation payment to physicians withheld by an HMO to create an incentive for efficient care. A physician who exceeds utilization norms does not receive the withheld amount. This system serves as a financial incentive for lower utilization. The withhold can cover all services or be specific to hospital care, laboratory usage, or specialty referrals. (TMA)

JAMA Theme Issue: Managed care

JAMA 1995 Jan 5 273(4).

Issue includes the AMA's CEJA report on the ethical issues present in a managed care environment (see above), plus editorials and an discussion of the patient-physician relationship.

Resources

American Association of Health Plans
1129 20th St NW, Ste 600, Washington, DC 20036
202-778-3200
Web address: http://www.aahp.org

Management

American Management Association
1601 Broadway, New York, NY 10019-7420
212 586-8100   Fax 212 903-8168

National Institute for Health Care Management
1225 19th St NW, Ste 710, Washington DC, 20036
202 296-4426   Fax 202 296-4319
E-mail: nihcm@aol.com
Web address: http://www.NIHCM.org

Management Services Organization (MSO)

An organization established to relieve the physicians of the administrative duties of running a practice while allowing them to retain ownership of their patient charts and records. The organization is set up by physicians, a hospital, or an independent party and furnishes services to a professional corporation of physicians for a monthly service fee.

There can be an exclusive contract with one professional corporation or a contract with more than one professional corporation. The physicians in the professional corporation can be independent contractors, employees, or partners in the corporation. The patient charts typically are retained by the physicians unless the physicians are employees of the corporation.

Most MSOs of not-for-profit hospitals are for-profit subsidiaries. It is hard to qualify an MSO as not-for-profit. Two examples of MSOs are Alta Bates MSO in Berkeley, Calif, and Mullikan Medical Group in Orange County, Calif. (MMCMP-1996)

Marijuana, Medical

What can you tell patients about pot? Calif. society releases guidelines; AMA pushes for clinical trials

Stephanie Stapleton
AM News Apr 7, 1997 p3

The California Medical Assn. has released guidelines to help physicians understand what they can and cannot tell patients about marijuana's potential therapeutic uses.

Meanwhile, the AMA is continuing to push for controlled clinical trials on marijuana's medical efficacy to generate the scientific data needed to formulate national public policy.

"What's at issue is state law and how it relates to federal law," said AMA Senior Health Counsel Bruce Blehart.

Released March 14, the CMA guidelines detail specific information physicians should provide to patients when asked about medical marijuana—including scientific evidence of potential risks and benefits, the lack of controlled clinical trials supporting such evidence, other patients' experiences, and the fact that, even if used for medical purposes, marijuana remains an illegal substance under federal law.

The guidelines also recommend that details of such conversations be documented in each patient's medical record.

CMA developed these parameters to quell confusion stemming from last November's election in which voters approved a state law legalizing marijuana for medical purposes if recommended by a doctor.

Voters in Arizona approved a similar proposal in November, but California has been center stage so far as the debate plays out.

Because marijuana remains a controlled substance under federal law, federal officials responded to the ballot

M

initiatives by threatening punitive action against physicians who prescribe pot to their patients.

At the urging of the AMA and the CMA, the Dept. of Justice and Dept. of Health and Human Services issued a clarification letter Feb. 27 to medical societies nationwide explaining that no gag rule exists on a physician's ability to discuss with patients marijuana's alleged medical benefits and health risks. Physicians cannot, however, recommend its use or take steps to help patients obtain it.

"We agreed with that legal standard," said Alice Mead, CMA legal counsel. The guidelines spell out what compliance to that standard involves.

However, the CMA's guidelines also may add a new wrinkle to a lawsuit filed in December by a group of California physicians.

The suit seeks to block federal officials from taking punitive actions against doctors who recommend the use of medical marijuana to their patients.

Although the plaintiffs view the guidelines as "a significant step in the right direction," a legal settlement is unlikely unless the federal government "commits" to them by assuring that doctors who follow the guidelines will not be prosecuted—a step it has so far not taken, said Graham Boyd, the physicians' attorney.

Without such an assurance, the positions outlined in the government's clarification letter could be changed, he said.

The CMA did not intend the document to play this role in the legal proceedings. Rather, the guidelines were intended as an information source for California physicians and do not require the federal government's approval, explained Mead.

The plaintiffs, however, will continue to seek a legally binding court order or regulatory mechanism, Boyd said.

Although neither the AMA nor the CMA is involved in the court action, the two organizations cosigned a letter March 14 to the Justice Dept. and the plaintiffs encouraging them to stop court proceedings.

"The government's [clarification] letter, particularly in conjunction with such [CMA] guidelines, appears to us to address the concerns expressed in the current lawsuit," the letter states.

"There is no assurance that a court opinion will be any more specific or protective of the patient-physician relationship; indeed, it could be less so," it continues.

The CMA and AMA also reiterated the federal government's bottom line: Though physicians may discuss the use of marijuana with patients, they cannot, under federal law, help them to obtain marijuana by providing written or oral recommendations for cannabis buyers' clubs, as outlined in the ballot proposal approved in November.

The two groups also emphasized that clinical trials, not ballot initiatives, are the proper venue by which marijuana's therapeutic efficacy should be determined.

To move toward this goal, the AMA will ask the National Institutes of Health to implement a set of specific policies to encourage clinical research on marijuana use for patients with conditions for which the bulk of anecdotal evidence suggests possible efficacy.

Though NIH is on record pledging fair evaluations of these types of research proposals, the AMA is concerned that such submissions, if channeled through the normal peer review process, may not receive scores sufficient to warrant funding and to obtain marijuana from the National Institute of Drug Abuse.

The AMA further recommends that NIH:
- Provide information to researchers on how they can incorporate marijuana into institutional review board and clinical research protocols.
- Earmark a pool of funds for medical marijuana research.
- Establish a special NIH review section for marijuana research.

How to 'talk pot' safely

The CMA recommends that physicians follow these guidelines in discussing "medical marijuana" with patients:
- Provide scientific evidence that reflects both the potential risks and benefits of marijuana for the patient's condition.
- Try to answer questions about risks and benefits while making clear that marijuana has not been fully tested in controlled clinical trials.
- Describe experiences of other similarly situated patients who have used marijuana.
- Counsel on possible ways to balance the risks and benefits, while also advising that you cannot lawfully recommend marijuana.
- Warn that, regardless of the new state law, cultivation, possession, and use of marijuana for any reason is illegal under federal law.
- State that you cannot take any action to enable a patient to obtain marijuana—including cooperating with a cannabis buyers' club, issuing a written marijuana "recommendation" as a potential legal defense, or offering in advance to testify for the patient in court.

Marketing

American Marketing Association
250 S Wacker Dr, Ste 200, Chicago, IL 60606
312 648-0536   Fax 312 993-7542

American Society for Healthcare Marketing & Public Relations
c/o American Hospital Association
1 N Franklin, Chicago, IL 60606
312 422-3737   Fax 312 422-4579

Marketing Research Information:
FIND SVP
625 Avenue of the Americas, New York, NY 10011
212 645-4500

Marriage

Today's medical marriage, Part 1

Wayne M. Sotile, PhD, Mary O. Sotile, MA
JAMA 1997 Apr 16; 277(15): 1180c

Based on insights gleaned from our 30 combined years of counseling physicians, we have found that married physicians with positive marital relationships cope better, remain more productive, and are happier overall than residents whose marriages are foundering.

Half of all medical students marry during medical school or residency training,[1] and more than 60% divorce within 10 years of completing residency training.[2] Approximately half of physicians claim that work-related stress contributes to discord in their marriages. Compared with other professionals, resident physicians are at special risk for work-related maladies that can lead to marital problems. Specifically, residents work longer hours, have more difficulty winding down after work,[3] suffer sleep deprivation, tend to be too tired to participate in social or leisure activities, and develop a form of learned helplessness when it comes to managing time.

This is not news. For years we have appreciated the uphill battle medical couples fight against work-related stress. The news is that the high-powered people physicians are now marrying bring their own brand of work-driven problems to the medical-related stressors.

While couples enter a medical marriage knowing that career demands will interfere, problems occur when partners become disillusioned with the reality of their marriage. If partners in a medical marriage can dispense with the notion that their lives will be well balanced, they will have overcome a critical hurdle. The expectation of having a thriving career, a loving family life, an especially intimate relationship, and sufficient personal time raises an impossible standard.

Residents who marry can either put their marriage on hold or try to find time to devote to the relationship. Couples who find the time have a better chance of keeping their marriage alive.[4] However, they must fully realize that this stage of their lives will be skewed by the excessive work commitments of both mates. Instead of harboring feelings of resentment toward each other, couples can increase the likelihood of sustaining their marriage by recognizing the heroic efforts each one makes to be together during what is often a time of extraordinary stress, challenge, and loneliness.

Overall, medical training is not a time for growth in a marriage; it is a time for personal survival without, one hopes, damaging the relationship. The analogy we suggest when working with couples, one or both of whom is a resident physician, is to think of themselves as if they were "on point" in a war zone, that is, in the lead position that bears the highest risk and stress of battle formation, and alter their expectations and dealings with each other accordingly. Quality-of-life concerns are not foremost in this setting; recognizing this helps couples realize that their reactions to their spouses are not due to their having married the wrong person but are normal reactions to excessive stress.

We remind partners in a resident physician marriage that just a small amount of change in the way you cope during these years can make a big difference in whether you keep your marriage alive. Relationships are shaped by the partners' most consistent behavioral and coping patterns. In our book, *The Medical Marriage: A Couple's Survival Guide*,[5] we elaborate on our clinical observations and discuss the effects a variety of coping habits can have on both a one- and two-physician marriage and outline strategies for effective emotional management.

References

1. Myers MF. Overview: the female physician and her marriage. *Am J Psychiatry*. 1984;141:1386-1391.

2. Marchand WR, Palmer CA, Gutmann L, Brogan WC. Medical student impairment: a review of the literature. *W V Med J*. 1985;81:244-248.

3. Arnetz BB. White collar stress: what studies of physicians can teach us. *Psychother Psychosom*. 1991;55:197-200.

4. Gabbard GO, Maninger RW. The psychology of postponement in the medical marriage. *JAMA*. 1989;261:2378-2381.

5. Sotile WM, Sotile MO. *The Medical Marriage: A Couple's Survival Guide*. New York, NY: Birch Lane Press, 1996.

Today's medical marriage, Part 2

Wayne M. Sotile, PhD, Mary O. Sotile, MA
JAMA 1997 Apr 23/30: 277(16); 1322

Maintaining harmony in a marriage is a challenge for any resident, but it proves to be especially difficult for female physicians. As we discussed in part 1 of this series, the high-powered people whom physicians marry bring their own kinds of work-driven problems that compound the stressors related to physician training. Ninety percent of female physicians marry men who are in occupations of the same status level, and 50% marry other physicians.[6] In contrast, only 20% of male physicians marry women of equal occupational status.[7] In a two-physician marriage, the woman is twice as likely to shape her career to accommodate her husband's career than if she is married to a nonphysician.[8] In other words, married female residents are much more likely than married male residents to experience career-related stress that can strain a marriage.

Another factor contributing to the challenges facing married female resident physicians involves child bearing and rearing. Since last reported, 68% of teaching hospitals had no formal policy offering maternity leave[9] and of the 32% that did, maternity leave averaged only two to six weeks.[10] More than 40% of female resident physicians who take maternity leave report they encounter hostility from their superiors and colleagues.[11] Yet, despite their demanding careers, virtually all women physicians oversee child care and household responsibilities.[12] One solution that would ease the burden of resident physician couples wanting to start a family during residency training would be for programs to institute part-time residencies and leave-of-absence policies for male and female physicians who want to raise a family. Until such changes occur, we counsel resident couples to postpone starting a family until after residency training, if possible.

The multiple roles required by married female resident physicians, that of spouse, physician-in-training, mother, and primary caregiver, promote a chronic hurriedness that fuels type A behavior, which female physicians are far more likely to develop than their male colleagues or than women in general.[13] Type A behavior can be particularly damaging to a marriage, especially when it is expressed through excessive work involvement. It is important that couples become aware of how type A behavior affects their marriage and learn to identify and modify such behavior.[14]

Many of the physician couples we have counseled have successfully negotiated the many obstacles that medical families encounter; some have not. Success requires both

M partners to maintain realistic expectations and a commitment to working together to manage the professional and relationship stresses that can imperil their marriage.

References

6. Gross EB. Gender differences in physician stress. *J Am Med Wom Assoc.* 1992;47:107-114.

7. Uhlenberg P, Cooney TM. Male and female physicians: family and cancer comparisons. *Soc Sci Med.* 1990;30:373-378.

8. Johnson CA, Johnson BE, Liese BS. Dual-doctor marriages: career development. *Fam Med.* 1992;24:205-208.

9. Silva BM. Pregnancy during residency: a look at the issues. *J Am Med Wom Assoc.* 1992;47:71-74.

10. Lenhard SA. Physician mothers: a conceptual model for planning and coping with motherhood and medical practice. *J Am Med Wom Assoc.* 1992;47:87-93.

11. Sayres M, Wyshak GF, Denterlein G, et al. Pregnancy during residency. *N Engl J Med.* 1986;314:418-423.

12. Tesch BJ, Osborne J, Simpson D, Murray SF, Spiro J. Women physicians in dual-physician relationships compared with those in other dual-career relationships. *Acad Med.* 1992;67:542-544.

13. Smith DF, Sterndorff B. Female physicians outscore male physicians and the general public on type A scales in Denmark. *Behav Med.* Winter 1991/1992;17:184-189.

14. Sotile WM, Sotile MO. *The Medical Marriage: A Couple's Survival Guide.* New York, NY: Birch Lane Press, 1996.

Resource

American Association of Marriage and Family Therapy
1100 17th St NW, 10th Fl, Washington, DC 20036
202 452-0109   Fax 202 223-2329

Massage Therapy

American Massage Therapy Association
820 Davis St, Ste 100, Evanston, IL 60201-4444
847 864-0123   Fax 847 864-1178

Matching Program

National Resident Matching Program
2450 N St NW, Ste 201
Washington, DC 20037-1141
202 828-0676

Residents who were not matched:
Neurology/Psychiatry
American Psychiatric Association
202 682-6000   Fax 202 682-6114

Obstetrics and Gynecology
American College of Obstetricians and Gynecologists
202 638-5577   Fax 202 484-8107

Otolaryngology
American Academy of Otolaryngology—Head and Neck Surgery
703 836-4444   Fax 703 683-5100

Plastic Surgery
University of Louisville
502 588-6880

All others, contact appropriate specialty society.

Maternal and Child Care

National Center for Education in Maternal and Child Health
2000 15th St N, Ste 701
Arlington, VA 22201-2617
703 524-7802   Fax 703 524-9335
E-mail: ncemch01@gumedlibdml.georgetown.edu

Maxillofacial Surgery

Oral and Maxillofacial Surgeon. Alternate title: oral surgeon. Performs surgery on mouth, jaws, and related head and neck structure. Executes difficult and multiple extraction of teeth. Removes tumors and other abnormal growths. Performs preprosthetic surgery to prepare mouth for insertion of dental prosthesis. Corrects abnormal jaw relations by mandibular or maxillary revision. Treats fractures of jaws. Administers general and local anesthetics. May treat patients in hospital. (DOT-1991)

Resource

American Society of Maxillofacial Surgeons
444 E Algonquin Rd, Arlington Heights, IL 60005
847 228-9900   Fax 847 228-6509

Mayo Clinic

Obituary

Mayo, Charles Horace 1865-1939
JAMA 1939 Jun 3; 112(22): 2342

Charles Horace Mayo, noted as a surgical genius, a great medical administrator, and a genial physician, died in Chicago of pneumonia May 26. The younger of the two world-famed Mayo brothers was born in Rochester, Minn., July 19, 1865, the son of William Worrall Mayo and Louise Wright Mayo. After an education in the Rochester high school and at the Niles Academy he attended Chicago Medical College, later known as Northwestern University, and received his degree in medicine in 1888. As a young boy he began, almost from childhood, to live in a medical atmosphere and to become inspired toward medicine as a career. After his graduation in medicine he returned to Rochester, where his urge toward research and his surgical genius led to innumerable investigations in medicine and in surgery. His first published statement entitled "Report of Clinic in St. Mary's Hospital, Rochester, Minnesota, January 19, 1891," was published in the Northwest *Lancet* in November of that year. From that time on hardly a year passed without a contribution by either Dr Charles H. Mayo alone or with his brother, or with some of the younger men who soon became attracted to them. These contributions cover every phase of medicine and surgery and in later years embrace as well the fields of philosophy, economics, and statesmanship.

In the field of scientific medical organizations Dr Charles H. Mayo was president of the Western Surgical Association in 1904, the Minnesota State Medical Association in 1905, the Society of Clinical Surgery in 1911, the Clinical Congress of Surgeons of North America in 1914, the American Medical Association in 1916, the American College of Surgeons in 1924, the American Surgical

Association in 1931 and the Minnesota Public Health Association from 1932 to 1936.

Dr William J. Mayo, Dr Charles Horace Mayo, and their distinguished father made a small village become one of the most notable medical centers of the world. Throughout their careers these distinguished leaders devoted themselves to the advancement of organized medicine. The medical society of the county in which they practiced was founded by Dr William Worrall Mayo. Dr Charles H. Mayo was widely known not only as a surgical genius, as a great surgical teacher, as an inspired organizer, as a leader in medical advancement and as a citizen of his city, county, state, and of the nation, but also as a warm-hearted, genial, faithful, true humanitarian, easily approachable, unostentatious, ready to trade wits and banter, always in the most kindly and sympathetic manner. Such men come but infrequently in any civilization and their places are not easily filled as the world moves on.

In 1915 Drs William J. and Charles H. Mayo established the Mayo Foundation for Medical Education and Research in Rochester, affiliating this organization with the University of Minnesota. Their first contribution was $1,500,000, which has now been increased to more than $2,650,000. In order to perpetuate this institution, the Mayo Properties Association was established in 1919 to hold all the property, endowments, and funds of the Mayo Clinic and to insure the permanence of the institution for public understanding that the moneys and property can never inure to the benefit of any individual.

Obituary

Mayo, William James 1861-1939
JAMA 1939 Aug 5; 113(6): 524

Dr William J. Mayo, former president of the American Medical Association, recognized throughout the world as a brilliant surgeon, a great organizer, and an esteemed leader in the field of medicine, died at his home in Rochester, Minn, July 28, at age 78; an operation for a perforating ulcer of the stomach had been performed April 22. But a few months have passed since the death of the younger of the two brothers, Dr Charles H. Mayo. Their careers were inseparable. Their passing this life so closely together was no doubt as they might have wished it.

The career of Dr William J. Mayo will be fully recorded in many biographies in which space will be available for proper consideration of its many facets. Since the 16th century, the Mayo family has been one closely associated with science. The father of the two boys, Dr William Worrall Mayo, was born in Manchester, England, May 31, 1819; after training as a physicist and chemist he came to the United States in 1845. In 1847 he removed to Lafayette, Ind., where he studied medicine with Dr Eleazar Deming. He then completed his medical studies in the University of Missouri and graduated in 1854. After practicing briefly in Laporte, Ind, Dr William Worrall Mayo removed to Minnesota, settling eventually in Rochester in 1863, where he was in charge of the draft board during the Civil War. The father of these boys was himself a competent surgeon, one of the first physicians in the West to use the microscope, founder of the Minnesota State Medical Association and its president in 1873. Dr William Worrall Mayo died in Rochester in 1911. He and Mrs William Worrall Mayo had three daughters and two sons.

The elder son, William James Mayo, was born in LeSueur, Minn, June 29, 1861. The family moved to Rochester when he was slightly more than one-and-a-half years old. The boy attended the public school and the high school in Rochester and thereafter spent 1 year in a private school for languages and science and 2 years in Nile's academy. During their youth, both William and Charles accompanied their father on his rounds and had an opportunity to observe both surgical operations and postmortem examinations. For a time, both clerked in the drugstore. With their father they learned to use the microscope. In 1880, William J. Mayo went to the University of Michigan, Ann Arbor, and completed a 3-year course which had just been established to replace the former 2-year medical course. In his medical education Dr William J. Mayo had an opportunity to be associated with the anatomist Ford and with Victor C. Vaughan, and his training in surgery was under Donald McLean, then professor of surgery. When he was 22, Dr William J. Mayo completed his medical studies in the university and received his degree.

From 1889 until 1905, the Drs Mayo carried on their work in St. Mary's Hospital in Rochester, an institution which they, with their father, had aided in establishing and one which is now known throughout the world largely because of their work. The record of surgical procedures performed indicate an early tendency toward selection of abdominal surgery by Dr Will, leaving many of the other fields to Dr Charles. As Dr Will himself said, "Charlie soon had me driven to cover by being a better surgeon, and I began to specialize in abdominal work and in operations on the ureters and kidneys." As the repute of their work spread, they soon began to associate with themselves younger men who had shown special predilection for surgical work, the first to be selected being Dr E. Starr Judd, who had charge of the third operating room in 1905. From that time on, the surgical developments in Rochester were so rapid that additional wings continued to be added to the hospital, an annex was opened and additional hospitals were built. As it became apparent that internal medicine and diagnosis, with the work of the laboratory, would be of prime importance, these developments were particularly encouraged. Throughout the record of the growth and development of this monumental institution to the proud position which it now occupies signs of the leadership of Dr William J. Mayo appear again and again. Early in his career Dr Will conceived the idea of a permanent endowed institution in Rochester to be connected with a university. He elaborated the concept of the Mayo Foundation and he gave freely of himself, of his funds and of his life for its perpetuation.

Dr William J. Mayo became associated early with medical organizations. He served as president of his county and state medical associations. He was chairman of the Section on Surgery and Anatomy of the American Medical Association, 1898-1899, and President of the American Medical Association, 1906-1907. He was also president of the American Surgical Association, of the American College of Surgeons, of the Congress of American Physicians and Surgeons, and of the Inter-State Postgraduate Medical Association of North America.

In 1915, Drs William J. and Charles H. Mayo donated $1,500,000 to establish the Mayo Foundation for Medical Education and Research in Rochester in affiliation with the University of Minnesota. In 1919 the brothers formed the Mayo Properties Association to hold all the properties, endowments and fund of the Mayo Clinic to insure the permanence of the institution for public service. Again in 1934 the Mayo Properties Association presented a gift of $500,000 to the University of Minnesota, making a total of $2,800,000 that the brothers had given to the Mayo Foundation. In sending this contribution, Dr William J. Mayo wrote, in part:

"Our father recognized certain definite social obligation. He believed that any man who had better opportunity than others; greater strength of mind, body, or character, owed something to those who had not been so provided; that is, that the important thing in life was not to accomplish for oneself alone, but for each to carry his share of collective responsibility....The fund which we had built up and which had grown far beyond our expectations had come from the sick, and we believed that it ought to return to the sick in the form of advanced medical education, which would develop better-trained physicians, and to research to reduce the amount of sickness....The people's money, of which we have been the custodians, is being irrevocably returned to the people from whom it came.... The practice of medicine in Rochester is carried on in the same manner as by other members of the regular medical profession throughout the state and nation. All classes of patients, without regard to race or creed, social or financial standing, receive necessary care without discrimination...."

These words reflect the great character, the human kindliness, the profound human sympathy that were part of Dr William James Mayo. It has been said that opportunity and great occasions make great men. Exception to this rule is present in the lives of Drs William J. and Charles H. Mayo. They made a small village into one of the most notable medical centers of the world wholly through a genius for surgery and for medical leadership. Throughout their careers they devoted themselves to the advancement of scientific medicine and of the medical profession which they served so nobly and which gloried so greatly in their achievements.

In 1906, when Dr William J. Mayo read his presidential address to the American Medical Association, he forecast and considered some of the great problems that concern medical practice today. He attacked abuses of medical care by public service corporations and the abuses of medical charity by those able to pay. He condemned all attempts by those not trained in the science and art of medicine to dominate its functions. To the very end he contended for this point of view. And in a note written just a few days before his death, he urges continued work for the advancement and stabilization of medical science and the traditions of medical practice.

All the world pauses in the midst of its turmoil and stress to give him honor and to pay him in his death the tribute that is so justly his due—a great physician, a superb surgeon, a magnificent leader, a beloved man!

Resource

Mayo Clinic
200 First St SW, Rochester, MN 55905
507 282-2511

Medicaid

Medicaid at 30: new challenges for the nation's health safety net (excerpt)

JAMA 1995 July 19; 274(3): 271-273

Since its enactment in 1965, Medicaid has been on the front lines in meeting the health needs of our nation's most vulnerable populations. It has evolved from the companion legislation to Medicare that provided health financing to states for coverage of their welfare population, to a program that now finances health and long-term care services for one in eight Americans. In its 30 years, Medicaid has enabled millions of low-income Americans to gain access to needed health services, helping to close the gaps in care between the poor and nonpoor, ease financial burdens, and provide a safety net for the most needy Americans.[1]

Today, Medicaid's role as a health insurer and safety net for vulnerable Americans is visible throughout the health care system. Medicaid finances care for one in four American children, pays for one third of the nation's births, assists 60% of people living in poverty, pays for half of all nursing home care, and accounts for 13% of all health care spending.[2,3] It is the source of insurance for 13% of the nonelderly population and supplements Medicare by paying premiums and cost sharing for one in 10 elderly and disabled Medicare beneficiaries.[4] Its funding is the major source of federal financial assistance to the states, accounting for 40% of all federal grant-in-aid payments to states.[5]

As it enters its 30th year, Medicaid is at a critical juncture. In its role as a medical safety net, Medicaid financed care for over 32 million of the poorest, sickest, and most disabled Americans at a cost of over $125 billion to federal and state governments in 1993.[6] As the number of Americans without health insurance continues to grow, Medicaid's role as the insurer of low-income Americans is particularly important. Expansions in Medicaid coverage of the low-income population over the last decade has mitigated the growth in America's uninsured population and has been the cornerstone of virtually all state health care system reform activities.[7]

But Medicaid has been a victim of its own success. At the same time as the program was broadening its reach in providing health insurance to the poor and becoming the mainstay of financing for long-term care, spending was rapidly rising. A doubling of program costs over the last 5 years has raised new questions about the ability of the federal and state governments to sustain such growth.

Proposals to restructure the program to limit federal spending, promote broadened use of managed care, and give states additional flexibility over program design are now under active consideration. Some proposals would convert the program from an entitlement that guarantees coverage to all eligible individuals, to a block grant providing states with federal funds for indigent care and few or no requirements on how those funds are used. By the end of its 30th year, Medicaid could be dramatically reshaped with a substantially reduced federal role and new responsibilities for states.

References

1. Rowland D, Feder J, Lyons B, Salganicoff A. *Medicaid at the Crossroads.* Washington, DC: The Kaiser Commission on the Future of Medicaid; November 1992.

2. Holahan J, Winterbottom C, Rajan S. *The Changing Composition of Health Insurance Coverage in the United States.* Washington, DC: The Kaiser Commission on the Future of Medicaid; January 1995.

3. Levit K, Sensenig A, Cowan C, et al. National health expenditures, 1993. *Health Care Financ Rev.* 1994;16:247-294.

4. Employee Benefit Research Institute. *Sources of Health Insurance and Characteristics of the Uninsured: Analysis of the March 1994 Current Population Survey.* Washington, DC: Employee Benefit Research Institute; February 1995.

5. National Association of State Budget Officers. *1993 State Expenditure Report.* Washington, DC: National Association of State Budget Officers; March 1994.

6. The Kaiser Commission on the Future of Medicaid. *Health Needs and Medicaid Financing: State Facts.* Washington, DC: The Kaiser Commission on the Future of Medicaid; April 1995.

7. Rowland D. Directions for health reform. Testimony before Senate Committee on Labor and Human Resources; March 15, 1995.

The Medicaid Program is a medical assistance program jointly financed by state and federal governments for eligible low-income individuals. Medicaid covers health care expenses for all recipients of Aid to Families With Dependent Children, and most states also cover the needy elderly, blind, and disabled who receive cash assistance under the Supplemental Security Income Program. Coverage also is extended to certain infants and low-income pregnant women and, at the option of the state, other low-income individuals with medical bills that qualify them as categorically or medically needy. (USG-1996)

Medicaid Offices, Statewide

Alabama Medicaid Agency
PO Box 5624
Montgomery, AL 36103-5624
334 242-5000   Fax 334 240-5097

Alaska Department of Health and Social Services
Division of Public Assistance
Alaska Office Bldg, Rm 309, PO Box 110640
Juneau, AK 99811-0610
907 465-2845   Fax 907 586-1877

Arizona Department of Economic Security
Division of Aging and Community Services
801 E Jefferson, Phoenix, AZ 85034
602 417-4000

Arkansas Department of Human Services
Division of Economic and Medical Services
Office of Economic Services
Section of Income Support
Donaghey Plaza S, PO Box 1437, Slot 100
Little Rock, AR 72203-1437
501 682-8292   Fax 501 682-1197

California Health and Welfare Agency
Department of Health Services
Medical Care Services
714 P St, #1253, Sacramento, CA 95814
916 657-5173   Fax 916 657-1156

Colorado Department of Human Services
Health Care Policy and Financing Division
1575 Sherman St, 8th Fl, Denver, CO 80203-1714
303 866-5678   Fax 303 866-4214

Connecticut Department of Social Services
Health Care Financing Division
25 Sigourney St, Hartford, CT 06106
203 424-5053   Fax 203 424-5129

Delaware Department of Health and Social Services
Division of Social Services, Medicaid Unit
1901 N Du Pont Hwy, New Castle, DE 19720
302 577-4900   Fax 302 577-4510

District of Columbia Department of Human Services
Social Services Commission Medicaid Unit
Income Maintenance Administration
645 H St NE, Washington, DC 20002
202 724-5035   Fax 202 727-1687

Florida Agency for Health Care Administration
Medicaid Office
2728 Ft Knox Blvd, Tallahassee, FL 32308
904 488-3560   Fax 904 488-0043

Georgia Department of Medical Assistance
2 Peachtree St NW, Atlanta, GA 30303
404 656-6359

Hawaii Department of Human Services
Medical QUEST Division
PO Box 339, Honolulu, HI 96809-0339
808 586-5390   Fax 808 586-4890

Idaho Department of Health and Welfare
Medicaid Division
450 W State St, 2nd Fl, PO Box 83720
Boise, ID 83720-0036
208 334-5747   Fax 208 334-6558

Illinois Department of Public Aid
Medicaid Programs Division
100 S Grand Ave E, 3rd Fl, Springfield, IL 62762
217 782-1214   Fax 217 785-5095

Indiana Family and Social Services Administration
Medicaid Policy and Planning Office
402 W Washington, Rm 341
Indianapolis, IN 46204
317 233-4455   Fax 317 233-4693

Iowa Department of Human Services
Medical Services Division Medicaid Program
Hoover State Office Bldg, Des Moines, IA 50319
515 281-8621   Fax 515 281-7791

Kansas Department of Social and
Rehabilitation Services
Adult/Medical Services Commission
915 SW Harrison, Topeka, KS 66612
913 296-3981   Fax 913 296-4813

Kentucky Human Resources Cabinet
Department for Medicaid Services
275 E Main St, Frankfort, KY 40621
502 564-4321   Fax 502 564-3232

Louisiana Department of Health and Hospitals
Services Financing Bureau
PO Box 91030, Baton Rouge, LA 70821-9030
504 342-5774

Maine Department of Human Services
Medical Services Bureau
Medicaid Policy and Program Division
State House, Sta 11, Augusta, ME 04333
207 287-3799   Fax 207 287-2675

Maryland Department of Health and Mental Hygiene
Medical Care Policy Administration
Medical Care Finance and Compliance Division
201 W Preston St, 2nd Fl, Baltimore, MD 21201
410 255-1582   Fax 410 333-5520

Massachusetts Executive Office of Health and
Human Services
Medical Assistance Division
600 Washington St, Boston, MA 02111
617 348-8400   Fax 617 348-8575

Michigan Department of Social Services
Medical Services Administration
Medicaid Operations Bureau
400 S Pine St, PO Box 30043
Lansing, MI 48909
517 335-5453   Fax 517 335-5007

Minnesota Department of Human Services
Health Care Administration Health Care
Strategies Division
444 Lafayette Rd, St Paul, MN 55155-3853
612 297-4113   Fax 612 282-9922

Mississippi Office of the Governor
Medicaid Division
PO Box 136, Jackson, MS 39215
601 359-6050   Fax 601 359-3741

Missouri Department of Social Services
Medical Services Division
0615 Howerten Ct, PO Box 6500
Jefferson City, MO 65109
314 751-3425   Fax 314 751-6564

Montana Department of Social and
Rehabilitation Services
Medicaid Services Division
PO Box 4210, Helena, MT 59604
406 444-4540

Nebraska Department of Social Services
Medical Services Division
301 Centennial Mall S, 5th Fl, PO Box 95026
Lincoln, NE 68509
402 471-9118   Fax 402 471-9449

Nevada Department of Human Resources
Medicaid Welfare Division Program
2527 N Carson St, Carson City, NV 89710
702 687-4354   Fax 702 687-5080

New Hampshire Department of Health and
Human Services
Human Services Division
Medical Services Bureau
6 Hazen Dr, Concord, NH 03301
603 271-4353   Fax 603 271-4727

New Jersey Department of Human Services
Medical Assistance and Health Services
Division Medical Care Administration
7 Quakerbridge Plaza, CN 712
Trenton, NJ 08625-0712
609 588-2611

New Mexico Department of Human Services
Medical Assistance Division
PO Box 2348, Santa Fe, NM 87504-2348
505 827-3100   Fax 505 827-6286

New York State Department of Social Services
Health and Long Term Care Division
40 N Pearl St, Albany, NY 12243
518 474-9132

North Carolina Department of Human Resources
Medical Assistance Division
PO Box 29529, Raleigh, NC 27626-0529
919 733-2060   Fax 919 733-6608

North Dakota Department of Human Services
Medical Services Division
600 E Blvd, State Capitol, 3rd Fl, Bismarck, ND 58505
701 328-2321   Fax 701 328-2359

Ohio Department of Human Services
Division of Claims Processing
Medicaid Services Bureau
30 E Broad St, 32nd Fl, Columbus, OH 43266-0423
614 644-0410   Fax 614 466-2815

Oklahoma Health Care Authority
4545 N Lincoln Blvd, Ste 124
Oklahoma City, OK 73125
405 530-3439   Fax 405 530-3405

Oregon Department of Human Resources
Medical Assistance Program Office
500 Summer St NE, Salem, OR 97310-1013
503 945-5772   Fax 503 373-7689

Pennsylvania Department of Public Welfare
Medical Assistance Office
Health and Welfare Bldg, PO Box 2675
Harrisburg, PA 17105
717 787-1870   Fax 717 772-2062

Rhode Island Department of Human Services
Medical Services Division
600 New London Ave, Cranston, RI 02920
401 464-3575   Fax 401 464-3350

South Carolina Health and Human Services Department
Medicaid Program
Health Services Bureau
1801 Main St, PO Box 8206
Columbia, SC 29202-8206
803 253-6100   Fax 803 253-4137

South Dakota Department of Social Services
Program Management Division
Medical Services Office
Kneip Bldg, 700 Governors Dr, Pierre, SD 57501
605 773-3495   Fax 605 773-4855

Tennessee Department of Finance and Administration
Teencare
729 Church St, Nashville, TN 37247-6501
615 741-0192   Fax 615 741-0882

Texas Department of Health Care Financing Division
Managed Care Bureau
1100 W 48th St, Austin, TX 78756
512 794-6838   Fax 512 338-6945

Utah Department of Health
Health Care Financing Division
Medicaid Policy and Planning Bureau
PO Box 14290, Salt Lake City, UT 84114-6478
801 538-9925   Fax 801 538-6478

Vermont Agency for Human Services
Social Welfare Department, Medicaid Division
State Complex, 103 S Main St
Waterbury, VT 05671-1201
802 241-2880   Fax 802 241-2830

Virginia Department of Health and Human Resources
Social Services Department Benefits Program Division
730 Broad St, Richmond, VA 23219-1849
804 642-1740   Fax 804 692-1949

Washington Department of Social
and Health Services
Medical Assistance Services
PO Box 45500, Olympia, WA 98504-5500
360 753-1777   Fax 360 586-5874

West Virginia Department of Health
and Human Resources
Human Resources Bureau Income Maintenance Office
State Capitol Complex, Bldg 6, Rm B-617
Charleston, WV 25305
304 558-8290   Fax 304 558-1008

Wisconsin Department of Health and Social Services
Health Division
Health Care Financing Bureau
PO Box 7850, Madison, WI 53707-7850
608 266-2522   Fax 608 267-2832

Wyoming Department of Health
Health Care Financing Division
Minimum Medical Program
117 Hathaway Bldg, Cheyenne, WY 82002-0710
307 777-7821   Fax 307 777-7439

Contact state or local Department of Public Aid.

Medical Assistant

Locating a medical assistant

There are many ways to find and hire a competent medical office assistant. It's important to select the right assistant, particularly if a physician is just starting a practice. An inexperienced or inefficient assistant could prove an expensive investment at a time when the physician can least afford financial mistakes. It is suggested that physicians do the following:

1. Check with the local medical society for possible job candidates; many run formal or informal placement services for such employees.

2. Contact the local chapter of the American Association of Medical Assistants (AAMA) for suggestions. It has chapters in nearly all states today.

3. Get in touch with schools in the area with accredited training programs for medical assistants and medical secretaries, whose graduates may be seeking positions. Some run rotating externship programs in physicians' offices.

4. If schools offering specialized training programs are not operating locally, call community college placement offices, other secretarial schools, or high schools to inquire about possible good applicants.

5. Talk with other physicians; they may know of suitable applicants.

6. Call the local hospital(s) personnel department for leads.

7. Get assistance in locating good job candidates when using a professional management consultant to help launch a practice.

8. Ask detail people and medical supply sales people if they know of assistants coming onto the job market.

9. Utilize the services of personnel agencies.

10. Advertise in local newspapers and professional journals. (BUS–1989, adaptation)

Medical Assistants

History

Since its founding in 1956, the American Association of Medical Assistants (AAMA) has been the only professional association devoted exclusively to the profession of medical assisting. The American Medical Association (AMA), an early supporter of the AAMA, still provides assistance, in recognition of the AAMA's important role in improving the educational preparation and continuing education opportunities for the medical assistant.

The first certification examination was administered in 1963, preceding the establishment of the accreditation program. In 1966, the AAMA began work on formal curriculum standards in collaboration with the AMA. A task force of physicians and medical assistants surveyed existing medical assistant programs and drew up tentative standards, which were adopted in 1969. About 3 years were spent in laying a solid groundwork for a 2-year associate degree program. In 1971, after 2 years of actual accreditation activity, the initial standards were revised to allow for the accreditation of 1-year educational programs.

Occupational description

Medical assisting is a multiskilled allied health profession; practitioners work primarily in ambulatory settings such as medical offices and clinics. Medical assistants function as members of the health care delivery team and perform administrative and clinical procedures.

Job description

Medical assistants are allied health professionals who assist physicians in their offices or other medical settings. In accordance with respective state laws, they perform a broad range of administrative and clinical duties, as indicated by the 1990 *Developing a Curriculum* (DACUM) occupational analysis.

Administrative duties include scheduling and receiving patients, preparing and maintaining medical records, performing basic secretarial skills and medical transcription, handling telephone calls and writing correspondence, serving as a liaison between the physician and other individuals, and managing practice finances.

Clinical duties include asepsis and infection control, taking patient histories and vital signs, performing first aid and CPR, preparing patients for procedures, assisting the physician with examinations and treatments, collecting and processing specimens, performing selected diagnostic tests, and preparing and administering medications as directed by the physician.

Both administrative and clinical duties involve maintenance of equipment and supplies for the practice. A medical assistant who is sufficiently qualified by education and/or experience may be responsible for supervising personnel, developing and conducting public outreach programs to market the physician's professional services, and participating in the negotiation of leases and of equipment and supply contracts.

Employment characteristics

More medical assistants are employed by practicing physicians than any other type of allied health personnel. Medical assistants are usually employed in physicians' offices, where they perform a variety of administrative and clinical tasks to facilitate the work of the physician. The responsibilities of medical assistants vary, depending on whether they work in a clinic, hospital, large group practice, or small private office. With a demand from more than 200,000 physicians, there are, and will probably continue to be, almost unlimited opportunities for formally educated medical assistants.

According to the AAMA, the average entry-level salary in 1995 was $18,000. (AHRP-1997)

Resources

AMA Division of Allied Health
312 553-9355

American Association of Medical Assistants
20 N Wacker Dr, Ste 1575, Chicago, IL 60606-2903
800 228-2262   312 899-1500   Fax 312 899-1259

Medical Associations

American Medical Association
515 N State St, Chicago, IL 60610
312 464-5000   Fax 312 464-4184
Web address: http://www.ama-assn.org

American Medical Women's Association
801 N Fairfax St, Ste 400, Alexandria, VA 22314
703 838-0500   Fax 703 549-3864

Australian Medical Association
42 Macquarie St
Barton, ACT (Australian Capital Territory) 2600
(06) 270-5400   Fax (06) 270-5499

British Medical Association
BMA House, Tavistock Square
London WC1H 9JP, England
171 387-4499   Fax 171 383-400

Canadian Medical Association
1867 Alta Vista Dr, Box 8650, Ottawa, Ontario K1G 3Y6
613 731-9331   Fax 613 731-9013
Web address: http://www.cna.ca

Christian Medical and Dental Society
PO Box 5, Bristol, TN 37321-0005
423 844-1000   Fax 423 844-1005
E-mail: 75364.331@compuserve.com

National Medical Association
1012 10th St NW, Washington, DC 20001
202 347-1895   Fax 202 842-3293

Pan American Medical Association
c/o Frederic C. Fenig, MD
745 5th Ave, Ste 403, New York, NY 10151
212 753-6033   Fax 212 308-6847

Royal College of Physicians
11 St Andrew's Pl, London NW1 4LE, England
171 935-174   Fax 171 487-218

Royal College of Surgeons
35-43 Lincoln's Inn Fields, London WC2A 3PN, England
171 405-474   Fax 171 831-438   TX 936573 RCSENG

Southern Medical Association
35 Lake Shore Dr, PO Box 190088
Birmingham, AL 35219-0088
205 945-1840
Web address: http://www.sma.org

World Medical Association
(Association Medicale Mondiale—AMM)
28, Ave des Alpes, F-01210 Ferney-Voltaire, France
50-40-7575   Fax 50-40-5937

Medical Illustration

Medical Illustrator

History

Formal educational programs for the medical illustrator date back to the early 1900s, with Max Broedel's school at Johns Hopkins University. The Association of Medical Illustrators (AMI) was established in 1945. Under the auspices of the AMI, standards were developed by which the organization has accredited medical illustration programs in this country since 1967.

In 1986, the AMI expressed a desire to have educational programs for the medical illustrator accredited by the Committee on Allied Health Education and Accreditation (CAHEA) of the American Medical Association (AMA). This desire stemmed from the recognition that professional medical illustrator programs were more closely related to allied health than to the visual arts.

An Ad Hoc Committee on Outside Accreditation of the AMI worked with staff of the AMA Division of Allied Health Education and Accreditation to modify the existing standards to comply with the format recommended by the CAHEA. The resulting *Essentials and Guidelines of an Accredited Educational Program for the Medical Illustrator* were adopted by the AMI and the AMA Council on Medical Education (CME) in 1987. Revised standards were adopted by the AMI and the AMA in 1992. Today, the standards are adopted by the Commission on Accreditation of Allied Health Education Programs (CAAHEP) in collaboration with the AMI.

Occupational description

The term "medical illustrator" applies to competent professionals in the discipline of medical illustration. Medical illustrators create visual material designed to facilitate the recording and dissemination of medical, biological, and related knowledge. The medical illustration profession not only embraces production of such material, but also functions in an administrative, consultive, and advisory capacity. Medical illustration employs a variety of artistic techniques, ranging from drawing, painting, sculpting, layout, design, and typography to computer graphics and electronic imaging.

With a strong foundation in biological sciences, anatomy, physiology, pathology, and general medical knowledge, combined with a high degree of proficiency in the visual arts, medical illustrators are able to depict subjects with extreme accuracy and realism or to interpret and reduce a complex idea to a simple explanatory diagram or schematic concept.

Job description

Through the medical graphics they create, medical illustrators are communicators and teachers. Although some medical illustrators specialize in a single art medium or confine their interest to one of the medical specialties, the majority handle an ever-changing variety of assignments. They work with many different media to produce the highly accurate and authentic illustrations used in the publication of medical books, journals, films, videotapes, exhibits, posters, wall charts, and computer programs. Materials prepared by medical illustrators may also be used for projection in the classroom or for professional group presentations.

A medical illustrator may also work as a member of a research team to provide illustrations or to participate directly in the research problem. Some specialize in preparing prosthetics or in preparing models for instructional purposes.

In addition to the production of graphics and three-dimensional works, medical illustrators may serve as producers/directors or designers in the development of instructional programs. They may also organize and administer biomedical communication centers or illustration services at major teaching hospitals, health science centers, or elsewhere.

Employment characteristics

The majority of medical illustrators are employed by medical schools and large medical centers that conduct teaching and research programs. Others are in private, state, and federal hospitals, clinics, and dental and veterinary schools. Many work independently on a freelance basis for medical publishers, pharmaceutical houses, and advertising agencies, in commercial settings, or for lawyers. Medical illustrators with appropriate background and professional experience are qualified to direct an illustration service unit or a biomedical communication center.

Entry level salaries for graduates of medical illustration schools range from $27,000 to $35,000. Experienced medical illustrators can earn an average of anywhere from $35,000 to $100,000. (AHRP-1997)

Resources

AMA Allied Health Department
312 553-9355

*Accreditation Review Committee for the
Medical Illustrator:*
CAAHEP
515 N State St, Ste 7530
Chicago, IL 60610-4377
312 464-4636

Association of Medical Illustrators
1819 Peachtree St NE, Ste 620
Atlanta, GA 30309
404 350-7900   Fax 404 351-3348

Medical Practice Acts

Code of Alabama
Title 34; Chapter 24: Physicians and Other Practitioners of the Healing Arts
sections 34-24-1 through 34-24-406

Alaska Statutes
Title 8; Chapter 64: Medicine
sections 08.64.010 through 08.64.380

Arizona Revised Statutes Annotated
Title 32; Chapter 13: Medicine and Surgery
sections 32-1401 through 32-1491

Arkansas Code of 1987 Annotated
Title 17; Chapter 93: Physicians and Surgeons
sections 17-93-101 through 17-93-505

West's Annotated California Codes
Division 2; Chapter 5: Medicine
sections 2.5.2000 through 2.5.2505

Colorado Revised Statutes
Title 12; Article 36: Medical Practice
sections 12-36-101 through 12-36-139

General Statutes of Connecticut
Title 20; Chapter 370: Medicine and Surgery
sections 20-8 through 20-14k

Delaware Code Annotated
Title 24; Chapter 17: Medical Practices Act
sections 1701 through 1795

District of Columbia Code
Title 2; Chapter 33: Health Occupations
sections 2-3301.0 through 2-3312.1

West's Florida Statutes Annotated
Title 32; Chapter 458: Medical Practice
sections 458.001 through 458.349

Official Code of Georgia Annotated
Title 43; Physicians, Physicians Assistants and Respiratory Care
sections 43-34-1 through 43-34-151

Hawaii Code Annotated
Title 25; Chapter 453: Medicine and Surgery
sections 453-1 through 453-33

Idaho Code
Title 54; Chapter 18: Physicians and Surgeons
sections 54-1801 through 54-1841

Smith Hurd Illinois Compiled Statutes Annotated
Medical Practice Act
Act 60/1 through 60/63

Burns Indiana Statues Annotated
Title 25; Article 22.5: Medicine, Physicians Surgeons and Osteopaths
sections 25-22.5-1-1.1 through 25-22.5-8-4

Code of Iowa
Title 4; Chapter 148: Medicine and Surgery
sections 148.1 through 148.13

Kansas Statutes Annotated
Chapter 65; Article 28: Healing Arts
sections 65-2801 through 65-28,122

Kentucky Revised Statutes
Title 26; Chapter 311: Physicians, Osteopaths and Podiatrists: Practice of Medicine and Osteopathy
sections 311.010 through *311.620*

Louisiana Statutes
Title 37; Chapter 15: Physicians, Surgeons, Osteopaths, and Midwives
sections 37:1261 through 37:1360.38

Maine Revised Statutes
Title 32; Chapter 48: Board of Licensure in Medicine
sections 3263 through 3300

Annotated Code of Maryland
Health Occupations: Title 14: Physicians
sections 14-101 through 14-702

Annotated Laws of Massachusetts
Title XVI; Chapter 112: Registration of Physicians and Surgeons
sections 112:2 through 112:12H

Michigan Statutes Annotated
Title 14; Part 170: Medicine
sections 14.15(17001) through 14.15(17088)

Minnesota Statutes Annotated
Chapter 147: Board of Medical Practice
sections 147.01 through 147.36

Mississippi Code Annotated
Title 73, Chapter 25: Physicians
sections 73-25-1 through 73-25-95

Revised Statutes for the State of Missouri
Title XXII; Chapter 334: Physicians and Surgeons, Therapists, Athletic Trainers—Health Care Providers
sections 334.010 through 334.748

Montana Code Annotated
Title 37; Chapter 3: Medicine
sections 37-3-101 through 37-3-405

Revised Statutes of Nebraska
Chapter 71: Practice of Medicine and Surgery
sections 71-1,102 through 71-1,107.30

Nevada Revised Statutes Annotated
Title 54; Chapter 630: Physicians and Assistants
sections 630-003 through 630-411

New Hampshire Revised Statutes Annotated
Title XXX; Chapter 329: Physicians and Surgeons
sections 329:1 through 329:31

New Jersey Statutes
Title 45; Chapter 9: Medicine and Surgery
sections 45:9-1 through 45:9-58

New Mexico Statutes of 1978 Annotated
Chapter 61; Article 6: Medicine and Surgery
sections 61-6-1 through 61-6-35

McKinney's Consolidated Laws of New York Annotated
Book 16, Title 8; Article 131: Medicine
sections 6520 through 6529

General Statutes of North Carolina
Chapter 90; Article 1: Practice of Medicine
sections 90-1 through 90-21.21

North Dakota Century Code Annotated
Title 43; Chapter 43-17: Physicians and Surgeons
sections 43-17-01 through 43-17-42

Page's Ohio Revised Code Annotated
Title 47; Chapter 4731: Physicians
sections 4731.01 through 4731.99

Oklahoma Statutes
Title 59; Chapter 11: Medicine
sections 481.1 through 536.11

Oregon Revised Statutes
Title 52; Chapter 677: Regulation of Medicine, Podiatry and Related Medical Services
sections 677.010 through 677.419

Purdon's Pennsylvania Statutes Annotated
Title 63; Chapter 12: Physicians and Surgeons
sections 422.1 through 422.45

General Laws of Rhode Island
Chapter 37: Board of Medical Licensure and Discipline
sections 5-37-1 through 5-37-32

Code of Laws of South Carolina
Title 40; Chapter 47: Physicians, Surgeons and Osteopaths
sections 40-47-5 through 40-47-660

South Dakota Codified Laws
Title 36; Chapter 36-4: Physicians and Surgeons
sections 36-4-1 through 36-4-41

Tennessee Code Annotated
Title 63; Chapter 6: Medicine and Surgery
sections 63-6-101 through 63-6-606

Vernon's Texas Annotated Civil Statutes
Chapter 6: Medicine
articles 4495b through 4512m

Utah Code Annotated
Title 58; Chapter 12: Practice of Medicine and Surgery and the Treatment of Human Ailments;
part 5: Medical Practice Act
sections 58-12-26 through 58-12-44

Vermont Statutes Annotated
Title 26; Chapter 23: Medicine and Surgery
sections 1311 through 1449

Code of Virginia
Title 54.1; Chapter 29: Medicine and Other Healing Arts
sections 54.1-2900 through 54.1-2993

West's Revised Code of Washington Annotated
Title 18; Chapter 18.71: Physicians
sections 18.71.002 through 18.71.941

West Virginia Code
Chapter 30; Article 3: West Virginia Medical Practice Act
section 30-3-1 through 30-3-17

West's Wisconsin Statutes Annotated
Chapter 448: Medical Practices
sections 448.01 through 448.40

Wyoming Statutes Annotated
Title 33; Chapter 26: Physicians and Surgeons
sections 33-26-101 through 33-26-511

Medical Records

The medical record

A well-documented, legible, structured medical record is the physician's first line of defense in the event of a malpractice suit. The medical record is a form of communication among health care professionals about the patient's condition. This documentation identifies the patient, supports the diagnosis, justifies the treatment, and documents the results of treatment.

The medical record is confidential. The information is private, should remain secure, and should not be made public. The record belongs to the physician, but the information belongs to the patient.

Authorization to release records

The patient has the *sole* authority to release information from his or her medical record.

The office should be prepared with a printed release form that the patient signs to release the medical record to a third party. The release form need not be complicated or full of legal language.

A word of caution: HIV/AIDS information is not included in a standard release form. The release form must *specifically* state that this information is included.

Any mention of HIV/AIDS testing or treatment is extremely sensitive and should be maintained in a separate part of the medical record. Some attorneys suggest it should be maintained in an envelope marked CONFIDENTIAL! DO NOT RELEASE.

Tip: Never release a patient record without the physician's approval.

Records are the heart of systematic patient care. Excellent record keeping is one of the most effective tools in patient care and in preventing claims. Following are the keys elements of a good medical record.

Uniform Records. Medical records should be uniform within the practice. Inserting dividers for lab, X ray, progress notes, etc, and using a problem list is an excellent way to structure charts in a format that organizes the record for easy scanning by all health care professionals who subsequently use the chart.

Secure Pages. Secure all pages of the record in chronological order with fasteners to prevent pages from being lost.

Organization. Organize records for easy accurate retrieval. Whatever system is used, it should be logical and clear to all staff members and physicians (active vs inactive patient, color coding for chronic problems or frequent diagnoses, etc).

Timeliness. Make all entries in the record, whether written or dictated, at the time of the patient contact. Include the date and the time of the exam or contact. The greater the time lapse between the exam and the entry, the less credible the medical record becomes.

Legible Records. Records must be legible. Health care professionals with illegible handwriting should dictate their notes. This helps to avoid misinterpretations that result in improper treatment.

Dictated Records. Dictated notes must be proofread and signed. The statement "dictated but not read" does not relieve the physician from responsibility for what was transcribed. At best, the statement alerts another health care professional that the note has not been proofed and may not be correct.

Accurate Records. It is important to record all information in objective and concise terms. Never include extraneous information or subjective assessments of the patient, such as "this patient is a jerk." Include direct quotations from the patient. However, reduce the essential information to the least possible number of words.

Corrections. Never improperly or unlawfully alter a medical record. If an error has been made, draw a single line through the inaccurate entry and enter the necessary correction. Date, time, and initial the correction in the margin. It is also acceptable to make an addendum to a medical record. It should be made after the last entry, noting the current date and time, and both entries should be cross-referenced. A record that appears to have been altered implies that a cover-up has occurred. Do not obliterate an entry with a marker or correction fluid.

Jousting. Never criticize or make derogatory comments about another health care professional or organization to the patient or in the medical record. A negative comment can undermine a patient's confidence in the previous health care worker and contribute to or cause a decision to pursue a legal claim regardless of causation and/or who was responsible.

Patient Telephone Calls. Document all patient telephone calls in the medical record. When the physician speaks to a patient while away from the office and the medical record is not available, notes regarding any prescriptions or medical advice given over the telephone can be recorded on a phone call pad. The sheet can be torn out and presented for entry into the chart when the physician returns to the office.

Conversations. Address and document all patient/family worries or concerns in the patient record. Record the source of the information, if other than the patient.

Always document important warnings and instructions given to the patient at the time of discharge. Documenting discharge instructions may help prove noncompliance. Juries are not as sympathetic to noncompliant patients.

To reinforce the signed informed consent form, always document information disclosed during the informed consent process.

Potential Complications. Document all possible complications that might occur. Failure to recognize a complication in time to prevent injuries is a common basis for lawsuit. Proving negligence is difficult if the record shows prior awareness that a complication might occur. (PHSPA-1996. See Exhibit 7-5 on page 137 for a Medical Records Checklist Form.)

Record retention

Whether retiring or selling the practice, a physician should start making arrangements for handling the office's medical records at least 3 months before closing. What are the rules for record retention after closing an office?

How long should medical records be kept?

There are no hard and fast rules. When there is no legal requirement, which is the case in most states, records should be kept for the period of the statute of limitations for professional liability (the length of time in which a suit can be filed).

The time period varies by state, but is usually under 10 years. The local or state medical society should be contacted to find out what the local laws are.

It should be noted, too, that the statute of limitations does not begin running for children until they reach the age of majority—usually 18. In many states, the statute of limitations is 2 years from the date of discovery. If the practice specialty is pediatrics or obstetrics, or otherwise involves treatment of children, some records should be retained a minimum of 30 years.

It may be advantageous to retain some records for a "reasonable amount of time" beyond the statute. Records should be available in the event that patients want them. Of course, only four or five patients in a couple of thousand may actually contact their physician for the record. But it may make a dramatic difference to that person if the record is available. For instance, women whose mothers took DES during their pregnancy have been grateful to physicians who retained records containing the information.

How to decide which records to keep

Unless unlimited storage space is available, it will be necessary to set some guidelines for which records to keep and which to purge. As a rule, the physician can discard records of patients seen only once for a routine checkup or procedure and of patients with uncomplicated problems who have not been seen in a number of years.

Deceased patients' records can be destroyed a few years after their deaths. Once the estate is closed, and any statute of limitations for wrongful death actions has run, no suits for professional liability can be brought.

The physician should retain records of active patients. How is active defined? Where is the cutoff in terms of the date of the last visit or the complexity of the case? Once again, the judgment call is the physician's to make.

Even if a physician is a part of a group practice or partnership that will retain the patient's records after the physician leaves, purging inactive records before terminating the business relationship is a good idea. Inactive files should not take up valuable space from colleagues.

In what form should a medical record be transferred?

The physician owns the original hard copy of the record and therefore should keep it. If a patient requests the forwarding of a file to a new doctor, the original physician has two options. Either he or she can photocopy the entire contents, letting the new physician decide what to retain, or a summary of the record can be made. The summary is preferable if there are notes in shorthand or if the physician's handwriting is illegible.

What if a patient owes on account? Is the physician obliged to transfer the patient's record if requested?

The physician cannot refuse to forward a record because a patient owes money. Nor should such information be in the medical record. If it is, it may be a violation of state or federal laws.

Should a copy of the record be given to the patient?

A number of states have passed laws granting patients the access to their medical records. Note, however, that you should provide a copy, not the original.

What are the options for storing medical records?

When closing a practice, the physician faces the decision of where to store medical records. There are several options:

1. The local medical society must be contacted. Some have storage centers or know of others in the community.

2. Is there room in the physician's basement, attic, or garage? Does the physician intend to stay in that location? Are these places dry and safe?

3. The physician should check out storage companies in the area and what they charge for retrieving a record.

What about microfilm?

Microfilming records may or may not be the answer to the physician's storage problems. The initial cost can be high, depending on the size and number of charts. The major cost is for labor to prepare the record for filming. The physician may want to select only certain material for filming, which will require review of each record. Then there is the removing of staples and paper clips and putting the papers in the proper sequence.

What can be done with X-ray film?

If the physician retains the report in the X ray, the information is probably sufficient. If, for any reason, the X ray might be needed later, it should be kept.

X rays may be turned in for their silver value. The physician should call the local medical society to find out who in the area might be interested in the films for their silver content.

How are records destroyed?

The physician should find a way in which the records will not fall into the hands of someone outside who might use them. If a refuse service picks up the records, the physician should make sure they will be burned. The records should be cut or torn in half before being disposed of. (CLO-1988; adaptation)

Medical records: getting yours:
Available for $5
Health Research Group, Publications Manager
2000 P St NW, Ste 700, Washington, DC 20036
202 833-3000

Resources

American Association for Medical Transcription
PO Box 576187, Modesta, CA 95357-6187
800 982-2182   209 551-0883   Fax 209 551-9317

American Health Information Management Association
919 N Michigan Ave, Ste 1400, Chicago, IL 60611-1683
800 621-6828   312 787-2672   Fax 312 787-9793
(Contact for "Your health information belongs to you")

Medical Information Bureau
160 University Ave, Westwood, MA 02090-2307
617 329-4500   Fax 617 329-3379

Medical Schools, US

Association of American Medical Colleges
2450 N St NW, Washington, DC 20037
202 828-0400   Fax 202 828-1125
E-mail: webmaster@aamc.org
Web address: http://www.aamc.org

Alabama
University of Alabama School of Medicine
813 6th Ave, UAB Station, Birmingham, AL 35233
205 934-4011   Fax 205 934-0333

University of South Alabama College of Medicine
307 University Blvd, Mobile, AL 36688
205 460-7174   Fax 205 460-6073
Web address: http://www.usouthal.edu/uas/library/
index.htm

Arizona
University of Arizona College of Medicine
Arizona Health Sciences Center
1501 N Campbell Ave, Tucson, AZ 85724
602 626-6214   Fax 602 626-4884
Web address: http://www.ahsc.arizona.edu/com.shtml

Arkansas
University of Arkansas College of Medicine
4301 W Markham St, Little Rock, AR 72205
501 686-5000   Fax 501 686-8160
Web address: http://amanda.uams.edu/uams.html

California
Loma Linda University School of Medicine
Loma Linda, CA 92350
909 824-4467   800 422-4558   Fax 909 824-4146
Web address: http://www.llu.edu/llu/medicine/

Stanford University School of Medicine
300 Pasteur Dr, Stanford, CA 94305
415 725-3900   Fax 415 725-7368
Web address: http://med.www.stanford.edu/
medCenter/MedSchool/MedSchool.html

University of California
Davis School of Medicine, Davis, CA 95616
916 752-0331   Fax 916 752-3517
Web address: http://edison.ucdmc.ucdavis.edu

University of California
Irvine College of Medicine, Irvine, CA 92717
714 856-6119   Fax 714 725-3517
Web address: http://www.com.uci.edu

University of California, Los Angeles
UCLA School of Medicine, 10833 Le Conte Ave
Los Angeles, CA 90024
310 825-9111   Fax 310 206-5046
Web address: http://www.mednet.ucla.edu/dept/som/
mnsom_default.htm

University of California, San Diego
School of Medicine, La Jolla, CA 92093
619 534-3713
Web address: http://cybermed.ucsd.edu

University of California, San Francisco
School of Medicine, 513 Parnassus Ave
San Francisco, CA 94143-0410
415 476-9000   Fax 415 476-0689
Web address: http://www.ucsf.edu

University of Southern California School of Medicine
1975 Zonal Ave, Los Angeles, CA 90033
213 342-1544   Fax 213 342-2722
Web address: http://www.usc.edu/hsc/med-sch/med-
home.html

Colorado
University of Colorado School of Medicine
4200 E Ninth Ave, Denver, CO 80262
303 399-1211   Fax 303 270-8494
Web address: http://www.hsc.colorado.edu

Connecticut
University of Connecticut School of Medicine
263 Farmington Ave, Farmington, CT 06030
203 679-2000   Fax 203 679-1282
Web address: http://www.uchc.edu

Yale University School of Medicine
333 Cedar St, PO Box 208055
New Haven, CT 06520
203 423-4771   Fax 203 785-7437
Web address: http://info.med.yale.edu

District of Columbia
George Washington University
School of Medicine and Health Sciences
2300 Eye St NW, Washington, DC 20037
202 994-3266

Georgetown University School of Medicine
3900 Reservoir Rd NW, Washington, DC 20007
202 687-1612   Fax 202 687-2792
Web address: http://www.dml.georgetown.edu/schmed

Howard University College of Medicine
520 W St NW, Washington, DC 20059
202 806-6270   Fax 202 806-7934
Web address: http://www.cldc.howard.edu/~bhlogan/
hucm-cat.html

Florida
University of Florida College of Medicine
J. Hillis Miller Health Center, Box 100215
Gainesville, FL 32610
904 392-5397   Fax 904 392-6482
Web address: http://www.med.ufl.edu

University of Miami School of Medicine
1600 NW 10th Ave, PO Box 016099 (R59)
Miami, FL 33101
305 547-6545   Fax 305 548-4888
Web address: http://www.med.miami.edu

University of South Florida College of Medicine
12901 Bruce B. Downs Blvd, MDC Box 2
Tampa, FL 33612-4799
813 974-2196   Fax 813 974-3886
Web address: http://www.med.usf.edu

Georgia
Emory University School of Medicine
Woodruff Health Sciences Center Administration Bldg
1440 Clifton Rd NE, Atlanta, GA 30322
404 727-5640   Fax 404 727-0473
Web address: http://www.cc.emory.edu/WHSC/MED/
med.html

Medical College of Georgia School of Medicine
1120 15th St, Augusta, GA 30912
404 721-0211   Fax 404 721-7035
Web address: http://www.mcg.edu

Mercer University School of Medicine
1550 College St, Macon, GA 31207
912 752-2600   Fax 912 752-2547
Web address: http://gain.mercer.peachnet.edu

Morehouse School of Medicine
720 Westview Dr SW, Atlanta, GA 30310-1495
404 752-1500   Fax 404 752-8443
Web address: http://www.msm.edu

M

Hawaii
University of Hawaii
John A. Burns School of Medicine
1960 East-West Rd, Honolulu, HI 96822
808 956-8287   Fax 808 956-5506
Web address: http://medworld.biomed.hawaii.edu/
jabson_mw.html

Illinois
Loyola University of Chicago
Stritch School of Medicine
2160 S First Ave, Maywood, IL 60153
708 216-9000   Fax 708 216-4305
Web address: http://www.meddean.luc.edu

Northwestern University Medical School
303 E Chicago Ave, Chicago, IL 60611-3008
312 503-8649
Web address: http://www.nwu.edu/academic/
schools.html

Rush Medical College of Rush University
600 S Paulina St, Chicago, IL 60612
312 942-6913   Fax 312 942-2828
Web address: http://www.rpslmc.edu/index.html

Southern Illinois University School of Medicine
801 N Rutledge, PO Box 19230
Springfield, IL 62794-9230
217 782-3318   217 524-0786
Web address: http://www.c-som.siu.edu

University of Chicago
Pritzker School of Medicine
5841 S Maryland Ave, Chicago, IL 60637
773 702-1000   Fax 773 702-1897
Web address: http://www.c-som.siu.edu

University of Health Sciences
Chicago Medical School
3333 Green Bay Rd, North Chicago, IL 60064
312 578-3000

University of Illinois College of Medicine (UIC)
1853 W Polk St (M/C 784), Chicago, IL 60680
312 996-3500   Fax 312 996-9006

UIC—College of Medicine at Peoria
1 Illini Dr, PO Box 1649, Peoria, IL 61656
309 671-3000

UIC—College of Medicine, Rockford
1601 Park Ave, Rockford, IL 61107
815 395-5600

Indiana
Indiana University School of Medicine
Indiana University Medical Center
1120 South Dr, Indianapolis, IN 46202-5114
317 274-8157
Web address: http://www.medlib.iupui.edu

Iowa
University of Iowa College of Medicine
200 Medical Administration Bldg
Iowa City, IA 52242-1101
319 335-8050   Fax 319 335-8049
Web address: http://www.medadmin.uiowa.edu

Kansas
University of Kansas Medical Center School of Medicine
39th and Rainbow Blvd, Kansas City, KS 66160-7300
913 588-5200   Fax 913 588-5299
Web address: http://www.kumc.edu

Kentucky
University of Kentucky College of Medicine
A. B. Chandler Medical Center
800 Rose St, Lexington, KY 40536-0084
606 233-5000   Fax 606 323-2039
Web address: http://www.uky.edu/College of Medicine

University of Louisville School of Medicine
Health Sciences Center, Louisville, KY 40292
502 852-5184   Fax 502 852-6849
Web address: http://kdp-sparc.kdp_baptist.louisville.
edu/index.html

Louisiana
Louisiana State University School of Medicine,
New Orleans
1542 Tulane Ave, New Orleans, LA 70112-2822
504 568-4007   Fax 504 568-4008
Web address: http://www.lsumc.edu

Louisiana State University School of
Medicine in Shreveport
PO Box 33932, Shreveport, LA 71130-3932
318 675-5000   Fax 318 675-5244
Web address: http://gopher/library./sumc.edu/WWW/
root.htm

Tulane University School of Medicine
1430 Tulane Ave, New Orleans, LA 70112
504 588-5263   Fax 504 584-2495
Web address: http://www.mci.tulane.edu

Maryland
Johns Hopkins University School of Medicine
720 Rutland Ave, Baltimore, MD 21205
410 955-5000   Fax 410 955-0495
Web address: http://infonet.welch.jhu.edu

JAMA Theme Issue: Johns Hopkins

JAMA 1989 June 2; 261(21)

A theme issue of *JAMA* that commemorates the centennial of this medical institution. Subjects range from DNA markers in Huntington's disease, to the attitudes and practices of medical students and house staff regarding alcoholism, to an essay about Johns Hopkins' first century. The cover features a 1906 portrait of the four founders of the institution by American painter John Singer Sargent.

Uniformed Services University of the Health Sciences
F. Edward Herbert School of Medicine
4301 Jones Bridge Rd, Bethesda, MD 20814-4799
301 295-3016   Fax 301 295-3542
Web address: http://www.usuhs.mil

University of Maryland School of Medicine
655 W Baltimore St, Baltimore, MD 21201
410 328-7410   Fax 410 706-0235
Web address: gopher://umabnet.ab.umd.edu:70/11/
.schools/.medicine

Massachusetts
Boston University School of Medicine
80 E Concord St, Boston, MA 02118
617 638-8000   Fax 617 638-5258
Web address: http://med-amsa.bu.edu/Main.html

Harvard Medical School
25 Shattuck St, Boston, MA 02115
617 432-1000   Fax 617 432-3907
Web address: http://www.med.havard.edu

Tufts University School of Medicine
136 Harrison Ave, Boston, MA 02111
617 956-7000   Fax 617 856-0375
Web address: http://polaris.nemc.org/tusm

University of Massachusetts Medical School
55 Lake Ave N, Worcester, MA 01655
508 856-0011   Fax 508 856-8181
Web address: http://www.ummed.edu

Michigan
Michigan State University
College of Human Medicine
A-110 E Fee Hall, East Lansing, MI 48824
517 353-1730   Fax 517 355-0342
Web address: http://omerad7.chm.msu.edu/Users/
~omerad

University of Michigan Medical School
Medical Sciences Bldg I, 1301 Catherine Rd
Ann Arbor, MI 48109-0624
313 763-9600   Fax 313 763-4936
Web address: http://www.med.umich.edu/medschool

Wayne State University School of Medicine
540 E Canfield, Detroit, MI 48201
313 577-1460   Fax 313 577-8777
Web address: http://www.phypc.med.wayne.edu

Minnesota
Mayo Medical School
200 First St SW, Rochester, MN 55905
507 284-3671   Fax 507 284-2634
Web address: http://www.mayo.edu/education/
education.html

University of Minnesota
Duluth School of Medicine
10 University Dr, Duluth, MN 55812
218 726-7571   Fax 218 726-6235
Web address: http://www.d.umn.edu/medweb

University of Minnesota Medical School—Minneapolis
UMHC Box 293, 420 Delaware St SE
Minneapolis, MN 55455
612 624-1188   Fax 612 626-6800
Web address: http://www.med.umn.edu

Mississippi
University of Mississippi School of Medicine
2500 N State St, Jackson, MS 39216
601 984-1000   Fax 601 984-0011
Web address: http://fiona.umsmcd.edu

Missouri
St Louis University School of Medicine
1402 S Grand Blvd, St Louis, MO 63104
314 577-8200   Fax 314 577-8214
Web address: http://www.slu.edu/slumed

University of Missouri
Columbia School of Medicine
MA204 Medical Sciences Bldg
1 Hospital Dr, Columbia, MO 65203
314 882-2923   Fax 314 884-4808
Web address: http://www.miaims.missouri.edu/
index.html

University of Missouri
Kansas City School of Medicine
2411 Holmes St, Kansas City, MO 64108-2792
816 235-1800   Fax 816 235-5277
Web address: http://www.research.med.umkc.edu

Washington University School of Medicine
660 S Euclid Ave, St Louis, MO 63110
314 362-5000   Fax 314 362-9862
Web address: http://medicine.wastl.edu/wums

Nebraska
Creighton University School of Medicine .
California at 24th St, Omaha, NE 68178
402 280-2900   Fax 402 280-2599
Web address: http://medicine.creighton.edu

University of Nebraska at Omaha
College of Medicine
600 S 42nd St, Omaha, NE 68198
402 559-4000   Fax 402 559-4148
Web address: http://www.unmc.edu/unmc.html

Nevada
University of Nevada-Reno, School of Medicine
Savitt Medical Sciences Bldg
Reno, NV 89577-0046
702 784-6001   Fax 702 784-6096
Web address: http://www.scs.unr.edu/unr/med.html

New Hampshire
Dartmouth Medical School
Hanover, NH 03756
603 646-1471   Fax 603 650-1614
Web address: http://usl.dhmc.dartmouth.edu

New Jersey
University of Medicine and Dentistry of New Jersey
New Jersey Medical School
185 S Orange Ave, Newark, NJ 07103-2714
201 982-4300   Fax 201 982-7104
Web address: http://hjmsa.umdnj.edu/umdnj.html

University of Medicine and Dentistry of New Jersey
Robert Wood Johnson Medical School
675 Hoes Ln, Piscataway, NJ 08854-5635
908 235-5600   Fax 908 235-4006
Web address: http://www2.umdnj.edu/rwjms.html

New Mexico
University of New Mexico School of Medicine
Albuquerque, NM 87131
505 277-2413   Fax 505 277-6851
Web address: http://www.unm.edu/medicine.html

New York
Albany Medical College
47 New Scotland Ave, Albany, NY 12208
518 445-5582   Fax 518 262-5029
Web address: http://www.aecom.yu.edu

Albert Einstein College of Medicine of
Yeshiva University
1300 Morris Park Ave, Bronx, NY 10461
212 430-2000   Fax 212 430-2488
Web address: http://www.aecom.yu.edu

Columbia University College of
Physicians and Surgeons
630 W 168th St, New York, NY 10032
212 305-3592   Fax 212 305-3545
Web address: http://cpmcnet.columbia.edu

Cornell University Medical College
1300 York Ave, New York, NY 10021
212 746-5454   Fax 212 746-0931
Web address: http://www.med.cornell.edu

Mount Sinai School of Medicine of
the City University of New York
1 Gustave L. Levy Pl, New York, NY 10029-6574
212 241-6500   Fax 212 410-6111
Web address: http://www.cuny.edu/about_cuny/
mtsinai.html

New York Medical College
Administration Bldg, Valhalla, NY 10595
914 993-4000   Fax 914 993-4565
Web address: http://www.nymc.edu

New York University School of Medicine
550 First Ave, New York, NY 10016
212 263-7300   Fax 212 725-2140
Web address: http://www.med.nyc.edu/HomePage.html

State University of New York
Health Science Center at Brooklyn College of Medicine
450 Clarkson Ave, PO Box 97, Brooklyn, NY 11203
718 270-1000   Fax 718 270-4074
Web address: http://hallux.medschool.hscbklyn.edu

State University of New York at Buffalo
School of Medicine and Biomedical Sciences
3435 Main St, Buffalo, NY 14214
716 829-2775   Fax 716 829-3395
Web address: gopher://wing.buffalo.edu:3000/7/
medicalschool

State University of New York at Stony Brook
Health Sciences Center
School of Medicine, Stony Brook, NY 11794-8430
516 444-2080   Fax 516 444-2202
Web address: http://www.informatics.sunysb.edu/som

State University of New York
Health Science Center of Syracuse College of Medicine
750 E Adams St, Syracuse, NY 13210
315 464-5540   Fax 315 464-5564
Web address: http://www.hscsyr.edu

University of Rochester School of Medicine and Dentistry
601 Elmwood Ave, Rochester, NY 14642-7181
716 275-7181   Fax 716 256-1131
Web address: http://wwwminer.lib.rochester.edu

North Carolina
Bowman Gray School of Medicine of
Wake Forest University
Medical Center Blvd, Winston-Salem, NC 27157-1040
910 716-2011   Fax 910 716-5139
Web address: http://pandoras-box.bgsm.wfu.edu

Duke University School of Medicine
PO Box 3005, Durham, NC 27710
919 684-8111   Fax 919 684-2593
Web address: http://medschl-www.mc.duke.edu

East Carolina University School of Medicine
Greenville, NC 27858-4354
919 816-2201   Fax 919 816-3192
Web address: http://www.med.ecu.edu

University of North Carolina at Chapel Hill
School of Medicine, Chapel Hill, NC 27599
919 966-4161   Fax 919 966-7564
Web address: http://www.med.unc.edu

North Dakota
University of North Dakota School of Medicine
501 N Columbia Rd, PO Box 9037
Grand Forks, ND 58203-9037
701 777-2514   Fax 701 777-3527
Web address: http://www.med.und.nodak.edu

Ohio
Case Western Reserve University
School of Medicine
10900 Euclid Ave, Cleveland, OH 44106-4915
216 368-2000   Fax 216 368-3013
Web address: http://mediswww.meds.cwru.edu

Medical College of Ohio
Caller Service #10008, Toledo, OH 43699-0008
419 381-4172   Fax 409 382-1319
Web address: http://www.mco.edu

Northeastern Ohio Universities College of Medicine
4209 State Route 44, PO Box 95
Rootstown, OH 44272
216 325-2511   Fax 216 325-7943
Web address: http://www.neoucom.edu

Ohio State University College of Medicine
370 W Ninth Ave, Columbus, OH 43210
614 292-5674   Fax 614 292-1544
Web address: http://www.osu.edu/units/cancer/
healthsc/html

University of Cincinnati College of Medicine
PO Box 670555, Cincinnati, OH 45267-0555
513 558-7391   Fax 515 558-3512
Web address: http://www.med.uc.edu/htdocs/
medicine/uccom.html

Wright State University School of Medicine
PO Box 927, Dayton, OH 45401-0927
513 873-3010   Fax 513 873-3672
Web address: http://www.med.wright.edu

Oklahoma
University of Oklahoma College of Medicine
PO Box 26901, Oklahoma City, OK 73190
405 271-2265   Fax 405 271-3032
Web address: http://www.tulsa.uokhsc.edu

Oregon
Oregon Health Sciences University
School of Medicine
3181 SW Sam Jackson Park Rd
Portland, OR 97201-3098
503 494-8311   Fax 503 494-3400
Web address: http://www.ohsu.edu

Pennsylvania
Hahnemann University School of Medicine
Broad and Vine Sts, Mail Drop 440
Philadelphia, PA 19102
215 448-7604

Jefferson Medical College of Thomas Jefferson
University
1025 Walnut St, Philadelphia, PA 19107-5083
215 928-6000   Fax 215 923-6939
Web address: http://www.tju.edu

Medical College of Pennsylvania and
Hahnemann University
2900 Queen Ln, Philadelphia, PA 19129
215 842-6000   Fax 215 991-8202
Web address: http://www.mcphu.edu

Pennsylvania State University College of Medicine
500 University Dr, PO Box 850, Hershey, PA 17033
717 531-8521   Fax 717 531-5351
Web address: http://www.hmc.psu.edu

Temple University School of Medicine
3400 N Broad St, Philadelphia, PA 19140
215 204-7000   Fax 215 707-2940
Web address: http://eclipse.hsclib.temple.edu

University of Pennsylvania School of Medicine
36th and Hamilton Walk, Ste 100, Edward J. Stemler Hall
Philadelphia, PA 19104-6087
215 898-8034   Fax 215 898-5607
Web address: http://www.med.upenn.edu

University of Pittsburgh School of Medicine
Alan Magee Scaife Hall of the Health Professions
Pittsburgh, PA 15261
412 648-9891   Fax 412 648-1236
Web address: http://www.upmc.edu

Puerto Rico
Ponce School of Medicine
PO Box 7004, Ponce, PR 00732
809 844-3710   Fax 809 840-9756

Universidad Central del Caribe School of Medicine
Call Box 60-327, Bayamon, PR 00960-6032
809 798-3001   Fax 809 798-6836

University of Puerto Rico School of Medicine
Medical Sciences Campus G, PO Box 365067
San Juan, PR 00936-5067
809 758-2525   Fax 809 751-6389

Rhode Island
Brown University Program in Medicine
97 Waterman St, Providence, RI 02912
401 863-3330   Fax 401 863-3431
Web address: http://biomedcs.biomed.brown.edu

South Carolina
Medical University of South Carolina
College of Medicine
171 Ashley Ave, Charleston, SC 29425
803 792-2300   Fax 803 792-2967
Web address: http://www.musc.edu

University of South Carolina School of Medicine
Columbia, SC 29208
803 733-3200   Fax 803 733-3335
Web address: http://www.med.sc.edu

South Dakota
University of South Dakota School of Medicine
2501 W 22nd St, Sioux Falls, SD 57117-5046
605 339-6648   Fax 605 357-1311
Web address: http://sunbird.usd.edu/med

Tennessee
East Tennessee State University
James H. Quillen College of Medicine
PO Box 70694, Johnson City, TN 37614
615 929-4112   615 929-6433
Web address: http://etsu.east-tenn-st.edu/~medcom

Meharry Medical College School of Medicine
1005 D. B. Todd Jr Blvd, Nashville, TN 37208
615 327-6337   Fax 615 327-6568

University of Tennessee, Memphis
College of Medicine
800 Madison Ave, Memphis, TN 38163
901 448-5529   Fax 901 448-7683
Web address: http://planetree1.utmem.edu/
StudentPages/first.html

Vanderbilt University School of Medicine
21st Ave S at Garland Ave, Nashville, TN 37232
615 322-2145   Fax 615 343-7286
Web address: http://vumclib.mc.vanderbilt.edu/
medschool

Texas
Baylor College of Medicine
1 Baylor Plaza, Houston, TX 77030
713 798-4951   Fax 713 790-0055
Web address: http://www. bcm.tmc.edu

Texas A&M University College of Medicine
147 Joe H. Reynolds Medical Bldg
College Station, TX 77843-1114
409 845-7743   Fax 409 847-8663
Web address: http://thunder.tamu.edu

Texas Tech University
Health Sciences Center, School of Medicine
3601 4th St, Lubbock, TX 79430
806 743-1000   Fax 806 743-3021
Web address: http://www.ttuhsc.edu

University of Texas
Southwestern Medical School
5323 Harry Hines Blvd, Dallas, TX 75235
214 648-3111   Fax 214 648-8690
Web address: http://www.swmed.edu

University of Texas Medical Branch
301 University Blvd, Galveston, TX 77550
409 772-1011   Fax 409 722-9598
Web address: http://www.utmb.edu/newhome.html

University of Texas Medical School at Houston
6431 Fannin, Houston, TX 77030
713 792-2121   Fax 713 796-8570
Web address: http://www.med.uth.tmc.edu

University of Texas Medical School at San Antonio
7703 Floyd Curl Dr, San Antonio, TX 78284-7790
210 567-4420   Fax 210 567-6962
Web address: http://www.uthscsa.edu

Utah
University of Utah School of Medicine
50 N Medical Dr, Salt Lake City, UT 84132
801 581-7201   Fax 801 585-3300
Web address: gopher://medstat.med.utah.edu

Vermont
University of Vermont College of Medicine
School of Medicine, Burlington, VT 05405
802 656-2150   Fax 802 656-8584
Web address: http://salus.uvm.edu

Virginia
Eastern Virginia Medical School
Medical College of Hampton Roads
PO Box 1980, Norfolk, VA 23501
804 446-5600   Fax 804 640-0311
Web address: gopher://picard.evms.edu

Virginia Commonwealth University
Medical College of Virginia, School of Medicine
Box 565 MCV Station, Richmond, VA 23298
804 786-9793   Fax 804 371-7628
Web address: http://views.vcu.edu/html/
mcvhome.2.html

University of Virginia School of Medicine
Medical Center Box 395
Charlottesville, VA 22908
804 924-0211   Fax 804 982-0874
Web address: http://www.med.virginia.edu

Washington
University of Washington
School of Medicine, Seattle, WA 98195
206 543-1060   Fax 206 543-3639
Web address: http://www.hslib.washington.edu/hsc

West Virginia
Marshall University School of Medicine
1801 6th Ave, Huntington, WV 25755
304 696-7000   Fax 304 696-7243
Web address: http://musom.mu.wvnet.edu

West Virginia University School of Medicine
Morgantown, WV 26506
304 293-4511   Fax 304 293-4973
Web address: http://www.hsc.wvu.edu

Wisconsin
Medical College of Wisconsin
8701 Watertown Plank Rd
Milwaukee, WI 53226
414 257-8296   Fax 414 257-0449
Web address: http://www.mcw.edu

University of Wisconsin Medical School
1300 University Ave, Madison, WI 53706
608 263-4900   Fax 608 262-2327
Web address: http://www.biostat.wisc.edu/
homepage.html

Medical Science Knowledge Program

Medical School Entrance Exam (MSKP)
Registration:
Association of American Medical Colleges
202 828-0400   Fax 202 828-1125

Test centers:
National Board of Medical Examiners
215 590-9500   Fax 215 590-9555

Medical Students

JAMA Article of Note: Educational programs in US medical schools, 1996-1997

JAMA 1997, Sept 3; 278(9): 750-754

Includes statistical tables on medical school students and graduates during a 20-year period, and of the racial and ethnic background of medical students.

Resource

American Medical Students Association
1902 Association Dr, Reston, VA 22091
800 767-2266   703 620-6600   Fax 703 620-5873

Medicare

The Medicare program provides health insurance coverage for people aged 65 and over, younger people who are receiving Social Security disability benefits, and persons who need dialysis or kidney transplants for treament of end-stage kidney disease. As a Medicare beneficiary, one can choose how to receive hospital, doctor, and other health care services covered by Medicare. Beneficiaries can receive care either through the traditional fee-for-service delivery system or through coordinated care plans, such as health maintenance organizations and competitive medical plans that have contracts with Medicare. (USG-1996)

Policy Perspectives
Medicare at 30; preparing for the future

JAMA 1995 July 19; 274(3): 259

Medicare's 30th anniversary is an appropriate time for celebration. Few programs, public or private, have had so demonstrably beneficial an impact on so many Americans as Medicare. But it is also a time both to reflect on Medicare's role in our society at large and to think strategically about how Medicare can fulfill its missions in the years ahead. In the increasingly contentious political environment, Medicare has been called a dinosaur—a program that is too costly, is too inefficient, and has outlived its usefulness. In the view of Medicare's critics, radical restructuring is the only cure. Although improvements can and should be made to Medicare, those calling for the end of Medicare as we know it are most charitably described as misguided. Medicare is responsible for major improvements in the health of elderly and disabled citizens, is well managed, and provides the financial underpinning for much of the US health care system.

Medicare insures 37 million elderly and disabled people

Before Medicare's enactment, 50% of elderly people had no health insurance. Now more than 97% of senior citizens are insured by Medicare, as are more than 90% of those who have end-stage renal disease and 3.6 million disabled people. Medicare has relieved elderly people of the terrible anxiety they suffered when they did not have health insurance and could not pay for their own care.

Medicare has dramatically increased access to health care. In 1964, just before Medicare's enactment, there were 190 hospital discharges per 1000 elderly people. By 1973, that number had increased to 350 discharges—one indication that Medicare helps elderly people get the health care they need at the time of their lives they need it most.[1-3] Although it is difficult to prove a causal relationship, Medicare—and the increased access to health care it provides—has undoubtedly contributed to increased longevity among the elderly. In 1960, men who survived to 65 years of age could expect to live to 78 years of age; by 1992, they could expect to reach 81 years of age. Women achieved similar gains.

Most Medicare beneficiaries rely on the financial security and access to health care that Medicare provides. In 1992, 83% of Medicare spending was on behalf of beneficiaries with annual incomes less than $25,000. Fully 20% of beneficiaries are either 85 years of age and older (most of whom are women) or persons with disabilities or end-stage renal disease (Office of the Actuary, Health Care Financing Administration [HCFA], unpublished data from the Medicare Current Beneficiary Survey, 1992). Providing health care to our most vulnerable citizens is a significant accomplishment of which all Americans should be justly proud.

Most beneficiaries think that Medicare is valuable to them. Nearly 90% of beneficiaries are satisfied with the overall quality of their health care, have a regular source of health care, and have great confidence in their physicians (Office of the Actuary, HCFA, data from the Medicare Current Beneficiary Survey, 1992).

References

1. Gornick M. Ten years of Medicare: impact on the covered population. *Soc Secur Bull.* July 3-21, 1976:3-21.

2. Gornick M, Greenberg JN, Eggers PW, et al. Twenty years of Medicare and Medicaid: covered populations, use of benefits, and program expenditures. *Health Care Financing Rev.* 1985;annual suppl:13-59.

3. Moon M. *Medicare Now and in the Future.* Washington, DC: Urban Institute Press; 1993.

Glossary of Terms

Actual charge—The physician's billed or submitted charge, which is the amount Medicare will pay if it is lower than the Medicare payment schedule amount.

Adjusted historical payment basis (AHPB)—The weighted average of all 1991 Medicare approved amounts for a service in a locality updated to 1992 and adjusted for the transition asymmetry. The AHPB reflects the average prevailing charge for a service for each specialty, weighted by the frequency with which each specialty provided the service, as well as physician customary charge levels.

AMA/Specialty Society RVS Update Committee (RUC)—The RUC was established by the AMA and national medical specialty societies in 1991 and makes annual recommendations to the Health Care Financing Administration (HCFA) on the work relative value units (RVUs) to be assigned to new and revised Current Procedural Terminology (CPT) codes as they are adopted by the AMA CPT Editorial Panel.

Approved amount—Physician payment for a service that includes the Medicare payment amount and the patient's 20% copayment.

Assignment—When a physician accepts the Medicare approved amount (including the 80% Medicare payment and 20% patient copayment) as payment in full, it is called "accepting assignment." The physician submits a claim to Medicare directly and collects only the appropriate deductible and the 20% copayment from the patient.

Balance bill—That portion of a physician's charge exceeding the Medicare approved amount, which is billed to the patient. When a physician balance bills, the patient is responsible for the amount of the physician's charge that exceeds the Medicare approved amount up to the limiting charge, as well as the 20% copayment. Only nonparticipating physicians may balance bill their Medicare patients.

Baseline adjustment—A 6.5% reduction to the conversion factor to maintain budget neutrality that was adopted in the 1991 Final Rule to account for volume increases due to patient demand, physician responses to the RBRVS payment system, and other factors projected by the Health Care Financing Administration (HCFA). This adjustment replaced an initial 10% "behavioral offset" proposed in the Notice of Proposed Rulemaking (NPRM) that reflected anticipated increases in physician services. The HCFA adopted the term "baseline adjustment" due to concerns of the AMA and others that the term "behavioral offset" was misleading. No such offsets were included in the budget neutrality adjustments again until 1997.

Behavioral offset—A reduction in the conversion factor proposed in the Notice of Proposed Rulemaking (NPRM) to compensate for the Health Care Financing Administration (HCFA) assumption that physicians would increase the volume of services in response to decreases in payment. The NPRM included a 10% volume or "behavioral" offset in 1992 payments, but it was replaced in the 1991 Final Rule with a 6.5% baseline adjustment to maintain budget neutrality during the full transition period. A –0.9% behavioral offset was applied to the 1997 conversion factors.

Budget neutrality—A provision of OBRA 89, the legislation creating the Medicare RBRVS payment system, that required 1992 expenditures to neither increase nor decrease from what they would have been under a continuation of customary, prevailing, and reasonable (CPR). A similar limitation continues to apply, specifying that changes in the relative value units (RVUs) resulting from changes in medical practice, coding, new data, or addition of new services may not cause Part B expenditures to differ by more than $20 million from the spending level that would occur in the absence of these adjustments.

The HCFA has applied a budget neutrality adjustment each year since implementation of the RBRVS payment system, although its form has varied. Two separate budget neutrality adjustments were applied for the 1997 payment schedule. First, to adjust for changes in payments resulting from the 5-year review of the RBRVS, HCFA reduced the RVUs for physician work by 8.3% through a budget neutrality adjuster applied to the work RVUs. A separate budget neutrality adjustment was made through a reduction to the conversion factors of 1.5%. This adjustment was due to new payment policies and changes in RVUs from CPT coding changes (–0.6%), as well as anticipated changes in the volume and intensity of physicians' services (–0.9%). For the 1996 RVS, HCFA applied a –0.36% budget neutrality adjustment to the conversion factors. In previous years, however, the adjuster was applied to the relative values.

Carrier—A private contractor to HCFA that administers claims processing and payment for Medicare Part B services.

Conversion factor (CF)—The factor that transforms the geographically adjusted relative value for a service into a dollar amount under the physician payment schedule. The current conversion factors for 1997 are $40.603 for surgical services, $35.7671 for other nonsurgical services, and $33.8454 for primary care services.

Current Procedural Terminology (CPT)—System for coding physician services developed by the American Medical Association to file claims with Medicare and other third-party payers; level 3 of the HCFA Common Procedure Coding System (HCPCS).

Customary charge—The physician's median charge for a service that is based on data collected during the July-June period preceding the current calendar year. One of the factors considered in determining a physician's Medicare payment under the customary, prevailing, and reasonable (CPR) system.

Customary, prevailing, and reasonable (CPR)—The payment system used to determine physician payment under the Medicare program prior to implementation of the Medicare RBRVS payment system on January 1, 1992. The CPR system paid the lowest of the physician's actual charge for a service, that physician's customary charge, or the prevailing charge in the locality. Due to diversity in physicians' charges for the same services, the CPR system allowed for wide variation in Medicare payment levels across specialties and geographic areas.

Deductible—A specified amount of covered medical expenses a beneficiary must pay before receiving benefits. Medicare Part B has an annual deductible of $100 in 1997.

Department of Health and Human Services (HHS)—Department within the US government that is responsible for administering health and social welfare programs.

Evaluation and management (E/M) services—Patient evaluation and management services that a physician provides during a patient's office, hospital, or other visit or consultation. New codes for visits and consultations, developed by the AMA CPT Editorial Panel and adopted by Health Care Financing Administration (HCFA) for implementation under the Medicare program beginning January 1, 1992, improved the coding uniformity for these services, and their appropriateness for use in an RBRVS-based payment schedule. The E/M codes utilize a more precise method of describing services. This method is based primarily on type of history, examination, and medical decision making.

Final Notice—A portion of the November 25, 1992, *Federal Register* containing a summary of the comments received on the 1991 "interim" relative values, a description of the Health Care Financing Administration (HCFA) refinement methodology, and a table of the resulting 1993 relative values for physician services; a table of the codes included in the refinement process; a table of the AMA/Specialty Society RVS Update Committee's (RUC's) recommendations for new and revised codes with HCFA's decisions; and a budget neutrality adjustment to all RVUs of –2.8%. No changes to the geographic practice cost indexes (GPCIs) were included in this Final Notice.

Final Rule—A portion of the *Federal Register* that contains a summary of the final regulations for implementing the Medicare RBRVS payment schedule. It generally includes updated relative value units for all physician services payable under the payment schedule, revised payment rules, analyses of comments on the previous proposed rule and HCFA's response, updated geographic practice cost indexes, and an impact analysis of the new rules on physicians and beneficiaries.

Five-year review—A review process mandated by OBRA 89 requiring HCFA to conduct a review of all work relative values no less often than every 5 years. Activities for this first 5-year review were initiated in 1995 and included work RVUs for all codes on the 1995 RBRVS payment schedule. The AMA/Specialty Society RVS Update Committee (RUC) plays a key role in the review process. Final RVUs were published by HCFA in the 1996 Final Rule, effective for the 1997 Medicare relative value scale (RVS).

Geographic adjustment factor (GAF)—The adjustment made to a service included in the resource-based relative value scale (RBRVS) to account for geographic cost differences across Medicare localities, which are based on the geographic practice cost indexes (GPCIs).

Geographic practice cost index (GPCI)—An index reflecting differences across geographic areas in physicians' resource costs relative to the national average: cost of living, practice costs, and professional liability insurance (PLI). Three distinct GPCIs are used to calculate the payment schedule amount for a service in a Medicare locality.

Global charge—The sum of the professional component and technical component of a procedure when provided and billed by the same physician.

Global service—A payment concept defined by Medicare as a surgical "package" that includes all intraoperative and follow-up services, as well as some preoperative services, associated with the surgery for which the surgeon receives a single payment. The initial evaluation or consultation is excluded from the global package under the Medicare payment schedule.

Health Care Financing Administration (HCFA)—Agency within the Department of Health and Human Services (HHS) that administers the Medicare program.

HCFA Common Procedure Coding System (HCPCS)—Coding system, required for billing Medicare, that is based on Current Procedural Terminology (CPT) but supplemented with additional codes for nonphysician services.

Health professional shortage areas (HPSAs)—Urban or rural areas identified by the Public Health Service (PHS) as medically underserved. The PHS may also designate population groups and public nonprofit medical facilities as medically underserved. Physicians in designated HPSAs who furnish covered services to Medicare patients receive a 10% bonus payment in addition to the payment schedule amount.

Limiting charge—Statutory limit on the amount a nonparticipating physician can charge for services to Medicare patients. The limiting charge replaced the maximum allowable actual charge (MAAC), effective January 1, 1991. The limiting charge in 1993 and subsequent years is 115% of the Medicare approved amount for nonparticipating physicians.

Locality—Geographic areas defined by HCFA and used to establish payment amounts for physician services. The HFCA fundamentally revised the methodology for establishing localities effective for 1997 payments, reducing the number to 89 from 211. The new methodology increased the number of statewide localities and generally combined others into counties and groups of counties.

Maximum allowable actual charge (MAAC)—Under the customary, prevailing, and reasonable (CPR) system, a limit on the amount nonparticipating physicians could charge their Medicare patients above the Medicare approved amount. The MAACs were different for each physician because they were based on the individual physician's customary charges. During a transition period from January 1, 1991, through December 31, 1992, MAACs were phased out and replaced by limiting charges.

Medicare economic index (MEI)—An index introduced in 1976 that is intended to measure the annual growth in physicians' practice costs and general inflation in the cost of operating a medical practice. Under the Medicare payment schedule, the MEI is a factor in updating the conversion factor. Under the customary, prevailing, and reasonable (CPR) payment system, the MEI was a limitation on increases in a physician's prevailing charges.

Medicare payment schedule—A payment schedule adopted by the Health Care Financing Administration (HCFA) for payment of physician services effective January 1, 1992, replacing the customary, prevailing, and reasonable (CPR) system. This payment schedule is based on the resource costs of physician work, practice overhead, and professional liability insurance, with adjustments for differences in geographic practice costs. The payment schedule for a service includes both the 80% that Medicare pays and the patient's 20% copayment.

Medicare volume performance standard (MVPS)—A spending goal for Medicare Part B services. It is established either by Congress, based upon recommendations submitted by the Department of Health and Human Services (HHS) and Physician Payment Review Commission (PPRC) or by a statutory default formula, if Congress chooses not to act. The MVPS is intended to encompass all factors contributing to the growth in Medicare spending for physicians' services, including changes in payment levels, size and age composition of Medicare patients, technology, utilization patterns, and access to care. The conversion factor update default formula, which becomes automatically effective if Congress fails to act by October 31 of each year, is linked to changes in the medical economic index (MEI) as adjusted for the amount by which actual expenditures the preceding year were greater or less than the MVPS-established goals.

Model fee schedule—A payment schedule the Health Care Financing Administration (HCFA) developed in 1990, as required in OBRA 89. The narrative portion of the model fee schedule included the statutory requirements of OBRA 89 as well as technical and policy issues not prescribed by statute; preliminary estimates of the relative values for approximately 1400 services studied under Phase I of the Harvard study; and preliminary geographic practice cost indexes (GPCIs) for all Medicare localities.

Nonparticipating physician—A physician who has not signed a participation agreement with Medicare and, therefore, is not obligated to accept the Medicare ap-

proved amount as payment in full for all cases. Their Medicare patients are billed directly, including the balance of the charge that is not covered by the Medicare approved amount, but this balance cannot exceed the limiting charge. Nonparticipating physicians may still accept assignment on a case-by-case basis.

Notice of Proposed Rulemaking (NPRM)—The proposed rules to implement the Medicare payment schedule and relative values for 4000 services studied under Phase II of the Harvard study; published by the Health Care Financing Administration (HCFA) for public comment on June 5, 1991.

OBRA 89 (Omnibus Budget Reconciliation Act of 1989)—The congressional legislation creating Medicare physician payment reform that provided for a payment schedule based on a resource-based relative value scale (RBRVS), which included three components: physician work, practice expense, and professional liability insurance (PLI) costs.

OBRA 93—The congressional legislation that included a number of revisions to Medicare physician payment under the RBRVS. These provisions include the elimination of payment reductions for "new" physicians, the repeal of the ban on payment for interpretation of electrocardiograms, and several changes to the default payment update and MVPS.

Participating physician—A physician who has signed a participation agreement with Medicare; the physician is bound by the agreement to accept assignment on all Medicare claims for the calendar year.

Physician Payment Review Commission (PPRC)—An advisory body created by Congress in 1986 to recommend reforms in the methods Medicare uses to pay for physicians' services. The PPRC's charge is now broadened to include recommendations for health system reforms to the private as well as public sectors.

Physician work—The physician's individual effort in providing a service, which includes time, technical difficulty of the procedure, severity of patient's condition, and the physical and mental effort required to provide the service; one of three resource cost components included in the formula for computing payment amounts under the Medicare payment schedule.

Practice expense—The cost of physician practice overhead, including rent, staff salaries and benefits, medical equipment, and supplies; one of three resource cost components included in the formula for computing Medicare payment schedule amounts.

Prevailing charge—One of the factors under the CPR system used to determine physician payment for a particular service. The prevailing charge for a service was an amount set high enough to cover the full customary charges of the physicians in a locality whose billings accounted for at least 75% of the charges for that service. Increases in prevailing charges were capped by increases in the Medicare economic index (MEI).

Primary care services—The HCFA restricts its definition of primary care services to the following: Office or other outpatient services (99201-99215); Emergency department services (99281-99285); Nursing facility services (99301-99313); Domiciliary, rest home, or

M custodial care services (99321-99333); Home services (99341-99355); Eye exam, new patient (92002-92004); Prolonged services, office (99354-99355); and Care plan oversight services (99375). For the 1996 relative value scale, the primary care services category was expanded to include end-stage renal disease (ESRD) services (90935-90947). The OBRA 93 requires that this definition be used to determine those services included in the primary care update.

Professional component—In coding for physician services, that portion of the service that denotes the physician's work and associated overhead and professional liability insurance (PLI) costs.

Professional liability insurance (PLI)—Insurance to protect a physician against professional liability; one of three resource cost components included in the formula developed by HCFA for computing Medicare payment schedule amounts.

Relative value scale (RVS)—An index of physicians' services ranked according to "value," with value defined according to the basis for the scale. In a charge-based RVS, services are ranked according to the average fee for the service or some other charge basis. A resource-based RVS ranks services according to the relative costs of the resources required to provide them.

Relative value unit (RVU)—The unit of measure for the Medicare resource-based relative value scale. The RVUs must be multiplied by a dollar conversion factor to become payment amounts.

Resource-based practice expense—A methodology for determining practice expense relative values based on physicians' practice overhead costs, including rent, staff salaries, and medical equipment and supplies. The Social Security Act Amendments of 1994 contain provisions mandating development of resource-based practice expense relative values for implementation on January 1, 1998.

Resource-based relative value scale (RBRVS)—A relative value scale based on the resource costs of providing physician services; adopted in OBRA 89 as the basis for physician payment for Medicare Part B services effective January 1, 1992. The relative value of each service is the sum of relative value units (RVUs) representing physician work, practice expense, and professional liability insurance (PLI) adjusted for each locality by a geographic adjustment factor and converted into dollar payment amounts by a conversion factor.

Social Security Act Amendments of 1994—Technical corrections legislation adopted by Congress that contains a number of provisions relative to the Medicare RBRVS. These provisions include development of resource-based practice expense relative values, HCFA authority to enforce balance billing requirements, study of needed data refinements to update the geographic practice cost indexes (GPCIs), and development and refinement of relative values for the full range of pediatric services.

Specialty differential—Under the customary, prevailing, and reasonable (CPR) system, some Medicare carriers paid different amounts to physicians, according to specialty, for providing the same service. The OBRA 89 required that such payment differentials be eliminated.

Sustainable growth rate (SGR)—A spending goal for Medicare Part B services proposed in the December 1995 Congressional Conference Report as an alternative to the Medicare volume performance standard (MVPS). Provisions in the Conference Report, which was vetoed by President Clinton, would have abolished the MVPS in favor of a sustainable growth rate that would allow for annual updates to the conversion factor based on a volume allowance of growth in the real gross domestic product (GDP) per capita plus 2 percentage points.

Technical component—In coding for physician services, the portion of a service or procedure that includes cost of equipment, supplies, and technician salary. Payment for the technical component of a service is composed of relative values for practice expense and professional liability insurance (PLI).

Transition asymmetry—The effect of payments for evaluation and management (E/M) services increasing at a faster rate than payments for other services decrease during the 1992 through 1995 transition to the full payment schedule, causing total oulays in 1992 to exceed what they would have been had the CPR system been retained. To allow payments for services during the transition period to increase and decrease at about the same rate and maintain budget neutrality, Health Care Financing Administration (HCFA) made a one-time 5.5% reduction to the adjusted historical payment basis (AHPB).

Transition offset—To maintain budget neutrality during the transition to the full payment schedule, given the transition asymmetry, a 5.5% adjustment was adopted in the 1991 Final Rule and applied to the adjusted historical payment basis (AHPB) instead of the conversion factor, as proposed in the Notice of Proposed Rulemaking (NPRM). By applying this adjustment to the AHPBs, permanent cuts to the conversion factor were prevented. (MPP-1997)

Medicare RBRVS: The Physicians' Guide. Chicago, Ill: American Medical Assocation; 1997.
ISBN 0-89970-860-9 OP059697

Physicians' Medicare Guide
(Looseleaf manual for Medicare Part B—includes full descriptions of the CPT codes from the AMA's CPT book including RBRVS and is updated 10 times a year.) From:

Commerce Clearing House
4025 W Peterson Ave, Chicago, IL 60646
312 583-8500

Resources

Physician Payment Review Commission
2120 L St NW, Ste 510, Washington, DC 20037
202 653-7220

Complaints regarding fraud, waste, abuse, etc:
Department of Health and Human Services
(Inspector General's Hotline)
800 368-5779; 301 597-0724 (in MD)

Contact local Medicare office or state department of public aid.

Contact Medicare Carrier or AMA Members Service Center for Unique Physician Identification Number. (UPIN).

Medicare Carriers

Medicare Part B carriers

Listed below are Medicare Part B carriers according to state. Physicians may need to contact their carrier for more specific information on payment policies and procedures than that provided in the *Physicians' Guide*. Such requests can be made over the telephone using the numbers provided below, although in some instances physicians may find that a written communication provides important documentation if a dispute with a carrier should arise.

The number of insurance companies contracting with Medicare for Part B claims processing has declined over the past few years as a number of companies have chosen not to renew their Medicare contracts. As a result, a single carrier may process claims from a number of different states.

Effective October 1, 1997, all claims processing and other carrier functions performed by Aetna Life Insurance Company were transferred to other contractors, as indicated below. In addition, carrier services were split between two contractors in the following states: Alaska, Arizona, Hawaii, Nevada, Oregon, and Washington. Blue Cross and Blue Shield of North Dakota process physician claims for these states, while other carrier services, including medical review, fraud and abuse, and Medicare secondary payer, are performed by Transamerica Occidental Life Insurance Company. The Health Insurance Portability and Accountability Act of 1996 allows the separation of payment integrity functions from other carrier services.

Alabama
Medicare B
Blue Cross-Blue Shield of Alabama
450 Riverchase Pkwy E, Birmingham, AL 35298
205 988-2100   Fax 205 733-7255

Alaska
Medicare B
Blue Cross-Blue Shield of North Dakota
4510 13th Ave SW, Fargo, ND 58121
701 282-1100   Fax 701 282-1002

Arizona
Medicare B
Blue Cross-Blue Shield of North Dakota
4510 13th Ave SW, Fargo, ND 58121
701 282-1100   Fax 701 282-1002

Arkansas
Medicare B
Arkansas Blue Cross and Blue Shield
601 Gaines St, Little Rock, AR 72203
501 378-2000   Fax 501 378-2804

California
Medicare B
State of California (North)
National Heritage Insurance Company
5400 Legacy Dr, H3-3A-05, Plano, TX 75024
916 896-7025   Fax 916 896-7182

State of California (South)
Transamerica Occidental Life Insurance Company
Medicare Operations
PO Box 54905, Los Angeles, CA 90054-0905
213 748-2311   Fax 213 741-6803

Colorado
Medicare B
Blue Cross-Blue Shield of North Dakota
4510 13th Ave SW, Fargo, ND 58121
701 282-1100   Fax 701 282-1002

Connecticut
Medicare B
Metrahealth Insurance Company
450 Columbus Blvd—5GB, PO Box 15045
Hartford, CT 06115-0450
860 702-6668   Fax 860 702-6587

Delaware
Medicare B
Highmark
PO Box 890065, Camp Hill, PA 17089-0065
717 763-3151   Fax 717 975-7045

District of Columbia
Medicare B
Highmark
PO Box 890065, Camp Hill, PA 17089-0065
717 763-3151   Fax 717 975-7045

Florida
Medicare B
Blue Cross and Blue Shield of Florida, Inc
532 Riverside Ave, PO Box 2078
Jacksonville, FL 32231-0048
904 791-8155   Fax 904 791-8378

Georgia
Medicare B
Blue Cross-Blue Shield of Alabama
450 Riverchase Pkwy E
Birmingham, AL 35298
205 988-2100   Fax 205 733-7255

Hawaii
Medicare B
Blue Cross-Blue Shield of North Dakota
4510 13th Ave SW, Fargo, ND 58121
701 282-1100   Fax 701 282-1002

Idaho
Medicare B
Connecticut General Life Insurance Company (CGLIC)
Hartford, CT 06152
615 782-4576   Fax 615 244-6242

Illinois
Medicare B
Health Care Service Corp
233 N Michigan Ave, Chicago, IL 60601
312 938-8000   Fax 312 861-0319

Indiana
Medicare Part B
Administar Federal, Inc
8115 Knue St, Indianapolis, IN 46250-2804
317 841-4400   Fax 317 841-4691

Iowa
Medicare B
IASD Health Services Corp
636 Grand Ave, Station 28, Des Moines, IA 50309
515 245-4618   Fax 515 245-3984

Kansas
Medicare B
Blue Cross and Blue Shield of Kansas, Inc
1133 Topeka Ave, PO Box 239
Topeka, KS 66601
913 291-7000   Fax 913 291-8532

Kentucky
Medicare B
Administar Federal, Inc
8115 Knue St, Indianapolis, IN 46250-2804
317 841-4400   Fax 317 841-4691

Louisiana
Medicare B
Arkansas Blue Cross and Blue Shield
601 Gaines St, Little Rock, AR 72203
501 378-2000   Fax 501 378-2804

Maine
Medicare B
Blue Cross and Blue Shield of Massachusetts, Inc
100 Summer St, Boston, MA 02110
617 741-3122   Fax 617 741-3211

Maryland
Medicare B
Blue Cross Blue Shield of Texas, Inc
PO Box 660156, Dallas, TX 75266-0156
214 766-6900   Fax 214 766-7612

Counties of Montgomery, Prince Georges
Medical Service Association of Pennsylvania
PO Box 890065, Camp Hill, PA 17089-0065
717 763-3151   Fax 717 975-7045

Massachusetts
Medicare B
Blue Cross and Blue Shield of Massachusetts, Inc
100 Summer St, Boston, MA 02110
617 741-3122   Fax 617 741-3211

Michigan
Medicare B
Health Care Service Corp
233 N Michigan Ave, Chicago, IL 60601
312 938-6360   Fax 312 861-0319

Minnesota
Medicare B
Metrahealth Insurance Company
450 Columbus Blvd—5GB, PO Box 15045
Hartford, CT 06115-0450
860 702-6668   Fax 860 702-6587

Mississippi
Medicare B
Metrahealth Insurance Company
450 Columbus Blvd—5GB, PO Box 15045
Hartford, CT 06115-0450
860 702-6668   Fax 860 702-6587

Missouri
Medicare B (Western Missouri)
Blue Cross and Blue Shield of Kansas, Inc
1133 Topeka Ave, PO Box 239
Topeka, KS 66601
913 291-7000   Fax 913 291-7824

Medicare B (Eastern Missouri)
General American Life Insurance Co
PO Box 505, St Louis, MO 63166
314 525-5441   Fax 314 525-5593

Montana
Medicare B
Blue Cross and Blue Shield of Montana, Inc
PO Box 4310, 2501 Beltview
Helena, MT 59601
406 791-4000   Fax 406 442-9968

Nebraska
Medicare Part B
Blue Cross and Blue Shield of Kansas, Inc
1133 Topeka Ave, PO Box 239
Topeka, KS 66601
913 291-7000   Fax 913 291-7824

Nevada
Medicare B
Blue Cross-Blue Shield of North Dakota
4510 13th Ave SW, Fargo, ND 58121
701 282-1100   Fax 701 282-1002

New Hampshire
Medicare B
Blue Cross and Blue Shield of Massachusetts, Inc
100 Summer St, Boston, MA 02110
617 956-3445   Fax 617 350-4555

New Jersey
Medicare B
Highmark
PO Box 890065, Camp Hill, PA 17089-0065
717 763-3151   Fax 717 975-7045

New Mexico
Medicare B
Arkansas Blue Cross and Blue Shield
601 Gaines St, Little Rock, AR 72203
501 378-2000   Fax 501 378-2804

New York
Medicare B
Blue Cross and Blue Shield of Western New York, Inc
7-9 Court St, Binghamton, NY 13901-3197
716 887-6900   Fax 716 887-8548

Empire Blue Cross and Blue Shield
Counties of Bronx, Columbia, Delaware, Dutchess,
Greene, Kings, Nassau, New York, Orange, Putnam,
Richmond, Rockland, Suffolk, Sullivan, Ulster, and
Westchester
622 Third Ave, New York, NY 10017
212 476-1000   Fax 212 682-5746

North Carolina
Medicare B
Connecticut General Life Insurance Company (CGLIC)
Hartford, CT 06152
615 782-4576   Fax 615 244-6242

North Dakota
Medicare B
Blue Cross-Blue Shield of North Dakota
4510 13th Ave SW, Fargo, ND 58121
701 282-1100   Fax 701 282-1002

Ohio
Medicare B
Nationwide Mutual Insurance Company
PO Box 16788 or 16781
Columbus, OH 43216
614 249-7111   Fax 614 249-3732

Oklahoma
Medicare B
Arkansas Blue Cross and Blue Shield
601 Gaines St, Little Rock, AR 72203
501 378-2000   Fax 501 378-2804

Oregon
Medicare B
Blue Cross-Blue Shield of North Dakota
4510 13th Ave SW, Fargo, ND 58121
701 282-1100   Fax 701 282-1002

Pennsylvania
Medicare B
Medical Services Association of Pennsylvania
PO Box 890065, Camp Hill, PA 17089-0065
Express Mail: 1800 Center St
Camp Hill, PA 17089
717 763-3151   Fax 717 975-7045

Puerto Rico
Medicare B
Triple-S, Inc
Box 363628, San Juan, PR 00936-3628
809 749-4080   Fax 809 749-4092

Rhode Island
Medicare B
Blue Cross and Blue Shield of Rhode Island
444 Westminster St
Providence, RI 02903-3279
401 459-1000   Fax 401 459-1709

South Carolina
Medicare B
Blue Cross and Blue Shield of South Carolina
300 Arbor Lake Dr, Ste 1300
Columbia, SC 29223
803 735-1034   Fax 803 691-2188

South Dakota
Medicare Part B
Blue Cross-Blue Shield of North Dakota
4510 13th Ave SW, Fargo, ND 58121
701 282-1100   Fax 701 282-1002

Tennessee
Medicare B
Connecticut General Life Insurance Company (CGLIC)
Hartford, CT 06152
615 782-4576   Fax 615 244-6242

Texas
Medicare B
Blue Cross and Blue Shield of Texas, Inc
901 S Central Expressway
Richardson, TX 75080
214 766-6900   Fax 214 766-7612

Utah
Medicare B
Blue Cross and Blue Shield of Utah
1455 Parley's Way, PO Box 30270
Salt Lake City, UT 84130
801 487-6441   Fax 801 481-6994

Vermont
Medicare B
Blue Cross and Blue Shield of Massachusetts, Inc
100 Summer St, Boston, MA 02110
617 956-3445   Fax 617 350-4555

Virginia
Medicare B
Metrahealth Insurance Company
450 Columbus Blvd—5GB, PO Box 15045
Hartford, CT 06115-0450
860 702-6668   Fax 860 702-6587

Washington
Medicare B
Blue Cross-Blue Shield of North Dakota
4510 13th Ave SW, Fargo, ND 58121
701 282-1100   Fax 701 282-1002

West Virginia
Medicare B Nationwide Mutual Insurance Co
PO Box 16788, Columbus, OH 43216
614 249-7111   Fax 614 249-3732

Wisconsin
Medicare B
Wisconsin Physicians' Service Insurance Corp
PO Box 1787, Madison, WI 53701
608 221-4711   Fax 608 223-3614

Wyoming
Medicare B
Blue Cross-Blue Shield of North Dakota
4510 13th Ave SW, Fargo, ND 58121
701 282-1100   Fax 701 282-1002
(MPP-1997)

Medicare Reform

Three problems

To preserve the Medicare program, at least three distinct Medicare problems must be addressed. The most familiar has been publicized perennially in annual reports of the trustees of the Medicare trust funds. The report issued in June of 1996 projected that the Medicare hospital trust fund (Part A) will be exhausted in 2000 or 2001. Current law does not allow deficit spending from the Part A trust fund; unless the law is changed and other sources of funds are tapped, payments to hospitals for services provided to Medicare beneficiaries will cease.

The second problem is that Medicare's expenditure growth cannot be sustained. The high growth rates for many of the services are due to a combination of factors, including increased beneficiary demand for new services, slow program response to known flaws in payment rules that encourage high-volume growth in some categories of service, insulation of most beneficiaries from cost considerations, and ineffective approaches to cost control.

The methods used by government to try to control the growth have not worked. Price controls have been one of the main approaches; they have been used since 1983 in Part A, and since 1975 in various forms in Part B. Budget cuts have been another heavily used attempt to control growth. Seventy distinct budget cuts in Medicare payments to physicians have been taken since the program began, resulting in a cumulative reduction in Part B outlays of $39 billion. Budget cuts of $59 billion have also been made to Part A.

Despite the budget-cutting and holding payment rates to providers below private sector levels and rates of inflation, Medicare expenditures grew from 3.7% of the federal budget in 1970 to 13% in 1995. If the rates of spending in both parts of Medicare are not slowed, spending is projected to grow rapidly from 2.6% of gross domestic product in 1995 to 7.8% in 2035.

The third problem is a longer-term problem: the number of workers contributing payroll taxes to finance the hospital trust fund is declining. In 1965 when Medicare was enacted, there were 5.5 working-age Americans for every individual over 65. Today, there are only 3.9. In the coming decades, as the "baby boom" generation continues to age, the number will fall more rapidly. By the year 2030 there will be only 2.2 working-age Americans for each individual over age 65. By that time, 20% of the population will be covered by Medicare, compared with 12.8% now.

Medicare's problem involves its promises, its financing, and the way it is run. The program has severe structural problems dating from its original design. Medicare must be restructured so that it can continue to achieve its objectives in the 21st century without large tax increases or benefit reductions. The AMA's proposal to transform Medicare is a comprehensive approach to addressing all of Medicare's problems.

What is Medicare?

Most think of Medicare as a government insurance program covering health care for Americans who are age 65 and older. However, because Medicare benefits are somewhat meager compared with the employer-sponsored benefits that many covered beneficiaries enjoyed during their working years, most beneficiaries are covered by various supplements to Medicare that they or their former employers purchase, or that are provided by other government programs such as Medicaid. Seventy-eight percent of Medicare beneficiaries are covered by private Medicare supplemental policies (called "medigap"), which essentially convert Medicare into first-dollar coverage by paying Medicare's cost-sharing (ie, deductibles and copayments) requirements. Another 12% are eligible for Medicaid, which also covers Medicare's cost-sharing requirements.

In all, almost 90% of Medicare beneficiaries have coverage beyond basic Medicare benefits. Therefore, Medicare must be viewed as more than a public program. It is a combination of insurance coverage, both public and private. The fact that it is a combination of coverages expands the scope of Medicare's problems far beyond those that would prevail if Medicare were not supplemented by other coverage. It also magnifies the practical and political difficulty of dealing with Medicare's problems.

Because the term *trust fund* is officially used to describe the financing of Medicare, many people think that the payroll taxes they pay are saved and accumulate interest to pay for their medical needs in retirement. In fact, the Part A program is financed on a pay-as-you-go basis, with taxes paid into the program being used to pay for the benefits received by current retirees, and the excess used to purchase unfunded federal debt. Part B is financed mostly out of general revenues, with the premiums that retirees pay calculated to cover only about 25% of the outlays. Part B is modeled after a private sector health plan, but whereas premiums in private plans cover

100% of outlays, taxpayers fund 75% of the cost of providing Part B services to beneficiaries.

Most retirees have received many more benefits than their contributions to the program could purchase. The pay-as-you-go financing of Part A of Medicare is often likened to a chain letter. The similarity lies in the promise of future benefits to those who fund services for current beneficiaries, and the need for a growing number of new contributors to fund the growing number of beneficiaries. Chain letters must eventually collapse due to insufficient influx of new participants. Theoretically, Medicare need not collapse if the Congress is willing to use its power to tax to make up for the falling ratio of Medicare contributors to beneficiaries as well as the growth in the cost per beneficiary. Medicare actuaries estimate that the tax would have to be increased immediately from its current level of 2.9% to 7.4%. This would bring the current combined tax rate of Social Security and Medicare to 19.8%. However, a tax increase would also be necessary to bring the Social Security trust fund into future actuarial balance. The Social Security trustees have estimated that the payroll tax would have to be raised from the current 12.4% to 18.8%. Thus, the payroll tax rate for a tax-based bailout of Social Security and Medicare is 26.2%. Increasing taxes has not been considered a politically feasible option. Congress has looked for other ways to save Medicare.

Proposals to save Medicare

The 104th Congress made a serious attempt to reform Medicare in its first session. In the budget debate between the President and congressional Republican leadership following passage of the Omnibus Budget Reconciliation Act of 1995 (OBRA 95) and its veto by the President, both sides claimed that their version of the budget "saved" Medicare.

OBRA 95 contained several major changes to Medicare. The most significant was the addition of a "Medicare Plus" program, which would have enabled beneficiaries to purchase various forms of private health insurance with a defined government contribution. The MedicarePlus program was very similar to the current Federal Employee Health Benefit Program that was proposed as a model for Medicare by the AMA and the Heritage Foundation. The President's proposal also expanded the types of plans available to beneficiaries, but retained the current system Medicare uses for paying HMOs—rather than a defined contribution—to pay for them. Both proposals retained the traditional fee-for-service Medicare program essentially in its current form.

Would either of these two approaches "save" Medicare? Although there is some potential for containing the growth of expenditure by expanding private health plan offerings to beneficiaries, the Congressional Budget Office predicted only 24% of beneficiaries would have joined MedicarePlus plans by 2002. Thus, in the short run, most beneficiaries would have remained in the traditional program where the problems that have led to the current crises remain untouched by either proposal.

Like the alternatives of the President and the Republican Congress, many of the other proposals for comprehensive reform of Medicare would have extended the choices of beneficiaries to a variety of private health plans, but would have preserved the current program as one of the options. However, if the traditional Medicare program were retained, significant reforms would have to be made in its structure and administration to contain costs and save Medicare. The AMA has a proposal to fix the traditional program to correct its serious design flaws that does not limit beneficiary access and choice. We propose an approach to reconfiguring the traditional Medicare to include coverage equivalent to that which most beneficiaries purchase privately, but in a way that costs most beneficiaries less than they pay now, and that saves the government money as well. This extra savings to the government can be used to expand benefits or reduce beneficiary costs even further.

The 105th Congress
A solid consensus seems to have formed that expanding choice for Medicare beneficiaries is the favored approach to reform. The 104th Congress preferred to provide a defined contribution toward beneficiary purchase of private plans, while the president's approach preserved the defined benefit method. The defined contribution approach provides a direct way of limiting government's cost, but the schedule of increases to the annual contribution Congress offered was less than the rate of inflation projected by the Congressional Budget Office, leading to charges that they were cutting benefits. As proposed by some research organizations, the market price of a basic benefit package could be used to determine the defined contribution to guarantee that basic benefits would not be cut.

It is likely that the attempt that the 105th Congress makes to save Medicare will keep the traditional program as an option for beneficiaries. We strongly believe that it should. If it is kept, its structure must be significantly changed to increase its efficiency and remove the built-in incentives for cost growth. If not, continued budget cuts and price regulation will make participation increasingly problematic for physicians, hospitals, and other health care providers, so that patient access to care will be compromised. To prevent that result, the AMA has suggested a set of reforms for the traditional program based on sound economic principles to improve efficiency and save money for both beneficiaries and the government.

Few detailed proposals have been made for saving Medicare for the long term. Consequently, there has been much talk of a Presidential Commission to consider the problem.

Increasing the age of eligibility and reducing the subsidy for high-income beneficiaries, rather than tax increases, have been proposed. Such measures are only the initial steps in light of the magnitude of the future expenditures that will have to be financed. Furthermore, they would not correct the perverse incentives built into the structure of the program that discourage efficiency.

As a long-run approach to the Medicare financial problem, some have proposed that strong incentives be provided to the current working-age population to save enough during their working years so that they do not plan to rely on the Medicare program for medical care needs in retirement. Some would provide the savings incentives through Medical Savings Accounts (MSAs) that would also be used for preretirement medical needs. Others have suggested a separate program of private saving be mandated by the government as an approach to

funding health care for retirees in the long run. We support increasing the age of eligibility to match that scheduled to occur for Social Security. We support reducing the subsidy for high-income beneficiaries using income-related premiums. We believe that private savings during working years for health care in retirement should be part of the solution to Medicare's financial health over the long term. (TM-1995)

Meetings, Medical
World Meetings Publications
Macmillan Publishing Company
866 3rd Ave, New York, NY 10022

World Meetings: Medicine
ISSN 0161-2875 (2-year listing of upcoming medical meetings updated quarterly)

World Meetings: United States and Canada
ISSN 0043-8693 (2-year listing of upcoming scientific, technical, and medical meetings)

World Meetings: Outside United States and Canada
ISSN 0043-8693 (2-year listing of upcoming scientific, technical, and medical meetings)

Scientific Meetings Publications
PO Box 81662, San Diego, CA 92138
619 270-2910

Scientific Meetings
ISSN 0487-8965 (quarterly listing of future meetings of technical, scientific, medical, and management organizations and universities)

The Laux Company
63 Great Rd, Maynard, MA 01754

Medical Meetings
ISSN 0093-1314
(bimonthly publication to aid in the planning of medical meetings)

Mental Health

AMA Policy

Mental Health Consequences of Interpersonal and Family Violence (H-515.976) CSA Rep B, A-93

Implications for the Practitioner: The AMA encourages physicians to: (1) routinely inquire about the family violence histories of their patients as this knowledge is essential for effective diagnosis and care; (2) make appropriate referrals to address intervention and safety needs as a matter of course upon identifying patients currently experiencing abuse or threats from intimates; (3) screen patients for psychiatric sequelae of violence and make appropriate referrals for these conditions upon identifying a history of family or other interpersonal violence; and (4) become aware of local resources and referral sources that have expertise in dealing with trauma from victimization.

A Piece of My Mind

The surprise party

Harold I. Eist, MD

JAMA 1983 June 24; 249(24):2632

In understanding the experience of mentally ill individuals, we should recognize the courage they often exhibit even while engaging in superficial ordinary human interactions. Unless we appreciate this, their responses of isolation and withdrawal because of interpersonal terror will seem inexplicable. Two clinical examples help to clarify this point.

An alcoholic woman began talking about her son, who had been psychotic since childhood, and I wondered if there would ever be any end to her grief. Alcohol had destroyed her liver, but it had not washed away the grief. She mentioned with a slight smile that finally she was beginning to accept the many losses her son's illness represented.

"We had him home from the hospital Sunday, and Mary, the friend I told you about who also has a schizophrenic son, brought him over. The two boys have known each other since they were kids and there they were, both of them on the couch, acting like the other and one didn't exist."

Her remark took me back 17 years to a medication group I had run for chronically schizophrenically ill patients at a Veterans Administration hospital. During my weekly sessions with the group, as each of the 10 assiduously avoided eye contact with the other, I often thought, "You guys don't need a psychiatrist—you need an air traffic control operator."

Six weeks prior to my leaving this group, I announced I was moving on to another service. Each patient responded by firmly fixing his eyes on a distant point. I wondered if there was any concern on the part of the group members at my leaving, but I couldn't tell for sure.

As the group assembled at the last meeting, one of the members, who was uncharacteristically well groomed, emptied a bag of doughnuts in the center of the group-room table. Each member of the group filed to the table and took a doughnut.

"The last one's for you, Doc," one of them said. "It's a surprise party." Suddenly it hit me that these terribly isolated men had gotten together in spite of their fearfulness and had planned a party for me. Furthermore, in the face of crippling illness, they had carried it off.

We ate our doughnuts silently, no one looking at anyone else, and then we discussed medications. I shook hands with each of them, and someone said, "Hope you enjoy your new job."

"Me too," I answered, full of sadness, gratitude, and new-found understanding.

JAMA Article of Note: Utility of a new procedure for diagnosing mental disorders in primary care: The PRIME-MD 1000 Study.

JAMA 1994;272(22):1749-1756

Resources

National Alliance for the Mentally Ill
200 N Glebe Rd, Ste 1015, Arlington, VA 22203-3728
800 950-NAMI   703 524-7600   Fax 703 524-9094
Web address: http://www.cais.com/vikings/nami

National Depressive and Manic Depressive Association
730 N Franklin, Ste 501, Chicago, IL 60610
800 82-NDMDA   312 642-0049   Fax 312 642-7243

National Institute of Mental Health
Office of Scientific Information
Public Inquiries Section
5600 Fishers Ln, Rm 15C-17, Rockville, MD 20857
301 443-4513
Web address: http://www.nimh.nih.gov

National Mental Health Association
1021 Prince St, Alexandria, VA 22314-2971
800 969-NMHA (800 969-6642)
703 684-7722   Fax 703 684-5968
Web address: http://www.worldcorp.com/dc-online/nmha

Mental Retardation

American Association on Mental Retardation
444 N Capital St NW, Ste 846
Washington, DC 20001-1512
800 424-3688   202 387-1968   Fax 202 387-2193

Mergers

Mergers: Don't jump in without doing your homework

Michael Weinstein
AM News Nov 7, 1994 pp50-1

During the past two years, some appalling mergers have occurred among medical groups, independent practice associations, and health plans throughout the United States. In many instances it appears that strong medical groups and IPAs are merging because they are in a state of panic.

This panic is being caused by two factors: Many physicians are experiencing anxiety about the push for national health system reform. And plans are reacting to mergers and alliances that are occurring in their marketplace.

What is most disturbing about these quick mergers of medical groups and independent practice associations is that often assets are literally being given away.

Medical groups and IPAs are being acquired and/or merged on the basis that the organizations will be granted stock options or other compensations based upon future group earnings. In addition, many health plans and hospitals are purchasing practices at what first appears to be very attractive offers, but which actually are well below the practice's true value.

It is important for medical groups and IPAs to realize that their organizations are an extremely valuable asset and have built up significant equity. Even if the organization itself is not showing a bottom-line profit, it can still be a valuable asset with restructuring and revamped management.

Most of the time the acquiring organizations realize the immediate and future earnings potential of these groups. If you're considering a sale or merger, you should realize these potentials, too.

Ask for help
When a medical group and/or IPA is considering the sale of their assets, a merger, or a joint venture management service organization, it should seek professional assistance to develop a short- and long-term strategic plan.

Look for consultants with a proven track record and an understanding of health system reform, particularly managed care. Select legal counsel with a proven track record in developing these mergers and/or joint ventures.

With many merger and/or sale arrangements, the acquiring party will pick up all or part of the costs associated with assessing the value of your practice, developing your strategic plan, identifying the best organizations to align with, and obtaining the legal services to complete these transactions.

Before you proceed, you must clearly understand the value of the assets and the equity that you have built within your organization. This equity is not only your current earnings, but your future earnings potential.

Professional assistance can help you end up with more successful alignments, receive better financial terms, and develop options that are tailor designed to meet both parties' needs.

Meet your potential partners
Meet with all the possible entities—groups, IPAs, physician-hospital organizations, medical staff organizations, hospitals—that you are considering linking with through merger or sale. Don't draw preconceived conclusions on who the suitable partners are. Many times, a group does not immediately recognize the best potential partner.

Also, meet with the various health plans with which you have and/or would like to have an affiliation. Health plans are a good resource and can provide excellent insight about the organizations they feel your group will benefit through an alignment. They can help you categorize the medical groups from a quality and cost-effectiveness basis, and be candid as to how they would react if you were to align with the various entities in your marketplace.

Don't underestimate your assets
Many times medical groups and/or IPAs will have not only capital assets but also receivables and future earnings potential. These organizations may not be financially successful, but will have the capability of turning this around and significantly improving their cash flow through improved management and reimbursement (which might occur through an alignment with another medical group and/or IPA).

As a result, it is important that you do a detailed financial analysis of your corporation so that you do not give away assets that may have significant future earnings potential to the acquiring and/or merging entity.

Learn the corporate culture
Meet with prospective alliances to get a clear understanding of their corporate culture. The policies and philosophies of the various evolving mega-medical groups vary greatly.

Some groups look at truly making the merged organization part of the founding organizations, while others clearly are taking over complete control of your organization and you are now "the hired help."

Align yourself with an organization that has a philosophy you are comfortable with.

Who has the clout?
As you are assessing an alignment, consider the leverage that each organization could bring to your group. Some groups will bring an infusion of capital, other groups will bring in strong management systems, others will have better negotiated contracts with the health plans.

If a group is bringing in management expertise, meet with the individuals who will be actually responsible for working with your organization. Make sure the management companies have the management expertise and depth that they profess to have.

Will the cash flow?
Look at the cash-flow projections in each of the proposals presented. Have your current and future practice professionally appraised so that you have a clear understanding of the current and future earnings value of your practice.

This is important not only if you are selling your assets, but when you are negotiating joint ventures such as a medical service organization or merger agreement. Understand the tax consequences of the deal you are contemplating.

In summary, medical groups and IPAs must exert a great deal of due diligence to avoid giving their practices away. Plan, don't panic. It will pay off handsomely in both the short and long term.

Note: Michael Weinstein is president of Managed Care Planning Associates, a national consulting firm that specializes in managed care strategic planning for integrated health care delivery systems, medical groups, IPAs, and major health care corporations and systems. MCPA's principals include a physician, a medical group chief executive officer, and a hospital chief executive officer.

Midwives
American College of Nurse-Midwives
1522 K St NW, Ste 1000, Washington, DC 20005
202 728-9860   Fax 202 289-4395

Informed Homebirth Informed Birth and Parenting
PO Box 3675, Ann Arbor, MI 48106
313 662-6857

Planned Parenthood Federation of America
810 Seventh Ave, New York, NY 10019
212 541-7800   Fax 212 245-1845

Position on Midwifery:
American College of Obstetricians
and Gynecologists
409 12th St SW, Washington, DC 20024
202 638-5577   Fax 202 484-8107

Military Medicine

AMA Policy

Elimination of Anti-Personnel Landmines (H-520.989)
Res 424, I-96

(1) The AMA urges the US government to (*a*) renounce its claimed exceptions to a ban on antipersonnel landmines, (*b*) effectuate through the United Nations an international ban on the product, stockpiling, sale, transfer, or export of these weapons, (*c*) establish a hemispheric landmine free zone in support of the Organization of American States position, and (*d*) sign the Ottawa Treaty banning all antipersonnel landmines by December 1997.

(2) The AMA encourages the US government and all members of the United Nations, as well as other interested charitable and medical organizations, to contribute funds for the care, treatment, and rehabilitation of landmine trauma victims.

Poetry and Medicine

Arlington Cemetery, Virginia

E. Cameron Ritchie, MD
JAMA 1996 October 16; 276(15): 1202b

General Lee's garden:
purpled shoots rise;
jackets open, kids
race down the paths;
tombstones settle in
snow melt and March wind.

Stone crosses parade the slopes:
soldiers fallen in battle
or faded in nursing homes.
Snow highlights graves
with translucent peace.

Kennedy's eternal flame,
fire blue and gold,
burns flanked by cameras.

Tall soldiers with shined brass
stamp, black shoes click heels,
change arms, honor a rock box,
Tomb of the Unknown Soldier.
Skulls and armbones tumble,
souls riding the gusts.

We tromp to the ridge
where physician soldiers lie,
surveying the Potomac.

Walter Reed rests here,
"Conqueror of Yellow Fever,"
enabler of the Panama Canal.

General Rumbaugh died
parachuting into Honduras,

airdropping a hospital.

I remember: bugles calling Taps,
sharp rifle cracks,
the long line of mourners.

His epitaph: "He did not
merely exist in our world; he
roared through it, carrying
the rest of us in his vortex."

The breeze blows, flags snap.
So many grieve here.

Next, we seek my grandfather:
small headstone with Russian
cross. He fought in three wars,
and died at 85, demented.
No tourists.

Daffodils spurt upwards.
More bugles sound.
Trees dream of bloom.

Gulf War Mystery

Bill Clements
AM News Jan 6, 1997 p18

The symptoms plaguing thousands of Operation Desert Storm veterans continue to baffle health experts. Meanwhile, suspicion over the way the military has dealt with their claims has kept many former soldiers from seeking help in Veterans Affairs health centers. (excerpt)

Military health facilities may be the best places for Persian Gulf War veterans to get medical help for health problems associated with "Gulf War syndrome."

Yet, Gulf War veterans are not exactly flocking to the 160 Veterans Affairs Medical Centers. Experts say many vets are distrustful of military-run facilities because they are dissatisfied with the way the Dept. of Defense has handled information regarding possible chemical and pesticide exposure during Operation Desert Storm.

According to the VA, of the nearly 700,000 men and women who served in the Gulf War in 1991, only 70,000 have sought medical assistance at VA sites, which include four major regional referral centers—Birmingham, Ala; Houston; Los Angeles; and Washington, DC. About 10,000 of those vets were found to be healthy.

Officials say about 85% of the Gulf War vets found to be sick have been diagnosed with known illnesses—among them, connective tissue disorder and chronic fatigue syndrome—and have received or are receiving appropriate care, many under a VA medical compensation plan.

But VA physicians have not been able to diagnose the health complaints of the other 10,000 vets (about 15% of the total)—health problems that must have appeared either during Gulf War service or within two years of leaving Southwest Asia to be covered by the VA health benefits plan.

The undiagnosed problems fall into 13 categories: fatigue; signs or symptoms involving skin; headache; muscle pain; joint pain; neurologic signs or symptoms; neuropsychological signs or symptoms; signs or symptoms involving the respiratory system (upper or lower); sleep disturbances; gastrointestinal signs or symptoms;

cardiovascular signs or symptoms; abnormal weight loss; and menstrual disorders.

What to ask Gulf War veterans

AM News Jan 6, 1997 p 18

These are sample questions taken from the questionnaire developed by Claudia Miller, MD, at the Houston Veterans Affairs Medical Center. The questionnaire asks the vets to rate the severity of their symptoms to these exposures—from both before and since the Gulf War—on a scale of 1 to 10.

Q: Do you feel sick or experience any symptoms when you are exposed to:
Diesel or gas engine exhaust?
Tobacco smoke?
Insecticides?
Gasoline, like at a service station while filling the gas tank?
Paint or paint thinner?
Fresh tar or asphalt?
Nail polish, nail polish remover, or hairspray?
New furnishings, such as new carpeting, a new soft plastic shower curtain, or the interior of a new car?

Q: Are there any particular foods that make you feel ill, such as candy, pizza, milk, fatty foods, meats, barbecue, onions, garlic, or spicy foods?

Q: Do you feel ill after meals?

Q: Do you feel ill if you drink beverages that contain caffeine, such as coffee, tea, cola drinks, Big Red, Dr. Pepper, or Mountain Dew? Or if you eat chocolate?

Q: Do any fabrics, metal jewelry, creams, cosmetics, or other items that touch your skin cause problems for you?

Q: Does drinking a small amount of certain alcoholic beverages make you feel ill?

War zone telemedicine

AM News Jan 22/29, 1996

Army Surgeons in Bosnia will soon use portable satellite dishes and miniature television cameras to communicate with specialists elsewhere, as the result of a $9 million Defense Dept. program to adapt telemedicine to battlefield conditions. In February (1996), the Army will install gear linking hospitals and clinics in Hungary and Bosnia with hospitals in the United States and Europe. The equipment is designed for use in small, transportable operating rooms.

Traumatic stress (posttraumatic stress disorder)

While people are most likely to be familiar with posttraumatic stress disorder as an aftereffect of combat, it can occur in anyone who has suffered some form of overwhelming trauma. This includes experiencing or even witnessing a life-threatening incident, rape, natural disaster such as an earthquake or hurricane, or accident. It is not uncommon, for example, to read or see newspaper or TV news coverage of an anniversary of a disaster where, 1 year later, survivors are still affected by nightmares, tension headaches, or terrible fears.

The effects of posttraumatic stress disorder are very real. They include:
• Flashbacks (intrusive memories of events that are related to the trauma) and frequently remembering the event.
• Emotional numbness or loss of feeling.
• Extreme emotional outbursts and feeling pain, anxiety, rage, guilt, or grief.
• Sleeping problems.
• Feeling isolated or unable to fit in with other people, including those with whom you would normally feel close.

People also develop problems:
• Concentrating.
• Controlling their impulses.
• Making decisions.
• Remembering things.
(CS-1996)

JAMA Theme Issue: Gulf War Syndrome

JAMA 1997 Jan 15: 277(3)

This issue presents several articles discussing different medical aspects of the Gulf War: a factor analysis of the symptoms of the Gulf War syndrome, general illness in Gulf War veterans, and exposure to chemical combinations during the Gulf War.

Resources

Association of Military Surgeons of the United States
9320 Old Georgetown Rd, Bethesda, MD 20814
301 897-8800   Fax 301 530-5446

The Society of Medical Consultants to the Armed Forces
PO Box 2700, Kensington, MD 20891-2700
301 295-3903   Fax 202 726-3616

Missing Children

Childfind Hotline
800 I-AM-LOST

Missing Child Hotline
National Center for Missing and Exploited Children
800 843-5678 9 am to midnight

MEDWATCH
800 I-AM-LOST (800 426-5678)
(Sponsored by Wyeth Laboratories)

Multiple Births

Center for Study of Multiple Birth
333 E Superior St, Ste 464, Chicago, IL 60611
312 266-9093

National Organization of Mothers of Twins Club
PO Box 23188, Albuquerque, NM 87112-1188
505 275-0955

Twinline
2131 University Ave, Ste 234, Berkeley, CA 94704
415 644-0861

Muscle Disorders

The most common muscle disorder is injury, followed by symptoms caused by a lack of blood supply to a muscle (including the heart). In addition, there are a number of other rarer disorders of muscle.

Genetic disorders
The muscular dystrophies cause progressive weakness and disability. Some types appear at birth, some in infancy, and some develop as late as the fifth or sixth decade. One type of cardiomyopathy, a general term for disease of the heart muscle, is inherited.

Infection
The most important infection of muscle is gangrene, which may complicate deep wounds (especially those contaminated by soil). Tetanus is acquired in a similar way, causing widespread muscle spasm through the release of a powerful toxin.

Viruses
Viruses (especially influenza B) may infect muscles (causing myalgia), as may the organism causing toxoplasmosis. Trichinosis is an infestation of muscle with the worm *Trichinella spiralis,* which is acquired by eating undercooked meat (usually pork).

Injury
Muscle injuries, such as tears and sprains, are very common; they cause bleeding into the muscle tissue. Healing leads to formation of a scar in the muscle, which shortens its natural length. Blunt muscle injury may result in hematoma formation from bleeding into the muscle. Rarely, bone may form in the hematoma, causing myositis ossificans.

Tumors
Primary muscle tumors may or may not be cancerous. Noncancerous tumors are called myomas, those affecting smooth muscle are leiomyomas, and those affecting skeletal muscle are rhabdomyomas. Myomas of the uterus are among the most common of all tumors. Cancerous tumors are called myosarcomas and are very rare; cancers of the skeletal muscle are known as rhabdomyosarcomas.

Secondary tumors, which spread from a primary site of cancer elsewhere in the body, very rarely involve muscle.

Hormonal and metabolic disorders
Muscle contraction depends on the maintenance or proper levels of sodium, potassium, and calcium in and around muscle cells. Any alteration in the concentration of these substances affects muscle function. For example, a severe drop in the level of potassium (hypokalemia) causes profound muscle weakness and may stop the heart. A drop in blood calcium (hypocalcemia) causes increased excitability of muscles and, occasionally, spasms.

Thyroid disease is often associated with muscle disorders, the most common being a swelling of the small muscles that move the eyes, causing a bulging eyeball. Adrenal failure causes general muscle weakness.

Impaired blood supply
Muscles depend on a good blood supply for normal function. Cramp is usually caused by a lack of blood flow, sometimes associated with severe exertion. Peripheral vascular disease, which restricts the blood supply, causes claudication (muscle pain on exercise). Angina pectoris (chest pain caused by lack of blood supply to heart muscle) occurs in coronary heart disease.

The compartment syndrome is pain in muscles as a result of swelling that limits the blood supply. It is brought on by injury or exercise, occurring often in athletes with well-developed muscles.

Poisons and drugs
Several toxic substances can damage muscle. They include alcohol, which can cause damage following a prolonged drinking bout. Other substances that may cause muscle damage include aminocaproic acid, chloroquine, clofibrate, emetine, and vincristine.

Autoimmune disorders
Myasthenia gravis is a disorder of transmission of nerve impulses to muscles; it usually begins by causing drooping of the eyelids and double vision. Other diseases with an autoimmune basis that may affect muscles are lupus erythematosus, rheumatoid arthritis, scleroderma, sarcoidosis, and dermatomyositis.

Investigation
Muscle disorders are investigated by EMG (electromyography), which measures the response of muscles to electrical impulses, and by muscle biopsy. (ENC-1989)

Resources
Muscular Dystrophy Association
3300 E Sunrise Dr, Tucson, AZ 85718
800 223-6666 520 529-2000 Fax 520 529-5300

Myasthenia Gravis Foundation
222 S Riverside Pl, Ste 1540, Chicago, IL 60606
800 541-5454 312 427-6252 Fax 312 427-8437

National Multiple Sclerosis Society
733 Third Ave, New York, NY 10017
800 624-8236 212 986-3240 Fax 212 986-7981
E-mail: mmss.org
Web address: http://www.nmss.org

Museums, Medical
Historical Museum of Medicine and Dentistry
230 Scarborough St, Hartford, CT 06105
203 236-5613
Weekday hours 10 am to 4 pm

International College of Surgeons
1516 N Lake Shore Dr, Chicago, IL 60610
312 642-3555 Fax 312 787-1624
E-mail: exd@aol.com
Tuesday through Saturday 10 am to 4 pm
Sunday 11 am to 5 pm

Museum of Ophthalmology
655 Beach St, San Francisco, CA 94133
415 561-8500
Weekday hours 8 am to 5 pm

Musuem of Questionable Medical Devices
201 Main St SE, Minneapolis, MN 55416
612 379-4046
Web address: http://www.mtn.org.quack/

National Museum of Health and Medicine
(Walter Reed Army Medical Center)
Dahlia and 14th Sts NW
Washington, DC 20306-6000
202 782-2200
Weekday hours 9:30 am to 4:30 pm
Weekend hours 11:30 am to 4:30 pm.

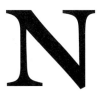

N

Narcolepsy

American Narcolepsy Association
1255 Post St, E F Towers, Ste 404
San Francisco, CA 94109
415 788-4793

Narcotics

Narcotics Anonymous
PO Box 9999, Van Nuys, CA 91409
818 773-9999   Fax 818 700-0700
Web address: http://www.wsoinc.com

Narcotic Educational Foundation of America
24509 Walnut St, Ste 201
Santa Clarita, CA 91321-2846
805 287-0198

National Institutes of Health

A reorganization order, signed by the Secretary on October 31, 1995, and published in the *Federal Register* on November 9, 1995, established the National Institutes of Health (NIH) as an operating division within the Department. The Institute is the principal biomedical research agency of the federal government. Its mission is to employ science in the pursuit of knowledge to improve human health conditions. To accomplish this goal, the Institute seeks to expand fundamental knowledge about the nature and behavior of living systems, to apply that knowledge to extend the health of human lives, and to reduce the burdens resulting from disease and disability. In the quest of this mission, NIH supports biomedical and behavioral research domestically and abroad, conducts research in its own laboratories and clinics, trains promising young researchers, and promotes acquiring and distributing medical knowledge. Focal points have been established to assist in developing NIH-wide goals for health research and research training programs related to women and minorities, coordinating program direction, and ensuring that research pertaining to women's and minority health is identified and addressed through research activities conducted and supported by the NIH. Research activities conducted by NIH will determine much of the quality of health care for the future and reinforce the quality of health care currently available. (USG-1996)

National Institutes of Health
9000 Rockville Pike, Bethesda, MD 20892
301 496-5787
Web address: http://www.nih.gov

Specific institutes are listed below, and their Web presence is accessible via the home page for NIH.

National Cancer Institute

Research on cancer is a high-priority program as a result of the National Cancer Act, which made the conquest of cancer a national goal. The Institute developed a National Cancer Program to expand existing scientific knowledge on cancer cause and prevention as well as on the diagnosis, treatment, and rehabilitation of cancer patients.

Research activities conducted in the Institute's laboratories or supported through grants or contracts include many investigative approaches to cancer, including chemistry, biochemistry, biology, molecular biology, immunology, radiation physics, experimental chemotherapy, epidemiology, biometry, radiotherapy, and pharmacology. Cancer research facilities are constructed with Institute support, and training is provided under university-based programs. The Institute, through its cancer control element, applies research findings in preventing and controlling human cancer as rapidly as possible.

The Institute sponsors extensive programs to disseminate cancer information and supports the Cancer Information Service, which responds to 600,000 callers a year at 800 422-6237.

For further information, call 301 496-5585; public inquiries, 301 496-5583. (USG-1996)

National Eye Institute
301 496-4583

National Heart, Lung, and Blood Institute

The Institute provides leadership for a national program in diseases of the heart, blood vessels, blood, and lungs, and in the use of blood and the management of blood resources.

It plans, conducts, fosters, and supports an integrated and coordinated program of basic research, clinical investigations and trials, and observational studies. It conducts research on clinical use of blood and all aspects of the management of blood resources.

The Institute plans and directs research in the development, trials, and evaluation of interventions (including emergency medical treatment) and devices related to prevention, treatment, and rehabilitation of patients suffering from such diseases and disorders. It conducts research in its own laboratories and supports scientific institutions and individuals by research grants and contracts.

The Institute also supports and conducts research training and coordinates with other research institutes and all federal health programs relevant to activities in the areas of heart, blood vessels, lung, and blood, sleep disorders,

N and blood resources. It maintains continuing relationships with institutions and professional associations, and with international, national, state, and local officials, as well as voluntary organizations working in the above areas.

For further information, call 301 496-2411; public inquiries, 301 496-4236. (USG-1996)

National Institute on Aging
301 496-1752

National Institute of Alcohol Abuse and Alcoholism
301 443-3885

National Clearinghouse for Alcohol Information
301 443-3860

National Institute of Allergy and Infectious Diseases
Public Response
301 496-5717

National Institute of Arthritis and Musculoskeletal and Skin Diseases
301 496-4353

National Institute of Child Health and Human Development
Public Information
301 496-5133

National Institute of Dental Research
Information
301 496-6621

National Institute of Diabetes and Digestive and Kidney Diseases
301 496-3583

National Institute on Drug Abuse & National Clearinghouse for Drug Abuse

The Institute's mission is to lead the nation in bringing the power of science to bear on drug abuse and addiction, through the strategic support and conduct of research across a broad range of disciplines, and the rapid and effective dissemination and use of the results of that research to significantly improve drug abuse and addiction prevention, treatment, and policy. 301 443-6480 (USG-1996)

National Institute of General Medical Sciences
301 594-7811

National Institute of Neurological Disorders and Stroke
301 496-5751

National Institute of Mental Health
Public Communication
301 443-4515

National Library of Medicine

The Library, which serves as the nation's chief medical information source, is authorized to provide medical library services and online bibliographic searching capabilities, such as MEDLINE, TOXLINE, and others, to public and private agencies and organizations, institutions, and individuals. Through grants and contracts, the Library administers programs of assistance to the nation's medical libraries that include support of a National Network of Libraries of Medicine, research in the field of medical library science, establishment and improvement of the basic library resources, and supporting biomedical scientific publications of a nonprofit nature.
301 496-6308 (USG-1996)

Office of Alternative Medicine
301 402-2466

Natural Childbirth
American Society for Psychoprophylaxis in Obstetrics (ASPO Lamaze)
1200 19th St NW, Ste 300
Washington, DC 20036-2422
800 368-4404   202 857-1128   Fax 202 223-4579
E-mail: aspo@sba.com

International Childbirth Education Association
c/o Encyclopedia of Association
PO Box 20048, Minneapolis, MN 55420
612 854-8660

Naturopathy

Doctor, Naturopathic. Diagnoses, treats, and cares for patients, using system of practice that base treatment of physiological functions and abnormal conditions on natural law governing human body. Utilizes physiological, psychological, and mechanical methods, such as air, water, light, heat, earth, phytotherapy, food and herb therapy, psychotherapy, electrotherapy, physiotherapy, minor and orificial surgery, mechanotherapy, naturopathic corrections and manipulation, and natural methods or modalities, together with natural medicines, natural processed foods, and herbs and nature's remedies. Excludes major surgery, therapeutic use of X rays and radium, and use of drugs, except those assimilable substances logically compatible to body processes for maintenance of life. (DOT-1991)

Resource
American Association of Naturopathic Physicians
2366 Eastlake Ave E, Ste 322, Seattle, WA 98102
206 323-8510   Fax 206 323-7612
E-mail: 74602.3715@compuserve.com
Web address: http://healer.infinite.org/
Naturopathic.Physician

Nephrology
American Society of Nephrology
1200 19th St NW, Ste 300
Washington, DC 20036
202 857-1190   Fax 202 223-4579
E-mail: Asn@sba.com

Board Certification:
American Board of Internal Medicine
3624 Market St, Philadelphia, PA 19104
800 441-2246   215 243-1500   Fax 215 382-4702

Neurofibromatosis

National Neurofibromatosis Foundation
95 Pine St, New York, NY 10005
800 323-7938   212 344-6633   Fax 212 529-6094
E-mail: nnf@aol.com

Neurological Surgery

(for use of the profession only, please)
American Academy of Neurological Surgery
2128 Taubman, University Hospital
Ann Arbor, MI 48109
313 936-5015   Fax 313 936-9294

American Association of Neurological Surgeons
22 S Washington, Park Ridge, IL 60068
847 692-9500   Fax 847 629-2589
E-mail: info@aans.org

American Board of Neurological Surgery
6550 Fannin St, Ste 2139, Houston, TX 77030-2722
713 790-6015

Congress of Neurological Surgeons
The Emory Clinic, c/o Daniel L. Barrow
1365 Clifton Rd NE, Atlanta, GA 30322
404 248-4369   Fax 404 248-3791

Neurology

Neurologist. Alternate title: nerve specialist. Diagnoses and treats organic diseases and disorders or nervous systems. Orders and studies results of chemical, microscopic, biological, and bacteriological analyses of patient's blood and cerebrospinal fluid to determine nature and extent of disease or disorder. Identifies presence of pathological blood conditions or parasites and prescribes and administers medications and drugs. Orders and studies results of electroencephalograms or X rays to detect abnormalities in brain wave patterns, or indications of abnormalities in brain structure. Advises patient to contact other medical specialist, as indicated. (DOT-1991)

Resources

American Academy of Neurology
2221 University Ave SE, Ste 335
Minneapolis, MN 55414
612 623-8115   Fax 612 623-3504

American Board of Psychiatry and Neurology
500 Lake Cook Rd, Ste 335, Deerfield, IL 60015
847 945-7900   Fax 847 945-1146

New England Journal of Medicine

New England Journal of Medicine
ISSN 0028-4793

Massachusetts Medical Society
1440 Main St, Waltham, MA 02154-1649
617 893-4610   Fax 617 893-3481
Web address: http://www.nejm.org

Nuclear Medicine

American Board of Nuclear Medicine
900 Veteran Ave, Rm 12-200
Los Angeles, CA 90024-1786
310 825-6787   Fax 310 825-9433

American College of Nuclear Medicine
PO Box 175, Landisville, PA 17538
717 898-6006   Fax 717 898-0713

American College of Nuclear Physicians
1200 19th St NW, Ste 300, Washington, DC 20036
202 857-1135   Fax 202 223-4579

The Society of Nuclear Medicine
1850 Samuel Morse Dr, Reston, VA 22090
703 708-9000   Fax 703 708-9015

Nuclear Medicine Technologist

History

The Joint Review Committee on Educational Programs in Nuclear Medicine Technology was formed by the Society of Nuclear Medicine, Society of Nuclear Medical Technologists, American College of Radiology, American Society of Clinical Pathologists, American Society for Medical Technology, and American Society of Radiologic Technologists. The first meeting of the Joint Review Committee was held in January 1970.

The Society of Nuclear Medical Technologists, one of the original sponsors, terminated its corporate status as a professional organization in 1975. The American Society for Medical Technology and the American Society of Clinical Pathologists relinquished sponsorship in 1994. Current representation of collaborating sponsors on the review committee includes two public members and three members appointed from each of the following organizations: the American College of Radiology, American Society of Radiologic Technologists, Society of Nuclear Medicine, and Society of Nuclear Medicine—Technologist Section. The current sponsorship maintains a balance between physicians and technologists.

The responsibilities of the Joint Review Committee include coordinating the preparation and revision of educational standards for adoption by collaborating organizations and conducting program reviews. The committee meets twice annually to review educational programs and determine accreditation status.

The first *Essentials of an Accredited Educational Program for the Nuclear Medicine Technologist* were adopted by the collaborating organizations in 1969. The *Essentials* were substantially revised in 1976, 1984, and 1991.

Occupational description
Nuclear medicine is the medical specialty that uses the nuclear properties of radioactive and stable nuclides to make diagnostic evaluations of the anatomic or physiologic conditions of the body and to provide therapy with unsealed radioactive sources. The skills of the nuclear medicine technologist complement those of the nuclear medicine physician and of other professionals in the field.

Job description
Nuclear medicine technologists perform a number of tasks in the areas of patient care, technical skills, and

administration. When caring for patients, they acquire adequate knowledge of the patients' medical histories to understand and relate to their illnesses and pending diagnostic procedures for therapy, instruct patients before and during procedures, evaluate the satisfactory preparation of patients before commencing a procedure, and recognize emergency patient conditions and initiate lifesaving first aid when appropriate.

Nuclear medicine technologists apply their knowledge of radiation physics and safety regulations to limit radiation exposure, prepare and administer radiopharmaceuticals, use radiation detection devices and other kinds of laboratory equipment that measure the quantity and distribution of radionuclides deposited in the patient or in a patient specimen, perform in vivo and in vitro diagnostic procedures, use quality control techniques as part of a quality assurance program covering all procedures and products in the laboratory, and participate in research activities.

Administrative functions may include supervising other nuclear medicine technologists, students, laboratory assistants, and other personnel; participating in procuring supplies and equipment; documenting laboratory operations; participating in departmental inspections conducted by various licensing, regulatory, and accrediting agencies; and participating in scheduling patient examinations.

Employment characteristics

The employment outlook in nuclear medicine technology is good. Opportunities may be found in major medical centers, smaller hospitals, and independent imaging centers. Opportunities are also available for obtaining positions in clinical research, education, and administration. Salaries vary depending on the employer and geographic location.

According to a 1994 survey of 1514 nuclear medicine technologists by the Society of Nuclear Medicine, 32% earn between $31,000 and $40,000 per year, 27% earn between $40,000 and $49,000, and 26% earn $50,000 or more. (AHRP-1997)

Resources

AMA Allied Health Department
312 553-9355

American Registry of Radiologic Technologists
1255 Northland Dr, Mendota Heights, MN 55120
612 687-0048

American Society of Radiologic Technologists
15000 Central Ave SE, Albuquerque, NM 87123
505 298-4500   Fax 505 298-5063

Joint Review Committee on Educational Programs in Nuclear Medicine Technology
350 S 400 East, Ste 200
Salt Lake City, UT 84111-2938
801 364-4310   Fax 801 364-9234

Nuclear Medicine Technology Certification Board
2970 Clairmont Rd NE, Ste 610
Atlanta, GA 30329-1634
404 315-1739   Fax 404 315-6502

Society of Nuclear Medicine—Technologist Section
1850 Samuel Morse Dr, Reston, VA 22090-5316
703 708-9000   Fax 703 708-9015

Nuclear War

JAMA Theme Issue: Weapons of destruction

JAMA 1994 Aug 3; 272(5)

Since the early 1980s, JAMA regularly commemorates the August 6, 1945, bombing of Hiroshima by printing details from the *Hiroshima Murals* of Iri and Toshi Maruki on the cover. Occasionally, the issue reflects concerns of the use of these weapons, both the environment that favors and the technology that supports them, on society. This issue specifically presents material on the mental health of torture survivors, the Persian Gulf experience, and the mortality and morbidity assessment methods applied during the recent famine in Somalia.

Nurse Anesthetist

Nurse Anesthetist. Administers local, inhalation, intravenous, and other anesthetics prescribed by anesthesiologist to induce total or partial loss of sensation or consciousness in patients during surgery, deliveries, or other medical and dental procedures. Fits mask to patient's face, turns dials and sets gauges of equipment to regulate flow of oxygen and gases to administer anesthetic by inhalation method, according to prescribed medical standards. Prepares prescribed solutions and administers local, intravenous, spinal, or other anesthetic, following specified methods and procedures. Notes patient's skin color and dilation of pupils and observes video screen and digital display of computerized equipment to monitor patient's vital signs during anesthesia. Initiates remedial measures to prevent surgical shock or other adverse conditions. Informs physician of patient's condition during anesthesia. (DOT-1991)

Resource

American Association of Nurse Anesthetists
222 S Prospect, Park Ridge IL 60068-4001
847 708 692-7050   Fax 847 692-6968

Nurse Attorneys

American Association of Nurse Attorneys
3525 Ellicott Mills Dr, Ste N
Ellicott City, MD 21043-4547
410 418-4800   Fax 410 418-4805

Nurse Midwife

Nurse Midwife. Provides medical care and treatment to obstetrical patients under supervision of obstetrician, delivers babies, and instructs patients in prenatal and postnatal health practices. Participates in initial examination of obstetrical patient, and is assigned responsibility for care, treatment, and delivery of patient. Examines patient during pregnancy, using physical findings, laboratory test results, and patient's statements to evaluate condition and ensure that patient's progress is normal. Discusses case with obstetrician to ensure observation of specified practices. Instructs patient in diet and prenatal health practices. Stays with patient during labor to reassure patient and to administer medication. Delivers infant and performs postpartum examinations and treatments to ensure that patient and infant are responding normally. When deviations from standard are encountered during pregnancy or delivery, administers stipulated emergency measures, and arranges for immediate contact of obstetrician. Visits patient during postpartum period in hospital and at home to instruct patient in care of self and infant and examine patient. Maintains records of cases for inclusion in establishment file. Conducts classes for groups of patients and families to provide information concerning pregnancy, childbirth, and family orientation. May direct activities or other workers. May instruct in midwifery in establishment providing such training. (DOT-1991)

Resource

American College of Nurse-Midwives
1522 K St NW, Ste 1000, Washington, DC 20005
202 728-9800   Fax 202 289-4395

Nursing

AMA Policy

Professional Nurse Staffing in Hospitals (H-360.986)
BOT Rep 11, I-96

The AMA:

(1) encourages medical and nursing staffs in each facility to closely monitor the quality of medical care to help guide hospital administrations toward the best use of resources for patients;

(2) encourages medical and nursing staffs to work together to develop and implement in-service education programs and promote compliance with established or pending guidelines for unlicensed assistive personnel and technicians that will help assure the highest and safest standards of patient care;

(3) encourages medical and nursing staffs to use identification mechanisms, eg, badges, that provide the name, credentials, and/or title of the physicians, nurses, allied health personnel, and unlicensed assistive personnel in facilities to enable patients to easily note the level of personnel providing their care;

(4) encourages medical and nursing staffs to develop, promote, and implement educational guidelines for the training of all unlicensed personnel working in critical care units, according to the needs at each facility; and

(5) encourages medical and nursing staffs to work with hospital administrations to assure that patient care and safety are not compromised when a hospital's environment and staffing are restructured.

Nurses, physicians reconsider relationships

Leigh Page
AM News Dec 5, 1994 pp 3, 59, 63.

"In the future," the American Nurses Association proclaimed last year, "your family doctor may be a nurse."

At that time, it wasn't only rhetoric. President Bill Clinton's health reform plan hinted at more independence and responsibilities for advanced practice nurses, especially nurse practitioners.

But with the demise of comprehensive reform plans, nurses' future roles seem murky. No one is expecting a

quick resolution to the tensions between organized medicine and nursing. Both groups have been debating how they should relate to each other for at least 20 years.

Managed care may decide
With nurses and doctors at an impasse and federal action unlikely in the near future, managed care looks to be the most important influence on how the two groups will relate.

HMOs long have followed their own standards for use of nonphysician providers, particularly nurse practitioners. Physician assistants have similar training and often are given the same privileges as nurse practitioners, but as a group are not interested in independent practice.

For example, Kaiser Northern California and Harvard Community Health Plan, two large, respected HMOs, say they have used nurse practitioners for many routine services for years and that most patients are satisfied.

Now, as price wars among plans heat up, some leading players in managed care networks are using less costly nurse practitioners for more than just routine services.

In Minneapolis, a leading managed care market, nurse practitioners under physician supervision perform endoscopic exams at Park Nicollet Medical Center, a large physician group. Such procedures are rarely done by nonphysicians, Dr. Jacott reports.

And in New York City, which is seeing the formation of managed care networks around major hospitals, Columbia Presbyterian Medical Center granted nurse practitioners admitting privileges this year. Hospital President William T. Speck, MD, said the decision was based on "a major paradigm shift" further blurring the line between what nurses and doctors do.

The legacy of reform
Managed care does not, however, speak with one voice. It took national policymakers working on federal health reform plans to propose basic strategies for expanded use of nurse practitioners.

At the time, such strategies made some sense. Since the late 1980s, more medical students had been fleeing primary care careers. Some policymakers predicted medicine one day would be almost completely specialized, leaving primary care to nurses.

Such predictions remain open to debate; medical students have shown new interest in primary care careers lately. But policy statements from physician still show the impact of the push to give nurses a greater role in health care delivery.

One such statement was published by the American College of Physicians in the Nov. 1 *Annals of Internal Medicine*. It recommends that nurse practitioners and PAs be given expanded roles, such as the power to prescribe, but only "under systems that ensure accountability to a physician."

The ACP warns that if this is not done, generalist physicians won't be able to meet the growing demand for primary care. This also was a basic assumption of the Clinton plan, whose call for universal coverage heightened the projected need for primary care even more.

But these assumptions no longer seem to hold. The demise of comprehensive reform means universal coverage is probably unreachable in the near future, suggesting that demand for primary care services may not rise significantly.

Many groups, including the AMA, say there is still a need for more primary care physicians. But some experts question even this assumption. An independent study simulating projected growth of managed care, based on HMO staffing patterns, recently concluded that primary care supply would be adequate through the turn of the century. In the report, published in the July 20 *Journal of the American Medical Association,* Jonathan Weiner, DSc, of the Johns Hopkins School of Public Health, predicts rather that there will be a huge surplus of specialists.

With the need for more nonphysician caregivers now in doubt, groups like the AMA and American Academy of Family Physicians, which have not called for expanded privileges for nonphysician practitioners, may have more credibility with federal policymakers.

In contrast, the ACP statement calls for expanded privileges. But the differences between AMA and ACP policies may be mostly rhetorical. For example, the ACP endorses NPs prescribing under physician supervision, while AMA policy does not address prescribing directly but insists on physician supervision generally. Also, both groups agree that studies have not proved that advanced practice nurses are just as qualified as physicians to provide primary care.

Nurse, General Duty. Alternative title: nurse, staff. Provides general nursing care to patients in hospital, nursing home, infirmary, or similar health care facility. Administers prescribed medications and treatments in accordance with approved nursing techniques. Prepares equipment and aids physician during treatments and examinations of patients.

Observes patient, records significant conditions and reactions, and notifies superior or physician of patient's condition and reaction to drugs, treatments, and significant incidents. Takes temperature, pulse, blood pressure, and other vital signs to detect deviations from normal and assess condition of patient. May rotate among various clinical services of institution, such as obstetrics, surgery, orthopedics, outpatient and admitting, pediatrics, and psychiatry. May prepare rooms, sterile instruments, equipment and supplies, and hand items to surgeon, obstetrician, or other medical practitioner. May make beds, bathe, and feed patients. May serve as leader for group of personnel rendering nursing care to number of patients. (DOT-1991)

Nurse Practitioner. Alternate title: primary care nurse practitioner. Provides general medical care and treatment to patient in medical facility, such as clinic, health center, or public health agency, under direction of physician. Performs physical examinations and preventive health measures within prescribed guidelines and instructions of physician. Orders, interprets, and evaluates diagnostic tests to identify and assess patient's clinical problems and health care needs. Records physical findings, and formulates plan and prognosis, based on patient's condition. Discusses case with physician and other health professionals to prepare comprehensive patient care plan. Submits health care plan and goals of individual patients for

periodic review and evaluation by physician. Prescribes or recommends drugs or other forms of treatment such as physical therapy, inhalation therapy, or related therapeutics procedures. May refer patients to physician for consultation or to specialized health resources for treatment. May be designated according to field of specialization as pediatric nurse practitioner. Where state law permits, may engage in independent practice. (DOT-1991)

Nurse, Licensed Practical. Provides prescribed medical treatment and personal care services to ill, injured, convalescent, and handicapped persons in such settings as hospitals, clinics, private homes, schools, sanitariums, and similar institutions. Takes and records patients' vital signs. Dresses wounds, gives enemas, douches, alcohol rubs, and massages. Applies compresses, ice bags, and hot water bottles. Observes patients and reports adverse reactions to medication or treatment to medical personnel in charge. Administers specified medication, orally or by subcutaneous or intermuscular injection, and notes time and amount on patients' charts. Assembles and uses such equipment as catheters, tracheotomy tubes, and oxygen suppliers. Collects samples, such as urine, blood, and sputum, from patients for testing and performs routine laboratory tests on samples. Sterilizes equipment and supplies, using germicides, sterilizer, or autoclave. Prepares or examines food trays for prescribed diet and feeds patients. Records food and fluid intake and output. Bathes, dresses, and assists patients in walking and turning. Cleans rooms, makes beds, and answers patients' calls. Washes and dresses bodies of deceased persons. Must pass state board examination and be licensed. May assist in delivery, care, and feeding of infants. May inventory and requisition supplies. May provide medical treatment and personal care to patients in private homes and be designated home health nurse, licensed practical nurse. (DOT-1991)

Resources

American Academy of Nurse Practitioners
LBJ Building, PO Box 12846, Capital Station
Austin, TX 78711
512 442-4262   512 442-6469

American Association of Colleges of Nursing
1 Dupont Circle NW, Ste 530
Washington, DC 20036
202 463-6930   202 785-8320

American Nurses Association
600 Maryland Ave SW, Ste 100W
Washington, DC 20024-2571
202 651-7000   Fax 202 651-7001

National Institute of Nursing Research
Bldg 31, Rm 5B13
31 Center Dr, Mail Stop Code 2176
Bethesda, MD 20892
301 496-0207

National League of Nursing
350 Hudson St, New York, NY 10014
800 669-1656   212 989-9393   Fax 212 989-9256

Nursing Associations, Statewide

Alabama State Nurses' Association
360 N Hull St, Montgomery, AL 36104-3658
334 262-8321   334 262-8578

Alaska Nurses' Association
237 E Third Ave, Ste 3, Anchorage, AK 99501
907 274-0827   Fax 907 272-0292

Arizona Nurses' Association
1850 E Southern Ave, Ste 1, Tempe, AZ 85282-5832
602 831-0404   Fax 602 839-4780

Arkansas Nurses' Association
117 S Cedar St, Little Rock, AR 72205
501 664-5853   Fax 501 664-5859

California Nurses' Association
1145 Market St, Ste 1100, San Francisco, CA 94103
415 864-4141   Fax 415 252-9083

Colorado Nurses' Association
5453 E Evans Pl, Denver, CO 80222
303 757-7483   Fax 303 757-2679

Connecticut Nurses' Association
377 Research Pkwy, Ste 2D, Meriden, CT 06450
203 238-1207   Fax 203 238-3437

Delaware Nurses' Association
2634 Capitol Trail, Ste A, Newark, DE 19711
302 368-2333   Fax 302 366-1775

District of Columbia Nurses' Association
5100 Wisconsin Ave NW, Ste 306
Washington, DC 20016
202 244-2705   Fax 202 362-8285

Florida Nurses' Association
PO Box 536985, Orlando, FL 32853-6985
407 896-3261   Fax 407 896-9042

Georgia Nurses' Association
1362 W Peachtree St NW, Atlanta, GA 30309
404 876-4624   Fax 404 876-4621

Guam Nurses' Association
PO Box CG, Agana, GU 96910
671 477-6877   Fax 671 472-1350

Hawaii Nurses' Association
677 Ala Moana Blvd, #301, Honolulu, HI 96813
808 521-8361   Fax 808 524-2760

Idaho Nurses' Association
200 N Fourth St, Ste 20, Boise, ID 83702-6001
208 345-0500   Fax 208 345-1163

Illinois Nurses' Association
300 S Wacker Dr, Ste 2200, Chicago, IL 60606
312 360-2300   Fax 312 360-9380

Indiana State Nurses' Association
2915 N High School Rd, Indianapolis, IN 46224-2969
317 299-4575   Fax 317 297-3525

Iowa Nurses' Association
1501 42nd St, Ste 471, Des Moines, IA 50266
515 225-0495   Fax 515 225-2201

Kansas State Nurses' Association
700 SW Jackson, Ste 601, Topeka, KS 66603-3731
913 233-8638   Fax 913 233-5222

Kentucky Nurses' Association
1400 S 1st St, PO Box 2616, Louisville, KY 40201
502 637-2546   Fax 502 637-8236

Louisiana State Nurses' Association
712 Transcontinental Dr, Metairie, LA 70001
504 889-1030   Fax 504 888-1158

Maine State Nurses' Association
283 Water St, PO Box 2240, Augusta, ME 04338-2240
207 622-1057   Fax 207 623-4072

Maryland Nurses' Association
849 International Dr, Airport Square 21, Ste 255
Linthicum Heights, MD 21090
410 859-3000   Fax 410 859-3001

Massachusetts Nurses' Association
340 Turnpike St, Canton, MA 02021
617 821-4625   Fax 617 821-4445

Michigan Nurses' Association
2310 Jolly Oak Rd, Okemos, MI 48864
517 349-5640   Fax 517 349-5818

Minnesota Nurses' Association
1295 Bandana Blvd N, Ste 140
St Paul, MN 55108-5115
800 647-5301   612 646-4807   612 647-5301

Mississippi Nurses' Association
135 Bounds St, Ste 100, Jackson, MS 39206
601 982-9182   Fax 601 982-9183

Missouri Nurses' Association
1904 Bubba Ln
Jefferson City, MO 65109
573 636-4623   Fax 573 636-9576

Montana Nurses' Association
104 Broadway, Ste 62, PO Box 5718
Helena, MT 59601
406 442-6710   Fax 406 442-6738

Nebraska Nurses' Association
1430 South St, Ste 202, Lincoln, NE 68508-2446
402 475-3859   Fax 402 475-3961

Nevada Nurses' Association
3660 Baker Ln, Ste 104, Reno, NV 89509
702 825-3555   Fax 702 825-3555

New Hampshire Nurses' Association
48 West St, Concord, NH 03301
603 225-3783   Fax 603 225-3783

New Jersey State Nurses' Association
320 W State St, Trenton, NJ 08618
609 392-4884   Fax 609 396-2330

New Mexico Nurses' Association
909 Virginia NE, Ste 101, Albuquerque, NM 87108
505 268-7744   Fax 505 268-7711

New York State Nurses' Association
2113 Western Ave, Guilderland, NY 12084
518 456-5371   Fax 518 456-0697

North Carolina Nurses' Association
103 Enterprise St, Box 12025
Raleigh, NC 27605-2025
919 821-4250   Fax 919 829-5807

North Dakota Nurses' Association
212 N Fourth St, Bismarck, ND 58501
701 223-1385   Fax 701 223-0575

Ohio Nurses' Association
4000 E Main St, Columbus, OH 43213-2950
614 237-5414   Fax 614 237-6074

Oklahoma Nurses' Association
6414 N Santa Fe, Ste A, Oklahoma City, OK 73116
405 840-3476   Fax 405 840-3013

Oregon Nurses' Association
9600 SW Oak St, Ste 550, Portland, OR 97223
503 293-0011   Fax 503 293-0013

Pennsylvania Nurses' Association
2578 Interstate Dr, PO Box 68525
Harrisburg, PA 17105-8525
717 657-1222   Fax 717 657-3796

Colegio de Professionales de la Enfermeria
de Puerto Rico
PO Box 363647, San Juan, PR 00936-3647
809 753-7197

Rhode Island State Nurses' Association
550 S Water St, Unit 540 B, Providence, RI 02903-4861
401 421-9703   Fax 401 421-6793

South Carolina Nurses' Association
1821 Gadsden St, Columbia, SC 29201
803 252-4781   Fax 803 779-3870

South Dakota Nurses' Association
1505 S Minnesota, Ste 6, Sioux Falls, SD 57105
605 338-1401   Fax 605 338-0516

Tennessee Nurses' Association
545 Mainstream Dr, Ste 405, Nashville, TN 37228-1201
615 254-0350   Fax 615 254-0303

Texas Nurses' Association
7600 Burnet Rd, Ste 440, Austin, TX 78757-1292
512 452-0645   Fax 512 452-0648

Utah Nurses' Association
455 E 400 S, Ste 402, Salt Lake City, UT 84111
801 322-3439   Fax 801 322-3430

Vermont State Nurses' Association
Champlain Mill, Box 26, 1 Main St
Winooski, VT 05404-2230
802 655-7123   Fax 802 655-7187

Virgin Islands Nurses' Association
Christiansted, PO Box 583, St Croix, VI 00821-0583
809 773-2323

Virginia Nurses' Association
7311 Three Chopt Rd, Ste 204, Richmond, VA 23226
804 282-1808   Fax 804 282-4916

Washington State Nurses' Association
2505 Second Ave, Ste 500, Seattle, WA 98121
206 443-9762   Fax 206 728-2074

West Virginia Nurses' Association
101 Dee St, PO Box 1946, Charleston, WV 25327
304 342-1169   Fax 304 345-1538

Wisconsin Nurses' Association
6117 Monona Dr, Madison, WI 53716
608 221-0383   Fax 608 221-2788

Wyoming Nurses' Association
1603 Capitol Ave, Rm 305, Cheyenne, WY 82001
307 635-3955   Fax 307 635-2173

Nursing Homes

Poetry and Medicine

I was once
Cynthia Lelos
JAMA 1992 Oct 21; 268(15): 2018

I was once

Ruler of the World
he said

No kidding
she said adjusting her bifocals

when I was Lord trees flew
and gold dripped down from the sky

I remember seeing
a tree like that she said

He leaned over his wheelchair
and balanced on the edge
of her walker   God came to me
this morning and said   He's going
to cure my diverticulitis   Wow

she said Could you ask Him to fix
this arthritis   It's killing me

He glanced around (to be sure
no one could overhear him) I could
do it myself he said but I wouldn't
want the others to know my special
Powers

I understand she said   Once I was
the most famous most breathtaking
Model in the Universe   My legs were
spears that pierced men's hearts
My lips were perfectly pink
But I had to give it up before
my beauty blinded men's eyes

You're still Something he said

Together they sat holding hands
watching the sun set
beyond the Rest Home courtyard

Resources
American Health Care Association
1201 L St NW, Washington, DC 20005
202 842-4444   Fax 202 842-3860

American Association Homes and Services for the Aging
901 E St NW, Ste 500
Washington, DC 20024-2037
202 783-2242   Fax 202 783-2255

Accreditation:
Joint Commission on Accreditation of
Healthcare Organizations
1 Renaissance Blvd, Oakbrook Terrace, IL 60181
630 792-500   Fax 630 792-5001
Web address: http://www.jcaho.org/

Contact state or local department of public health for complaints regarding nursing homes.

Referrals are made by a personal physician.

Nutrition

American College of Nutrition
301 E 17th St, New York, NY 10003
212 777-1037   Fax 212 777-1103

American Society for Parenteral and Enteral Nutrition
8630 Fenton St, Ste 412
Silver Spring, MD 20910-3805
301 587-6315   Fax 301 587-2365
E-mail: aspen@access.digex.net

Food and Nutrition Information Center
National Agricultural Library Bldg, Rm 304
Beltsville, MD 20705
301 504-5414
E-mail: fnic@nal.usda.gov
Web address: http://www.nal.usda.gov

Food safety:
US Department of Agriculture
Meat and Poultry Hotline (Food safety)
800 535-4555

Four basic food groups:
Human Nutrition Information Service
US Department of Agriculture
6505 Bellcrest Rd, Hyattsville, MD 20782
301 436-8617

Nutrition programs in medical schools:
American Society for Clinical Nutrition
9650 Rockville Pike, Bethesda, MD 20814
301 530-7110

O

Obesity

What to tell patients

AM News Mar 3, 1997 p 28

The right approach to counseling is vital in helping patients reach and maintain healthy weight.

Set realistic goals. The first step may be to prevent further weight gain. Weight losses of 5% to 10% may be enough to achieve health benefits.

Make lifestyle changes. To prevent gain and maintain losses, establish a healthy diet and exercise plan that can last a lifetime.

Don't focus on lost pounds. Instead, focus on improvements in measurable risk factors, such as blood pressure and cholesterol levels.

Consider drug therapy. Patients with a BMI of 30 or higher, or who have comorbidities, are candidates for weight-loss medication.

Stay on track. Annual checkups and other visits help track progress and reinforce positive health messages. They're also an opportunity to catch gradual weight gains that can add up over time.

Advice for physicians

AM News Mar 3, 1997 p 28

Former Surgeon General C. Everett Koop, MD, founder of the nonprofit group Shape Up America!, says physicians "are in a unique position to reduce the distress" many overweight patients experience. To do that, doctors should:

Examine their own feelings about obesity and the obese. Doctors may unknowingly harbor feelings that influence their patient interactions.

View each patient as a unique, competent individual worthy of time and respect. The reasons for their obesity will differ from patient to patient, as will its impact on their lives.

Encourage patients to discuss their weight and their efforts to reduce or maintain it. Listen and empathize with their concerns and frustrations.

Encourage patients to be partners in making decisions about treatment strategies and options.

Learn to recognize and comment on positive changes in health status, weight loss, and eating and exercise efforts.

JAMA Article of Note: Long-term pharmacotherapy in the management of obesity

JAMA 1996 Dec 18; 276(23): 1907-1915

Abstract: The objectives of the study were to examine the rationale for long-term use of medications in the management of obesity, to provide an overview of published scientific information on their safety and efficacy, and to provide guidance to patients and practitioners regarding risks and benefits of treatment. The conclusions were that pharmacotherapy for obesity, when combined with appropriate behavioral approaches to change diet and physical activity, helps some obese patients lose weight and maintain weight loss for at least one year. There is little justification for the short-term use of anorexiant medications, but few studies have evaluated their safety and efficacy for more than one year. Until more data are available, pharmacotherapy cannot be recommended for routine use in obese individuals, although it may be helpful in carefully selected patients.

Resources

American Society of Bariatric Physicians
5600 S Quebec, Ste 109A, Englewood, CO 80111
303 779-4833   Fax 303 779-4834

Gastroplasty Support Group
c/o Lumbomyr Kuzmak, MD
657 Irvington Ave, Newark, NJ 07106
201 374-1717

National Association to Advance Fat Acceptance
PO Box 188620, Sacramento, CA 95818
800 442-1214   916 558-6880   Fax 916 558-6881
E-mail: naafa@world.std.com

Obsessive Compulsive Disorder

Obsessive Compulsive Foundation
PO Box 70, Milford, CT 06460-0070
203 878-5669   Fax 203 847-3843   Fax 203 847-2826
E-mail: jphs23A@prodigy.com
Web address: http://www.iglou.com/fairlight/ocd

Obstetrics and Gynecology

Obstetrician. Treats women during prenatal, natal, and postnatal periods. Examines patient to ascertain condition, utilizing physical findings, laboratory results, and patient's statements as diagnostic aids. Determines need for modified diet and physical activities, and recommends plan. Periodically examines patient, prescribing medication or surgery, if indicated. Delivers infant, and cares for mother for prescribed period of time following childbirth. Performs cesarean section or other surgical

...ded to preserve patient's health and ...fely. May treat patients for diseases of ...ans. (DOT-1991)

...

Board of Obstetrics and Gynecology
...e St, Dallas, TX 75204-1069
...1-1619   Fax 214 871-1943

...can College of Obstetricians and Gynecologists
409 12th St SW, Washington, DC 20024-2188
202 638-5577   Fax 202 484-8143
Web address: http://www.acog.com

American Association of Gynecologic Laparoscopists
13021 E Florence Ave, Santa Fe Springs, CA 90670
800 554-2245   562 946-8774   Fax 562 946-0073
E-mail: generalmail@aagl.com
Web address: http://www.aagl.com

Occupational Medicine

Occupational Physician. Alternate titles: company doctor; physician, industrial. Diagnoses and treats work-related illnesses and injuries of employees, and conducts fitness-for-duty physical examinations. Attends patients in plant or hospital, and reexamines disability cases periodically to verify progress. Oversees maintenance of case histories, health examination reports, and other medical records. Formulates and administers health programs. Inspects plant and makes recommendations regarding sanitation and elimination of health hazards. (DOT-1991)

Nurse, Staff, Occupational Health Nursing. Alternate title: nurse, staff, industrial. Provides nursing service and first aid to employees or persons who become ill or injured on premises of department store, industrial plant, or other establishment. Takes patient's vital signs, treats wounds, evaluates physical condition of patient, and contacts physician and hospital to arrange for further medical treatment, when needed. Maintains record of persons treated, and prepares accident reports and insurance forms. Develops employee programs, such as health education, accident prevention, alcohol abuse counseling, curtailment of smoking, and weight control regimens. May assist physician in physical examination of new employees. (DOT-1991)

Guidelines for physicians contracting occupational health services

Physicians providing occupational health care, either as an employee or as a contractor, must negotiate certain basic rules with the management at the onset of the relationship. As in most contractual relationships, the physician's requests and preferences are more likely to be heard and respected prior to the signing of a contract. Parkinson[1] has outlined several areas for discussion between the physician and the employer:

a) **Physician visibility and accessibility.** Physicians who agree to provide medical consultation in the workplace must inspect the workplace at regular intervals. Workers must have access directly to the physician, either individually or through a joint health and safety committee of workers and management, if the industry is large enough to have such a committee.

b) **Industrial hygiene.** If a full-time industrial hygienist is not available, the physician must alert management to the need for periodic industrial hygiene consultation, in order to correct deficient work practices and maintain effective hygiene at the work site.

c) **Workers' compensation education and prevention.** The physician has an obligation to inform a worker if a disease possibly is related to the worker's occupation. If necessary, the physician must assist the worker or representative in filing the documentation necessary for establishment of a claim.

d) **Education and prevention.** The physician should participate actively in illness prevention at the workplace and should have access to the workplace for programs of education and health promotion. Also, the physician must maintain skills in occupational medicine and have the support of the company for continuing his or her education. In addition to NIOSH educational resource centers, the American Occupational Medical Association offers a "basic curriculum" in occupational medicine. The program involves a three-part course offered in two-day segments on a yearly rotating basis.

e) **Communication.** The physician should establish the right to communicate directly with individual workers and with labor representative on matters affecting health and safety. Health and safety should not become matters that are resolved by confrontations of labor and management.

f) **Record keeping.** Thorough and confidential records should be kept, preferably in a standardized format that is amenable to easy extraction of data by hand or computer. The data should be available for use in epidemiologic studies. An annual or periodic report should be prepared using information gathered from employee medical examinations that are either preventive or illness related. When combined with industrial hygiene data, such reports may uncover relationships between workplace exposures and illnesses or injuries.

g) **Preplacement examinations.** The employer must furnish a description of the physical and mental requirements of the job under consideration. The physician will furnish the prospective employer with a statement of the patient's suitability for placement based on these requirements. No other information should be supplied. Only the patient, not the potential employer, should be notified of medical conditions that require follow-up. The employers should receive no information about medical diagnoses or laboratory evaluations. Of course, the decision to hire rests with the employer.

h) **Periodic government-mandated examinations.** Employers as well as employees should be notified of evidence indicating adverse effects of occupational exposures. Recommendations concerning maintenance of health through elimination of exposure should be made to both. Only the employee should be given information regarding medical follow-up that may be necessary.

i) **Chief executive officer support.** As part of any employment contract, physicians offering occupational health services should have an agreement with the company's chief executive officer about guidelines (preferably this agreement would be in writing). In addition, all physician-worker-management interactions should be guided by the American Occupational Medical Association's Code of Ethical Conduct for Physicians.

Conclusions

Several aspects of family medicine coincide with providing occupational health care. The continuity of care provided by family physicians increases the likelihood of detecting delayed or chronic health effects due to occupational exposures. Training in behavioral skills allows for better recognition of disturbed biorhythms due to shift work, substance abuse, or job stress. The care of other family members provides an opportunity to identify health effects among family members due to agents brought home by an employee. Worker-related effects involving children or spouse may be detected more readily when the entire family is seen by the same physician. The traditional advocacy role of the family physician may encourage greater confidence among workers if the same physician is seen at the workplace.

An awareness of community resources, such as visiting nurses, public welfare agencies, industrial health coalitions, local health departments, other medical practitioners, and voluntary health agencies, is necessary for optimal patient care by both the occupational and the family physician. Cooperative health ventures between industries and physicians may be important resources in communities where industries do not have large corporate medical departments but do have an active interest in the well-being of working people.

Reference

1. Parkinson DHK. Occupational health in family medicine education. Address presented at the National Conference on Occupational and Environmental Health Education in Family Medicine, Kansas City, Mo, Sept 13, 1983.

(FAM-1984)

Resources

American College of Occupational and
Environmental Medicine
55 W Seegers, Arlington Heights, IL 60005
847 228-6850   Fax 847 228-1856

Board Certification:
American Board of Preventive Medicine
9950 W Lawrence Ave, Ste 106
Schiller Park, IL 60176
847 671-1750   Fax 847 671-1751

Occupational Health and Safety

How to deal with requirements of OSHA safety rules

Mike Mitka
AM News May 18, 1992 pp 23-26

OSHA's bloodborne pathogen standards, implemented in June of 1992, were put in place to protect all workers who could be "reasonably anticipated" to face contact with blood and other potentially infectious materials.

Physicians appear willing to meet these standards, but confusion still remains. Below find a list of key points that physicians should be aware of.

Exposure control plan. Physicians must complete an exposure control plan, which is designed to document what risks are present in the workplace and what protective measures are being utilized.

The plan must contain an exposure determination list, a schedule, and methods for implementing the OSHA regulations and protocols for evaluation of exposure incidents.

Exposure determination list. The list cites the job classifications in which all employees risk exposure, that is, unprotected contact with blood or other potentially infectious material. It also lists job classifications in a facility in which some employees risk exposure and procedures performed on site in which occupational exposures can occur. The list of jobs and procedures should be based on risks incurred without use of personal protective equipment.

Schedule and methods for implementation. These must include brief descriptions of how a facility complies with regulations on workplace and engineering controls, personal protective equipment, housekeeping, hepatitis B vaccination, postexposure evaluation and follow-up, labels, signs, and recordkeeping.

- For workplace and engineering controls, the standard emphasizes hand washing and procedures for minimizing needlesticks and the splashing and spraying of blood. It also requires appropriate packaging and labeling of specimens, regulated wastes, and contaminated equipment.
- Personal protective equipment, such as gloves, gowns, masks, mouthpieces, and resuscitation bags, must be provided at no cost to employees, and its appropriate use required.
- A written housekeeping schedule must be maintained noting that employees are responsible for ensuring that equipment and surfaces are cleaned with an appropriate disinfectant and decontaminated immediately after a spill or leakage occurs and at the end of a work shift.
- A hepatitis B vaccination must be made available at no cost to all employees within 10 working days of an assignment involving potential occupational exposure to blood. The OSHA-approved waiver form must be signed by any employee declining the vaccine.
- Post-exposure evaluation and follow-up requires that specific procedures will be made available at no cost to all employees who have had an exposure incident. The follow-up must include a confidential medical evaluation.
- Labels and signs must be used on all hazardous items.
- Recordkeeping requires that confidential medical records will be kept for all employees with occupational exposure for at least 30 years after the person leaves employment. Training records of workers at risk to occupational exposure must also be kept for at least three years following the date of the training sessions.

Protocols for evaluation of exposure incidents

A written procedure must be maintained that includes four key elements. They are:
- The name of the contact person for exposure accidents.
- The name of the person who will evaluate the exposure incident to determine if any procedures should be changed.

- A requirement for written documentation of the incident that includes the name of the exposed individual, the source of exposure, a description of what happened, and the date and time.
- A requirement for written evaluation of the exposure incident including any suggestions for procedure changes and a record of how these changes were implemented.

Physicians and employers seeking more detailed information about the standards should contact their OSHA area office.

Periodic updating needed

The exposure control plan is the most important document to be maintained by physicians regarding the Occupational Safety and Health Administration bloodborne pathogens standard.

In the unlikely event of an OSHA inspection, the exposure control plan will be used by the inspector as a key to how well a physician is complying.

The plan is not a passive document. It will need periodic updating:
- At least annually.
- When new tasks and procedures that affect occupational exposure are added.
- When tasks and procedures affecting occupational exposure are changed or modified.
- When new employee positions with occupational exposure risk are added or when employee positions are changed to include the exposure.

Resources

Clearinghouse for Occupational Safety and Health Information
4676 Columbia Pkwy, Cincinnati, OH 45226
800 356-4674 513 533-4674

Occupational Safety and Health Administration
Department of Labor
200 Constitution Ave NW, Washington, DC 20210
202 523-1452
Web address: http://www.osha.gov

OSHA Regional Offices

Region I
CT, MA, ME, NH, RI, VT
133 Portland St, 1st Fl, Boston, MA 02114
617 565-7164

Region II
NJ, NY, PR, VI
201 Varick St, Rm 670, New York, NY 10014
212 337-2378

Region III
DC, DE, MD, PA, VA, WV
Gateway Building
3535 Market St, Ste 2100, Philadelphia, PA 19104
215 596-1201

Region IV
AL, FL, GA, KY, MS, NC, SC, TN
1375 Peachtree St NE, Ste 587, Atlanta, GA 30367
404 347-3573

Region V
IL, IN, MI, MN, OH, WI
230 S Dearborn St, Rm 3244, Chicago, IL 60604
312 353-2220

Region VI
AR, LA, NM, OK, TX
525 Griffin St, Rm 602, Dallas, TX 75202
214 767-4731

Region VII
IA, KS, MO, NE
911 Walnut St, Rm 406, Kansas City, MO 64106
816 426-5861

Region VIII
CO, MT, ND, SD, UT, WY
Federal Bldg, 1961 Stout St, Rm 1576
Denver, CO 80294
303 844-3061

Region IX
AS, AZ, CA, GU, HI, NV
71 Stevenson St, Rm 415
San Francisco, CA 94105
415 744-6670

Region X
AK, ID, OR, WA
1111 Third Ave, Ste 715, Seattle, WA 98101
206 553-5930

Occupational Therapy

History

In 1933, the American Occupational Therapy Association (AOTA) requested that the Council on Physical Therapy of the American Medical Association (AMA) undertake review and evaluation of occupational therapy programs. The AMA Board of Trustees referred the request to the Council on Physical Therapy and the Council on Medical Education and Hospitals.

The Council on Physical Therapy had been created in 1925 "to investigate and report on the value and merits of all non-medicinal apparatus and contrivances offered for sale to physicians and hospitals, and to publish in the *Journal* from time to time the results of its investigations." The Council on Medical Education and Hospitals was selected as the proper body to undertake the reviews because of its experience in all phases of medical education, including the investigation of medical schools, teaching hospitals, and programs for the education of technicians in specialties that are closely allied to medical service. The review of occupational therapy programs, which began in 1933, was carried out in conjunction with the other activities of the Council.

In 1934 and 1935, joint meetings were held with representatives of the AOTA, the AMA Council on Physical Therapy, and the Council on Medical Education and Hospitals to establish *Essentials* for educational programs. The *Essentials* were adopted by the AMA House of Delegates in 1935. The *Essentials* were revised in 1938, 1943, 1949, 1965, 1973, 1983, and 1991. The 1991 *Essentials* have been updated to reflect ACOTE as the accrediting body and to comply with US Department of Education (ED) requirements.

During the 1950s, educational programs for assistant-level personnel in occupational therapy were developed. In 1958, AOTA formalized the implementation of a plan for the Certified Occupational Therapy Assistant (COTA), approved educational standards, and assumed responsibility for review and approval of the educational programs. There were originally two sets of educational standards for the occupational therapy assistant. One set was for the certificate programs, generally hospital-based, that were a year or less in length. The second was for the associate degree programs at community and junior colleges. In 1975, the *Essentials and Guidelines of an Approved Educational Program for the Occupational Therapy Assistant* (modeled after the *Essentials* established for the professional-level programs) were established and adopted, and hospital-based programs were discontinued. Educational standards were revised in 1983 and again in 1991. During 1990, at the request of the AOTA, CAHEA and the AOTA developed a process to bring OTA programs into the CAHEA accreditation system.

The Accreditation Committee of the AOTA was established in 1935 and was sponsored by the Association. The collaboration in accreditation activities with the CAHEA/AMA continued until January 1, 1994.

The Accreditation Council for Occupational Therapy Education (ACOTE) was established January 1, 1994. On March 1, 1994, all accredited and approved educational programs, and all developing programs as of that date, were grandfathered into ACOTE with their accreditation status as of that date.

ACOTE is recognized by the Commission on Recognition of Postsecondary Accreditation (CORPA) and ED. ACOTE places emphasis on objectivity and consistency in its accreditation process. Accreditation activities in addition to program review include sponsoring workshops, promoting the development of new programs in underserved areas and providing guidance during the development process, and publishing newsletters for the academic community and the evaluator pool. Further efforts are directed toward decreasing time and costs for both the institution and the committee and toward continually improving the selection and training of on-site evaluators. (AHRP-1997)

Occupational therapist

Occupational description
Occupational therapy is the use of purposeful activity and interventions to achieve functional outcomes. "Achieving functional outcomes" means to maximize the independence and the maintenance of health of any individual who is limited by a physical injury or illness, a cognitive impairment, a psychosocial dysfunction, a mental illness, a developmental or learning disability, or an adverse environmental condition.

Job description
Occupational therapy services are based on assessment methods, including the use of skilled observation or the administration and interpretation of standardized or nonstandardized tests and measurements to identify areas for occupational therapy services.

Occupational therapy services include, but are not limited to, the assessment, treatment, and education of, or consultation with, the individual, family, or other persons; interventions directed toward developing daily living skills, work readiness or work performance, play skills or leisure capacities, or enhancing educational performances skills; or providing for the development of sensorimotor, perceptual or neuromuscular functioning, or range of motion, or emotional, motivational, cognitive, or psychosocial components of performance.

Occupational therapy services may require assessment of the need for and use of interventions such as the design, development, adaptation, application, or training in the use of assistive technology devices; the design, fabrication, or application of rehabilitative technology such as selected orthotic devices; training in the use of assistive technology, orthotic, or prosthetic devices; the application of physical agent modalities as an adjunct to or in preparation for purposeful activity; the use of ergonomic principles; the adaptation of environments and processes to enhance functional performance; or the promotion of health and wellness.

Employment characteristics
The wide population served by occupational therapists is located in a variety of settings, such as hospitals, clinics, rehabilitation facilities, long-term care facilities, extended care facilities, schools, camps, and the patients' own homes. Occupational therapists both receive referrals from and make referrals to the appropriate health, educational, or medical specialists.

AOTA studies indicate that the average entry-level salary in 1995 for occupational therapists was $38,300. (AHRP-1997)

Occupational therapy assistant

Occupational description
Under the direction of an occupational therapist, the occupational therapy assistant directs an individual's participation in selected tasks to restore, reinforce, and enhance performance; to facilitate learning of those skills and functions essential for adaptation and productivity; to diminish or correct pathology; and to promote and maintain health. The occupational orientation of the assistant is that of guiding the individual's goal-directed use of time, energy, interest, and attention. A fundamental concern is the development and maintenance of the capacity throughout the life span to perform with satisfaction to self and others those tasks and roles essential to productive living and to the mastery of self and the environment.

Under the therapist's direction, the assistant participates in the development of adaptive skills and performance capacity and is concerned with factors that promote, influence, or enhance performance, as well as those that serve as barriers or impediments to the individual's ability to function. The occupational therapy assistant provides service to those individuals whose abilities to cope with tasks of living are threatened or impaired by developmental deficits, the aging process, poverty and cultural differences, physical injury or illness, or psychological and social disability.

Job description
Entry-level occupational therapy assistant technical education prepares the individual to:

1. Collaborate in providing occupational therapy services with appropriate supervision to prevent deficits and to maintain or improve functions in the activities of daily living, work, and play/leisure and in the underlying components, including sensorimotor, cognitive, and psychosocial.
2. Participate in managing occupational therapy service.
3. Direct activity programs.
4. Incorporate values and attitudes congruent with the profession's standards and ethics.

Employment Characteristics

COTAs assist in the planning and implementation of treatment of a diverse population in a variety of settings such as nursing homes, hospitals and clinics, rehabilitation facilities, long-term care facilities, extended care facilities, sheltered workshops, schools and camps, private homes, and community agencies. AOTA studies indicate that the average entry-level salary in 1995 for certified occupational therapy assistants was $27,400. (AHRP-1997)

Resources

American Occupational Therapy Association
4720 Montgomery Ln, PO Box 31220
Bethesda, MD 20824-1220
301 652-2682   301 652-6611   Fax 301 652-7711

National Board for Certification in Occupational Therapy (NBCOT)
800 S Frederick Ave, Ste 200
Gaithersburg, MD 20877-4150
301 990-7979
E-mail: NatBdCrtOT@AOL.COM

Office Laboratories

Commission on Office Laboratory Assessment (COLA)
8701 Georgia Ave, Ste 610, Silver Spring, MD 20910
301 588-5882

Oncology

American Society of Clinical Oncology
435 N Michigan Ave, Ste 1717
Chicago, IL 60611-4067
312 644-0828   Fax 312 644-8557

American Society for Therapeutic Radiology and Oncology
1891 Preston White Dr, Reston, VA 22091
800 962-7876   703 716-7588   Fax 703 476-8167

Society for Oral Oncology
c/o Carol S. Beckert, DDS
Affiliated Pediatric Dental Specialists
3901 Beaubien Blvd, Detroit, MI 48201

Board Certification in Medical Oncology:
American Board of Internal Medicine
3624 Market St, Philadelphia, PA 19104
800 441-ABIM (800 441-2246)
215 243-1500   Fax 215 382-4702

Board Certification in Gynecologic Oncology, Maternal and Fetal Oncology:
American Board of Obstetrics and Gynecology
2915 Vine St, Dallas, TX 78504
214 871-1619   Fax 214 871-1943

Board Certification in Radiation Oncology:
American Board of Radiology
5255 E Williams Cir, Ste 6800, Tucson, AZ 85711-7401
520 790-2900   Fax 520 790-3200

Ophthalmic Medical Technician

History

Established in 1969, the Joint Commission on Allied Health Personnel in Ophthalmology (JCAHPO) represents all segments of ophthalmology, including representatives of the American Academy of Ophthalmology, the Association of University Professors in Ophthalmology, the Contact Lens Association of Ophthalmologists, the Society of Military Ophthalmologists, the Canadian Ophthalmological Society, the American Ophthalmological Society, the Association of Technical Personnel in Ophthalmology (ATPO, formerly AACAHPO), the American Orthoptic Council, the American Society of Ophthalmic Registered Nurses, the American Association of Certified Orthoptists, the Association of Veterans Affairs Ophthalmologists, and the Canadian Orthoptic Society. JCAHPO and ATPO are the agencies jointly designated to collaborate with the Commission on Accreditation of Allied Health Education Programs (CAAHEP) in the accrediting of educational programs.

In February 1974, the AMA Council on Health Manpower approved the concept of the ophthalmic medical assistant and agreed that a need for a single category of ophthalmic assistant had been demonstrated. To develop educational *Standards (Essentials)*, the AMA Council on Medical Education (CME) worked with representatives of the American Association of Certified Allied Health Personnel in Ophthalmology (AACAHPO), the American Association of Medical Assistants (AAMA), the American Association of Ophthalmology (AAO), the American Academy of Ophthalmology and Otolaryngology (AAOO), the Association of University Professors in Ophthalmology (AUPO), the Contact Lens Association of Ophthalmologists (CLAO), the COA-OMP, and the Society of Military Ophthalmologists (SMO).

It was agreed that in the establishment of *Standards* and the accreditation of educational programs for the ophthalmic medical assistant, the interests of ophthalmological medicine would be represented by COA-OMP and the interests of the allied health occupations by AACAHPO and AAMA. These three organizations developed and adopted the *Standards and Guidelines of an Accredited Educational Program for the Ophthalmic Medical Assistant,* which were then adopted by the AMA House of Delegates at its June 1975 meeting. The Joint Review Committee for the Ophthalmic Medical Assistant changed its name to the Joint Review Committee for Ophthalmic Medical Personnel in 1988, then to the Committee on Accreditation for Ophthalmic Medical Personnel (CoA-OMP) in 1995. AACAHPO also changed its name in 1988 to "Association of Technical Personnel in Ophthalmology." Under the *Standards* approved in 1988, "ophthalmic medical assistant" was omitted and no longer accredited by the Committee on Allied Health Education and Accreditation (CAHEA). The *Standards* now include two levels of programs, "ophthalmic medical technician" and "ophthalmic medical technologist," that are accredited by CAAHEP.

Occupational description
Ophthalmic medical technicians and technologists are skilled persons qualified by academic and clinical training to perform ophthalmic procedures under the direction or supervision of the ophthalmologist.

Job description
Ophthalmic medical technicians and technologists assist ophthalmologists by performing tasks delegated to them, such as collecting data and administering treatment ordered by ophthalmologists. They are qualified to take a medical history, administer diagnostic tests, take anatomical and functional ocular measurements, test ocular functions (including visual acuity, visual fields, and sensorimotor functions), administer topical ophthalmic and oral medications, and instruct the patient (as in home care and in use of contact lenses). Duties include caring for and maintaining ophthalmic instruments, sterilizing surgical instruments, assisting in ophthalmic surgery in the office or hospital, taking optical measurements, assisting in the fitting of contact lenses, and adjusting and making minor repairs on spectacles. Ophthalmic medical technicians and technologists may also maintain ophthalmic and surgical instruments as well as office equipment.

Ophthalmic medical technologists perform all duties performed by technicians, but are expected to do so at a higher level of expertise and to exercise considerable technical clinical judgment. Additionally, technologists may be expected to perform ophthalmic clinical photography and fluorescence angiography, ocular motility and binocular function tests, and electrophysiological and microbiological procedures, as well as to provide instruction and supervision of other ophthalmic personnel and patients. (Ophthalmic medical technologist programs are designated with an asterisk in the program listing.)

Employment characteristics
Ophthalmic medical technicians and technologists render supportive services to the ophthalmologist. They are employed primarily by ophthalmologists, but may be employed by medical institutions, clinics, or physician groups and assigned to an ophthalmologist who is responsible for their direction. They may be involved with patients of an ophthalmologist in any setting for which the ophthalmologist is responsible. Salaries vary depending on employer and geographic location. (AHRP-1997)

Resources
AMA Department of Allied Health
312 553-9355

Joint Commission on Allied Health Personnel
in Ophthalmology
2025 Woodlane Dr, St Paul, MN 55125-2995
800 284-3937   612 731-2944   Fax 612 731-0410
Web address: http://www.jcaho.org

Ophthalmic-Related Occupations

History
The Commission on Opticianry Accreditation was formed in 1979 with the sole purpose of accrediting ophthalmic dispensing and ophthalmic laboratory technician educational programs, formerly a function of the National Academy of Opticianry. In 1985, the US Department of Education recognized the commission as the accrediting body for 2-year ophthalmic dispensing and 1-year ophthalmic laboratory technology programs.

Ophthalmic dispensing optician
Occupational description
Ophthalmic dispensing opticians adapt and fit corrective eyewear, including eyeglasses and in some cases contact lenses, as prescribed by an ophthalmologist or optometrist. They help customers select appropriate and attractive frames, then prepare work orders for ophthalmic laboratory technicians, who grind and insert lenses into frames. The dispensing optician then adjusts the finished eyewear to fit customer needs.

Job description
The ophthalmic dispensing optician combines an understanding of the human eye and vision with customer service skills to order the production of corrective eyewear, aid the patient/customer in selecting appropriate, aesthetically pleasing frames, and adjust the frames to fit the customer's face.

Chief duties of the dispensing optician include:
- Identifying eye structure, function, and pathology, and determining facial and eye measurements.
- Assisting the customer in selecting frames and lenses that match the customer's physical features and aesthetic desires.
- Using an ophthalmologist's or optometrist's prescription to prepare work orders for the ophthalmic laboratory technician.
- Delivering prescription eyewear/vision aids and instructing customers in use and care.
- Maintaining patient/customer records and addressing complaints.
- Providing follow-up services, including eyewear adjustment, repair, and replacement.
- Operating and maintaining equipment, and demonstrating proficiency in lens finishing techniques.
- Adapting, dispensing, and fitting contact lenses.
- Assisting in various business duties, including frame and lens inventory, supply and equipment maintenance, and patient insurance/claim forms submission and record-keeping.

Employment characteristics
Most dispensing opticians work 40-hour weeks in retail stores, some of which may offer one-stop eye examinations, frames, and on-the-spot lens grinding and fitting.

According to the Commission on Opticianry Accreditation, the average salary for ophthalmic dispensing opticians varies depending on region: Northeast, $30,615-32,927; Southeast, $26,958-27,044; Upper Midwest, $26,520-$26,271; Northwest, $25,743-$26,601; Southwest, $26,762-$26,738; and Pacific, $26,889-$27,272.

Employment outlook
As the percentage of middle-aged and elderly people increases, so will these individuals' need for corrective eyewear. Eyewear as fashion—more and more people today now own two or more pairs of eyeglasses for different occasions—also translates into strong future demand for ophthalmic dispensing opticians, as do the many new vision products, such as photochromic lenses (glasses that turn into sunglasses outdoors), now available in plastic and glass; tinted lenses; and bifocal, extended-wear, and disposable contact lenses. (AHRP-1997)

Ophthalmic laboratory technician

Occupational description

Ophthalmic laboratory technicians cut, grind, edge, and finish lenses and fabricate eyewear. Duties include transcribing prescriptions, selecting appropriate lens forms, and processing the materials to meet the prescription.

Job description

Working from a prescription written by an ophthalmologist or optometrist, the ophthalmic laboratory technician uses various types of equipment and machines, including grinders, polishers, and lensometers, to ensure that the finished lenses match the specifications. The technician also assembles the lens and frame parts into a finished set of eyeglasses.

Chief duties of the ophthalmic laboratory technician include:
• Safely and effectively operating and maintaining equipment needed to produce lenses and make eyewear.
• Performing basic mathematical and algebraic operations required on the job.
• Tinting and coating lenses and performing minor frame repair.
• Performing impact resistance treatment and testing.
• Working with ophthalmic dispensing opticians to address and rectify customer/patient complaints.
• Providing follow-up services, including eyewear adjustment, repair, and replacement.
• Discussing prescription eyewear/vision aids and consumer/patient-related information with the prescriber.
• Assisting in various business duties, including frame and lens inventory, supply and equipment maintenance, and record keeping.

Employment characteristics

Most ophthalmic laboratory technicians work 40-hour weeks, either in retail stores that make and sell prescription glasses or for optical laboratories. Some technicians work for optometrists or ophthalmologists. Depending on the size of the business, the technician may either handle every phase of lenses and frame production or work with other technicians, assembly-line style.

According to the Opticians Association of America, the average salary for ophthalmic laboratory technicians varies depending on region.

Employment outlook

As the percentage of middle-aged and elderly people increases, so will these individuals' need for corrective eyewear. Much of the growth in this profession will occur in retail optical chain stores that make prescription eyewear on the premises and offer quick turnaround time. (AHRP-1997)

Resources

Commission on Opticianry Accreditation
10341 Democracy Ln
Fairfax, VA 22030-2121
703 352-8028   Fax 703 691-3929

Contact Lens Society of America
441 Carlisle Dr, Reston, VA 22070
703 437-5100

National Academy of Opticianry
National Federation of Opticianry Schools
10111 Martin Luther King Jr Hwy, Ste 112
Bowie, MD 20720-4299
301 577-4828

Optical Laboratories Association
PO Box 2000, Merrifield, VA 22116-2000
703 849-8550

Optical Manufacturers Association
6055-A Arlington Blvd, Falls Church, VA 22044
703 237-8433

Opticians Association of America
10341 Democracy Ln, Fairfax, VA 22030-2521
703 691-8355   Fax 703 691-3929

Ophthalmology

Ophthalmologist. Alternate titles: eye specialist, oculist. Diagnoses and treats diseases and injuries of eye. Examines patients for symptoms indicative of organic or congenital ocular disorders, and determines nature and extent of injury or disorder. Performs various tests to determine vision loss. Prescribes and administers medications, and performs surgery, if indicated. Directs remedial activities to aid in regaining vision, or to utilize sight remaining, by writing prescriptions for corrective glasses, and instructing patient in eye exercises. (DOT-1991)

Resources

American Academy of Ophthalmology
655 Beach, San Francisco, CA 94109
415 561-8500   Fax 415 561-8533

American Board of Ophthalmology
111 Presidential Blvd, Ste 241
Bala Cynwyd, PA 19004
215 664-1175

Optometric Associations, Statewide

Alabama Optometric Association
400 S Union St, Ste 435, Montgomery, AL 36104
205 834-1057

Alaska Optometric Association
Eagle River Vision Center
2211 E Northern Lights, Ste 202, Anchorage, AK 99508
907 276-2080

Arizona Optometric Association
3625 N 16th St, Ste 119, Phoenix, AZ 85016
602 279-0055

Arkansas Optometric Association
University Tower Bldg
100 S University, Ste 311, Little Rock, AR 72205-5216
501 661-7675

California Optometric Association
801 12th St, Ste 2020, Sacramento, CA 95814
916 441-3990

Colorado Optometric Association
410 17th St, Ste 2060, Denver, CO 80202-4433
303 892-8898

Connecticut Optometric Association
638 Prospect Ave, Hartford, CT 06105-4298
203 586-7508

Delaware Optometric Association
419 Market St, Wilmington, DE 19801
302 654-6490

District of Columbia Optometric Society
7705 Cayuga Ave, Bethesda, MD 20817
301 229-4990

Florida Optometric Association
PO Box 13429, Tallahassee, FL 32317
904 877-4697

Georgia Optometric Association
2175 Northlake Pkwy, Ste 128, Tucker, GA 30084
404 908-0208

Hawaii Optometric Association
1580 Makaloa St, Ste 590, Honolulu, HI 96814
808 947-0111

Idaho Optometric Association
9077 Maple Hill Dr, Boise, ID 83709
208 378-7700

Illinois Optometric Association
304 W Washington St, Springfield, IL 62701
217 525-8012

Indiana Optometric Association
201 N Illinois St, Ste 1920
Indianapolis, IN 46204-4236
317 237-3560

Iowa Optometric Association
1454 30th St, Ste 304
West Des Moines, IA 50266-1312
515 222-5679

Kansas Optometric Association
1266 SW Topeka Blvd, Topeka, KS 66612
913 232-0225

Kentucky Optometric Association
PO Box 572, Frankfort, KY 40602
502 875-3516

Louisiana State Association of Optometrists
PO Box 13451, Alexandria, LA 71315-3451
318 449-9467

Maine Optometric Association
RR 1, Box 2675, Gardiner, ME 04345
207 582-9910

Maryland Optometric Association
720 Light St, Baltimore, MD 21230
301 727-7800

Massachusetts Society of Optometrists
101 Tremont St, Rm 608, Boston, MA 02108
617 542-9200

Michigan Optometric Association
530 W Ionia St, Ste A, Lansing, MI 48933
517 482-0616

Minnesota Optometric Association
1821 University Ave, Ste 492N, St Paul, MN 55104
612 646-2883

Mississippi Optometric Association
5420 I-55 N, Ste D, PO Box 16441
Jackson, MS 39236-0441
601 956-7412

Missouri Optometric Association
417 E High St, Jefferson City, MO 65101-3274
314 635-6151

Montana Optometric Association
36 S Last Chance Gulch, Ste A, Helena, MT 59601
406 443-1160

Nebraska Optometric Association
201 N 8th St, Ste 400, PO Box 81706
Lincoln, NE 68501-1706
402 474-7716

Nevada Optometric Association
9230 W Sahara, Las Vegas, NV 89117
702 228-8644

New Hampshire Optometric Association
195 Hanover St, Portsmouth, NH 03801
603 431-6814

New Jersey Optometric Association
652 Whitehead Rd, Trenton, NJ 08648
609 695-3456

New Mexico Optometric Association
10131 Coars Rd NW, Ste 227, Albuquerque, NM 87114
505 898-6885

New York State Optometric Association
90 S Swan St, Albany, NY 12210
518 449-7300

North Carolina State Optometric Association
114 N Pine St, PO Box 1206, Wilson, NC 27894-1206
919 237-6197

North Dakota Optometric Association
204 W Thayer Ave, Ste 302, Bismarck, ND 58501
701 258-6766

Ohio Optometric Association
169 E Livingston Ave, Columbus, OH 43215
614 224-2600

Oklahoma Optometric Association
Lincoln Plaza Office Center
4545 N Lincoln Blvd, Ste 105, Oklahoma City, OK 73105
405 524-1075

Oregon Optometric Association
6901 SE Lake Road, Ste 26
Milwaukie, OR 97267-2195
503 654-5036

Pennsylvania Optometric Association
PO Box 3312, Harrisburg, PA 17105
717 233-6455

Rhode Island Optometric Association
PO Box 8400, Warwick, RI 02888-0400
401 461-7550

South Carolina Optometric Association
2730 Devine St, Columbia, SC 29205
803 799-6721

South Dakota Optometric Association
116 N Euclid, PO Box 1173, Pierre, SD 57501
605 224-8199

Tennessee Optometric Association
3200 West End Ave, Ste 402, Nashville, TN 37203
615 269-9092

Texas Optometric Association
1503 S IH35, Austin, TX 78741
512 707-2020

Utah Optometric Association
230 W 200 South, Ste 2110
Salt Lake City, UT 84101-3409
801 364-9103

Vermont Optometric Association
26 State St, PO Box 1531, Montpelier, VT 05601
802 233-1197

Virginia Optometric Association
118 N 8th St, Richmond, VA 23219-2305
804 643-0309

Washington Optometric Association
555 116th NE, Ste 166, Bellevue, WA 98004-5274
206 455-0874

West Virginia Optometric Association
Morrison Bldg, 815 Quarrier St, Ste 215
Charleston, WV 25301-2616
304 345-4710

Wisconsin Optometric Association
5721 Odana Rd, Madison, WI 53719
608 274-4322

Wyoming Optometric Association
520 Randall St, Cheyenne, WY 82001
307 632-8819

Optometry

Optometrist. Examines eye to determine nature and degree of vision problem or eye disease and prescribes corrective lenses or procedures. Examines eyes and performs various tests to determine visual acuity and perception and to diagnose diseases and other abnormalities, such as glaucoma and color blindness. Prescribes eyeglasses, contact lenses, and other vision aids or therapeutic procedures to correct or conserve vision. Consults with and refers patients to ophthalmologist or other health care practitioner if additional medical treatment is determined necessary. May prescribe medications to treat eye diseases if state laws permit. May specialize in type of services provided, such as contact lenses, low vision aids or vision therapy, or in treatment of specific groups, such as children or elderly patients. May conduct research, instruct in college or university, act as consultant, or work in public health field. (DOT-1991)

Optometric assistant. Performs any combination of following tasks to assist optometrist: Obtains and records patient's preliminary case history, maintains records, schedules appointments, performs bookkeeping, correspondence, and filing. Prepares patient for vision examination, assists in testing for near and far acuity, depth perception, macula integrity, color perception, and visual field, utilizing ocular testing apparatus. Instructs patient in care and use of glasses or contact lenses. Works with patient in vision therapy. Assists patient in frame selection. Adjusts and repairs glasses. Modifies contact lenses. Maintains inventory of materials and cleans instruments. Assists in fabrication of eyeglasses or contact lenses. (DOT-1991)

Resource

American Optometric Association
243 N Lindbergh Blvd, St Louis, MO 63141
314 991-4100   Fax 314 991-4101

Organ Donations

A Piece of My Mind

Custodian

Victor T. Wilson, MD
JAMA 1987 Oct 9; 258(14): 1898

This patient, this beautiful four-year old boy, was brought in by helicopter from the scene of a head-on auto collision. The nurse recounts the familiar story: an unrestrained back-seat passenger, found under the front dash in the crushed plastic and steel mess. He was extracted with pneumatic jaws and immobilized on a board. Ringer's lactate brought the blood pressure up. Oxygen through an endotracheal tube pinkened his lips. He did not move then and does not now. His pupils do not shrink from light. His skull is in pieces and his brain on CT scan is distorted, cut by white jags of hemorrhage. The flurry of deep-line placements, roentgenograms, burr holes, and blood tests have settled into routine intensive care. Pressor drips infuse. His vital signs are stable now.

Bandaged and crying, his parents are led to him. Their shock, guilt, and grief are the same as they are every time, with every child like him, but still I must turn away from it. I think of my own sweet son and feel dread.

The neurological examination remained barren throughout the night: no reflexes, no tone, and no brain-stem signs. I remove his ventilator briefly and wait for him to breathe. He does not. This morning the unassailable judgment of a cerebral perfusion scan is accomplished. The boy is dead.

This is where my job usually ends. Tubing would be disconnected, machines turned off. The coroner would come. But now we ask gently and urgently of his parents that they give a great gift. Would they donate his organs? At first they are repulsed. Then their anger melts and they see in it a hope and a comfort. They whisper, and embrace, and agree.

I check on the other patients in the unit. The teenager with asthma is better. I kid him about his tattoo and he grins. The baby recovering from repair of a heart defect is not ventilating well. After some adjustments, she breathes easier and grabs my finger.

A curious feeling takes me: as physician to these other children, I continue to work, hoping they will get better, that we will best the disease. But for the dead boy there is no hope and no struggle. For him I am now merely custodian of organs.

The transplant surgeons arrive. Is the heart still good? A last diagnostic flourish of echocardiogram, Swan-Ganz catheter, and isoenzymes suggests it is. The ward clerk wonders how to bill the child's supplies, now that he is no longer a patient. His blood pressure falls slowly. A little fluid, a little more pressor drip, and he is nudged back to a tenuous homeostasis. I stand at the bedside and touch his warm toes. "He is gone, isn't he?" his mother asks. I tell her yes.

Potential recipients rush to the hospital. Heart, kidneys, eyes, and pancreas will be harvested. His parents have said their good-byes and have gone. I sit in his room and watch him, looking for the difference, but he still looks like a live little boy. In midafternoon he is wheeled past me to the operating room, the beautiful dead boy I cared for today. His vital signs are stable.

How organs are donated

Deborah Shelton Pinkney
AM News June 6, 1994 p 20

Rules on which hospital personnel get involved, and standards for donor suitability and family consent, vary slightly from hospital to hospital and among the dozens of procurement agencies. In general, the process goes as follows:

- A hospital nurse or physician identifies potential donor—a brain-dead patient with healthy organs—and notifies local procurement agency.
- The donor is kept on a respirator to keep tissues and organs viable.
- The nurse, physician, or procurement official approaches the family about donation. Most states have "required request" laws, making it mandatory for the hospital to ask. If agreeable, the family signs the donor-consent form. Family permission is needed even when patient has signed a donor card.
- The organ-procurement agency or hospital donor coordinator evaluates the potential donor. Coordinator arranges for surgical team.
- Retrieval surgery takes place. Complete operating room staff is needed for multiple organ retrieval, and a special surgical team usually is required to remove heart, liver, or pancreas.
- A preservationist arranges transport of organs to local agency, where they are matched to potential recipients and distributed. Tissue typing, when needed, takes 8 to 12 hours.
- The recipient gets a preoperative work-up.
- Transplant surgery takes place.
- The procurement agency handles follow-up, including letters to the donor family, staff physician, and nurses about transplanted organs.

What doctors can do

AM News June 6, 1994 p 21

If you're a primary care physician:
- Encourage patients to decide about organ donation while healthy, and to make wishes known to family.
- Explain organ donation and transplantation, including definition of brain death.
- Include pamphlets about donation in mailings with medical bills or in office waiting room.
- Refer patients for more information to local procurement agency or advocacy groups like the National Kidney Foundation and American Heart Association.

If you're hospital-based:
- Make sure local procurement agency is contacted so that process can begin.
- Use this agency's expertise: Talking to families and requesting donor organs is their specialty. Let them do it.
- Separate notification of death from request for donation, to give survivors time to comprehend their loss.
- Be prepared to explain medical procedures and tests, repeating information as often as needed.

JAMA Article of Note: The use of anencephalic neonates as organ donors

JAMA 1995 May 24; 273(20): 1614-1618.

JAMA Article of Note: Strategies for cadaveric organ procurement. AMA Council on Ethical and Judicial Affairs

JAMA 1994 Sept 14; 272(10):809-812.

Resources

Association of Organ Procurement Organizations
1250 24th St NW, Ste 280, Washington, DC 20037
202 466-4353
(Contact if donating party is mistakenly billed)

Living Bank
PO Box 6725, Houston, TX 77265
800 528-2971 713 961-9431   Fax 7013 961-0979
800 527-2971 (donor registration)

Medic Alert Organ Donor Program Foundation
2323 Colorado Ave, Turlock, CA 95380
209 668-3333 (only for ID bracelets)

National Kidney Foundation
30 E 33rd St, 11th Fl, New York, NY 10016
800 622-9010 212 889-2210   Fax 212 689-9261

Organ Transplant Fund
1027 S Yates Rd, Memphis, TN 38119
800 489-3863   Fax 901 684-1128

National Society to Prevent Blindness
500 E Remington Rd, Schaumburg, IL 60173
800 331-2020   847 843-2020   Fax 847 843-8458

Entire Body:
Anatomical Gift Association
2240 W Fillmore, Chicago, IL 60612
312 733-5283

Eye Donor Registry:
Lions Club International
300 22nd St, Oak Brook, IL 60521
630 571-5466   Fax 630 571-8890

Uniform Donor Cards:
United Network for Organ Sharing
PO Box 13770, 1100 Boulder Pkwy, Ste 5000
Richmond, VA 23225
800 243-6667   804 330-8500
Fax 804 330-8517
Web address: http://www.ew3.att.net/unos

Orphan Drugs

In 1982, the Office of Orphan Products Development was established within the Food and Drug Administration, an agency of the Department of Health and Human Services. The Orphan Drug Act (Public Law 97-414) to encourage the development of drugs to treat rare diseases became law in 1983 and was amended in 1984, 1985, and 1988. The Act defines an orphan drug as one used for the diagnosis, treatment, or prevention of a disease or condition affecting fewer than 200,000 people in the United States. If more than 200,000 people are affected, a drug has orphan status when the cost of developing and making it available would not be expected to be covered by sales in the United States. Application for an orphan designation must be made prior to filing a New

Drug Application or Product License Application. More than 400 products have been given orphan designations. (DEA-1995)

Resources

National Information Center for Orphan Drugs and Rare Diseases
PO Box 1133, Washington, DC 20013
800 336-4797

National Organization for Rare Disorders
PO Box 8923, New Fairfield, CT 06812-1783
800 999-6673   203 746-6518   Fax 203 746-6481
E-mail: orphan@nord-edb.com
Web address: http://www.pcnet.com/~orphan

Office of Orphan Drugs
Food and Drug Administration
5600 Fishers Ln, Rockville, MD 20857
301 443-3170

Pharmaceutical Manufacturers Association
Commission on Drug for Rare Disorders
1100 15th St NW, Ste 900, Washington, DC 20005
202 835-3400

Orthomolecular Medicine

Orthomolecular Medical Society
Huxley Institute for Biosocial Research
900 N Federal Hwy, Boca Raton, FL 33432
800 847-3802

Orthopaedics

American Academy of Orthopaedic Surgeons
6300 N River Rd, Rosemont, IL 60018-4226
800 346-AAOS   847 823-7186   Fax 847 823-8125
Web address: http://www.aaos.org

American Board of Orthopaedic Surgery
400 Silver Cedar Ct, Chapel Hill, NC 27514
919 929-7103   Fax 919 942-8988

American Orthopaedic Foot and Ankle Society
1216 Pine St, Ste 201, Seattle, WA 98101
206 223-1120   Fax 206 223-1178
E-mail: aofas@aofas.org
Web address: http://www.aofas.org

American Orthopaedic Association
6300 N River Rd, Rosemont, IL 60018-4226
847 318-7330   Fax 847 318-7339

American Orthopaedic Society for Sports Medicine
6300 N River Rd, Ste 200, Rosemont, IL 60018
847 292-4900   Fax 847 292-4905

Orthotics

Orthotics/Prosthetics

History

The Educational Accreditation Commission (EAC) was created in August 1972 by the American Board of Certification in Orthotics and Prosthetics, Inc (ABC) to meet the orthotics and prosthetics profession's need for an institutional accreditation program. That same year the EAC set out to establish criteria to assess and compare orthotics and prosthetics curricula. These criteria *Stan-*

dards (Essentials) were developed and revised to meet the profession's needs in training orthotists and prosthetists.

In 1991, the EAC was reorganized and renamed the National Commission on Orthotic and Prosthetic Education (NCOPE). NCOPE's primary mission and obligation is to ensure that educational programs meet the minimum standards of quality to prepare individuals to enter the orthotics and prosthetics profession.

During 1992, the NCOPE and its collaborating organizations, the American Orthotic and Prosthetic Association (AOPA) and the American Academy of Orthotists and Prosthetists (AAOP), applied to the American Medical Association (AMA) Council of Medical Education (CME) for recognition of orthotics and prosthetics as an allied health profession. Recognition was granted in August 1992.

In February 1993, the NCOPE reformatted its existing *Standards* to meet the requirements of the Committee on Allied Health Education and Accreditation (CAHEA) Recommended Format for *Standards and Guidelines.* The *Standards* were adopted by AOPA in April 1993. The AMA CME adopted the *Standards* in August 1993, and the AAOP adopted the *Standards* in September 1993.

Occupational description

Orthotics and prosthetics are applied physical disciplines that address neuromuscular and structural skeletal problems in the human body with a treatment process that includes evaluation and transfer of forces using orthoses and protheses to achieve optimum function, prevent further disability, and provide cosmesis.

The orthotist and prosthetist work directly with the physician and representatives of other allied health professions in the rehabilitation of the physically challenged. The orthotist designs and fits devices, known as orthoses, to provide care to patients who have disabling conditions of the limbs and spine. The prosthetist designs and fits devices, known as prostheses, for patients who have partial or total absence of a limb.

Job description

In 1990 and 1991, a role delineation study was conducted by the profession to study the primary tasks performed by the entry-level orthotist and prosthetist. It focused on which tasks are performed on the job, how important each task is, how frequently the task is performed, and how critical the task is. The study concluded that the role of the orthotist and prosthetist includes, but may not be limited to, five major domains: clinical assessment, patient management, technical implementation, practice management, and professional responsibility.

Employment characteristics

Orthotists and prosthetists typically provide their services in one or more of the following settings: private facilities, hospitals and clinics, colleges and universities, and medical schools.

According to the NCOPE, the salary for board-certified orthotists and prosthetists averaged between $36,000 and $59,000 in 1995. (AHRP-1997)

Orthotist. Provides care to patients with disabling conditions of limbs and spine by fitting and preparing orthopedic braces, under direction of and in consultation with physician. Assists in formulation of specifications for braces. Examines and evaluates patient's needs in relation to disease and functional loss. Formulates design of orthopedic brace. Selects materials, making cast measurements, model modifications, and layouts. Performs fitting, including static and dynamic alignments. Evaluates brace on patient and makes adjustments to ensure fit, function, and quality of work. Instructs patient in use of orthopedic brace. Maintains patient records. May supervise orthotics assistants and other support personnel. May supervise laboratory activities relating to development of orthopedic braces. May lecture and demonstrate to colleagues and other professionals concerned with orthotics. May participate in research. May perform functions of prosthetist and be designated orthotist-prosthetist. (DOT-1991)

Orthotics Assistant. Assists orthotist in providing care and fabricating and fitting orthopedic braces to patients with disabling conditions of limbs and spine. Under guidance of and in consultation with orthotist, makes assigned casts, measurements, model modifications, and layouts. Performs fitting, including static and dynamic alignments. Evaluates orthopedic braces on patient to ensure fit, function, and workmanship. Repairs and maintains orthopedics braces. May be responsible for performance of other personnel. May also perform functions of prosthetics assistant and be designated orthotics-prosthetics assistant. (DOT-1991)

Resources

American Academy of Orthotists and Prosthetists
E-mail: aaopline@aol.com

American Board for Certification in Orthotics & Prosthetics, Inc
E-mail: lanceabc@aol.com

National Commission on Orthotic and Prosthetic Education
E-mail: opncope@aol.com

All located at:
1650 King St, Ste 500, Alexandria, VA 22314
703 836-7118   Fax 703 836-0838

Osteopathic Medicine

Osteopathic Physician. Alternate titles: doctor, osteopathic; osteopath. Diagnoses and treats diseases and injuries of human body, relying upon accepted medical and surgical modalities. Examines patient to determine symptoms attributable to impairments in musculoskeletal system. Corrects disorders and afflictions of bones, muscles, nerves, and other body systems by medicinal and surgical procedures, and, when deemed beneficial, manipulative therapy. Employs diagnostic images, drugs, and other aids to diagnose and treat bodily impairments. May practice medical or surgical specialty. (DOT-1991)

Resource

American Osteopathic Association
142 E Ontario, Chicago, IL 60611
800 621-1773   312 280-5800   Fax 312 280-3860
Web address http://www.am-osteo-assn.org

Osteopathic Specialty Boards

American Osteopathic Board of Anesthesiology
17201 E US Hwy 40, S 204
Independence, MO 64055-6427
816 373-4700   Fax 816 373-1529

American Osteopathic Board of Dermatology
25510 Plymouth Rd, Redford, MI 48329
313 937-1200

American Osteopathic Board of Emergency Medicine
142 E Ontario St, Ste 217, Chicago, IL 60611
312 335-1065

American Osteopathic Board of Family Physicians
330 E Algonquin Rd, Ste 2, Arlington Heights, IL 60005

American Osteopathic Board of Internal Medicine
5200 S Ellis Ave, Chicago, IL 60615
312 947-4880

American Osteopathic Board of Neurology and Psychiatry
2250 Chapel Ave, Cherry Hill, NJ 08002
609 482-9000   Fax 609 482-1159

American Osteopathic Board of Nuclear Medicine
5200 S Ellis Ave, Chicago, IL 60615
312 947-4490   Fax 312 947-4575

American Osteopathic Board of
Obstetrics and Gynecology
5200 S Ellis Ave, Chicago, IL 60615
312 947-4630

American Osteopathic Board of Ophthalmology
and Otorhinolaryngology
3 MacKoil Ave, Dayton, OH 45403
513 252-0868

American Osteopathic Board of Orthopedic Surgery
450 Powers Ave, Ste 105, Harrisburg, PA 17109
717 561-8560   Fax 717 561-8562

American Osteopathic Board of Pathology
13355 E Ten Mile Rd, Warren, MI 48089
810 759-7565   Fax 810 759-2291

American Osteopathic Board of Pediatrics
142 E Ontario St, 6th Fl, Chicago, IL 60611
312 280-7434

American Osteopathic Board of Preventive Medicine
411 Stoneridge Ct, Grand Junction, CO 80840
970 245-4533

American Osteopathic Board of Proctology
104 American Kings Way W, Sewell, NJ 08080
609 582-7900

American Osteopathic Board of Radiology
119 E 2nd St, Milan, MO 63556-1331
816 265-4011   Fax 816 265-3494

American Osteopathic Board of Rehabilitation Medicine
9058 W Church St, Des Plaines, IL 60016
847 699-0048

American Osteopathic Board of Special Proficiency in Osteopathic Manipulative Medicine
3500 Depauw Blvd, Ste 1080
Indianapolis, IN 46268-1139
317 879-1881   Fax 317 879-0563

American Osteopathic Board of Surgery
3 MacKoil Ave, Dayton, OH 45403
513 252-0868

Osteopathic Schools

California
College of Osteopathic Medicine of the Pacific
309 E College Plaza, Pomona, CA 91766-1889
909 623-6116

Florida
Nova Southeastern University Health
Professional Division
College of Osteopathic Medicine
1750 NE 167th St, North Miami Beach, FL 33162-3097
305 949-4000

Illinois
Midwestern University
Chicago College of Osteopathic Medicine
555 31st St, Downers Grove, IL 60515-1235
630 515-6060

Iowa
University of Osteopathic Medicine and Health Sciences
College of Osteopathic Medicine and Surgery
3200 Grand Ave, Des Moines, IA 50312
515 271-1400

Maine
University of New England
College of Osteopathic Medicine
11 Hills Beach Rd, Biddeford, ME 04005
207 283-0171

Michigan
Michigan State University
College of Osteopathic Medicine
E Fee Halls, East Lansing, MI 48824
517 355-9611

Missouri
University of Health Sciences
College of Osteopathic Medicine
2105 Independence Blvd, Kansas City, MO 64124
816 283-2000

Kirksville College of Osteopathic Medicine
800 W Jefferson St, Kirksville, MO 63501
816 626-2121

New Jersey
University of Medicine and Dentistry of New Jersey
School of Osteopathic Medicine
40 East Laurel Rd, Ste 100, Stratford, NJ 08084
609 346-6990

New York
New York Institute of Technology
New York College of Osteopathic Medicine
Wheatley Rd, Box 170, Old Westbury, NY 11568
516 626-6900

Ohio
Ohio University College of Osteopathic Medicine
Grosvenor & Irvine Halls, Athens, OH 45701-2979
614 593-2500

Oklahoma
College of Osteopathic Medicine of
Oklahoma State University
1111 W 17th St, Tulsa, OK 74107
918 582-1972

Pennsylvania
Philadelphia College of Osteopathic Medicine
4150 City Ave, Philadelphia, PA 19131
215 871-6100

Texas
University of North Texas Health Science Center
Texas College of Osteopathic Medicine
3500 Camp Bowie, Fort Worth, TX 76107
817 735-2000

West Virginia
West Virginia School of Osteopathic Medicine
400 N Lee St, Lewisburg, WV 24901
304 645-6270

Osteopathic Associations, Statewide

Alabama Osteopathic Medical Association
PO Box 240248, Montgomery, AL 36124-0248
334 272-1002   Fax 334 272-1002

Alaska Osteopathic Medical Association
PO Box 870470, Wasilla, AK 99687
907 376-2006

Arizona Osteopathic Medical Association
5057 E Thomas Rd, Phoenix, AZ 85018
602 840-0460   Fax 602 840-0480

Arkansas Osteopathic Medical Association
412 Union Train Station, Little Rock, AR 72201
501 374-8900

Osteopathic Physicians and Surgeons of California
455 Capitol Mall, Ste 230, Sacramento, CA 95814
916 447-2004   Fax 916 447-4828

Association of Military Osteopathic Physicians
and Surgeons
32077 Stenzel Dr, Conifer, CO 80433
303 670-8789

Colorado Society of Osteopathic Medicine
50 S Steele St, Ste 440, Denver, CO 80209
303 322-1752   Fax 303 322-1956

Connecticut Osteopathic Medical Society
225 Main St, Manchester, CT 06040
203 646-6969   Fax 203 643-6112

Delaware State Osteopathic Medical Society
PO Box 845, Wilmington, DE 19899
302 764-6120   Fax 302 475-5160

Osteopathic Association of the District of Columbia
4001 N 9th St, Ste 216, Arlington, VA 22203
703 522-8404   Fax 703 522-2692

Florida Osteopathic Medical Association
The Hull Building
2007 Apalachee Pkwy, Tallahassee, FL 32301
904 878-7364   904 942-7538

Georgia Osteopathic Medical Association
1900 The Exchange, Ste 160, Atlanta, GA 30339
404 953-0801

Hawaii Association of Osteopathic Physicians
and Surgeons
122 Oneawa St, Kailua, HI 96734
808 261-6105

Idaho Osteopathic Medical Association
522 W Main St, Grangeville, ID 83530
208 983-1133

Illinois Association of Osteopathic Physicians
and Surgeons
PO Box 1037, Ottawa, IL 61350
815 434-5576   Fax 815 434-2540

Indiana Association of Osteopathic Physicians
and Surgeons
3520 Guion Rd, #202, Indianapolis, IN 46222
317 926-3009   Fax 317 926-3984

Iowa Osteopathic Medical Association
1113 Locust St, Ste 2B, Des Moines, IA 50309
515 283-0002   Fax 515 283-0355

Kansas Association of Osteopathic Medicine
1260 SW Topeka Blvd, Topeka, KS 66612
913 234-5563   Fax 913 234-5564

Kentucky Osteopathic Medical Association
c/o Association Professionals
1501 Twilight Trail, Frankfort, KY 40601
502 223-5322   Fax 502 223-4937

Louisiana Association of Osteopathic Physicians
6018 Colbert St, New Orleans, LA 70124
504 488-6743

Maine Osteopathic Association
RR 2, Box 1920, Manchester, ME 04351
207 623-1101   Fax 207 623-4228

Massachusetts Osteopathic Society
100 Concord St, Framingham, MA 01701
508 872-8900   Fax 508 872-8998

Michigan Association of Osteopathic Physicians
and Surgeons
33100 Freedom Rd, Farmington, MI 48336
800 626-7736   810 476-2800   Fax 810 476-1834

Minnesota Osteopathic Medical Society
2912 80th Circle N, Brooklyn Park, MN 55444
612 560-3346

Mississippi Osteopathic Medical Association
89 Jeff St, Oxford, MS 38655
601 234-6551   Fax 601 234-0468

Missouri Association of Osteopathic Physicians
and Surgeons
1423 Randy Ln, Jefferson City, MO 65102
314 634-3415   Fax 314 634-5635

Montana Osteopathic Association
Montana Bldg, Ste 401, Lewistown, MT 59457
406 538-7721

Nebraska Association of Osteopathic Physicians
and Surgeons
Box 24744, W Omaha Sta, Omaha, NE 68124
402 333-2744

Nevada Osteopathic Medical Association
3950 E Flamingo Rd, Ste E-4, Las Vegas, NV 89121
702 731-0304   Fax 702 732-2079

New Hampshire Osteopathic Association
PO Box 1624, Derry, NH 03038
603 625-1254

New Jersey Association of Osteopathic Physicians
and Surgeons
1212 Stuyvesant Ave, Trenton, NJ 08618
609 396-0466

New Mexico Osteopathic Medical Association
PO Box 90396, Albuquerque, NM 87199-0396
505 828-1905   Fax 505 821-1050

New York State Osteopathic Medical Society
87 A Lake Ave, Albany, NY 12203
800 841-4131   518 663-8812   Fax 518 663-8170

North Dakota Association of Osteopathic Physicians
and Surgeons
1714 S Ninth St, Fargo, ND 58103

Ohio Osteopathic Association
53 W Third St, PO Box 8130, Columbus, OH 43201
614 299-2107   Fax 614 294-0457

Oklahoma Osteopathic Association
4848 N Lincoln Blvd
Oklahoma City, OK 73105-3321
800 522-8379   405 528-4848   Fax 405 528-6102

Ostopathic Physicians and Surgeons of Oregon
2121 SW Broadway, Portland, OR 97201
503 244-7592   Fax 503 244-8009

Pennsylvania Osteopathic Medical Association
1330 Eisenhower Blvd, Harrisburg, PA 17111
800 544-7662   717 939-9318   Fax 717 939-7255

Rhode Island Society of Osteopathic Physicians
and Surgeons
1763 Broad St, Cranston, RI 02905
401 781-3940   Fax 401 781-3940

South Carolina Osteopathic Medical Assocation
401 N 5th St, Hartville, SC 29550

South Dakota Society of Osteopathic Physicians
and Surgeons
c/o MASSA-Berry Clinic, Sturgis, SD 57785
605 347-3616   Fax 605 347-4713

Tennessee Osteopathic Medical Association
530 Church St, Ste 700, Nashville, TN 37219
615 242-3032   Fax 615 254-7047

Texas Osteopathic Medical Association
1 Financial Center Ste, 100, IH35
Round Rock, TX 78664-2901
800 444-8662   512 388-9400   Fax 512 388-5957

Utah Osteopathic Medical Association
70 E 1100 North, Richfield, UT 84701
801 896-8254

Vermont State Association of Osteopathic Physicians
and Surgeons
28 School St, Montpelier, VT 05602
800 229-5619   802 229-9418

Virginia Osteopathic Medical Association
11900 Hull St Rd, Midlothian, VA 23112-2904
804 288-6414

Washington Osteopathic Medical Association
PO Box 16486, Seattle, WA 98116-0486
206 937-5358   Fax 206 933-6529

West Virginia Society of Osteopathic Medicine
PO Box 5266, Charleston, WV 25361-0266
304 345-9836   Fax 304 345-9865

Wisconsin Association of Osteopathic Physicians
and Surgeons
34615 Rd E, Oconomowoc, WI 53066
414 567-0520

Wyoming Association of Osteopathic Physicians
and Surgeons
625 Albany Ave, Torrington, WY 82240
307 532-2107   Fax 307 532-5206

Osteoporosis

National Institute of Arthritis and Musculoskeletal
and Skin Diseases
9000 Rockville Pike, Bethesda, MD 20892
301 496-4000

National Osteoporosis Foundation
1150 17th St NW, Ste 500, Washington, DC 20037
800 464-6700   202 223-2226   Fax 202 223-2237
Web address: http://www.nof.org

Ostomy

United Ostomy Association
36 Executive Park, Ste 120, Irvine, CA 92714
800 826-0826   714 660-8624   Fax 714 660-9262

Otolaryngology

Otolaryngologist. Alternate title: otorhinolaryngologist.
Diagnoses and treats diseases of ear, nose, and throat.
Examines affected organs, using equipment such as
audiometers, prisms, nasoscopes, microscopes, x-ray
machines, and fluoroscopes. Determines nature and
extent of disorder, and prescribes and administers medications, or performs surgery. Performs tests to determine
extent of loss of hearing due to aural or other injury, and
speech loss as a result of diseases or injuries to larynx.
May specialize in treating throat, ear, or nose and be
designated laryngologist; otologist; rhinologist.
(DOT-1991)

Resources

American Academy of Otolaryngology-
Head and Neck Surgery
1 Prince St, Alexandria, VA 22314-3357
703 836-4444   Fax 703 683-5100

American Academy of Otolaryngic Allergy
8455 Colesville Rd, Ste 745
Silver Spring, MD 20910-9988
301 588-1800   Fax 301 588-2454

American Board of Otolaryngology
2211 Norfolk, Ste 800, Houston, TX 77098-4044
713 528-6200

American Otological Society
Loyola University Medical School
2160 S First Ave, Bldg 105, #1870
Maywood, IL 60153
708 216-8526   Fax 708 216-4834

P

Paget's Disease

Paget Foundation for Paget's Disease of Bone and
Related Disorders
200 Varick St, Ste 1004, New York, NY 10014-4810
800 23-PAGET   212 229-1582   Fax 212 229-1502

Palliative Care

How you can improve pain management

(excerpt)
Flora Johnson Skelly
AM News Mar 3, 1994 p 19

Experts say pain management could be improved for
many patients if health professionals would take the
following steps:
• Believe the patient. People vary in their perception of
pain and response to medications.
• Use a pain scale."Give the patient a simple scale—from
'0,' which means 'no pain,' to '10,' which means 'pain
as bad as you can imagine,' " said Charles Cleeland,
PhD, director of the University of Wisconsin medical
school's Pain Research Group.
• Assess pain repeatedly.
• Make pain control a priority. "The first priority for the
care of patients facing severe pain as a result of a
terminal illness or chronic condition should be the
relief of their pain," according to a 1993 report of the
AMA Council on Ethical and Judicial Affairs.
• Give adequate medication. States the AMA report,
"Pain control medications should be employed in
whatever dose necessary, and by whatever route
necessary, to fully relieve the patient's pain."
• Take a multidisciplinary approach.
• Educate patients. Patients often need to be educated
about how to take analgesics. They often have questions or fears that need to be addressed.
• Don't let fear of legal repercussions or sanctions by
licensing boards prevent you from giving appropriate
treatment.

JAMA Article of Note: Good care of the dying
patient. Council on Scientific Affairs, American
Medical Association

JAMA. 1996;275:474-478

Article of Note: Consultation in palliative medicine

Arch Intern Med. 1997;157:733-737

Abstract: Palliative medicine is an emerging medical
discipline in the United States, modeled after similar
efforts in Great Britain, Australia, and Canada. Increasingly, academic medical centers are starting clinical
programs in palliative medicine, including inpatient
consultation services. A description of the essential components of a palliative medicine consultation is presented,
based on the author's experience of more than 600
patient encounters at the Medical College of Wisconsin
in Milwaukee. A palliative medicine consultation consists
of six features: assessment and management of physical
symptoms; assisting patients to identify personal goals for
end-of-life care; assessment and management of psychological and spiritual needs; assessment of the patient's
support system; assessment and communication of estimated prognosis; and assessment of discharge planning
issues.

Resources

American Academy of Hospice and Palliative Medicine
PO Box 14288, Gainesville, FL 32604-2288
352 377-8900 Fax 352 377-2349
Web address: http://www.aahpm.org

American Academy of Pain Medicine
4700 W Lake St, Glenview, IL 60025-1485
847 375-4731   Fax 847 375-4777
E-mail: aapm@dial.cic.net

American Pain Society
4700 W Lake St, Glenview, IL 60025-1485
847 375-4715   Fax 847 975-4777

Board Certification:
American Board of Anesthesiology
4101 Lake Boone Trail, Ste 510
Raleigh, NC 27607-7506
919 881-2570   Fax 919 881-2575

Pain Management Guidelines:
Agency for Healthcare Policy Research
PO Box 8547, Silver Spring, MD 20907
800 358-9295

Pancreas

American Pancreatic Association Surgical Service
VA Hospital, 16111 Plummer St, #112
Sepulveda, CA 91343
818 895-9461   818 895-9462   Fax 818 895-9535

Panic Attack

Panic Attack Sufferers' Support Group
1042 E 105th St, Brooklyn, NY 11236
718 763-0190

Paralysis

American Paralysis Association
500 Morris Ave, Springfield, NJ 07081
800 225-0292   201 379-2690 (in NJ)
Fax 201 912-9433
Web address: http://teri.bio.uci.edu/paralysis

Parkinson's Disease

American Parkinson's Disease Association
1250 Hyland Blvd, Staten Island, NY 10305
800 223-2732   718 981-8001   Fax 718 981-4399

Pathology

AMA Policy

Autopsies (H-85.989) CSA Rep G, I-86; Reaffirmed:
Sunset Report, I-96

The AMA (1) endorses the efforts of the Institute of
Medicine and other national organizations in formulating
national policies to modernize and promote the use of
autopsy to meet present and future needs of society;
(2) promotes the use of updated autopsy protocols for
medical research, particularly in the areas of cancer,
cardiovascular, occupational, and infectious diseases;
(3) promotes the revision of standards of accreditation
for medical undergraduate and graduate education programs to more fully integrate autopsy into the curriculum and require postmortems as part of medical educational programs; (4) encourages the use of a national
computerized autopsy data bank to validate technological
methods of diagnosis for medical research and to validate
death certificates for public health and the benefit of the
nation; (5) requests the JCAHO to consider amending
the *Accreditation Manual for Hospitals* to require that
the complete autopsy report be made part of the medical
record within 30 days after the postmortem; (6) endorses
the formalization of methods of reimbursement for
autopsy in order to identify postmortem examinations as
medical prerogatives and necessary medical procedures;
(7) promotes programs of education for physicians to
inform them of the value of autopsy for medical legal
purposes and claims processing, to learn the likelihood of
effects of disease on other family members, to establish
the cause of death when death is unexplained or poorly
understood, to establish the protective action of necropsy
in litigation, and to inform the bereaved families of the
benefits of autopsy; and (8) promotes the incorporation
of updated postmortem examinations into risk management and quality assurance programs in hospitals.

Pathologist. Alternate title: medical pathologist. Studies
nature, cause, and development of diseases, and structural and functional changes caused by them. Diagnoses,
from body tissue, fluids, secretions, and other specimens,
presence and stage of disease, utilizing laboratory procedures. Acts as consultant to other medical practitioners.
Performs autopsies to determine nature and extent of
disease, cause of death, and effects of treatment. May
direct activities of pathology department in medical
school, hospital, clinic, medical examiner's office, or
research institute. May be designated according to specialty as clinical pathologist; forensic pathologist; neuro-
pathologist; surgical pathologist. (DOT-1991)

Pathologist assistant

Occupational description
Anatomic pathologists are physicians who examine tissue
specimens from patients and perform autopsies to diagnose the disease processes involved. Pathologists' assistants participate in autopsies and in the examination,
dissection, and processing of tissue specimens. They
function as physician extenders.

Job description
The following services are provided under the direct
supervision of a licensed and board-certified pathologist,
and should include, but are not limited to:

Surgical pathology. Assisting in the preparation and performance of surgical specimen dissection by ensuring
appropriate specimen accessioning, obtaining pertinent
clinical information and studies, describing gross anatomic features, dissecting surgical specimens, preparing
and submitting tissue for histologic processing, obtaining
and submitting specimens for additional analytic procedures (immunostaining, flow cytometry, image analysis,
bacterial and viral cultures, toxicology, etc), and assisting
in photographing gross and microscopic specimens.

Autopsy pathology. Assisting in the performance of postmortem examination by ascertaining proper legal authorization; obtaining and reviewing the patient's chart and
other pertinent clinical data and studies; notifying involved personnel of all special procedures and techniques
required; coordinating special requests for specimens;
notifying involved clinicians and appropriate authorities
and individuals; assisting in the postmortem examination;
selecting and preparing tissue for histologic processing
and special studies; obtaining specimens for biological
and toxicologic analysis; assisting in photographing gross
and microscopic specimens and photomicrography; and
participating in the completion of the autopsy report.

Additional duties. Assuming duties as may be assigned
relative to teaching, administrative, supervisory, and
budgetary functions in anatomic pathology.

Employment characteristics
Pathologists' assistants are employed in a variety of settings, including community and regional hospitals, university medical centers, private pathology laboratories,
and medical examiners'/coroners' offices. Most work
40-55 hours per week. Salaries vary with geographic
location and type of employing institution. Entry-level
salaries are between $45,000 and $50,000.
(AHRP-1997)

Resources
American Association of Pathologists' Assistants
8030 Old Cedar Ave S, #225
Bloomington, MN 55425
800 532-AAPA

American Society for Investigative Pathology
9650 Rockville Pike, Bethesda, MD 20814-3993
301 530-7130   Fax 301 571-1879

American Board of Pathology
5401 W Kennedy Blvd, PO Box 25915
Tampa, FL 33622
813 286-2444   Fax 813 289-5279

American Society of Clinical Pathologists
2100 W Harrison St, Chicago, IL 60612-3798
800 621-4142   312 738-1336   Fax 312 738-1619
E-mail: info@asco.org *or* info@ascp.org
Web address: http://www.ascp.org

College of American Pathologists
325 Waukegan Rd, Northfield, IL 60093-2750
800 323-4040   847 446-8800   Fax 847 446-8807

National Association of Medical Examiners
1402 S Grand Blvd, St Louis, MO 63104
314 577-8298   Fax 314 268-5124

United States and Canadian Academy of Pathology
3643 Walton Way, Augusta, GA 30909
706 733-7550   Fax 706 733-8033

Patient Rights

AMA's Patient Bill of Rights

The AMA is concerned about patients as well as physicians. The AMA feels a great responsibility to the people it serves. The AMA *Principles of Medical Ethics* for physicians is an example of this commitment. The AMA *Patient Bill of Rights* is another. Both help ensure the rights of the patient. Physicians who belong to the AMA support these six rights:

1. The patient has the right to receive information from physicians and to discuss the benefits, risks, and costs of appropriate treatment alternatives.

2. The patient has the right to make decisions regarding the health care that is recommended by his or her physician.

3. The patient has the right to courtesy, respect, dignity, responsiveness, and timely attention to his or her needs.

4. The patient has the right to confidentiality.

5. The patient has the right to continuity of health care.

6. The patient has a basic right to have available adequate health care. (CHO)

Patient Education
National Council on Patient Information and Education
666 11th St NW, Ste 810
Washington, DC 20001
202 347-6711   Fax 202 638-0773

ODPHP National Health Information Center
PO Box 1133, Washington, DC 20013-1133
800 336-4797   301 565-4167
301 468-1273   Fax 301 984-4256
Web address: http://nhic-nt.health.org

Pediatrics

A Piece of My Mind

The ins and outs of outies

Howard J. Bennett
JAMA 1993 Oct 6; 270(13): 1508

I was putting alcohol on my newborn's umbilical cord the other day when my wife asked me if Molly had an innie or an outie. Since she was three weeks old at the time and her cord looked like it might hang around 'til kindergarten, I told Jan that it was too soon to tell.

"The reason I'm asking," she said, "is that half the babies who came to my mother's group today showed up without their cords, and the other half had gooey ones that were two breaths from the floor."

Although I felt vaguely responsible for this tardiness on Molly's part, I reassured Jan that like so much else in our daughter's life, we would have to pray a lot and keep our fingers crossed.

Over the next few days, Molly's cord finally yielded to peer pressure and dropped off during a middle of the night feeding. Unlike some parents, however, we tossed the purple glob into the diaper pail instead of pasting it in her baby book. After all, given the 22 hours we spent in labor, coupled with all the complications you'd expect at a doctor's delivery, we had all the memories we needed of Molly's birth.

The next morning, Jan queried me again about the status of Molly's belly button. Although I could think of better things to do at 6 am, I agreed to take a look. (Examining a baby's navel on 3 hours' sleep is not as easy as it sounds. In fact, it's a lot like trying to find an abnormality on a CT scan before the radiologist shows you where to look: "Oh sure, now I see it.") Anyway, as I examined Molly's belly, I discovered a granuloma the size of a small cranberry. When I presented the diagnosis to the patient's mom, I could see that she was disappointed. I told her not to worry, however, because I'd take care of it with a little silver nitrate. Unfortunately, the jury was still out on the innie/outie thing.

I fell back into bed hoping to catch an additional 4000 winks when, much to my surprise, I actually began thinking about innies and outies. I lay awake, in a groggy sort of way, and couldn't get the topic out of my head. I tried counting sheep, but that didn't work. I tried counting lawyers too (it helps if you imagine them jumping off a long pier), but that didn't work either. So there I was, curled up on my side, thinking about my daughter's belly button. As my mind drifted back to both medical school and my hospital training, I realized that no one had addressed this topic in depth. In fact, no one had addressed this topic at all. For example, I attended no lectures called "The Functional Significance of Outies" and of all the Grand Rounds I skipped out on as a resident, not one of them had anything to do with belly buttons.

Over the next few days, I decided to look into this area a little further. After all, I'm a resourceful fellow. If someone had written a definitive treatise on belly buttons, I should be able to find it. Unfortunately, after a review of the literature, a search through my pediatric texts, and a discussion with all the grandparents I know, I was unable to find any scientific information about what makes an outie an outie.

Although I could not find anything in print, that does not mean I was short on opinion, however. While some of my colleagues were convinced that umbilical hernias are the culprit, others chimed in with such helpful comments as "Search me" and "Don't you have better things to do with your time?" In addition, Jan reminded me that her own belly button not only disappeared during her pregnancy, but actually popped out in the last few weeks before Molly's birth. While this might be construed as some sort of outie variant, it still did not explain the big picture.

After mulling this over for a while, I realized that despite 15 years in practice, I have never actually seen an outie. Although a handful of parents have asked me the same question that Jan did, to the best of my knowledge, all of my patients have had innies. Was this really true? Or was it possible that I have seen outies, but that I've been calling them something else? Then it struck me. Perhaps outies are a consequence of umbilical granulomas that have been epithelialized. This would explain why an outie persists. It would also explain why I haven't seen any as a doctor—ie, I cauterize all my granulomas with silver nitrate, thereby nipping them in the proverbial bud.

When I presented this theory to Jan, I could see that she had gained new confidence in me as a doctor, a husband, and (more importantly) as a father. However small, we had survived the first medical crisis with our daughter!

As I applied the final dose of silver nitrate to Molly's belly button, I felt a degree of satisfaction that not only would she have an innie, but that her dad, the pediatrician, was in part responsible for the cute little dimple in her midriff.

Pediatrician. Plans and carries out medical care program for children from birth through adolescence to aid in mental and physical growth and development. Examines patients to determine presence of disease and to establish preventive health practices. Determines nature and extent of disease or injury, prescribes and administers medications and immunizations, and performs variety of medical duties. (DOT-1991)

Resources
Ambulatory Pediatric Association
6728 Old McLean Village Dr, McLean, VA 22101
703 556-9222   Fax 703 556-8729
E-mail: ambpeds@aol.com

American Academy of Pediatrics
141 Northwest Point Blvd, Box 927
Elk Grove Village, IL 60007-0927
800 433-9016 (outside IL)   847 228-5005 (in IL)
Fax 847 228-5097
E-mail: kidsdocs@aap.org
Web address: http://www.aap.org/dogl/dogl.html

American Board of Pediatrics
111 Silver Cedar Ct, Chapel Hill, NC 27514
919 929-0461   Fax 919 929-9255

American Pediatric Surgical Association
826 S Gretta Ave, West Covina, CA
Wilshire Park, Needham, MA 02192
617 482-2915

Children in Hospitals
300 Longwood Ave, Boston, MA 02115
617 355-6000   Fax 617 355-7429

Perfusionist

History
The field of cardiovascular perfusion emerged in the mid-1960s, with most of its practitioners trained on the job until the mid-1970s. Trainees often come from other disciplines: nursing, respiratory therapy, biomedical engineering, surgical technology, monitoring technicians, and the laboratory sciences.

In 1972, the American Society of Extra-Corporeal Technologists (AmSECT) began a program of certification for perfusionists. In 1975, this program was turned over to a new agency established to conduct certification as an independent activity: the American Board of Cardiovascular Perfusion (ABCP). The ABCP also adopted minimum standards for training programs as developed by AmSECT and began evaluation and accreditation activities. AmSECT, with the cosponsorship of the American Association of Thoracic Surgeons (AATS) and the Society of Thoracic Surgeons (STS), petitioned the American Medical Association (AMA) for recognition of the occupation in January 1975. The petition was amended on several occasions, and in December 1976 the Committee on Emerging Health Manpower recommended approval; the AMA Council on Medical Education (CME) granted recognition in that same month.

In 1977, four collaborating organizations sponsored the formation of the Joint Review Committee for Perfusion Education (JRC-PE)—the AATS, ABCP, AmSECT, and STS. From 1978 to 1979, the JRC-PE and others developed the *Standards (Essentials) and Guidelines for an Accredited Educational Program for the Perfusionist*. The *Standards* were adopted in 1980 and accreditation of programs began in 1981. The *Standards* were revised in 1984 and 1989. In 1984, the Perfusion Program Directors Council became an additional sponsor, as did the Society of Cardiovascular Anesthesiologists in 1989. In 1991, the review committee became known as the Accreditation Committee for Perfusion Education (AC-PE). In 1996, the American Academy of Cardiovascular Perfusion became an additional sponsor of the review committee.

Occupational description
A perfusionist is a skilled person, qualified by academic and clinical education, who operates extracorporeal circulation and autotransfusion equipment during any medical situation where it is necessary to support or temporarily replace the patient's circulatory or respiratory function. The perfusionist is knowledgeable concerning the variety of equipment available to perform extracorporeal circulation functions and is responsible, in consultation with the physician, for selecting the appropriate equipment and techniques to be used.

Job description
Perfusionists conduct extracorporeal circulation and ensure the safe management of physiologic functions by monitoring the necessary variables. Perfusion (extracorporeal circulation) procedures involve specialized instrumentation and/or advanced life-support techniques and may include a variety of related functions. The perfusionist provides consultation to the physician in the selection of the appropriate equipment and techniques to be used during extracorporeal circulation.

During cardiopulmonary bypass, the perfusionist may administer blood products, anesthetic agents, or drugs through the extracorporeal circuit on prescription and/or appropriate protocol. The perfusionist is responsible for the monitoring of blood gases and the adequate anticoagulation of the patient, induction of hypothermia, hemodilution, and other duties, when prescribed. Perfusionists may be administratively responsible for purchasing supplies and equipment, as well as for personnel and departmental management. Final medical responsibility for extracorporeal perfusion rests with the surgeon-in-charge.

Employment characteristics

Perfusionists may be employed in hospitals, by surgeons, and as employees of a group practice. They typically work during the week and are frequently on call for emergency procedures on weekends and nights. They may also work in an on-call system, depending on the number of perfusionists employed by the institution.

According to the AmSECT, the average base salary for a recently graduated perfusionist is $40,000; for a certified perfusionist with 2 to 5 years' experience, $55,000 to $60,000; 5 to 10 years' experience, $60,000 to $100,000; and chief perfusionist, $100,000 and higher. (AHRP-1997)

Resources

AMA Allied Health Department
312 553-9355

Accreditation Committee for Perfusion Education
7108C at S Alton Way, Englewood, CO 80112
303 694-9262   Fax 303 694-9169

American Academy of Cardiovascular Perfusion
PO Box 468, Pell City, AL 35125
205 338-6355
E-mail: OfficeAACP@aol.com
Web address: http://users.aol.com/OfficeAACP

American Board of Cardiovascular Perfusion
207 N 25th Ave, Hattiesburg, MS 39401
601 582-3309

American Society of Extra-Corporeal Technologists
11480 Sunset Hills Rd, Ste 210E
Reston, VA 22090-9955
703 435-8556   Fax 703 435-0056

Pesticides

National Coalition Against the Misuse of Pesticides
701 E St SE, Ste 200, Washington, DC 20003
202 543-5450   Fax 202 543-4791

National Pesticide Telecommunication Network
Agricultural Chemistry Extension
Oregon State University, 333 Weninger Hall
Corvallis, OR 97331-6502
800 858-7378   Fax 503 737-0761

Rachel Carson Council, Inc
8940 Jones Mill Rd, Chevy Chase, MD 20815
301 652-1877   Fax 301 951-7179
E-mail: rccouncil@aol.com

Pharmacology

American Society for Pharmacology and
Experimental Therapeutics
9650 Rockville Pike, Bethesda, MD 20814-3995
301 530-7060

American Society for Clinical Pharmacology
and Therapeutics
1718 Gallagher Rd, Norristown, PA 19401-2800
610 825-3838   Fax 610 834-8652
E-mail: ASCPT@aol.com

Pharmacy

Pharmacist. Alternate title: druggist. Compounds and dispenses prescribed medications, drugs, and other pharmaceuticals for patient care, according to professional standards and state and federal legal requirements. Reviews prescriptions issued by physician, or other authorized prescriber to ensure accuracy and determine formulas and ingredients needed. Compounds medications, using standard formulas and processes, such as weighing, measuring, and mixing ingredients. Directs pharmacy workers engaged in mixing, packaging, and labeling pharmaceuticals. Answers questions and provides information to pharmacy customers on drug interactions, side effects, dosage, and storage of pharmaceuticals. Maintains established procedures concerning quality assurance, security of controlled substances, and disposal of hazardous waste drugs. Enters data, such as patient name, prescribed medication and cost, to maintain pharmacy files, charge system, and inventory. May assay medications to determine identity, purity, and strength. May instruct interns and other medical personnel on matters pertaining to pharmacy, or teach in college of pharmacy. May work in hospital pharmacy and be designated pharmacists, hospital. (DOT-1991)

Pharmacist Assistant. Mixes and dispenses prescribed medicines and pharmaceutical preparations in absence of or under supervision of pharmacist. Compounds preparations according to prescriptions issued by medical, dental, or veterinary officers. Pours, weighs, or measures dosages and grinds, heats, filters, or dissolves and mixes liquid or soluble drugs and chemicals. Procures, stores, and issues pharmaceutical materials and supplies. Maintains files and records and submits required pharmacy reports. (DOT-1991)

Pharmacy Technician. Alternate title: pharmacy clerk. Performs any combination of following duties to assist pharmacist in hospital pharmacy or retail establishment. Mixes pharmaceutical preparations, fills bottles with prescribed tablets and capsules, and types labels for bottles. Assists pharmacist to prepare and dispense medication. Receives and stores incoming supplies. Counts stock and enters data in computer to maintain inventory records. Processes records of medication and equipment dispensed to hospital patient, computes charges, and enters data in computer. Prepares intravenous (IV) packs, using sterile technique, under supervision of hospital pharmacist. Cleans equipment and sterilizes glassware according to prescribed methods. (DOT-1991)

Resources

American Pharmaceutical Association
Academy of Pharmacy Practice and Management
c/o Susan C. Winckler
2215 Constitution Ave NW, Washington, DC 20037
800 237-APHA   202 628-4410   Fax 202 783-2351

Pharmaceutical Research and Manufacturers of America
1100 15th St NW, Washington, DC 20005
202 835-3400   Fax 202 835-3429

Phobias

A persistent, irrational fear of, and desire to avoid, a particular object or situation. Many people have minor phobias, experiencing some anxiety when unable to avoid contact with spiders, for example. However, these phobias do not impair the ability to cope with day-to-day life. It is only when a fear causes significant distress and interferes with normal social functioning that it is considered a psychiatric disorder.

Types

Simple phobias, also known as specific phobias, are the most common. They may involve fear of particular animals (most often dogs, snakes, spiders, or mice) or of particular situations, such as enclosed spaces (claustrophobia), heights, or air travel. Animal phobias usually start in childhood, but other forms may develop at any time. Treatment is not usually required, unless the feared object is so common that it is not easily avoided (eg, fear of elevators in a person who lives in a large city).

Agoraphobia (fear of open spaces or entering public places) is a more serious type of phobia, often causing severe impairment and disruption of family life.

It is the most common phobia for which treatment is sought. The disorder usually starts in the late teens or early 20s.

Social phobia, which is relatively rare, is fear of being exposed to the scrutiny of others. Examples include fear of eating, speaking, or performing in public, using public toilets, or writing in the presence of others. The disorder usually begins in late childhood or early adolescence. (ENC-1989)

Resource

Anxiety Disorders Association of America
6000 Executive Blvd, Ste 200, Rockville, MD 20852
301 231-9350   Fax 301 231-7392

Photographs, Medical

Historical:
National Library of Medicine
Prints and Photographs Collection
Bethesda, MD 20209
301 496-5961
Web address: http://lovell.nlm.nih.gov/top_level.dir/nlm_online_info.html

Bettman Archive, Inc
902 Broadway, 5th Fl, New York, NY 10010
212 777-6200

Smithsonian Institution
National Museum of History and Technology
14th St & Constitution Ave NW
Washington, DC 20560
202 357-1960

World Health Organization
525 23rd St NW, Washington, DC 20037
202 861-3200
Web address: http://www.who.com

Physical Examination

JAMA Article of Note: Physical examination guidelines, or Medical evaluation of healthy persons. Council on Scientific Affairs

JAMA 1983 Mar 25; 249(12): 1626-1633

For Pilots:

JAMA Article of Note: A review of the medical standards for civilian airmen

JAMA 1986 Mar 28; 255 (12): 1589-1599

Physical Medicine

Physiatrist. Alternate title: physical medicine specialist. Specializes in clinical and diagnostic use of physical agents and exercises to provide physiotherapy for physical, mental, and occupational rehabilitation of patients. Examines patient, utilizing electrodiagnosis and other diagnostic procedures to determine need for and extent of therapy. Prescribes and administers treatment, using therapeutic methods and procedures, such as light therapy, diathermy, hydrotherapy, iontophoresis, and cryotherapy. Instructs physical therapist and other personnel in nature and duration or dosage of treatment, and determines that treatments are administered as specified. Prescribes exercises designed to develop functions of specific anatomical parts or specific muscle groups. Recommends occupational therapy activities for patients with extended convalescent periods and for those whose disability requires change of occupation. (DOT-1991)

Resources

American Academy of Physical Medicine
and Rehabilitation
1 IBM Plaza, 25th Fl, Chicago, IL 60611-3604
312 464-9700   Fax 312 464-0227

American Board of Physical Medicine
and Rehabilitation
Northwest Center, 21 First St SW, Ste 674
Rochester, MN 55902
507 282-1776   Fax 507 282-9242

Association of Academic Physiatrists
7100 Lakewood Bldg
5987 E 71st St, Ste 112, Indianapolis, IN 46220
317 845-4200   Fax 317 845-4299
E-mail: aap@indy.net
Web address: http://al.com/aap/index.html

Physical Therapy

Physical Therapist. Alternate title: physiotherapist. Plans and administers medically prescribed physical therapy treatment for patients suffering from injuries, or muscle, nerve, joint, and bone diseases, to restore function, relieve pain, and prevent disability. Reviews physician's referral (prescription) and patient's condition and medical records to determine physical therapy treatment required. Tests and measures patient's strength, motor development, sensory perception, functional capacity, and respiratory and circulatory efficiency, and records findings to develop or revise treatment programs. Plans and prepares written treatment program based on evaluation of patient data. Administers manual exercises to improve and maintain function. Instructs, motivates, and assists patient to perform various physical activities, such as nonmanual exercises, ambulatory functional activities, daily-living activities, and in use of assistant and supportive devices, such as crutches, canes, and prostheses. Administers treatments involving application of physical agents, using equipment, such as hydrotherapy tanks and whirlpool baths, moist packs, ultraviolet and infrared lamps, and ultrasound machines. Evaluates effects of treatment at various stages and adjusts treatments to achieve maximum benefit. Administers massage, applying knowledge of massage techniques and body physiology. Administers traction to relieve pain, using traction equipment. Records treatment, response, and progress in patient's chart or enters information into computer. Instructs patient and family in treatment procedures to be continued at home. Evaluates, fits, and adjusts prosthetic and orthotic devices and recommends modification to orthotist. Confers with physician and other practitioners to obtain additional patient information, suggest revisions in treatment program, and integrate physical therapy treatment with other aspects of patient's health care. Orients, instructs, and directs work activities of assistants, aides, and students. May plan and conduct lectures and training programs on physical therapy and related topics for medical staff, students, and community groups. May plan and develop physical therapy research programs and participate in conducting research. May write technical articles and reports for publications. May teach physical therapy techniques and procedures in educational institutions. May limit treatment to specific patient group or disability or specialize in conducting physical therapy research. In facilities where assistants are also employed, may primarily administer complex treatment, such as certain types of manual exercises and functional training, and monitor administration of other treatments. May plan, direct, and coordinate physical therapy program and be designated director, physical therapy. Must comply with state requirement for licensure. (DOT-1991)

Physical Therapist Assistant. Alternate titles: physical therapy assistant; physical therapy technician. Administers physical therapy treatments to patients, working under direction of and as assistant to physical therapist. Administers active and passive manual therapeutic exercises, therapeutic massage, and heat, light, sound, water, and electrical modality treatments, such as ultrasound, electrical stimulation, ultraviolet, infrared, and hot and cold packs. Administers traction to relieve neck and back pain, using intermittent and static traction equipment.

Instructs, motivates, and assists patients to learn and improve function activities, such as preambulation, transfer, ambulation, and daily-living activities. Observes patients during treatments and compiles and evaluates data on patients' responses to treatments and progress and reports orally or in writing to physical therapist. Fits patient and supportive devices, such as crutches, canes, walkers, and wheelchairs. Confers with members of physical therapy staff and other health team members, individually and in conference, to exchange, discuss, and evaluate patient information for planning, modifying, and coordinating treatment programs. Gives orientation to new physical therapist assistants and directs and gives instructions to physical therapy aides. Performs clerical duties, such as taking inventory, ordering supplies, answering telephone, taking messages, and filling out forms. May measure patient's range of joint motion, length and girth of body parts, and vital signs to determine effects of specific treatments or to assist physical therapist to compile data for patient evaluations. May monitor treatments administered by physical therapy aides. (DOT-1991)

Resource

American Physical Therapy Association
1111 N Fairfax St, Alexandria, VA 22314
703 684-2782
Web address: http://apta.edoc.com/apta

Physicians

American College of Physicians
Independence Mall West, Sixth St at Race
Philadelphia, PA 19106-1572
800 523-1546   215 351-2400   Fax 215 351-2448
Web address: http://www.acponline.org

Association of American Physicians
PO Box 4000, Princeton, NJ 08543
609 252-4404   Fax 609 252-6609

Doctors Ought to Care (DOC)
5615 Kirby Dr, Houston, TX 77005
713 528-1487   713 528-1127   Fax 713 528-2146
E-mail: esolberg@bcm.tmc.edu
Web address: http://www.bcm.tmc.edu/doc

Physician Assistant

The concept of the physician assistant arose in the mid-1960s and early 1970s when a number of institutions and creative members of their faculty and staff began exploring new territory in American medical education. Their goal was to assist physicians in patient care. In the process, they developed curricula that taught individuals a body of clinical knowledge and skills that previously had largely been limited to the professional preserve of the physician.

In its restricted meaning, "physician assistant" is the title used since the late 1970s to identify a person prepared in the clinical knowledge and skills that are common to primary care medicine. Initially, this person was identified as an assistant to the primary care physician.

In its general meaning, "physician assistant" is used to encompass the primary care physician assistant, as described above, but it has also been applied to personnel

P such as surgeon assistants, anesthesiologist assistants, pathologists' assistants, radiologist assistants, urologist assistants, and others. While several of these types of physician assistants are very small in number, two occupations with listings in this Directory have obtained recognition from the American Medical Association: anesthesiologist assistant and physician assistant.

History

The profession of physician assistant originated in the mid-1960s with leadership from Duke University, the University of Colorado, the University of Washington, and Wake Forest University. The early 1970s brought a rapid growth in the number of such educational programs, which were supported initially with $6.1 million appropriated under the authority of the Health Manpower Act of 1972. This funding also supported some of the initial organization and administration of the national program for the accreditation of educational programs in this field, specifically those designed to prepare individuals as assistants to primary care practitioners.

Interest in the development of national accreditation standards for the education of assistants to primary care physicians was first expressed by the American Society of Internal Medicine.

By 1971, standards had been developed collaboratively by a committee composed of representatives from the American Academy of Family Physicians (AAFP), the American Academy of Pediatrics (AAP), the American College of Physicians (ACP), the American Medical Association (AMA), the Association of American Medical Colleges (AAMC), the American College of Obstetrics and Gynecology (ACOG), the American Society of Internal Medicine (ASIM), the nursing profession, and educators of the physician assistant. These standards were adopted in that year by the AMA, AAFP, AAP, ACP, and ASIM. (The ASIM withdrew its sponsorship of accreditation in September 1981.)

Early in 1972, the medical specialty organizations that had adopted the new educational standards established the Joint Review Committee on Educational Programs for the Assistant to the Primary Care Physician. A principal function of the committee was to assess the extent to which applicant programs were in compliance with the *Standards (Essentials) and Guidelines for the Assistant to the Primary Care Physician* and to formulate recommendations for accreditation to the AMA Council on Medical Education (CME). This committee was composed of three representatives from each of the four sponsoring organizations. In April 1973, the committee appointed three graduate physician assistants to serve as members-at-large for 1-year terms. By March 1974, the sponsors of the committee and the AMA had recognized the American Academy of Physician Assistants as the fifth sponsor of the review committee.

Standards for the surgeon assistant were adopted by the American College of Surgeons in 1973 and by the AMA in 1974. Originally, the American College of Surgeons Committee on Allied Health Personnel reviewed applicant programs' compliance with these standards.

As a result of discussions initiated in 1975, the review committees for the assistant to the primary care physician and surgeon assistant were brought together in 1976 into a unified accreditation review committee. On petition from the Association of Physician Assistant Programs, the collaborating sponsoring organizations of the accreditation review committee and the AMA recognized it as the seventh sponsor of the committee in 1978. The AMA became a sponsor of the review committee in 1994 following the dissolution of CAHEA. The committee was renamed the Accreditation Review Committee on Education for the Physician Assistant in 1988.

Following a 2-year consultation with accredited educational programs, sponsors of the accreditation service, and other interested parties, revised *Standards* were adopted for the education of assistants to primary care physicians in 1978. Following a similar consultation, the revised *Standards* were adopted in 1985 as standards for the education of physician assistants. In 1990, the accreditation standards were consolidated for physician assistant and surgeon assistant education and training, to ensure that both received a comparable base of knowledge and skill in primary care medicine. The *Standards* were last revised in 1997.

Accreditation was offered from 1970 through 1975 for orthopedic and urologic physician assistants. Unlike the *Standards* for the education of the surgeon assistant and the physician assistant, the standards for education of the orthopedic and urologic assistants did not require education and training for competence in eliciting a comprehensive health history and in performing a comprehensive physical examination. Accreditation for these programs was discontinued owing to the withdrawal of support by the American Academy of Orthopaedic Surgeons and the American Urological Association.

Occupational description

The physician assistant (PA) is academically and clinically prepared to practice medicine with the supervision of a licensed doctor of medicine or osteopathy. Within the physician/PA relationship, physician assistants exercise autonomy in medical decision making and provide a broad range of diagnostic and therapeutic services. The clinical role of physician assistants includes primary and specialty care in medical and surgical practice settings in both urban and rural areas. Physician assistant practice is centered on patient care and may include educational, research, and administrative activities. Physician assistants are accountable for their own actions as well as being accountable to their supervising physicians. The supervising physician is ultimately responsible for the patient care rendered by the physician assistant.

The specific tasks performed by individual physician assistants cannot be delineated precisely because of the variations in practice requirements mandated by geographic, political, economic, and social factors. At a minimum, however, physician assistants are educated in areas of basic medical science, clinical disciplines, and discipline-specific problem solving.

Job description

The role of the physician assistant demands intelligence, sound judgment, intellectual honesty, appropriate interpersonal skills, and the capacity to react to emergencies in a calm and reasoned manner. An attitude of respect for oneself and others, adherence to the concepts of privilege and confidentiality in communicating with patients, and a commitment to the patient's welfare are essential attributes.

Physician assistant practice is characterized by clinical knowledge and skills in areas traditionally defined by family medicine, internal medicine, pediatrics, obstetrics, gynecology, surgery, and psychiatry/behavioral medicine. Physician assistants practice in ambulatory, emergency, inpatient, and long-term care settings. Physician assistants deliver health care services to diverse patient populations of all ages with a range of acute and chronic medical and surgical conditions. They need knowledge and skills that allow them to function effectively in a dynamic health care environment.

Services performed by physician assistants while practicing with physician supervision include but are not limited to the following:

1. *Evaluation.* Elicit a detailed and accurate history; perform an appropriate physical examination; order, perform, and interpret appropriate diagnostic studies; delineate problems; develop management plans; and record and present data.
2. *Monitoring.* Implement patient management plans, record progress notes, and participate in the provision of the continuity of care.
3. *Therapeutic.* Perform therapeutic procedures and manage or assist in the management of medical and surgical conditions, which may include assisting surgeons in the conduct of operations and taking initiative in performing evaluation and therapeutic procedures in response to life-threatening situations.
4. *Patient Education.* Counsel patients regarding issues of health care management to include compliance with prescribed therapeutic regimens, normal growth and development, family planning, and emotional problems of daily living.
5. *Referral.* Facilitate the referral of patients to other health care providers or agencies as appropriate.

Licensure

Forty-nine states, the District of Columbia, and Guam have enacted legislation or regulations affecting physician assistants. Forty-two of these jurisdictions allow physicians to delegate prescriptive authority to PAs they supervise.

Employment characteristics

The 1995 *Census Report of Physician Assistants,* published in 1996 by the American Academy of Physician Assistants, indicates that of the more than 25,700 practicing physician assistants, almost half are practicing in primary care. Family practice is the most common specialty for physician assistants (37%), followed by surgery and surgical subspecialties, general internal medicine, emergency medicine, orthopedics, occupational medicine, pediatrics, and subspecialties of internal medicine, such as cardiology.

The majority of physician assistants practice in ambulatory care settings. Solo and group practices employ 40% of all physician assistants. The number of physician assistants employed by hospitals is 23%, due in part to the number of physician assistants working as house staff. The government employs almost 15% of the physician assistant workforce, primarily in the military and the Department of Veterans Affairs. The remaining members of the profession are practicing in managed care organizations, rural and urban clinics, correctional facilities, and other settings.

Physician assistants in outpatient settings work an average of 40 hours per week, while those in inpatient facilities work 43 hours. The number of patient visits for physician assistants in outpatient settings averages 21 per day; in inpatient settings the average is 16 patient visits per day. More than one third of physician assistants have on-call responsibilities that average 29 hours per week.

Salaries vary depending on the experience of the individual, the practice specialty, job responsibilities, and the regional cost of living. The median starting salary for new physician assistant graduates is $50,770. Experienced physician assistants working full-time commonly earn more than $60,000, and the upper salary range exceeds $100,000. It is anticipated that the demand for PAs will continue to increase. (AHRP-1997)

Resources

AMA Allied Health Department
312 553-9355

Accreditation Review Committee on Education for the Physician Assistant
1000 N Oak Ave, Marshfield, WI 54449-5788
715 389-3785   Fax 715 389-3131

American Academy of Physician Assistants
950 N Washington St, Alexandria, VA 22314-1552
703 836-2272   Fax 703 684-1924

Association of Physician Assistant Programs
950 N Washington St, Alexandria, VA 22314
703 548-5538

National Commission on Certification of Physician Assistants
2845 Henderson Mill Rd NE, Atlanta, GA 30341
404 493-9100   Fax 404 493-7316

National Commission on Certification of Physician Assistants (general public mailings)
6849-B2 Peachtree Dunwoody Rd, Atlanta, GA 30328
770 399-9971
Web address: http://www.social.com/health/nhic/hr1300/hr1334.html

Physician Broadcasters

National Association of Physician Broadcasters
515 N State St, Chicago, IL 60610
312 464-5484

Physician Credentials

For Professionals:
American Medical Accreditation Program
515 N State St, Chicago, IL 60610
312 464-4521

Data Bank (Information prior to 1990)
Federation of State Medical Boards of the United States
6000 Western Pl, Ste 707, Fort Worth, TX 76107
817 735-8445   Fax 817 738-6629

National Practitioner Data Bank
(Established under the Health Care Quality Improvement Act)
UNISYS Corporation
8301 Greensboro Dr, Ste 1100, McLean, VA 22102
800 767-6732

P

P

For Public:
Send stamped self-addressed envelope to:
AMA Department of Physician Data Services
515 N State St, Chicago, IL 60610
(To receive a free biography of an MD; requests must be in writing.)

Doctor Certification Line
American Board of Medical Specialties
800 776-2378
(information on board certification)
Certified Doctor from ABMS
Web address: http://www.certifieddoctor.org

Directory of Medical Specialists
Marquis Who's Who, Macmillan Directory Division
3002 Glenview Rd, Wilmette, IL 60091
800 621-9669 (outside IL) 847 441-2387

Physician Select from AMA
Web address: http://www.ama-assn.org

Physician Earnings

Why the AMA releases income data

Mike Mitka
AM News Dec 12, 1994 p17-8

Some physicians think that by releasing salary information, the AMA does a disservice to the profession by giving the media a weapon to portray doctors as members of an overpaid special interest group.

The Michigan delegation to the AMA Interim Meeting even introduced a resolution calling for an end to the salary survey because "the results are invariably used by the media to cast physicians in a negative light."

That position is also shared by other physicians out in the trenches.

"Physicians aren't the only ones who read *AM News*," says Lee S. Anderson, MD, a Ft. Worth, Tex, ophthalmologist. "It seems like we're fighting battles on all fronts with reform, the corporate practice of medicine and managed care. And then for the AMA to come out and announce that incomes are up doesn't make sense to me."

But the reality is that physician income is also tracked by other organizations. Eliminating the AMA's report would force the media to rely on numbers produced by others—numbers that may be used to fulfill another group's agenda.

And other organizations may compile data that isn't as reflective of the physician population as the AMA has through its Socioeconomic Monitoring System. As examples, the AMA cites income figures compiled by two other organizations.
- *Medical Economics* has reported a drop of 8.3% in median net income for physicians in 1993, with primary care physicians experiencing small gains while specialists saw earnings fall substantially, the AMA reports.
- The Medical Group Management Association (MGMA) reported that primary care physicians had income increases of about 8%, with specialists seeing declines or small increases in earnings.

But both of those surveys have response rates of 20% or less, while the SMS has response rates typically between 65 and 70%, the AMA says.

Because of the low response rate, *Medical Economics* estimates are not as precise for any given year and result in volatile percentage swings between years. Over the 1986 to 1993 period, *Medical Economics* has reported percentage changes ranging from an increase of 12.5% to a decrease of 8.3%, the AMA says.

As for the MGMA, its survey covers only those physicians in its member group practices—in other words, less than a third of all practicing physicians. So its results would not be representative of the entire physician population.

The AMA has two important reasons for publishing income figures as part of its annual survey of medical practice characteristics.

"Since physician income data have been and will be used for policy-making purposes, it is crucial for organized medicine to conduct independent income data-collection efforts to ensure accuracy and fair treatment of physicians," says the AMA's James W. Moser, PhD.

Critics of the income-figures release may say that Dr. Moser's reason is fine and could be kept in-house, but then there is the second reason.

"It should be stressed that collecting, but not reporting, income information would have significant fiscal implications," Dr. Moser says. "It is estimated that at least half the revenues from the sale of data publications and public-use tapes would be lost if income data were not included."

Trends in physician income, 1985-1995

by James W. Moser

The financial rewards to medical practice are of interest not only to current and prospective physicians, but to health policymakers, researchers, patients, insurers, and those who employ or advise doctors. This article has two purposes: to report income levels and changes for various specialty, geographic, and other categories into which physicians fall; and to attempt to explain these changes by accounting for some of the measurable factors associated with physician income.

Several marketplace trends have been noted in recent years. Doctors are becoming increasingly likely to be associated with group practices and to be employees. The traditional model of solo, fee-for-service medicine, although it has by no means disappeared, continues to gradually decline. Physicians are becoming more involved with managed care plans and capitated reimbursement. Insurers and employers are becoming increasingly aggressive in holding down health care expenses. Doctors are still adapting to Medicare's fee schedule, introduced in 1992, while more private payers are adopting the fee schedule's methodology. They physician workforce is growing nearly three times as fast as the general population. These are just a few of the factors that might be expected to affect physician income.

For the purposes of this article, a physician is defined as a nonfederal MD typically involved at least 20 hours per week in patient care activities. Both office- and hospital-based physicians are included; however, residents, clinical fellows, and physicians whose primary activities are research or administration are excluded. Both members and nonmembers of the American Medical Association (AMA) are included.

Physician net income is defined as income after expenses but before taxes. Income comprises all earnings from medical practice, including fees, salaries, retainers, bonuses, and contributions into deferred compensation programs. Income from non–patient care activities is excluded.

All physician and medical practice data are drawn from Socioeconomic Monitoring System (SMS) core surveys between 1986 and 1996. The statistics are weighted to adjust for survey nonresponse bias to improve the accuracy of estimates for the physician population. Appendices to *Socioeconomic Characteristics of Medical Practice 1997* describe the SMS survey, weighting, and tabulation methods in detail. Adjustments to income for the effects of inflation use the all-items consumer price index for urban consumers, released by the US Bureau of Labor Statistics.

Income for 1995

Median physician net income increased 6.7% in 1995, offsetting a 3.8% decrease in 1994. These opposing results for the last 2 years illustrate the danger of projecting long-term trends based on change in 1 year alone. The 2-year change in income amounts to an average annual increase of 1.3% from 1993 to 1995 which, when adjusted for inflation, represents an average annual decline of 1.4% in real income. Since 1992, median income increases have averaged 2.2% annually. This is below inflation of 2.8% per year. For comparison purposes, national health expenditures increased 5.5% in 1995, according to the Health Care Financing Administration.[1]

Table 1 presents median income for several specialties, employment statuses, and geographic areas. Income differs considerably from one specialty to another. Average income is lowest among general/family practitioners and pediatricians and highest for radiologists and surgeons, among the specialties examined separately. The change in income from 1994 to 1995 varied substantially across specialties. Primary care specialties generally enjoyed increases that were greater than the average for all physicians; the exception was the broad category of internal medicine, for which median income was unchanged. Increases for surgical specialties were below the all-physician average. Pathology had the largest percentage increase in 1995, but that followed a year in which it had the largest decrease.

The long-term trend away from self-employment and toward employee status continued in 1995. The proportion of employee physicians grew from 36% to 39% from 1994 to 1995. Nearly all of these additional employees came from the ranks of self-employed physicians, whose market share dropped to 55% from 58%. Since employees generally earn less than the self-employed, the trend is one that would tend to restrain increases in average physician income. As shown in Table 1, the percentage increase in income for self-employed physicians was greater than the increase for employees in 1995.

Incomes of self-employed physicians are nearly 50% higher than those of employees. Part of the differential is a return on entrepreneurship and risk taking, over and

Table 1. **Median physician net income by specialty, employment status, and census division, 1995**

	1995 Median Income (in thousands)	Percentage Change From 1994
All physicians*	$160	6.7%
Specialty		
General/family practice	124	12.7
Internal medicine	150	0.0
Surgery	225	2.7
Pediatrics	129	17.3
Obstetrics/gynecology	200	9.9
Radiology	230	4.5
Psychiatry	124	3.3
Anesthesiology	203	1.5
Pathology	185	21.7
Employment Status		
Self-employed	199	13.1
Employee	136	4.6
Independent contractor	155	10.7
Census Division		
New England	140	3.7
Middle Atlantic	173	23.6
East North Central	164	0.0
West North Central	160	6.7
South Atlantic	164	2.5
East South Central	175	7.4
West South Central	173	5.5
Mountain	151	3.4
Pacific	165	10.0

* Includes physicians in specialties not listed separately.

Source: 1995 and 1996 Socioeconomic Monitoring System core surveys.

above compensation for providing physician services. Other factors contribute to the differential. For instance, self-employees tend to be older, have more years of experience, work more hours, and are more likely to be certified by one or more specialty boards, all of which are associated with higher earnings. Controlling for these factors, the income differential due solely to employment arrangement would be much less than 50% of income for employees.[2] Therefore, a comparison of total compensation would show that the differential would be narrower than one based on cash income alone.

Managed care contracting has increased markedly in recent year. In 1995, 83% of physicians had contracts with managed care organizations, compared with 77% in 1994. Further, the share of revenue from those contracts (among physicians with contracts) declined slightly, from 34% to 33%.[3] How these events correlate with changes in net income is a subject of ongoing study. Published research suggests that "managed care has shifted the demand for physician services toward primary care providers, while reducing utilization, fees, or both for all physicians."[4] These findings are consistent with income

Figure 1. **Year-to-year percentage change in median physician net income after expenses before taxes, 1985–1995**

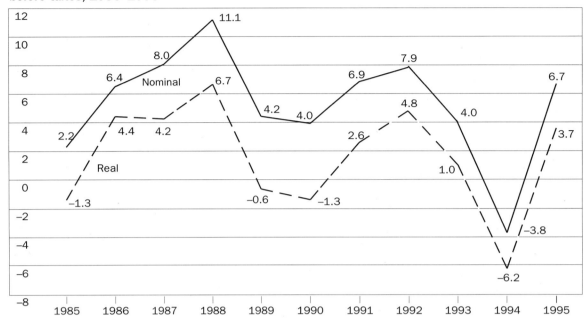

Note: Figures for 1992 and 1993 may differ from those published prior to 1995 because of a refinement in the calculation of income for 1992.

Source: 1986-1996 Socioeconomic Monitoring System core surveys.

patterns by specialty discussed here. It is important to keep in mind that managed care is not the only nor necessarily the most important factor affecting income changes from year to year.

Income tends to vary less across geographic areas than by specialty. Nevertheless, some notable variations occurred for 1994-1995 changes in income. Increases were well above average for physicians in the Middle Atlantic and Pacific areas, and well below average for those in the East North Central, South Atlantic, New England, and Mountain areas. The remaining regions did not differ much from the national average.

While median net income represents what the doctor at the 50th percentile earned, the distribution of physician income is very wide and many lie far below or above that figure. For example, among pediatricians, one fourth made $95,000 or less, compared with the median of $129,000. At the other extreme, one quarter of surgeons earned at least $316,000.

References

1. Levit KR., Lazenby HC, Braden BR, et al. National health expenditures, 1995. *Health Care Financing Rev* 1995;18 (fall):175-214.

2. Moser, JW. Employer-provided benefits for employee physicians. In: *Physician Marketplace Report 96-3*. Chicago, Ill: American Medical Association; April 1996.

3. Emmons DW, Simon CJ. Managed care. In: *Socioeconomic Characteristics of Medical Practice 1996*. Chicago, Ill: American Medical Association; 1996

4. Simon CJ, Born PH. Physician earnings in a changing managed care environment. *Health Affairs*. 1996;15(fall):124-133.

(SCM-1997)

Physician Fees

Fee discussions between physicians and patients

Patients who discuss specific fees for the services they receive from their doctors are the exception rather than the rule, and when discussions do occur with new patients, they are most likely to be with nonphysician staff. Those are two of the conclusions from a recent Socioeconomic Monitoring System survey by the American Medical Association. In 1993, nonfederal patient care physicians (excluding residents) were asked two question regarding fee discussions:

- "For what percentage of your services and procedures are fees discussed before initiating treatment?" and
- "How does your practice usually inform a new patient about the expected fee for a treatment plan—by discussion with the physician, by discussion with a nonphysician member of the staff, by letter prior to the appointment, or by some other means?"

Frequency of fee discussions

Using the responses to the first question, the percentage of all physicians who discussed fees at least 1% of the time was tabulated. Averaging over all physicians, fees were discussed prior to treatment by 44% of physicians, although physicians in the specialties of radiology, pathology, and emergency medicine were excluded from the analysis.

Highlights of the survey include:

- Psychiatrists (80%) and obstetricians/gynecologists (57%) are well above the average; the result for psychiatrists suggests that patients may be highly sensitive to price since these services are less likely to be covered under most health insurance plans; the result for OB/GYNs may be driven by obstetrical care, where expectant mothers are not critically ill and have some time to collect information on fees as well as other aspects of care associated with individual doctors.

- At the other end of the spectrum are anesthesiologists, less than 20% of whom discuss fees. This is not surprising given that they are often on the hospital staff and chosen by surgeons.

- The frequency of discussions varies less across geographic areas than among specialties. The percentage ranges from a low of 33% (in the West North Central census region) to a high of 52% (in the Middle Atlantic region).

- Fee discussions are more likely to occur, the larger and more metropolitan the area. This may reflect the distribution of specialties, as specialties with high discussion rates are more likely to be found in large metropolitan areas, whereas those with lower rates (eg, primary care specialties) are relatively more prominent in nonmetropolitan areas.

- Self-employed physicians discuss fees more frequently than employee physicians do. Employees are more likely to be salaried and less likely to be in a position to negotiate discounts than owners of the practice are, so this result is not surprising.

- Fee discussions decline steadily as the size of the practice (as given by the number of physicians in the practice) grows. This may reflect, at least in part, the finding by employment status: the smaller the practice, the more likely that the physician will have some ownership interest. It may also be because larger practices are more likely to have set policies with respect to fees to ensure consistency across all physicians.

Mode of fee discussions with new patients

Physicians who indicated that they had fee discussions were given several options from which to choose in responding to the question on mode of fee discussion with new patients: with the physicians, with a nonphysician staff member, by letter, or by some other unspecified means. A high majority (71%) of discussions take place with a nonphysician member of the staff. Most of the remainder are discussions directly with the physician. Some physicians who said they had fee discussions at least 1% of the time did not provide a usable response as to the mode of discussion.

Highlights of the survey include:

- Obstetrics/gynecology is the specialty with the highest incidence of discussions with staff, at nearly 85%. Anesthesiologists, on the other hand, are least likely to have a nonphysician staff member conduct the discussion (18%).

- Nearly one half of psychiatrists and anesthesiologists have the fee discussions themselves. OB/GYNs and pediatricians discuss fees directly with patients less than 10% of the time.

- Informing patient of fees by letter prior to the appointment is not particularly popular with any specialty.

- Some moderate differences among geographic regions exist. Aside from perhaps reflecting differences in practice styles, it is unclear exactly what accounts for the differences. The same is true across location types, in which physicians in large metropolitan areas are somewhat more likely to substitute direct discussions

for staff discussions, compared with those in nonmetropolitan areas.

- The results by size of practice are not linear. That is, solo practioners and physicians in the largest practices are the most likely to have fee discussions personally, and the least likely to have staff conduct the discussions; the tendencies are reversed for physicians in small groups. The explanation for this pattern is unclear.

Conclusions

One of the characteristics of an efficient, competitive market is the presence of customers who are well informed regarding prices. This study has shown that explicit fee discussions prior to treatment between patients and physicians occur slightly less than half of the time. Even in cases in which explicit discussions do not occur, however, it is unlikely that patients would enter into a course of treatment without having at least a general notion of the order of magnitude of fees. These notions could be formed, in part, by past experience with the physician, by information received from other patients, by a knowledge of the general level of fees in the area, or by having obtained fee information from a county medical society, an insurer, or a physician referral service. (PMR-1994)

Contact local medical society or state board of medicine.

Physician-Assisted Suicide

A Piece of My Mind

It's over, Debbie

Name withheld by request
JAMA 1988 Jan 8; 259(2): 272

The call came in the middle of the night. As a gynecology resident rotating through a large private hospital, I had come to detest telephone calls, because invariably I would be up for several hours and would not feel good the next day. However, duty called, so I answered the phone. A nurse informed me that a patient was having difficulty getting rest, could I please see her. She was on 3 North. That was the gynecologic-oncology unit, not my usual duty station. As I trudged along, bumping sleepily against walls and corners and not believing I was up again, I tried to imagine what I might find at the end of my walk. Maybe an elderly woman with an anxiety reaction, or perhaps something particularly horrible.

I grabbed the chart from the nurses' station on my way to the patient's room, and the nurse gave me some hurried details: a 20-year-old girl named Debbie was dying of ovarian cancer. She was having unrelenting vomiting, apparently as the result of an alcohol drip administered for sedation. Hmmm, I thought. Very sad. As I approached the room I could hear loud, labored breathing. I entered and saw an emaciated, dark-haired woman who appeared much older than 20. She was receiving nasal oxygen, had an IV, and was sitting in bed suffering from what was obviously severe air hunger. The chart noted her weight at 80 pounds. A second woman, also dark-haired but of middle age, stood at her right, holding her hand. Both looked up as I entered. The room seemed filled with the patient's desperate effort to survive. Her eyes were hollow, and she had suprasternal and intercostal retractions with her rapid inspiration. She had not eaten or slept in two days. She had not responded to chemotherapy and was being given supportive care only. It was a gallows scene, a cruel mockery of her youth and unfulfilled potential. Her only words to me were, "Let's get this over with."

I retreated with my thoughts to the nurses' station. The patient was tired and needed rest. I could not give her health, but I could give her rest. I asked the nurse to draw 20 mg of morphine sulfate into a syringe. Enough, I thought, to do the job. I took the syringe into the room and told the two women I was going to give Debbie something that would let her rest and say good-bye. Debbie looked at the syringe, than laid her head on the pillow with her eyes open, watching what was left of the world. I injected the morphine intravenously and watched to see if my calculations on its effect would be correct. Within seconds her breathing slowed to a normal rate, her eyes closed, and her features softened as she seemed restful at last. The older woman stroked the hair of the now-sleeping patient. I waited for the inevitable next effect of depressing the respiratory drive. With clocklike certainty, within four minutes the breathing rate slowed even more, then became irregular, then ceased. The dark-haired woman stood erect and seemed relieved.

Letters to the Editor

JAMA 1988 Apr 8; 259(14): 2095

To the Editor

I was deeply impressed by the article entitled, "It's Over, Debbie." I would like to extend my most enthusiastic congratulations to the author for having the courage to submit this account.

Faced with a similar situation as a resident some years ago, the morphine approach seemed to be the obvious situation. But I just didn't have the strength to relieve a young man's suffering in view of the possible repercussions of such an action. It is encouraging to learn that at least one of us risked his career to relieve the suffering of another.

Charles B. Clark, MD

To the Editor

I am outraged by the action of the physician in this case who served as jury, judge, and executioner of this young patient, and I believe that the vast majority of physicians feel the same way. I also strongly protest JAMA's publication of this article. It casts the medical profession in a very unfavorable light. Is it any wonder that most polls in recent years have shown that physicians are not held in as high esteem as they used to be?

John G. Manesis, MD

What do dying persons want most from their physicians

Excerpt from Doctor, I want to die. Will you help me?

Timothy E. Quill
JAMA 1993 Aug 18; 270(7): 872-873.

The views expressed in this article are those of the author and do not necessarily represent those of the University of Rochester or the Department of Medicine.

Most patients clearly do not want to die, but if they must, they would like to do so while maintaining their physical and personal integrity.[2] When faced with a patient expressing a wish for death, and a request for help, physicians (and others) should consider the following.

Listen and learn from the patient before responding
Learning as much as possible about the patient's unique suffering and about exactly what is being requested is a vital first step. Physicians tend to be action oriented, yet these problems only infrequently yield simple resolutions. This is not to say they are insoluble, but the patient is the initial guide to defining the problem and the range of acceptable interventions.

Be compassionate, caring, and creative
Comfort care is a far cry from not doing anything. It is completely analogous to intensive medical care, only in this circumstance the care is directed toward the person and his or her suffering, not the disease. Dying patients need our commitment to creatively problem-solve and support them no matter where their illness may go. The rules and methods are not simple when applied to real persons, but the satisfaction and meaning of helping someone find his or her own path to a dignified death can be immeasurable.

Promise to be there until the end
Many people have personally witnessed or in some way encountered "bad deaths," though what this might mean to a specific patient is varied and unpredictable. Patients need our assurance that, if things get horrible, undignified, or intolerable, we will not abandon them, and we will continue to work with them to find acceptable solutions. Usually those solutions do not involve directly assisting death, but they may often involve the aggressive use of symptom-relieving measures that might indirectly hasten death.[1,3] We should be able to reassure all our patients that they will not die racked by physical pain, for it is now accepted practice to give increasing amounts of analgesic medicine until the pain is relieved even if it inadvertently shortens life. Many patients find this promise reassuring, for it both alleviates the fear of pain, and also makes concrete the physician's willingness to find creative, aggressive solutions.

If asked, be honest about your openness to the possibility of assisted suicide
Patients who want to explore the physician's willingness to provide a potentially lethal prescription often fear being out of control, physically dependent, or mentally incapacitated, rather than simply fearing physical pain.[4] For many, the possibility of a controlled death if things become intolerable is often more important than the reality. Those who secretly hold lethal prescriptions or who have a physician who will entertain the possibility of such treatment feel a sense of control and possibility that, if things became intolerable, there will be a potential escape. Other patients will be adequately reassured to know that we can acknowledge the problem, talk about death, and actively search for acceptable alternatives, even if we cannot directly assist them.

Try to approach intolerable end-of-life suffering with an open heart and an open mind
Though acceptable solutions can almost always be found through the aggressive application of comfort care principles, this is not a time for denial of the problem or for

superficial solutions. If there are no good alternatives, what should the patient do? There is often a moment of truth for health care providers and families faced with a patient whom they care about who has no acceptable options. Physicians must not turn their backs, but continue to problem-solve, to be present, to help their patients find dignity in death.

Do not forget your own support
Working intensively with dying patients can be both enriching and draining. It forces us to face our own mortality, our abilities, and our limitations. It is vital to have a place where we can openly share our own grief, doubts, and uncertainties, as well as take joy in our small victories.[5] For us to deepen our understanding of the human condition and to help humanize the dying process for our patients and ourselves, we must learn to give voice to and share our own private experience of working closely with dying patients.

The patients with whom we engage at this level often become indelibly imprinted on our identities as professionals. Much like the death of a family member, the process that they go through and our willingness and ability to be there and to be helpful are often replayed and rethought. The intensity of these relationships and our ability to make a difference are often without parallel. Because the road is traveled by us all, but the map is poorly described, it is often an adventure with extraordinary richness and unclear boundaries.

In memory of Arthur Schmale, MD, who taught me how to listen, learn, and take direction from the personal stories of dying patients.

References

1. Council on Ethical and Judicial Affairs, American Medical Association. Decisions near the end of life. *JAMA.* 1992;267:2229-2233.

2. Cassel EJ. The nature of suffering and the goals of medicine. *N Engl J Med.* 1982;306:639-645.

3. Meier DE, Cassel CK. Euthanasia in old age: a case study and ethical analysis. *J Am Geriatr Soc.* 1983;31:294-298.

4. van der Maas PJ, van Delden JJM, Pijnenborg L, Looman CWN. Euthanasia and other medical decisions concerning the end of life. *Lancet.* 1991;338:669-674.

5. Quill TE, Williams PR. Healthy approaches to physician stress. *Arch Intern Med.* 1990;150:1857-1861.

JAMA 100 Years Ago

JAMA 1996 Oct 16; 276(15): 1222b

A slander in the medical profession

JAMA 1896 Oct 10;27:820-821

In a medico-legal congress a year or two ago it was asserted that it was the practice of reputable physicians to deliberately shorten life in cases of painful and incurable disease. A large portion of the public undoubtedly accepted this statement as gospel truth and possibly thought it nothing extraordinary. The superstition that the orthodox treatment of human rabies is of this character is held by many of the ignorant in the community, and even grosser errors of the same general nature may be occasionally met with among them.

The lawyer who made the statement referred to, defended and advocated the practice and his utterance was, without question, based on no knowledge but was offered as a part or support of the argument he was making before the congress. It is a pity his ideas of the ethics of another learned profession should have been so hazy, and also that he was not more scrupulous as to his facts. His ideas were noticed to some extent by the medical and secular press at the time; the public had at least a chance to be enlightened and it is probable that, on the whole, the utterances did little harm.

The notion, however, that incurable diseases should be cut short by an expeditious euthanasia is every little while advanced by some one-sided humanitarian. The latest comes from California, where a misguided clergyman offers an elaborate proposition of a law for the doing away with the victims of incurable disease. It provides that "a commission of eight persons of high character and unassailable reputation be appointed by the governor for the State, four to be physicians, and the others to be the district attorney, the chairman of the health board, and two public spirited citizens of pronounced humane tendencies. The sufferer should appeal to the commission with the consent of his family, then the case should be thoroughly investigated by the commission, and if the physicians are satisfied that every known remedy has been tried, and the case is absolutely incurable and the patient has suffered intolerable pain, and the relatives can show that they act from none but humane motives, and all these points have been settled to the satisfaction of the commission, it should be empowered gently and humanely to put an end to the misery of the affected person."

The above in its elaborate legal ordering of homicide is very reminiscent of an imaginative work of fiction by an English writer of note that appeared some ten or fifteen years back, and, like it, might be taken as a satire on certain extreme social and economic tendencies. The author of the present proposal, however, is accepted as in earnest, and is probably only one of a large number who in their ill-regulated philanthropy throw well known moral and social principles to the winds. It is easy to see to what consequences his line of reasoning would lead, if the idea of the sacredness of human life were abolished, as would be necessarily the case with the adoption of any such plan.

The medical profession owes to itself and to the public a duty in this matter. It is not that it is misunderstood and misrepresented; there are many respectable and even estimable people who are more or less demoralized by the publication of such propositions, and public sentiment, which ought to be on the highest plane, is degraded to a very material extent by them. Society needs all the safeguards it possesses and the belief in the absolute inviolability of human life is one of the most important of these. There is no need, of course, to say that regular physicians should not encourage any belief in popular impressions derived from such publications, but there may be a very positive utility in their actively denouncing them. At all events they should endeavor to correct any popular belief that our profession sanctions even the suggestion of the violation of human or moral laws. It ought to be unnecessary to say that this should be done, but if we grow familiar with such charges and consequently neglect or ignore them, we have no assurance that such neglect will not appear to the uninformed as a tacit acknowledgment of their truth. When clergymen make such propositions as the one here reported what wonder that a credulous public should think it possible that doctors might be ready to endorse them or carry them out. The commandment "Thou shall not kill," would seem to be binding even upon the clergy. The public knows little and misunderstands a great deal in regard to the ethics of our profession and it is not amiss therefore to occasionally correct a possible misapprehension that they are not in all respects strictly in accord with the highest ethical standards. There is little danger, judging from our past, that we will protest too much.

Resources

Choice in Dying
The National Council for the Right to Die
200 Varick St, 10th Fl, New York, NY 10014-4810
800 989-WILL   212 366-5540   Fax 212 366-5337

Hemlock Society, USA
PO Box 11830, Eugene, OR 97440-3900
800 247-7421   503 342-5748   Fax 503 345-2751

Physician-Patient Relations

A Piece of My Mind

The knee

Constance J. Meyd
JAMA 1982 Dec 24/31; 248(24): 403

We are on attending rounds with the usual groups: attending, senior resident, junior residents, and medical students. There are eight of us. Today we will learn how to examine the knee properly. The door is open. The room is ordinary institutional yellow, a stained curtain between the beds. We enter in proper order behind our attending physician. The knee is attached to a woman, perhaps 35 years old, dressed in her own robe and nightgown. The attending physician asks the usual questions as he places his hand on the knee: "This knee bothers you?" All eyes are on the knee; no one meets her eyes as she answers. The maneuvers begin—abduction, adduction, flexion, extension, rotation. She continues to tell her story, furtively, pushing her clothing between her legs. Her endeavors are hopeless, for the full range of knee motion must be demonstrated. The door is open. Her embarrassment and helplessness are demonstrated. More maneuvers and a discussion of knee pathology ensue. She asks a question. No one notices. More maneuvers. The door is open. Now the uninvolved knee is examined—abduction, adduction, flexion, extension, rotation. She gives up. The door is open. Now a discussion of surgical technique. Now review the knee examination. We file out through the open door. She pulls the sheet up around her waist. She is irrelevant.

How to use a patient satisfaction survey

If you want patients to complete a satisfaction survey, be proactive in your request. Do not simply leave it at the desk. The person who registers patients or schedules follow-up appointments should give a copy to the patient and ask them to complete it before leaving or send it soon. Include a stamped business-reply envelope to maximize the number of surveys returned. Consider amending the format to at least collect the zip code on patients who do not wish to reveal their name and home address. This will be useful in your geographic analysis.

- Distribute a significant number of surveys so a statistical analysis has some meaning.
- Determine if you will survey quarterly, bimonthly, or semiannually. Then select certain weeks or a full month in that time when all patients will be asked to complete surveys. This should give you a good cross section of your patient base.
- Have one person in charge of data gathering, analysis, and reporting of responses. This is often a role for the office manager.
- Be certain results are discussed in physician and full staff meeting within 60 days of the completion of the survey distribution. You will find it easier to recall and make changes on current data. Elicit change ideas from your staff.
- Number or otherwise code individuals who may be negatively referred to by name so the message is heard and the individual is protected. Share this information with that person or the lead physician so education can take place.
- Keep copies of the raw data and analysis for use in benchmarking progress and to better serve your patients in the future. Format the collected information in a way that it can be used for documenting results to your managed care plans.
- If your managed care organization requires a patient survey, try to combine your needs and theirs to one form so the data are useful to both.
- Be certain to follow up with unhappy patients by a phone call or in writing from the office manager or the physician. Dealing with dissatisfied patients forthrightly pays huge dividends in both the long and short run.
- Survey routinely to get the most from your efforts. Do not wait until there are problems or data deadlines. Develop and adhere to an annual schedule that meets your needs and that of your MCOs. (MMCMP-1996)

JAMA Article of Note: Calibrating the physician: personal awareness and effective patient care

JAMA 1997 Aug 13; 278(6): 502-509

Physicians, Employed

Doctor, employer deadlocked over union; Arizona physicians report intimidation, threats

Julie Johnson
AM News Feb 3, 1997 p 3

Doctors' battle to form a union at Tucson's Thomas-Davis Medical Centers has turned into a full-fledged war with the clinic's new owner.

The Arizona physicians say their organizing efforts have been stymied by threats, intimidation, and repeated appeals to the National Labor Relations Board by their employer, San Diego–based Family Associates Medical Management.

Ballots from the physicians' Dec. 5, 1996, union election have sat uncounted and impounded for nearly 2 months as a result of legal maneuvering by FPA, which purchased the 142-physician clinic from a California HMO in November (*AMNews,* Dec. 2, 1996).

The company also reportedly is investigating and considering legal action against some clinic physicians who briefly walked off the job earlier this month in a dispute with FPA over professional liability insurance.

But doctors have fired salvos of their own as the dispute with clinic management escalates.

Physicians' attorneys are studying the liability insurance contract to determine whether FPA limited doctors' coverage in retaliation for their unionization drive—potentially an unfair labor practice.

"The company has threatened those physicians who refused to see patients for a couple of hours with legal retaliation," says Robert Osborne, MD, a Tucson anesthesiologist who is leading the organizing drive. "Our interpretation is that it's just a continuation of their intimidation techniques."

The doctors' union also is seeking revenge in other forms: by organizing the clinic's 500 support staff, for starters. On Feb. 13, these health care workers will hold an NLRB-sanctioned vote on whether to join the Federation of Physicians and Dentists.

Dr. Osborne sees Tucson's flurry of union activity as the first step by physicians and providers to reclaim medical delivery from "administrators and accountants."

"Our ability to act as we have historically, as the patient advocate, is being severely compromised," he says. "The unionization of physicians, as protected by federal law, allows balance to be restored in a system that seems out of control."

Growing skirmishes

Skirmishes between employers and physicians bent on organizing are likely to become more common—more intense—as more doctors look to unions to protect their economic interests, labor experts say.

Employers "will threaten, coerce, intimidate, and begin to harass physicians, just like any other employees that attempt to organize for the purpose of collective bargaining," says Jack Sedsee, Fla.-based Federation of Physicians and Dentists, which has about 3000 members.

"Unlike many other employees, physicians are not prone to back down because of an employer's idle threats," he adds. "They're more prone, if threatened, to solidify into a force to take on the clinic or hospital."

The AMA may be willing to lend a hand to physicians contending with abusive employers, says Ed Hirshfeld, AMA vice president for health law. Current policy calls on the Association to provide guidance and expertise to physicians who are trying to engage in legal collective bargaining. "We're willing to assist, if they want help from us," he adds.

Labor battles are likely to intensify as more physicians turn to collective bargaining to challenge managed care companies and insurers, predicts Barry Liebowitz, MD, president of the Doctors Council, an independent New York union representing 3300 doctors. "I don't think anyone gives up power without a fight."

New interest

Fewer than 20,000 of the nation's 720,000 physicians belong to unions, according to some estimates. But physician interest in organized labor has surged recently, thanks to a spate of national publicity on the topic, the rapid emergence of employed doctors, and growing physician frustration with managed care.

"Based on the people I've been asked to speak to, I can tell you that interest has grown exponentially in the last six months," says Dr. Liebowitz, a pediatrician and a clinical professor at New York University. "It is no longer a fantasy that you'll have organized, unionized work forces in various institutions."

Seddon's union, which is affiliated with the AFL-CIO, also has seen physician interest peak in recent months. As a result, the federation is launching physician organizing drives in Seattle, New Mexico, and Las Vegas, he says.

Such organizing efforts largely have been limited to physicians employed by hospitals, universities, government, and HMOs.

That's because antitrust laws prohibit independent physicians who aren't part of an economically integrated joint venture from joining forces to set prices or divide markets. Violators face civil and criminal penalties, including prison sentences and steep fines.

This prohibition no longer poses as formidable a barrier to doctor unionization, thanks to the current rapid shift in physician practices. Between 1983 and 1995, the proportion of nonfederal physicians who are employed rose from 24.2% to 45.5% according to the AMA Council on Medical Service (*AMNews,* Jan. 20).

But even with this new strength in numbers, employed physicians should expect employers to fight to prevent them from forming an NLRB-sanctioned collective bargaining unit, Dr. Liebowitz warns.

"The organization campaigns are always difficult," says Dr. Liebowitz, who has headed the Doctors Council for 17 years. "It's only natural for employers to blanch at giving physicians more power," he adds. "Doctors have now become more powerful in an organization than they would be unorganized. You're a force to be reckoned with, with a whole host of laws and government to protect you.

But both sides always find a way to reconcile these differences—something that will eventually occur for physicians at Thomas-Davis Medical Centers, he adds.

"They all have mutual problems," Dr. Liebowitz notes. "Employers are caught in the same turmoil of the medical market. They're trying to survive—and they develop a cohesive partnership, productive to get together. The real issues aren't just doctors against the administration, but how to deal with this environment."

Ballots impounded

But the Tucson physicians and their California clinic owner seem far from any reconciliation.

The physicians were cleared to hold the Dec. 5 union election in a 27-page ruling Nov. 8, 1996, by Cornele Overstreet, a regional director for the NLRB.

Overstreet found that, after selling their practice to Foundation Health Plans in 1994, the physicians were

Pfrozen out of medical decision-making and stripped of control over their schedules and patient load. This loss of power showed that the staff physicians and the department chairs at the clinic were truly employees, not supervisors barred from unionization by federal labor law, Overstreet wrote.

The physicians' ballots were impounded the day after the election, however, when the clinic requested that the full NLRB review Overstreet's finding. The labor board rejected this request on Jan. 7.

FPA immediately requested another review, this time on the grounds that the labor practices in question occurred while Foundation owned the clinic, not after the San Diego company's Nov. 1 purchase.

But the clinic's administration has remained the same, Dr. Osborne counters, and FPA owned, the company at the time of the first review request. "These are just obstructionistic delaying tactics," he charges. At press time, the NLRB was expected to rule on the matter.

Liability insurance issue
Tensions between physicians and their new employers rose further after doctors discovered their new liability insurance policy for 1997 covered only FPA's liability.

Advised by private attorneys that they were no longer covered by the policy, some physicians refused to see nonemergency patients until the company corrected the situation. FPA issued a letter clarifying that physicians were, indeed, covered.

FPA didn't return phone calls from *AMNews*. But company spokeswoman Angela Rivera told the Associated Press that the physicians who walked off the job were under investigation.

"The doctors' actions did concern the company—our goal is quality for our patients, and they did disrupt that," she said. "We can't comment on what the discipline will be until we determine the extent of it. My understanding is that there have been no verbal threats to doctors of any kind."

The union also is reviewing this incident, Dr. Osborne says. "If it's related to physicians voting in a union, and if this were an intimidation technique, then it would be unfair labor practice."

In the meantime, physicians are determined to fight on for their elections and their union, he adds. "They've been very united and sincere in their efforts."

Physics

American Association for Physicists in Medicine
1 Physics Ellipse, College Park, MD 20740-3846
301 209-3350   Fax 301 209-0862
E-mail: strafi@aapm.acp.org
Web address: http://www.aapm.org

Health Physics Society
1313 Dolley Madison Blvd, Ste 402
McLean, VA 22101-3926
703 790-1745   Fax 703 790-9063

Physiology

American Physiological Society
9650 Rockville Pike, Bethesda, MD 20814-3991
301 530-7164   Fax 301 571-8305

Plastic Surgery

American Academy of Facial Plastic
& Reconstructive Surgery
1101 Vermont Ave NW, Ste 220
Washington, DC 20005
800 332-3223   202 842-4500   Fax 202 371-1514

American Association for Accreditation of Ambulatory
Surgery Facilities
1202 Allanson Rd, Mundelein, IL 60060
847 949-6058   Fax 847 566-4580

American Association of Plastic Surgeons
c/o R. Barrett Noone, MD
888 Glenbrook Ave, Bryne Mawr, PA 19010
610 527-4833   Fax 610 527-3568

American Board of Plastic Surgery
7 Penn Center, Ste 400, 1635 Market St
Philadelphia, PA 19103
215 587-9322

American Society of Plastic and Reconstructive Surgeons
444 E Algonquin, Arlington Heights, IL 60005
847 228-9900   Fax 847 228-9131
Referral Service 800 635-0635

Podiatrics and Podiatry

Podiatrist. Diagnoses and treats diseases and deformities of human foot. Diagnoses foot ailments, such as tumors, ulcers, fractures, skin or nail diseases, and congenital or acquired deformities, utilizing diagnostic aids, such as urinalysis, blood tests, and X-ray analysis. Treats deformities, such as flat or weak feet and foot imbalance, by mechanical and electrical methods, such as whirlpool or paraffin baths and short-wave and low-voltage currents. Treats conditions, such as corns, calluses, ingrowing nails, tumors, shortened tendons, bunions, cysts, and abscesses, by surgical methods, including suturing, medication, and administration of local anesthetics. Prescribes drugs. Does not perform foot amputations. Corrects deformities by means of plaster casts and strappings. Makes and fits prosthetic appliances. Prescribes corrective footwear. Advises patients concerning continued treatment of disorders and proper foot care to prevent recurrence. Refers patients to physician when symptoms observed in feet and legs indicate systemic disorders, such as arthritis, heart disease, diabetes, or kidney trouble. May treat bone, muscle, and joint disorders and be designated podiatrist, orthopedic; childrens' foot diseases and be designated podopediatrician; or perform surgery and be designated podiatric surgeon. (DOT-1991)

Podiatric Assistant. Assists podiatrist in patient care. Prepares patients for treatment, sterilizes instruments, performs general office duties, and assists podiatrist in preparing dressings, administering treatments, and developing X rays. (DOT-1991)

Resources

American Podiatric Medical Association
9312 Old Georgetown Rd, Bethesda, MD 20814
301 571-9200   Fax 301 530-2752

American Board of Podiatric Orthopedics and
Primary Medicine
401 N Michigan Ave, Chicago, IL 60611-4267
800 862-9589   312 321-5139   Fax 312 321-5144

American Board of Podiatric Public Health
9 Hansen Ct, Narberth, PA 19072
215 667-9183

American Board of Podiatric Surgery
1601 Dolores St, San Francisco, CA 94110-4906
415 826-3200   Fax 415 826-4640

Poison Control Centers

American Association of Poison Control Centers
3201 New Mexico Ave NW, Ste 310
Washington, DC 20016
202 362-7217
Web address: http://www.niu.edu/~pharmacy/
aapcc.html

Poison Control Branch, Food and Drug Administration
5600 Fishers Ln, Room 188-31, Rockville, MD 20857
301 443-6289

Polio

Polio, or poliomyelitis, is a viral infection that affects
muscle-controlling nerves. It used to be universally
feared, with parents dreading the "polio season," which
occurred in summer. This is because in a small proportion of cases the disease caused permanent paralysis or
death. But with modern preventive vaccination the disease has been almost eliminated in developed countries.
(FMG-1994)

Resources

Polio Survivors Association
12720 La Reina Ave, Downey, CA 90242
213 923-0034

Polio Society
PO Box 106273, Washington, DC 20016
202 897-8180   Fax 202 466-1911

Political Associations

American Association of Physicians for
Human Rights
273 Church St, San Francisco, CA 94114
415 255-4547

Physician Committee for Responsible Medicine
PO Box 6322, Washington, DC 20015
202 686-2210

Physicians for Human Rights
100 Boylston St, Ste 702, Boston, MA 02116
617 695-0041   Fax 617 695-0307
E-mail: peacenet.pnphrusa@igc.apc.org

Physicians for a National Health Program
332 S Michigan, Ste 500, Chicago, IL 60604
312 554-0382

Physicians for Social Responsibility
1101 14th St, 7th Fl, Washington, DC 20005
202 898-0150   Fax 202 898-0172

People's Medical Society
462 Walnut St, Allentown, PA 18102
800 624-8773   630 770-1670   Fax 610 770-0607
(advocates citizen involvement in public health issues)

Public Citizen Health Research Group (HRG)
2000 P St NW, 7th Fl, Washington, DC 20036
202 833-3000   Fax 202 463-8842
Publisher of *Public Citizen Health Resources Group
Health Letter,* the HRG monitors government health
agencies, analyzes proposed legislation, testifies at
hearings, and files lawsuits when it believes that
government agencies are too lax in protecting
consumers from dangerous foods, drugs, or medical
practices. Also investigates and issues reports on the
effectiveness of state licensing boards and on various
other ecomonic and quality-of-care issues. (ALT-1993)

Porphyria

American Porphyria Foundation
PO Box 22712, Houston, TX 77227
713 266-9617   Fax 713 871-1788

Practice Management

Practice management: The cornerstone of value

Although medical-practice marketing can be effective in
creating value, the best marketing available will not solve
problems if practice management is poor. Medical-
practice management is the single most important element in creating value. Medical-practice management
refers to both clinical and office operations. It is essential
that both of these be managed effectively and efficiently,
not only to provide good patient care but also to give the
practice the kind of economic value it strives toward.

All other things being equal, a well-managed medical
practice will always have a higher value than one that is
not well managed. This is because one of the key measurements of value is the ability to realize economic gains
in amounts correlated with professional effort. If a physician is working hard treating patients but is not realizing
the cash flow and collections from such treatment, the
practice value inevitably suffers. Although many physicians rightly focus most of their efforts on treating patients, practice management is important from the standpoint of creating value as well as providing effective
patient care. Medical practices that are well managed also
tend to provide a higher caliber of patient care and take
care of more patients. (ENH-1990)

Personnel policies

Developing one's own employee policy manual
The physician's own policies with regard to job descriptions, working hours, wages, and fringe benefits, which
will need to be established before hiring the first assistant
provide the basis for developing a policy manual—an
important and useful guidebook for present and future
employees. Here is a list of the policies a manual should
set forth:

What employees need and want to know

I. Introduction
   A. What's the purpose of this manual?
   B. How does it benefit me and my employer?
   C. Do I have any say if policies are revised?

II. The work week
   A. What are my working hours—daily, weekly?
   B. Explain my flex time arrangements or shifts.
   C. Do I get a paid lunch and breaks? How long? Will we close the office for lunch or do we have to stagger our times?
   D. What are your overtime policies?
   E. What type of time records does the office keep?
   F. When do I get my check? What happens when payday falls on a holiday? Can I get a salary advance if I need it?
   G. What about time paid for civic responsibilities, jury duty?
   H. Any exception to this because I'm a part-timer?

III. Sick leave policies
   A. How do I accumulate sick leave?
   B. When can I begin taking it?
   C. What if I don't use all the sick days I've earned?
   D. Can I carry over unused days until next year?
   E. What happens when I'm out for a long illness?
   F. If I'm a part-timer, do I get sick leave?
   G. Explain your "leave of absence" policies.

IV. Personal days
   A. What is a "personal day"? How many am I allowed?
   B. How much notice do you want if I'm going to use one?
   C. Can I use them in full- or half-day increments?

V. Holidays
   A. What holidays are we paid for?
   B. What happens when a holiday falls on a day when our office is normally closed?
   C. I'm a part-timer. Does the same apply to me?

VI. Vacations
   A. How is my vacation time computed?
   B. When can I take it? Can I take it a day at a time?
   C. When should I notify you of my vacation plans?
   D. Do we choose vacation preference based on seniority?
   E. Can I be paid in lieu of vacation not taken?
   F. Can I carry vacation time over to next year?
   G. What about part-timers?
   H. What if I'm sick during my vacation?
   I. What happens to earned vacation time if my employment is terminated?

VII. Benefits
   A. Do you offer any of the following?
      1. Medical insurance
      2. Dental insurance
      3. Life insurance
      4. Disability insurance
      5. Profit sharing and/or pension plan
      6. Credit union
      7. Other
   B. When do I become eligible to receive benefits?
   C. What do I contribute? What do you contribute?
   D. What about uniform allowance?

E. Do I receive educational reimbursement for such things as:
   1. Tuition—what kinds of courses?
   2. Dues and meetings—what kinds of association?
   3. Workshop and seminars?
F. Do you offer free parking?
G. Can I or my family receive free medical care in this office?
H. Can I use office medical supplies?

VIII. Employment responsibility
   A. How is my attitude important to the workings of this office?
   B. What are your ground rules for attendance and punctuality?
   C. Are personal phone calls allowed? What about long distance calls?
   D. Do you have dress code appearance standards?
   E. What about smoking and eating on the job?
   F. How should I report work-related injuries?

IX. Wage and job evaluation
   A. Is there a "probationary" period? What does this mean?
   B. How are salaries determined?
   C. When and how are they reviewed?
   D. Do you offer bonuses? Cost of living raises? Merit increases?
   E. How often is my job performance evaluated?
   F. Do I participate in this process?

X. Termination
   A. During the probationary period?
   B. How much notice should I give if I want to quit?
   C. If my work is unsatisfactory, do you have procedures for me to receive a second chance?
   D. Explain severance pay policies.
   E. What are grounds for immediate dismissal?
   F. Are there grievance procedures?

XI. Confidentiality
   A. What is the physician-patient relationship?
   B. What about the release of medical information?
   C. Are financial and other records confidential as well?
   D. What are "medical ethics?"

(BUS Adaptation-1989)

Here's how to avoid risk from answering machines

AM News Nov 14, 1994 p 45

Sometimes there's no alternative available to having an answering machine take your calls. If that's the case for you, you need to take steps to protect yourself, says David Karp, loss prevention manager for the Medical Insurance Exchange of California in Oakland. He recommends the following:

• Tell patients that when you are not available your calls will reach an answering machine. Provide written instructions for patients whose medical problems involve foreseeable complications or those who recently started new medications. Include basic drug information, including how to recognize side effects that may require medical attention.

• Record your taped message clearly and distinctly. Tell callers when the office will reopen. Direct them to an emergency department and tell them how to summon an ambulance.

- If you plan to direct patients to an emergency department, alert the emergency director. Request that patients be instructed to call your office when it reopens. Set limits on refills for chronic medications to discourage patients from delaying planned follow-up. To assist emergency physicians, complete operative reports and discharge summaries for recently discharged patients. Consider dispensing a wallet-size card that lists a patient's medication dosages and significant medical history.
- If the answering device can accept messages, give clear instructions to callers. Ask callers to state their name, the date and time, and a phone number where they can be reached. Your message should say when callers can expect a return call. Emphasize that if the patient's condition worsens, he or she should proceed to the emergency department immediately, rather than wait for your return call. The answering device should be able to handle a reasonable number of incoming calls. Avoid devices that rewind the tape and overwrite messages.
- Anticipate some patient dissatisfaction with not being able to reach you. Many people have a strong dislike or fear of answering machines and will not leave a message. Don't ridicule them because of their fear or distaste for talking to your answering device.
- You must decide for yourself if you are adequately protected from liability when relying on a backup "coverage" in the form of an answering machine that directs patients to an emergency department. Consult your liability carrier or a medical law attorney for advice and for review of your taped telephone message and backup policy.

Resources

Managing the Medical Practice. From the Practice Success Series. Chicago, Ill: American Medical Association; 1996. ISBN 0-89970-755-6 OP701295A

Financial Management of the Medical Practice. From the Practice Success Series. Chicago, Ill: American Medical Association; 1996. ISBN 0-89970-758-0 OP701195A

Personnel Management in the Medical Practice. From the Practice Success Series. Chicago, Ill: American Medical Association; 1996. ISBN 0-89970-756-4 OP700995

Practice Guidelines

HHS Press Release

AHCPR, AAHP, and AMA to develop national clinical guideline clearinghouse
May 28, 1997

HHS Secretary Donna E. Shalala today announced plans to develop a comprehensive Internet-based source for clinical practice guidelines. The new National Guideline Clearinghouse (NGC) will make available a full range of current guidance on treatments for specific medical conditions.

Under the plan, HHS's Agency for Health Care Policy and Research, the American Association of Health Plans and the American Medical Association will work jointly

to develop the new guideline clearinghouse. It is anticipated that AHCPR will award a contract later this year for the technical work to establish the NGC.

"Internet technology makes it possible to provide the rapid access to the latest information on medical treatments," Secretary Shalala said. "This clearinghouse will help professionals and patients alike to benefit from the growing volume of clinical practice information."

The target date for launching the new Internet clearinghouse site is fall 1998.

"The NGC will make clinical practice guidelines available to every physician, health plan, provider, purchaser, and consumer who can use a computer," said AHCPR Administrator John M. Eisenberg, MD. "It will provide access to the widest selection of guidelines available from public and private organizations by establishing an independent, interactive Website, accessible by using any standard Web browser or through the Websites of our three organizations."

The development and use of clinical practice guidelines have grown markedly in the past 5 years. However, many existing and potential guideline users have difficulty gaining access to and keeping abreast of the many clinical practice guidelines currently in use. In addition, existing guidelines often differ in their development and content, further complicating their use. To help address these issues, the NGC Website will:

1. Contain standardized information for thousands of guidelines such as title, sponsoring organization, author(s), and methodology used.
2. Provide guideline abstracts and, where possible, the full text of guidelines.
3. Compare and contrast the recommendations of guidelines on similar topics, with summaries covering major areas of agreement and disagreement.
4. Have topic-specific electronic mailing lists to enable registered users to communicate with one another on guideline development, dissemination, implementation, and use.

"Quality medical care is based on a combination of scientific knowledge, training, and experience," said Yank Coble, MD, AMA Trustee and Chair of AMA's Practice Parameters Partnership. "Scientifically based clinical practice guidelines are one invaluable aid to diagnosis and treatment. The AMA's medical guidelines evaluation process, coupled with the ease of access that the NGC will provide, should greatly enhance the value of clinical practice guidelines to physicians and their patients."

"The establishment of the NGC shows how our three organizations can work together to respond to the growing interest in improving quality of care, reducing uncertainty and unnecessary variation in health care decision making, and providing a solid scientific basis for allocation of health care resources," said AAHP's George Isham, MD, Chair of AAHP's Committee on Quality Health Care.

The Agency for Health Care Policy and Research, a part of the Department of Health and Human Services, is the lead agency charged with supporting research designed to improve the quality of health care, enhance access to essential services, and make this access to high-quality health care more affordable. To find out more about

AHCPR and its research findings and publications, visit AHCPR's home page on the World Wide Web at http://www.ahcpr.gov/

The American Medical Association strongly supports the development of scientifically sound and clinically relevant practice parameters as a method to improve the quality of medical care. Practice parameters are strategies for patient management developed to assist physicians in clinical decision making. Currently there are approximately 1800 practice parameters that have been developed by almost 75 physician organizations and other groups. (DIR & PPP-1997)

Directory of Clinical Practice Guidelines: Titles, Sources, and Updates, 1998 Edition. Chicago, Ill: American Medical Association; 1998. 200 pp
ISBN 0-89970-908-7 OP270397

Implementing Practice Parameters on the Local State Regional Level. Brochure. Chicago, Ill: American Medical Association; 1993. OP272793

Resources
Agency for Healthcare Policy Research
PO Box 8547, Silver Spring, MD 20907
800 358-9295
Web address: http://www.ahcpr.gov/

Preadmission Criteria:
Reference Criteria for Short-Stay Hospital Review
Order from NTIS (US Dept of Commerce):
5285 Port Royal Rd, Springfield, VA 22161
703 487-4650 (Order #PB81-179889)

Preferred Provider Organization

Definition
A preferred provider organization (PPO) is an entity representing a group of physicians and/or hospitals that contracts with employers, insurance carriers, or third-party administrators to provide comprehensive medical services on a fee-for-service basis to subscribers. The PPO contracts with physicians and hospitals to provide services at an established fee, generally at a discount from their usual charges. (DRS 1-1993)

How PPOs evolved
Although relatively new on the health care scene, PPOs have had a dramatic impact on health care delivery in this country. While use of the term "PPO" is recent, the concept of the PPO arrangement can be traced to the Foundations for Medical Care (FMCs) of the 1950s, which placed their emphasis on providing medical services within the traditional fee-for-service framework. PPOs in the early 1980s were loosely affiliated groups of providers who agreed to discount their services in exchanged for assurances of new patients. Discounted fees and utilization review were inherent in many PPOs at this time.

Initially, there was little regulation or control of PPOs by federal and or state governments. The first state PPO legislation can be traced to California, which in 1982 enacted statutes designed to eliminate existing regulatory obstacles inhibiting PPO development. According to the American Medical Care Review Association (AMCRA),

states had promulgated laws that could be interpreted as barring the channeling and selective contracting activities necessary to the effective operation of PPOs. These included the antidiscrimination and freedom-of-choice statutes often found in insurance codes; the antidiscrimination, freedom-of-choice, and "any willing provider" statutes found in legislation regulating health service corporations; and the various health maintenance organization acts. Because interpretation of these laws differed from state to state, the statutes tended to impose barriers to PPO development in about half the states and District of Columbia.

AMCRA also notes that states are attempting to encourage the development of PPOs through legislation and regulations. As of December 1986, 22 states had enabling provisions while only three states expressly prohibited the selective contracting and channeling activities essential to PPOs. Provisions in the new enabling measures, as well as preexisting regulations, protect consumers in PPOs, although it is still too early to assess their adequacy.

Because PPO arrangements are subject to the regulations that apply to the benefit plans they serve or to their sponsoring entities, they may be regulated in a variety of ways. These variations may create an imbalance between those that are less regulated and those that are subject to greater regulations. For example, a June 8, 1983, Federal Trade Commission advisory concluded that "the PPO program would likely improve competition in the health care sector and would not violate the Federal Trade Commission Act or any other antitrust statute." This opinion offered two important points—providers and payers must be free to participate in other programs, and competing providers and payers should not be involved in any agreement on PPO operations. In addition, according to the Justice Department, three key elements must be present to ensure that antitrust laws are not being violated. These are:
• no anticompetition purposes;
• the market share of the venture must not be so large that it forecloses effective competition; and
• provider agreements must be secondary to the cooperative activity that promotes competition.

Characteristics of PPOs
As contractual units, PPOs differ widely. In fact, there is no "typical" PPO. Yet, for their differences, most PPO designs share many of the following characteristics:
• A designated panel of health care professionals and/or institutions that serve as the contracted providers;
• an established fee schedule that generally results in a discount of as much as 15% to 20% from usual, customary, and reasonable reimbursements for the employers or insurance carriers who are the purchasers of care;
• medical services provided on a traditional fee-for-service basis;
• a strong emphasis on utilization review and control;
• usually no "lock-in" of the patient to specific health care providers; however, economic incentives such as the waiving or reducing of copayments or deductibles often are applied to encourage use of contracted providers;
• no formal risk-sharing arrangement by the physicians in a PPO as in the IPA model HMO; and

• a strong effort to pay providers within a designated time period.

In most cases, PPO enrollees are not required to receive care from contract physicians or hospitals but their out-of-pocket expenses are increased if they do not. A few PPOs may not provide any benefits if patients do not utilize PPO panel physicians and hospitals. These arrangements are called "exclusive provider organizations" (EPOs).

Most PPOs perform the functions of establishing a provider base of physicians and hospitals and marketing these providers to the payors. Utilization of review and claims processing usually are contracted out to third-party administrators, insurance companies, or professional review organizations. Some payers, however, process their own claims. Employers reimburse PPOs according to any one of several methods: an administrative fee, a monthly service fee, capitation, a percentage of claims, a per-claim fee, or a percentage of savings. (HDS-1993)

Resource
American Association of Preferred Provider Organizations
601 13th St NW, Washington, DC 20005
202 347-7600   Fax 202 347-7601

Pregnancy

JAMA Article of Note: Legal interventions during pregnancy: court-ordered medical treatments and their legal penalties for potentially harmful behavior by pregnant women

JAMA 1990 Nov 28; 264(20): 2663-2670

Resource
American College of Obstetricians and Gynecologists
409 12th St SW, Washington, DC 20024-2188
202 638-5577   Fax 202 484-8107

Premenstrual Syndrome

An estimated 20% to 40% of all women experience a range of physical and emotional symptoms in the 7 to 10 days preceding their period. This recurring cycle of symptoms is called premenstrual syndrome or PMS.

The nature and cause of PMS remain a mystery, but there is a growing recognition that it is a serious problem for many women. New treatments to lessen the symptoms of PMS are being developed. When seeking medical help for PMS, it is important for the patient to note the timing of symptoms because this information can help the provider track their cyclical nature and make a diagnosis.

PMS represents a wide variety of symptoms that can include any of the following: breast tenderness and swelling, weight gain, and bloating; emotional changes such as depression, crying, anxiety, nervous tension, mood swings, and irritability; and insomnia, headaches, food cravings (especially for sweets), increased appetite, and fatigue. These symptoms can range from mild to severe and vary among women. (WHG - 1996)

Resource
PMS Access Hotline
800 222-4767

Preventive Medicine

AMA Policy

Healthy People 2000—Challenges in Preventive Medicine (H.425.986) Amended BOT Rep B, I-90.

It is the policy of the AMA that (1) physicians should become familiar with and increase their utilization of clinical preventive services protocols; (2) individual physicians as well as organized medicine at all levels should increase communication and cooperation with and support of public health agencies. Physician leadership in advocating for a strong public health infrastructure is particularly important; (3) physicians should promote and offer to serve on local and state advisory boards; (4) physicians and medical societies should advocate for the adoption of local state health objectives for the year 2000; and (5) in concert with other groups, physicians should study local community needs, define appropriate health objectives, and work toward achieving health goals for the community.

Preventive medicine
The branch of medicine that deals with the prevention of disease by public health measures, such as the provision of pure water supplies; by health education aimed at discouraging smoking and the overuse of alcohol, promoting exercise, and giving advice about a prudent diet; by specific preventive treatments, such as immunization against infectious diseases; and by screening programs to detect diseases such as glaucoma, tuberculosis, and cancer of the cervix before they cause symptoms.

Most of the increase in the world's population during the 19th century was due to improvements in public health, particularly improvements in the overall standard of nutrition, and the provision of pure water supplies and proper sanitation. Today, these measures remain the priorities of preventive medicine in developing countries, and, along with a program of immunization in childhood, have been targeted as major objectives by the World Health Organization.

However, in developed countries, the primary objective is to persuade the adult population to adopt a healthier lifestyle. In the US, most premature death in adults (that is, deaths before the age of 65) are preventable, being due to accidents and/or linked to such factors as an unhealthy diet, smoking, and excessive drinking. Adoption of a healthier lifestyle, the wider use of screening for cancers, and measures to reduce accidents could lead to substantial improvements in the nation's health. (ENC-1989)

Resources
American Board of Preventive Medicine
9950 W Lawrence Ave, Ste 106
Schiller Park, IL 60176
847 671-1750   Fax 847 671-1751

American College of Preventive Medicine
1660 L St, Ste 206, Washington, DC 20036-5603
202 466-2044   Fax 202 466-2662
E-mail: info@acpm.org

Primary Care

Majority vote for primary care. Match continues move to generalist medicine.

Mike Mitka
AM News Apr 14, 1997 p 1

What was once a sea change is now the norm: More than half of graduating US medical school seniors will enter primary care residencies in 1997.

This interest in generalist medicine marks the third consecutive year primary care has garnered the majority of graduates, reinforcing theories that economics and curriculum changes are countering a long-standing bias toward specialty care training.

Results from the National Residency Matching Program find 7583 graduating US medical school seniors, or 56%, matching to a first-year residency position in internal medicine, family practice, or pediatrics. Last year, 54.4% matched into these specialties.

These results, however, do not mean the physician work force is nearing the 50-50 split between specialists and generalists that some advocate, since many internal medicine residents move into internal medicine subspecialties. Also, as US grads ignore specialty training, those slots continue to be filled by international medical graduates.

Market, curricula changes
Still, the Match results send encouraging signals to primary care advocates.

Jordan J. Cohen, MD, president of the Association of American Medical Colleges, said the shift reflects the current mood of the country.

"It's a combination of medical schools responding to the call from the public for more emphasis on primary care as well as the marketplace, which has sent strong signals for change," Dr. Cohen said.

Leaders of the American Academy of Family Physicians, who announced that a record 2905 family practice residency slots were filled, also were pleased with the national Match results.

"It's great news that increasing numbers of medical students are choosing family practice over subspecialty careers," said Douglas Henley, MD, chair of the AAFP's board of directors. "Medical students recognize the personal rewards of family practice's focus on treating the whole person and the entire family."

Growth in his specialty's residency programs, Dr. Henley added, helps resolve physician work force dilemmas.

"While there has been a great deal of discussion lately around the fact that we have too many doctors in this country, what tends to get lost in those discussions is that we have too few primary care doctors, especially family physicians," he said. "The oversupply of doctors is real, but that oversupply is of narrowly focused subspecialists."

As decision-makers ponder the great questions regarding the makeup of the physician work force, students still seem to be selecting residencies for personal reasons.

"I'm basically going into pediatrics because I enjoy working with kids," says Birute Wise, a fourth-year medical student at the University of Texas at Houston. "So the current environment stressing primary care didn't influence me."

But Christopher Cogle, chair of the AMA's Medical Student Section, echoed Dr. Cohen's remarks, noting the continued emphasis on primary care training.

"It shows that medical schools are responding to primary care initiatives by increasing the exposure of primary care in their curricula," said Cogle, a fourth-year medical student at the University of Florida. "Also, medical students are recognizing incentives for going into primary care whether they be monetary or practice characteristics—the challenge of having a wide breadth of issues to work on with patients."

The AMA's student section, he noted, advocates increasing primary care to meet the nation's needs while retaining students' freedom of choice of specialties.

Impact on oversupply
But this year's Match had little impact on another area of concern on the work force front: physician oversupply.

Advocates for fewer physicians want to achieve that result through a reduction in residency slots, with decreased Medicare funding for residency training. In the meantime, they hope teaching hospitals, forced by the changing health care marketplace, will voluntarily reduce those positions. The Match, however, shows that's not happening.

The NRMP reported that 20,209 first-year residency positions were offered in 1997—down slightly from 20,563 in 1996 and 20,751 in 1995.

And while the numbers have declined in the past three Matches, the percent of positions filled has risen; 89.9% were taken in 1997, up from 87.6% in 1996 and 86.1% in 1995.

It's interesting to track the source of these new residents.

A record 25,323 students from all countries applied, with 69% getting accepted. Of the US medical students, 13,554, or 92.7% of those applying, matched. Those numbers and percentages have remained fairly stable in the mid-1990s.

But that stability disappears when looking at international medical graduates.

The number of applications from US citizen IMGs rose from 735 in 1995 to 1467 this year. At the same time, the percentage accepted fell from 49.8% to 43.5%.

The numbers are more dramatic for non-US IMGs. Applications rose from 5675 in 1995 to 8090 this year, while the percentage matched plunged from 50.5% to 34.5%.

The percentage of slots filled by specialty also varies: emergency medicine, 97.8%; general surgery, 99.4% and pediatrics, 98.6%, along with several others that did quite well. In contrast, pathology only filled 69.1% of its offerings.

While flocking to primary care, US medical school graduates shied away from several specialties. Only 25.2% of the slots offered in anesthesiology were taken by US grads. Others with a small US presence: pathology, 39.3% and diagnostic radiology, 39.9%.

Resource

National Clearinghouse for Primary Care Information
8201 Greensboro Dr, Ste 600, McLean, VA 22102
703 821-8955

Product Safety

Consumer Product Safety Commission
Household Product Safety Hotline
800 638-2772

Professional Liability

What happens when a suit is filed?

The steps in the legal process involving a malpractice claim will vary from state to state, and from jurisdiction to jurisdiction, as well as with the insurance company by which the physician is covered. This is important to remember, since your experience will probably differ from the steps listed here.

Keep in mind, too, that the first few steps will happen almost simultaneously—the complaint will be filed, the insurance company contacted, an attorney appointed, meetings with the attorney. But while these activities may happen very quickly—in a matter of 2 weeks to 1 month—the next series of activities may stretch on into years.

These are some of the steps that may be encountered.

1. The patient consults a lawyer who will review the case. Most lawyers work on a contingency fee, which means there is no cost to the plaintiff unless the case is won. If the case is won, the lawyer collects an average of 30% to 50% of the award. So in the first step, the plaintiff's attorney will evaluate the case to see if it is worth the time and money to get involved. The lawyer may choose not to take the case if it appears it cannot be won or settled for a reasonable gain.

2. The plaintiff's attorney will draft a complaint and file it with the court. The physician will be served with a copy of the complaint and a summons to appear to answer the plaintiff's allegations. This is a critical time, because how the physician responds can influence the chances of a successful resolution. Many physicians react the wrong way. They get the notice of the complaint, comment to a colleague, "Can you believe this?" and throw the document away. There is a time frame in which the physician's attorney must file the physician's response to the allegations. That time frame in many jurisdictions is 20 to 30 days.

3. The physician should contact his or her insurance company, so an attorney can be assigned and the complaint can be answered, or a motion to dismiss can be filed. This is not the time to wait or hesitate. The plaintiff's lawyer has been working on the case for some time and has had access to the needed records to file the complaint. So in almost any situation, the physician's

attorney will be catching up in terms of the time spent on case research and preparation.

4. The physician's attorney will review the case to see how substantial it is, and how defensible it is. The strategy for defending against the claim begins here.

5. The physician should begin to research by pulling the records on the case and putting them in a special file where they can't be misplaced or tampered with. A file in the physician's desk drawer is often the best place for the attorney calls. The physician's attorney will obtain any records that may be needed from a hospital. It is vital that the records not be altered in any way.

The physician may want to search the literature for material pertinent to the case, such as an article that shows that the procedures used were acceptable or state-of-the-art for the patient's case. Material that will be helpful to the defense should be marked for future reference.

The physician will also want to think about the case so that honest, candid answers can be given to his or her attorney.

6. The physician will be working with the attorney during this time. Once again, it is vital that he or she be completely honest and candid about the case. The physician should ask for a thorough briefing about the case and the legal proceedings that will take place, as well as the physician's role in the proceedings. The physician will want to share with the attorney information gained from the research. He or she may help the lawyer formulate questions for the plaintiff's expert. Keep in mind a point made earlier—the lawyer knows the law; the physician knows medicine. Attorneys need physicians' help to win cases.

7. The physician will answer interrogatories, a written process designed to streamline court proceedings by getting the facts on the table—facts such as agreeing that the person is a physician who is licensed to practice, the sequence of events, and other things that will help clarify the case.

8. The physicians will attend a deposition. The deposition is similar to being in court. It usually occurs in a lawyer's office, where the parties come together, witnesses are sworn, and a court transcriber records the testimony. Since the transcript of the deposition may be used in the court proceedings, attorney will attempt to get witnesses to commit to as much as possible. If testimony is changed in court, the conflicting statements will weaken the case.

The physician will want, and will be advised, to answer questions calmly and succinctly, and not to volunteer information. In addition, the physician's attorney may not say much in terms of objecting to questions. And he or she may counsel the physician that if objections are made, they carry an important message for the physician.

Careful preparation for the deposition is vital. The physician may spend hours on this, reading records and background material. The attorney will be the coach, and will tell the physician who will be at the deposition, when to speak, what questions probably will be asked, and how to respond. This can be a very stressful time—one in which the spouse will want to be especially supportive and understanding, since it will take the physician away from the family.

The physician may want to take notes during the deposition that will be helpful to the attorney during the trial.

At this point, the attorney may meet with the spouse to explain the proceedings and how she or he can be involved.

9. A decision will have to be made on whether or not to settle. This decision can be made at any point in the process. Again, if there has been an injury caused by negligence, most attorneys will advise that the case be settled as quickly as possible for the sake of the patient. If a physician is clearly understood to have caused an injury, settlement may not be recommended.

The decision to settle, if the case is defensible, is a difficult one for physician. Many feel that they should "fight" and should have their day in court. Some have insisted on going to trial, even when the plaintiff was willing to settle for a very small amount of money. On the other hand, some physicians prefer to settle and put the whole matter behind them. This is a decision that can only be made by the physician and attorney.

Remember that most claims are settled out of court!

10. There may be a pretrial screening panel, consisting often of a physician, attorney, and judge. Generally, these panels review the case and listen to medical experts and presentations from the attorneys on both sides. The decision of the panel is not binding in most cases, but can be read into evidence at the trial. In some states, the panels become more significant, because those states have decided they should be used to weed out cases that are without legal merit.

11. If the decision is made to go to trial, the physician must be prepared to testify, and must review all of the research compiled for the deposition—the medical literature, patient charts and records, the testimony given at the deposition. Close contact will be kept with the defense counsel, who will advise on court procedures, strategies, and how to handle the cross-examination by the plaintiff's attorney. This cross-examination can be brutal, since the basis of a trial is to tear apart the opposing arguments.

The physician's presence at the trial will be extremely important, as will dress, demeanor, etc. Attorney and physician will work together, with the physician advising the attorney about possible errors on the part of the plaintiff's expert witness and the attorney alerting the physician to tactics by the plaintiff's counsel. When testifying, he or she will be advised to answer questions succinctly, and not to volunteer information. The physician will have the opportunity to tell his or her story when the defense counsel asks for it.

12. The case will be resolved. (SPP-1986)

Resources

Alliance of American Insurers
1501 Woodfield Rd, Ste 400W
Schaumburg, IL 60173-4980
847 330-8500   Fax 847 330-8602

American Insurance Assoc
1130 Connecticut Ave NW, Ste 1000
Washington, DC 20036
202 828-7100   202 828-7183   Fax 202 293-1219

American Medical Assurance Co (AMACO)
(only insures insurers)
303 E Wacker Dr, Ste 1330, Chicago, IL 60601
312 565-6463

American Tort Reform Association
1850 M St, Ste 1095, Washington, DC 20036-5803
202 682-1163   Fax 202 682-1022
E-mail: dswenson@atr.org
Web Address: http://www.atra.org/atra

*Harvard Medical Malpractice Study :
Patients, Doctors and Lawyers, Medical Injury,
Malpractice Litigation and Patient Compensation in New
York.* Cambridge, Mass: President and Fellows of
Harvard College; 1990.

Insurance Information Institute
110 William St, New York, NY 10038
212 669-9200   Fax 212 732-1916
E-mail: iiilibrary@aol.com

*Physician Insurers Association of America:
Membership Directory*
Physician Insurers Association of America
2 Princess Rd, Lawrenceville, NJ 08648
609 896-4131   609 896-2404 ext 258

Professional Liability—History
Tracing the history of the liability problem

Not until the 1930s did professional liability suits begin to materialize in any significant numbers—a development that paralleled the birth of modern medicine and its sophisticated technology. There was an upswing in numbers of claims until World War II and then there was a temporary decline.

After World War II, the problem began to surface again, increasing in the 1960s. The rising volume of claims against physicians and hospitals, with their growing impact upon health care costs, health manpower, and the delivery of health services—increasingly paid for by the government—prompted President Richard Nixon in 1971 to direct the Secretary of Health, Education, and Welfare to create a Commission on Medical Malpractice to gather current information on the problem and offer a set of recommendations.

In the introductory chapter of its final report issued in 1973, the Commission said, "The tempo of malpractice litigation again began to increase shortly after World War II. In part, this was due to the simple fact that many more people were able to afford, and received, medical care, automatically increasing the exposure to incidents that could lead to suits.

"At the same time, innovations in medical science increased the complexities of the health care system. Some of the new diagnostic and therapeutic procedures brought with them new risks of injury; as the potency of drugs increased, so did the potential hazards of using them. Few would challenge the value of these advances, but they did tend to produce a number of adverse results, sometimes resulting in severe disability...[and] thus the number of malpractice claims and suits increased."

The Commission, in one of the first detailed examinations of medical liability claims on a nationwide basis, surveyed claims closed in 1970 taken from a universe representing approximately 90% of the total in the nation. The Commission found that there were 15,000 claim files closed in 1970, representing 12,000 incidents and patients and 22,000 defendants—physicians, hospitals, nurses, drug companies, and equipment manufacturers. An estimated 10.6% more claims were opened in 1970 than were closed in that year, which, the Commission pointed out, "indicates that direction and some of the magnitude of this change."

The claims increase was not surprising. Numbers of claims were growing steadily and the rate of increase was clearly accelerating. Some areas of the country, as is the case today, were affected more than others. The Commission's 1970 study showed Tennessee leading the list of states in the rate of increase—40.9%—but that was partly due to the small base number of claims. California showed the greatest volume of change—up 26%. Upward blips were beginning to appear in Maryland, Texas, and Missouri and in 11 other states, while a few, such as Minnesota, actually showed a downturn.

The Commission's 1970 analysis, however, merely underscored a developing trend.

"Between 1935 and 1975—in that 40-year period—80 percent of all medical malpractice lawsuits were filed in the final five years of that period," Elvoy Raines, professional liability expert with the American College of Obstetricians and Gynecologists, told the Senate Committee on Labor and Human Resources on July 10, 1984. (LIA-1985)

Professional liability in the 1980s

Education and community action
The following recommendations are made in this area:

(1) Take the professional liability issue to the public. The public has a vital stake in the professional liability problem, from the standpoints of cost, quality, and access to medical care. The Task Force recommends that an intensive information campaign be conducted to improve public understanding and stress the need for legislative, judicial, and other actions.

(2) Arm state, local, and specialty medical societies with information to carry the professional liability message to the public. The Task Force will supervise the preparation of comprehensive informational materials, including background data, fact sheets, speech outlines and speeches, sample editorials, and letters to the editor. Display materials will be distributed throughout the federation and on request to individual members who will serve as advocates on this issue.

AMA will also hold periodic briefings on professional liability activities for state, county, and specialty societies. The AMA's Washington Office will brief medical specialty organizations' Washington representatives. The innovative and aggressive risk management programs that the societies have developed deserve wide publication and should be incorporated into the broad-based national effort.

(3) Publish a pamphlet for individual patients. The pamphlet will explain how the professional liability issue affects their own medical care, its costs, and its availability and will foster realistic expectations about medical care. It will be made available in quantity for distribution through physicians' offices.

(4) Develop an effective advocacy program on the professional liability problem. Physicians must have allies on this issue. An AMA action team composed of officers, trustees, and staff representatives will carry the professional liability message to organizations and individuals that are, or should be, concerned with the issue. The exact nature of the professional liability crisis, objectively and persuasively documented, must be presented at every appropriate forum. Business groups, labor organizations, public interest groups, legislators, legal organizations, judicial conferences, academic centers, the media, insurance groups, state and national agencies, organizations such as the American Association of Retired Persons, and others will be addressed at every opportunity. The reports of the Special Task Force will be bound into one volume and distributed throughout the nation. In short, the AMA will intensify its role as the physician's national spokesperson on this issue.

(5) Enlist the cooperation of health care coalitions composed of opinion leaders and policymakers to address the professional liability problem. The support of health care coalitions, involved in efforts to contain health care costs by reducing the professional liability problem, will be recruited. The Task Force will develop a handbook with the AMA's Department of Health Care Coalitions for this purpose. The AMA will elicit support from groups such as the Chamber of Commerce, the Business Roundtable, and other professional and civic groups.

(6) Expand the AMA's clearinghouse role. The AMA can also fulfill an essential role as a national clearinghouse, assembling data, legislative information, materials from other organizations, and other pertinent materials to share with physicians, medical organizations, legislators, policymakers, and other interested individuals and groups. Plans to share information will be effected with organizations such as the Physician Insurers Association of America, the National Association of Insurance Commissioners, research centers such as the Rand Corporation, and individual researchers actively involved in studies of professional liability. The Task Force will prepare and distribute to the federation, specialty societies, and other groups regular reports on new data, programs, and developments.

(7) Maintain professional liability as a critical priority.

The Special Task Force, with the resources of the AMA at its disposal, will be a permanent part of the AMA professional liability program. The research effort will not stop with the work already done and published by the Task Force. The Association's Center for Health Policy Research will focus on the effort to develop and publish reliable and current information on professional liability. AMA's Committee on Professional Liability will continue its studies of the costs and effects of professional liability of physicians, patients, and the nation.

Commentary: An effective national information campaign is essential to generate action on the professional liability problem. The perception persists, perpetuated by those who stand to gain most from the existing system, that there is no professional liability crisis, only a "pocketbook" concern of physicians. A similar misconception,

Preinforced by repetition, is that insurance companies are accumulating huge profits at physicians' expense and ample funds are available to pay claims. Those who hold these misconceptions also are convinced that physician negligence—"malpractice"—is the only reason for the professional liability crisis.

These views are wrong and must be refuted. Objective data on the numbers of claims, severity of claims, rapidly climbing costs of insurance premiums, and growing losses of professional liability insurers document a crisis far more serious than past ones.

The public pays for a large portion of professional liability costs in pass-throughs for physicians' increased overhead, in the enormous costs of defensive medicine—the ordering of tests and procedures primarily to protect against lawsuits—and in the staggering waste of an inefficient legal system. The public also pays for a system that is encouraging, almost forcing, physicians to avoid high-risk patients and specialties.

Physicians pay, too, not just in high insurance premiums, but in the personal anguish of claims and suits filed, especially if these actions are without merit. It is often not how the physicians practice, but the fact that they practice ever closer to the edges of technological frontiers that places them at greater legal risk. Physicians are among the nation's best and brightest. Highly educated, motivated for the most part by humanitarian concerns, yet they are held accountable for complex judgments made under pressure of life-and-death considerations. No other professionals are held to such standards. Though negligence does occur, physicians are too often sued for adverse events—bad results—beyond their control. Even when negligence exists, the system for compensating patients is being crushed by almost limitless awards and the costs of determining liability.

The realities of the professional liability situation must be brought to the public, to legislators, to lawyers, and to those in policymaking positions. The record must be set straight—the situation put into proper focus. (LIA-1985)

Liability reform in the 1990s

The Health Care Liability Alliance (HCLA), an advocacy coalition repesenting physicians, hospitals, blood banks, liability insurers, health device manufacturers, health care insurers, business, producers of medicines, and the biotechnology industry, represents many of the issues involved with professional liability reform today.

HCLA's goals for reform

1. Promoting patient safety and injury prevention programs in every medical setting. HCLA is proposing that state health care licensing fees should be used to promote patient safety, including disciplining health care professionals/practitioners, implementing quality assurance programs, producing public information on comparative quality of health plans, or encouraging volunteer services in medically underserved areas. In addition, HCLA itself, in partnership with outside groups, will be undertaking a consumer education program.

2. Implementing certain basic medical liability reforms nationwide, including:
- Placing a $250,000 ceiling on noneconomic damages. Ceilings on noneconomic damages do not keep people from recovering any amount necessary to pay for medical expenses, lost wages, rehabilitation costs, or any other economic loss suffered as the result of a health care injury. It limits only those damages awarded for pain and suffering, loss of enjoyment, and other intangible items. Limits on noneconomic damages are the single most effective reform in containing medical liability premiums, according to a report by the Office of Technology Assessment (OTA). California had the country's highest liability premiums before enacting a $250,000 ceiling on noneconomic damages; its premiums now are one-third to one-half those in states without such limits. No other country provides such an expansive benefit for noneconomic damages. Based on California's successful experience, HCLA supports a $250,000 limit.
- Holding each defendant responsible only for the portion of noneconomic damages attributable to his or her own acts or omissions. Under the current rules ("joint and several liability"), a defendant responsible for as little as 1% of the total fault may be required to pay the entire award. HCLA agrees that defendants should remain jointly liable for all economic losses, such as medical bills and lost wages, but should be held liable only for their own portion of the noneconomic and punitive damages.
- Applying liability reform provisions to all potential defendants in claims arising from health care-related injuries. The manufacturers of medical products, providers of blood and tissue services or products, HMOs, and other health care providers are all at risk of a lawsuit when a patient is injured. Addressing the liability problems in just one part of the health-care sector actually may stimulate litigation in other parts that are perceived to have "deeper pockets." The existing system increases defensive medicine and deters medical technology manufacturers from developing new innovative, cost-effective products.
- Limiting the amount of attorney contingency fees. HCLA supports setting limits for attorney contingency fees. The contingency fee is meant to enable those with less resources to obtain legal representation. However, the existing system is not serving this function well because it favors "big ticket" cases; consequently, most people with health care injury claims never get access to the civil justice system. Meanwhile, when they do, lawyers take large portions of claimants' awards.
- Halting double recovery. This reform would permit defendants to introduce to a jury evidence of any reimbursement to the claimant by health or disability insurers or others for losses resulting from an injury.
- Paying awards for future expenses or losses over time. Future expenses or losses over $50,000 should be paid periodically over time, while past and current expenses are paid in full lump-sum. Otherwise, claimants receive money, such as future lost wages, before they would have earned it. This reform also ensures that money is there when it is needed.
- Providing for a uniform statute of limitations. HCLA supports enacting a uniform statute of limitations. Standard rules should require that claims must be filed within 1 year from the date an injury is discovered, but should also provide an outside limit of 3 years from the date the injury occurred. Exceptions should allow extra

time for claims for children under age 6, who may not be able to communicate the existence of an injury, and for claims where something with no therapeutic purpose is left in a claimant's body and not discovered for many years.

- Encouraging alternative dispute-resolution methods. Alternative dispute resolution systems can save billions of health care dollars. The states should be given maximum flexibility to select a dispute resolution system that works best for them.
- Reforming punitive damages. Punitive damages should be awarded only if there is "clear and convincing" evidence that the injury meets the standard set by each jurisdiction. In those cases, damages should be limited to $250,000, or twice the compensatory damages (the total of economic plus noneconomic losses), whichever is greater. Manufacturers or distributors of medical products should not be held liable for punitive damages if their product received federal government approval or met FDA's "safe and effective" product requirements and there was no fraud in the approval process.

HCLA's programs include:
- Work for patient safety.
- Educate the public and elected officials about the need for comprehensive, effective health care liability reform.
- Coordinate HCLA members' lobbying on liability issues.
- Organize national and local support.
- Provide the media with information about medical liability reforms; place ads and op-eds for publication. (HCLA brochure-1995)

Tort reform glossary

Ad damnum clauses—The ad damnum clause is that part of a plaintiff's initial pleadings that states the amount of monetary damages and other relief requested by the plaintiff in a court action. Most of the legislation on this subject provides for the elimination of the ad damnum clause altogether; legislation also often provides that the defendant be apprised of the precise amount sought by the plaintiff through the normal course of pretrial discovery.

Arbitration—Arbitration statutes relate to voluntary procedures whereby patients and health care providers may enter into written agreements for the submission of any medical liability claims to binding arbitration. This procedure provides for limited judicial review of the arbitration decision.

Medical liability claims can currently be arbitrated in at least 30 states under the general arbitration statutes in those states. The chart only lists those states with arbitration legislation specifically for medical liability claims.

Most of the medical liability arbitration statutes provide that written arbitration agreements may cover present and future medical injury claims. All of the statutes generally provide that a person's right to treatment shall not be prejudiced in any way by the decision whether or not to enter into an agreement for arbitration of medical liability claims. In other words, the agreement must truly be voluntary to be binding. Also, most statutes that permit arbitration agreements to cover future medical

injury claims provide for a certain period of time, following either execution of the contract or provision of the services, in which the patient may reject the arbitration agreement.

Attorney fee regulation—The most common arrangement for payment of plaintiff attorney fees in medical liability cases is the "contingent fee." Under this type of arrangement the attorney receives as his or her fee an agreed upon percentage (commonly 30% to 50%) of any final award or settlement made to the plaintiff.

Legislation enacted during the last few years regulating attorney fees in medical liability cases has taken several different approaches: a sliding scale for the plaintiff attorney fees in terms of a percentage of the award; court review of the proposed fees and approval of what it considers to be a "reasonable fee," or limiting attorneys' fees to a certain percentage of the amounts recovered by the plaintiff.

Awarding costs, expenses, and fees—A few states have provisions designed to deter the pursuit of frivolous medical injury claims. These statutes generally provide that where one party to the action has been found to have acted frivolously in bringing the suit, the party may be found liable for payment of the other party's reasonable attorney and expert witness fees and court costs. These provisions differ from the usual civil trial situation in which attorney fees and expert witness fees are normally paid by the party who incurs them.

Collateral source provisions—The collateral source rule is a rule of evidence that prohibits the introduction into evidence at trial of any indication that a patient has been compensated or reimbursed for the injury from any source other than the defendant.

Legislation modifying the collateral source rule has taken several approaches: permitting consideration of compensation or payments received from some or all collateral sources; requiring the mandatory offset against any award in the amount of some or all collateral source payments received by the plaintiff; or allowing the defendant to introduce evidence of the plaintiff's compensation from collateral sources. The jury is instructed to make a mandatory reduction of the award for economic loss by a sum equal to the difference between the total benefits received and the total amount paid by the plaintiff to secure such benefits.

Expert witness—Expert witnesses are required to explain many of the complex and difficult issues in a medical negligence case. Legislation affects the qualifications and use of expert benefits.

Limits on liability—Some states have enacted legislation that limits the liability of defendants in medical lawsuits. These statutes limit liability in one of several ways: limiting recovery of a particular type of damages; placing an absolute cap on the amount of damages recoverable; or placing an absolute cap on physician liability under a patient compensation fund.

Patient compensation fund—A patient compensation fund is a governmentally operated mechanism established to pay that portion of any judgment or settlement against a health care provider in excess of a statutorily designated amount. A fund may pay the remainder of the award or it may have a statutory maximum (eg, 1 million dollars).

Patient compensation funds are generally funded through an annual surcharge assessed against health care providers, with such surcharge often being a specified percentage of the provider's annual insurance premium. Patient compensation funds are also known as "excess recovery funds."

Periodic payments—In most states, unless otherwise agreed on by the parties or mandated by the court, judgments can only be lump-sum awards. Under a periodic payments system, the payments are made over the actual lifetime of the plaintiff or for the actual period of disability.

Pretrial screening panels—Pretrial screening panels are prerequisites to trial. Procedures for panels usually require a mandatory pretrial to be conducted by a panel comprised of members as dictated by statute. In some states the pretrial hearing is voluntary. The composition of the panel and its scope of inquiry vary greatly from state to state.

All statutes establishing pretrial screening procedures provide that the panel's decision is not binding on the parties and that it does not preclude a plaintiff from initiating a lawsuit. Although some states permit the decision of the panel to be introduced into evidence in a subsequent lawsuit, the panel's decision is not binding upon a judge or jury.

Res ipsa loquitur—Res ipsa loquitur ("the thing speaks for itself") is a common law doctrine that applies when a plaintiff can demonstrate that the injury occurred while the instrumentality causing the injury was under the exclusive control of the defendant and that, if operated in a nonnegligent fashion, does not normally cause injury. In recent years, a number of state courts have expanded the application of res ipsa loquitur, and increased the effect of its applicability from that of a mere inference to that of a presumption that, if not rebutted, will allow the jury to reach no finding other than liability.

Legislation enacted in several states has codified the doctrine in regard to medical liability cases by delineating those circumstances when the doctrine may be applied, such as when a foreign object has been left in a body or the patient has suffered radiation burns. However, these statutes have sought to make it clear that the mere fact of injury is not sufficient to invoke the doctrine.

Standard of care—The standard of care in a medical negligence action is that level of care to which a health care provider is held accountable to a patient, and is based upon the prevailing level of care practiced within locality (community, state, or national).

Statute of limitations—A statute of limitations is a law that bars a cause of action after expiration of a specified time period. In many states the statute of limitations for medical liability actions begins to run only upon discovery of the injury. Injuries may be discovered several years after the treatment was provided, so the time period for filing an action may be uncertain. Some states have sought to eliminate the "long tail" by placing an absolute maximum time period within which medical liability suits may be brought. An exception to the time period is provided in some of these statutes where foreign objects are left in the body, or where the health care provider has fraudulently concealed the fact of injury.

Most state statutes of limitations provide that if an injury is incurred by a minor, the statute is tolled (ie, stops running) on the minor's cause of action until he or she reaches the age of majority. Changes in the statute of limitations for a minor's actions usually provide that the statute will begin running prior to the age of majority. (LIA-1985)

Project HOPE

Project HOPE
Health Science Education Center—Carter Hall
Millwood, VA 22646
800 544-HOPE   703 837-2100   Fax 703 837-1813
Web address: http://www.charity.org/phope

Prostate Cancer

JAMA 100 Years Ago

JAMA 1994 July 6 1994 272(1):26b

Diagnosis and treatment of prostatic enlargement

JAMA 1894; 23:61-62

The prostate of mammals in general is a purely sexual gland, often separated by a considerable space from the bladder, and entirely independent of this organ; in some animals (eg, the ram) the prostate is lacking; in others (the squirrel) it is entirely suburethral. In some mammals, notably man, the prostate presents an intimate anatomic relation with the bladder; its muscular fibers completely encircle the urethro-vesical orifice, and perform the function of a vesical sphincter. The human prostate lies at the junction of the genital and urinary channels, and it is intimately associated in function with both...

While the etiology of prostatic enlargement still remains a matter of speculation, it is certain that the earliest clinical symptoms are due to vascular engorgement of the prostate and by consequence of the bladder. The actual increase in the size of the gland should not obscure the other factors in producing the symptoms, which may be out of all proportion to the perceptible enlargement...

The most important as well as the most difficult task in diagnosis, is the differentiation among these various morbid states; for the prognosis as well as the treatment is determined by the predominance of one or another of them. For example a prostatic patient complains of frequent and painful urination; the chief trouble may be an aggravation of the usual venous congestion, in which case a brisk laxative, suppositories of icthyol and ergotin and strychnin internally will secure speedy relief. Again, the symptoms may be due to prostatic suppuration, in which event irrigation of the deep urethra with hot water containing hydrastin or silver nitrate is needed; or the frequent urination may be simply the overflow of a distended bladder, which is relieved by the cautious daily use of a clean catheter.

It would far transcend the allotted limits of this paper to discuss the differential diagnosis: I can only emphasize the statement that the symptoms clinically associated with prostatic hypertrophy depend upon several distinct morbid conditions, of which the mechanical impediment to the exit of urine may be the least; and that no routine treatment can be prescribed, the requirements varying with the case.

Our resources for meeting the needs of different patients may be thus summarized:

1. *Medical*

a. Improvement in the circulation through prostate and bladder is favored by proper diet and exercise, avoidance of constipation, massage of prostate between a sound in the bladder and finger in rectum, and by the daily use of a clean catheter; internally, ergotin and strychnin are certainly useful.

b. Suppuration in the bladder neck requires irrigation of the prostatic urethra with hot water, solutions of hydrastin, silver nitrate, in addition to the measures already mentioned.

c. Induration and distortion of the bladder neck may be improved by dilatation with large sounds or a special dilator.

In a certain percentage of cases the time arrives, sooner or later, when these measures fail to relieve, and more efficient and immediate aid must be rendered.

2. *Surgical Methods*

a. The simplest is a puncture of membranous urethra from the perineum, and introduction of a drain which is permitted to remain for a couple of weeks. The subsidence of congestion and edema, the cleansing of the bladder thus induced, sometimes makes an apparent cure for many months. Puncture with a trocar through the prostate... drainage of the bas fund behind the organ ... is even more desirable.

b. By a perineal urethrotomy the surgeon can secure not merely drainage but also thorough digital stretching of the prostate, and the incision or excision of obstructions at the orifice of the bladder.

c. More satisfactory excision of prostatic obstructions has been accomplished by a combination of suprapubic cystotomy with perineal urethrotomy now a standard operation.

Such are our resources, medical and surgical, for relieving the distress and preventing the fatal consequences of prostatic enlargement; and probably no other disease of the genito-urinary organs tests to an equal degree the knowledge, judgment and art of the surgeon. The day has long passed when the sole treatment for prostatics was the routine, sometimes careless and bungling, use of the catheter. While these patients commonly exhibit the impaired vitality of age and often the added effects of renal insufficiency, yet as a class they are far more amenable to treatment than our standard literature leads us to suppose.

JAMA Article of Note: Screening for prostate cancer: a decision analytic view

JAMA 1994, Sept 14; 272(10): 773-780.
Accompanying editorial. 272(10): 813-814

Resource
Us Too
1120 N Charles St, Ste 401, Baltimore, MD 21201
800 828-7866
(Information on support groups, diagnosis, and treatment options)

Prosthetics

Poetry and Medicine

Red Cross Orthopedic Hospital, Kabul

Barbara Seaman Lawrence
JAMA 1994, Aug 3; 272(5): 336B

White light bursting through a volley
of narrow windows. Backlit, five men benched,

khaki-skinned, a rubble of beards, one graying.
Eyes like caves, and for the everlasting

length of one shutter click
they stare at me. I stare back at five

unmatched pairs of legs lined up like columns
of newsprint in two different languages.

Right   right   left   right   left
are boned, fleshed, juiced, blood-warmed.

Left   left   right   left   right
shoulder-strapped, hinged, a riveted

prosthesis bare to the hip, on the end of each
thin strip that runs from knee

to floor: a shoe skewered like a kabob.
How to speak two languages at once.

Five men learning, a sixth sitting apart
in shadow, his unmatched pair dangling

mid-air. All of nine, he doesn't look at me
but stares instead at practice pairs

of footprints glued like a path
to the hospital floor. Bold yellow feet,

they strut across page thirty-six
left right left right out of the picture.

Prosthetist. Provides care to patients with partial or total absence of limb by planning fabrication of, writing specifications for, and fitting prothesis under guidance of and in consultation with physician. Assists physician in formulation of prescription. Examines and evaluates patient's prosthetic needs in relation to disease entity and functional loss. Formulates design of prosthesis and selects materials and components. Makes casts, measurements, and model modifications. Performs fitting, including static and dynamic alignment. Evaluates prosthesis on patient and makes adjustments to ensure fit, function, comfort, and workmanship. Instructs patient in prosthesis use. Maintains patient records. May supervise prosthetic assistants and other personnel. May lecture and supervise laboratory activities relating to development of prosthesis. May lecture and demonstrate to colleagues and other professionals concerned with practice of prosthetics. May participate in research. May also perform functions of orthotist. (DOT-1991)

Prosthetics Assistant. Assists prosthetist in providing care to and fabricating and fitting protheses for patients with partial or total absence of limb. Under direction of prosthetist makes assigned casts, measurements, and model modifications. Performs fitting, including static and dynamic alignments. Evaluates prosthesis on patient to ensure fit, function, and quality of work. Repairs and maintains prostheses. May be responsible for performance of other personnel. May also perform functions of orthotics assistant. (DOT-1991)

Resource

American Academy of Orthotists and Prosthetists
1650 King St, Ste 500, Alexandria, VA 22314
703 836-7118   Fax 703 836-0838
E-mail: aaopline@aol.com

Psychiatry

Editorial

Diagnosis and treatment of psychiatric disorders: a history of progress (excerpt)

Richard M. Glass, MD, Michael J. Veropil, MD
JAMA 1994 Dec 14; 272(22): 1792

Editorials represent the opinions of the authors and *The Journal* and not those of the American Medical Association.

The American Psychiatric Association (APA), the oldest national medical society in the United States, was established in 1844. Known then as the Association of Medical Superintendents of American Institutions for the Insane, the association was founded by 13 physicians from nine states who shared an interest in promoting research on mental illness and better treatment for the mentally ill.[1] The identity of psychiatry as a medical specialty emerged gradually during the second half of the 19th century. In 1892 the name of the organization was changed to the American Medico-Psychological Association.

The first half of the 20th century saw two parallel and sometimes conflicting developments: emphasis on descriptive diagnosis (especially the distinction between schizophrenia and affective disorders) and the growing influence of psychoanalysis. In 1921 the current name of the organization, the American Psychiatric Association, was adopted.

During the second half of the 20th century, dramatic developments in psychiatric knowledge have resulted in marked improvements in the reliability of psychiatric diagnoses and the efficacy of psychiatric treatments. Publication of the third edition of the APA's *Diagnostic and Statistical Manual of Mental Disorders*[2] (DSM-III) in 1980 signaled a major advance in psychiatric nomenclature and diagnosis, since it provided specific diagnostic criteria for each disorder. Subsequent empirical findings on the reliability and validity of psychiatric diagnoses were incorporated into the revised third edition[3] (DSM-III-R) in 1987 and the recently published fourth edition[4] (DSM-IV).

Patients can now benefit from a number of empirically validated biological and psychosocial treatments. Information regarding their effectiveness was summarized in a 1989 multivolume APA task force report.[5] The pace of developments continues to accelerate as illustrated by more recent therapeutic advances, including the introduction of two important drugs, clozapine and risperidone, for schizophrenia, and an entirely new class of drugs, serotonin-selective reuptake inhibitors, for depression. However, despite the fact that diagnosis and treatment of psychiatric disorders have come a long way, we still have a long way to go in overcoming policies that discriminate against appropriate care for persons with mental disorders.

References

1. Barton WE. *The History and Influence of the American Psychiatric Association*. Washington, DC: American Psychiatric Press Inc; 1987.

2. American Psychiatric Association. *Diagnostic and Statistical Manual of Mental Disorders, Third Edition*. Washington, DC: American Psychiatric Association; 1980.

3. American Psychiatric Association. *Diagnostic and Statistical Manual of Mental Disorders, Revised Third Edition*. Washington, DC: American Psychiatric Association; 1987.

4. American Psychiatric Association. *Diagnostic and Statistical Manual of Mental Disorders, Fourth Edition*. Washington, DC: American Psychiatric Association; 1994.

5. American Psychiatric Association. *Treatments of Psychiatric Disorders*. 3 vols. Washington, DC: American Psychiatric Association; 1989.

Psychiatrist. Diagnoses and treats patients with mental, emotional, and behavioral disorders. Organizes data concerning patient's family, medical history, and onset of symptoms obtained from patient, relatives, and other sources, such as nurse, general duty and social worker, psychiatric. Examines patient to determine general physical condition, following standard medical procedures. Orders laboratory and other special diagnostic tests and evaluates data obtained. Determines nature and extent of mental disorder, and formulates treatment program. Treats or directs treatment of patient, utilizing variety of psychotherapeutic methods and medications. (DOT-1991)

JAMA Theme Issue: Psychiatry and Mental Health.

JAMA 1994 Dec 14; 272(22)

This theme issue illustrates some current developments in psychiatry and provides practical guidance for physicians in recognizing and assessing patients with mental disorders, so that those patients will be more likely to receive needed treatment.

Resources

American Academy of Child and Adolescent Psychiatry
3615 Wisconsin Ave NW, Washington, DC 20016
800 333-7636   202 996-7300   Fax 202 966-2891
Web address: http://www.psch.med.umich.edu/web/aacap

American Academy of Clinical Psychiatrists
PO Box 3212, San Diego, CA 92163
619 298-0538

American Academy of Psychiatry and the Law
1 Regency Dr, PO Box 30, Bloomfield, CT 06002-0030
800 331-1389   860 242-5450   Fax 860 286-0787

American Board of Psychiatry and Neurology
500 Lake Cook Rd, Ste 335, Deerfield, IL 60015
847 945-7900   Fax 847 945-1146

American Psychiatric Association
1400 K St NW, Washington, DC 20005
202 682-6000   Fax 202 682-6114

Black Psychiatrists of America
c/o Dr Isaac Slaughter
2730 Adeline St, Oakland, CA 94607
510 465-1800   510 465-1508   Fax 510 465-1508

Psychoanalysis

Obituary

Sigmund Freud: 1856-1939

JAMA 1939 Oct 14; 113(6): 1494-1495

On September 22, in his eighty-third year, Sigmund Freud, founder of psychoanalysis, died in London. Men in the future may evaluate fully his contribution to medicine. No doubt much of his teaching will be modified and some of it will be discarded. Certain, however, is the revolutionary influence he has had on psychiatry. Freud was born in 1856 in Freiberg, a small provincial town of Moravia, then belonging to the Austro-Hungarian Empire, a son of simple Jewish parents. His nationality and his race influenced his career. He became a physician though later confessing that his secret desire had been to become a novelist. He was destined to be a profound student of human nature.

In his medical studies Freud was stimulated far more by Charcot and Bernheim in France than by his Viennese teachers. The Vienna Medical School was dominated by the mechanistic attitude of Virchow's cellular pathology. In the light of that concept the unity of the human being as manifested in the functioning of the highest integrating centers (personality) was lost. Freud began his medical career as a neurologist, with contributions on aphasia and on infantile cerebral palsy. Like many of his contemporaries, he soon became aware of the sterility, ineffectiveness and fundamental inadequacy of current neurologic practice in the care of the neuroses. In a search for more light he went to Charcot, whose fame was then at its peak. Charcot had demonstrated experimentally that ideas can produce bodily symptoms. By hypnotic suggestions he had succeeded in reproducing artificially in his patients hysterical symptoms similar to those of which they complained spontaneously.

From Bernheim's and Liebeault's post-hypnotic experiments in Nancy Freud learned that unconscious psychologic processes may influence overt behavior. Next came the observations of Joseph Breuer in Vienna, with whom Freud collaborated after his return from France. The real discoverer of psychoanalysis was Breuer's famous patient Anna, who began to talk freely under hypnosis of forgotten experiences. This reminiscing while under hypnosis was not simple remembering. It involved a dramatic display and expression of repressed emotions. This verbal outburst of emotions in hypnosis, which had such a beneficial effect on Anna's hysterical symptoms, Freud and Breuer called "cathartic hypnosis"; Anna herself gave it the name "talking cure."

These two factors, remembering of forgotten traumatic emotional experiences and the expression of pent up emotions, have remained two important therapeutic factors in psychoanalysis. Cathartic hypnosis, however, lacked one important element of modern psychoanalytic technic: insight, the intellectual digestion of the repressed forgotten emotional experiences. Under hypnosis the conscious personality of the patient was entirely eliminated. Freud recognized this defect of hypnotic therapy. He tried to reproduce without hypnosis and during these attempts discovered the most fundamental dynamic fact of psychology—the fact of repression and resistance. In the waking state patients could not face these repressed emotions which came to the surface in hypnosis. Our resistance toward the recognition of emotions, wishes, and tendencies which are painful and in conflict with accepted standards Freud called repression. During patient experimentation between 1895 and 1900 Freud discovered the method of free association by which he was able to circumvent the emotional resistance of patients against facing and recognizing their unconscious motive forces. In free association, conscious control is eliminated. The patient gives free course to his ideas, which drift, now converging toward, now receding from, the pathogenic repressed material. During this procedure, more and more of the unconscious repressed material becomes conscious. The physician's role is not active. His influence on this process of self revelation consists mainly in increasing the patient's courage and confidence to face his real self. Now sexual matters, which had been shunned by physicians and patients but which are nevertheless a significant part of our lives, began to become apparent as determining factors in some psychologic disorders. Challenging the hypocritical attitude of his time, Freud described sexual phenomena objectively. The first rejection with which his views were met was mainly due to the publication of these discoveries.

The aim of psychoanalysis, as Freud conceived it, was not to tell people unpleasant truths about themselves but to cure patients by giving the integrative powers of their rational and conscious personality an opportunity to deal with those psychologic forces which were excluded from their conscious mind. Most important was the discovery that repressions may go back to early childhood, when the infantile ego is too weak to deal with the onslaught of violent emotions. Under certain conditions, when these repressions are too excessive, the repressed impulses find a morbid outlet in neurotic and psychotic symptoms: irrational fears and ideas, depressions, delusions and the whole gamut of psychopathologic phenomena. Psychoanalytic therapy is based on the principle that the mature conscious ego can deal with repressed emotions which the childish ego cannot tolerate.

Most shocking to contemporary attitudes was the discovery of what Freud called the "family tragedy." Naturally, the first emotional difficulties in which the child becomes involved concern its parents. The typical combination of love and hate which the small child feels toward his parents Freud called the "Oedipus complex." More recently, the application of psychoanalysis to children had become a source of important information about early emotional and intellectual development.

P The emotional reactions to the freudian observations and formulations made objective evaluation extremely difficult. They permeated scientific discussions and developed strange accusations. Freud was accused of pansexualism, mysticism, dogmatism and unsound speculation. Moreover, Freud was held responsible for every vagary of his actual disciples and many a pseudoscientist who claimed to speak in his name. He was a pioneer working in an unknown territory—the dynamics of the mind; naturally his first generalizations were somewhat vague groping attempts. Nevertheless many of his observations have already passed the test of scientific scrutiny. The facts of repression, resistance, transference, infantile sexuality and its typical manifestations in family life, the unconscious emotional origin of psychoneurotic and many psychotic symptoms, the principal laws of psychodynamics as observed in such mechanisms as rationalization, projection and overcompensation form the basis of both normal and morbid psychology.

Sigmund Freud was 35 years old when he returned from Paris to Vienna and laid the foundations of psychoanalysis. Failing to be accepted and supported by his colleagues in Vienna, including at last even Breuer, he worked for 10 years entirely alone. Gradually a few students began to gather around him. Among these early followers were Karl Abraham, Sandor Ferenczi, Max Eitingon, Karl Jung, Alfred Adler, Wilhelm Steckel, Otto Rank, Hans Sachs, Ernest Jones, and others whose names did not become so well known. Some of these pupils were unwilling to follow completely along the untrodden paths into which Freud was leading them. Chief among these dissenters were Jung, Adler and Rank. Yet already psychoanalysis has become firmly established in psychology, in education and in medicine. The technic of psychoanalytic therapy has become standardized and is taught to psychiatrists in psychoanalytic institutes. A number of well trained psychoanalysts are united in scientific societies. The effects of emotional factors on physiologic and pathologic processes are being studied by adequate methods. Such generalities as worry, fear, and overwork as causes of physical disturbances are being replaced by precise descriptions of the emotional factors. By this pathway Freud's influence on general medicine will be most felt in the future. But his influence on our times cannot be evaluated by restricting attention to the medical implications of his teachings alone. All the scientific fields which deal with man's relation to man and all the social sciences have received a new impetus from his dynamic psychology.

Correction: *JAMA* 1939 Oct 28; 113(18)

Sigmund Freud's Age.—*The Journal*, October 14, page 1494, stated that Sigmund Freud died Sept. 22, 1939, in his eighty-third year. Dr. Freud was born May 6, 1856, and was therefore at the time of his death in his eighty-fourth year. Dr. Freud died about 3 a. m. September 23, London time and, thus figured, would make the date of death September 22.

Resource
American Academy of Psychoanalysis
47 E 19th St, 6th Fl, New York, NY 10003-1323
212 475-7980   Fax 212 475-8101
E-mail: miriam-paluba@jofi.com

Psychology
American Board of Professional Psychology
2100 E Broadway, Ste 313, Columbia, MO 65201
800 255-7792   573 875-1267   Fax 573 443-1199

American Psychological Association
750 1st St NE, Washington, DC 20002-4242
202 336-5500

Psychosomatic Medicine
Academy of Psychosomatic Medicine
5824 Magnolia, Chicago, IL 60660
773 784-2025   Fax 773 784-1304

Public Health
The evolution of public health
JAMA 1994 Nov 2; 272(17): 1315

When President Franklin Delano Roosevelt signed into law the Public Health Service Act of 1944, no one foresaw that 50 years later this act of Congress would be viewed as a farsighted law serving as a model for contemporary efforts at reinventing government.

Yet that kind of tribute to the law occurred recently when past officials of the US Public Health Service (PHS) gathered with current personnel in Washington, DC, to discuss history and share a gigantic birthday cake.

Some who attended the celebration said provisions of the Public Health Service Act reflect so many of the public's basic needs that it is difficult to imagine how the nation could do without it. The act started as a mere effort at housekeeping—straightening out who was responsible for what. But a closer look at its evolution reveals the substantial role the act played in shaping today's PHS.

The PHS originated in 1798 as a medical service for merchant seamen. The service expanded over the years, gradually adding public health functions, including research. But it was not until 1912 that it was given its current name to reflect this growing public health role.

In the 1930s, two significant pieces of legislation helped to further define the functions of the PHS. The Social Security Act of 1935 allowed it to distribute federal grants in aid to the states to control venereal diseases and tuberculosis and to support general public health functions. The National Cancer Institute Act of 1937 established the PHS role in funding biomedical research.

As the United States entered World War II, the PHS faced challenges from its own leadership, Congress, and the nation. Former senators Claude Pepper (D, Fla) and Elbert Thomas (D, Utah) and Rep Alfred L. Bulwinkle (D, NC) pressed the agency to address wartime health needs: malaria and venereal disease control, industrial hygiene, and environmental sanitation. At the same time, PHS Surgeon General Thomas Parran, MD, worked to establish the financing and provision of health care as an integral part of Roosevelt's New Deal.

Roosevelt and Parran saw the PHS as the natural choice to lead and coordinate the federal government's efforts in health affairs. But major legal and administrative changes were required to broaden the agency's scope beyond the missions of quarantine, service to federal beneficiaries, scientific research, and limited grants in aid to the states.

Although the nation was at war in 1944, public health received remarkable attention. Congress and the Roosevelt administration agreed on legislation that revamped the PHS in the following ways:

By expanding the agency's authority to make grants and contracts, Congress enabled the extramural programs of the National Institutes of Health, the Centers for Disease Control and Prevention, and other PHS agencies.

The act paved the way for the PHS to support state health department efforts in a continuing partnership.

The PHS personnel base was strengthened by commissioning nurses, sanitarians, and other specialists in scientific fields related to public health.

Expansion of the Office of the Surgeon General improved public education about good health habits.

Today, the PHS again faces a task of renewal during a time of great challenge. For more than a decade, local health departments have been struggling with the dual demands of providing medical care for the indigent and uninsured while coping with a serious erosion of the public health infrastructure. The health system reform debate has brought to the fore the need to reinvent public health.

Part of that reinvention involves finding ways to ensure that, regardless of changes in paying for and providing health care, the US Congress and state and local governments provide resources to support and improve the core missions of public health: protecting and promoting the health of all Americans, particularly through population-based prevention programs.

A year after the 1944 act was passed, the surgeon general gave an address on public health issues that is worth noting. His words demonstrate the need for continued vigilance in monitoring public health threats. In his day, Parran worried about typhus and plague transmitted by rats; today we contend with the dangers of rodent-borne hantavirus. He spoke of preventing venereal diseases; antibiotics have since come into widespread use, but we still grapple with treating and preventing many of the same sexually transmitted diseases in addition to acquired immunodeficiency syndrome. Soldiers fighting in World War II risked contracting malaria; today, we puzzle over Gulf War syndrome.

But there also has been great public health progress:
• Smallpox has been eradicated worldwide.
• Polio caused by wild virus has not been seen in the United States since 1979 or in the Americas since 1991.
• Diseases such as legionnaire's, toxic shock syndrome, and the hantavirus pulmonary syndrome have emerged—and have been identified and treated.
• Cardiovascular deaths have declined dramatically in part because of government campaigns warning of the dangers of cigarette smoking and in part because of its collaborative efforts in research, patient care, and public education on management of hypertension.
• Diabetes mellitus is under better control. Recent research has demonstrated that striking reductions in complications of type I diabetes are possible with effective management.

Since 1944 the average life span of 65.2 years has increased to 75.7. Infant mortality is down from 39.8 deaths per thousand births to 8.5 per thousand in 1992; more progress is possible.

Throughout the debate on health system reform, themes from Parran's 1945 speech still ring true: "The heavy cost of catastrophic disease falls unpredictably and unevenly upon the population. For the individual family, I believe that these risks should be met on a national basis, either through insurance, or through public taxes, or preferably through a combination of both. But," he added, "Social insurance in itself, no matter how inclusive, does not constitute a total health program."

The health system reform debate of 1994, like the deliberations 50 years ago that reshaped the PHS and gave it a leadership position in providing and protecting the public's health, must lead to a revitalization of public health at the local, state, and national levels.

How to do it is not a mystery. Whether and when we will do it remain the overriding questions.

Nurse, Staff, Community Health. Alternate title: public health nurse. Instructs individuals and families in health education and disease prevention in community health agency. Visits homes to determine patient and family needs, develops plan to meet needs, and provides nursing services. Instructs family in care and rehabilitation of patient, and in maintenance of health and prevention of disease for family members. Gives treatments to patient following physician's instructions. Assists community members and health field personnel to assess, plan for, and provide needed health and related services. Refers patients with social and emotional problems to other community agencies for assistance. Teaches home nursing, maternal and child care, and other subjects related to individual and community welfare. Participates in programs to safeguard health of children, including child health conferences, school health, group instruction for parents, and immunization programs. Assists in preparation of special studies and in research programs. Directs treatment of patient by nurse, licensed practical and home attendant. Cooperates with families, community agencies, and medical personnel to arrange for convalescent and rehabilitation care of sick or injured persons. May specialize in one phase of community health nursing, such as clinical pediatrics or tuberculosis. (DOT-1991)

Public Health Dentist. Plans, organizes, and maintains dental health program of public health agency. Analyzes dental needs of community to determine changes and trends in patterns of dental disease. Instructs community, school, and other groups on preventive oral health care services. Produces and evaluates dental health educational materials. Provides clinical and laboratory dental care and services. Instigates methods for evaluating changes in dental health status and needs of community. (DOT-1991)

Public Health Physician. Plans and participates in medical care or research program in hospital, clinic, or other public medical facility. Provides medical care for

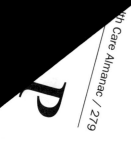

and institutes program of preventive
...ounty, city, or other government or civic
...vaccinations, imposes quarantines, and
...dards for hospitals, restaurants, and other
...ole danger. May conduct research in par-
...of medicine to aid in cure and control of
... be designated medical officer. (DOT-1991)

...on

The Public Health Service was established by an act of
July 16, 1798 (ch 77, 1 stat 605), authorizing marine
hospitals for the care of American merchant seamen.
Subsequent legislation has vastly broadened the scope of
its activities. Major organizational changes have occurred
within the Public Health Service since its inception to
support its mission to promote the protection and advancement of the nation's physical and mental health.

The Public Health Service Act of July 1, 1944 (42 USC
201), consolidated and revised substantially all existing
legislation relating to the Public Health Service. Legal
responsibilities have been broadened and expanded many
times since 1944. Major organizational changes have
occurred within the Public Health Service to support its
mission to promote the protection and advancement of
the nation's physical and mental health. This is accomplished by:
- coordinating with the states to set and implement
  national health policy and pursue effective intergovern-
  mental relations;
- generating and upholding cooperative international
  health-related agreements, policies, and programs;
- conducting medical and biomedical research;
- sponsoring and administering programs for the
  department of health resources, prevention and control
  of diseases, and alcohol and drug abuse;
- providing resources and expertise to the states and
  other public and private institutions in the planning,
  direction, and delivery of physical and mental health
  care services; and
- enforcing laws to ensure the safety and efficacy of drugs
  and protection against impure and unsafe foods,
  cosmetics, medical devices, and radiation-producing
  projects.

The Office of the Assistant Secretary for Health consists
of general and special staff offices that support the Assistant Secretary for Health and the Surgeon General to
plan and direct the activities of the Public Health Service.
(USG-1996)

Resources

American Association of Public Health Physicians
Department of Family Practice
c/o Armand Start, MD
777 S Mills St, Madison, WI 53715
608 263-1326   Fax 608 263-5813

American Public Health Association
1015 15th St NW, Washington, DC 20005
202 789-5600   Fax 202 789-5681

Association of the Schools of Public Health
1660 L St NW, Ste 204, Washington, DC 20036
202 296-1099   Fax 202 296-1252

United States Public Health Service (USPHS)
200 Independence Ave SW, Washington, DC 20201
202 690-6867

*Contact county/state public health department for local
programs and assistance.*

Public Health Departments, Statewide

Alabama Department of Public Health
434 Monroe St, Montgomery, AL 36130-3017
334 613-5200   Fax 334 240-3387

Alaska Department of Health and Social Services
Public Health Division
PO Box 110610, Juneau, AK 99811-0610
907 465-3090   Fax 907 586-1877

Arizona Department of Public Health
1740 W Adams, Phoenix, AZ 85007
602 542-1025   Fax 602 542-1062

Arkansas Department of Public Health
PO Box 3278, Little Rock, AR 72203-3278
501 661-2111   Fax 501 671-1450

California Health and Welfare Agency
Health Services Department
Public Health Division
714 P St, #1253, Sacramento, CA 95814
916 657-1425   Fax 916 657-1156

Colorado Public and Environment Department
Health Office
4300 Cherry Creek Dr S, Denver, CO 80222-1530
303 692-2100   Fax 303 692-0095

Connecticut Department of Public Health
150 Washington St, Hartford, CT 06106
203 566-2038   Fax 203 566-3302

Delaware Department of Health and Social Services
Division of Public Health, Jesse Cooper Bldg
802 Silver Lake Blvd, PO Box 637
Dover, DE 19903
302 739-4701   Fax 302 739-6659

District of Columbia Department of Human Services
Public Health Commission
1660 G St NW, Washington, DC 20001
202 727-0014   Fax 202 727-0379

Florida Department of Health and Rehabilitative Services
Health Program Office, Bldg 2, Room 429
1317 Winewood Blvd, Tallahassee, FL 32399-0700
904 487-2945   Fax 904 922-2993

Georgia Department of Human Resources
Public Health Division
2 Peachtree St NW, Atlanta, GA 30303
404 657-2700   Fax 404 657-2715

Hawaii Department of Health
1250 Punchbowl St, PO Box 3378
Honolulu, HI 96813
808 586-4410   Fax 808 586-4444

Idaho Department of Public Health and Welfare
Division of Health
450 W State St, Boise, ID 83720-0036
208 334-5945   Fax 208 334-6558

Illinois Department of Public Health
535 W Jefferson St, Springfield, IL 62761
217 782-4977   Fax 217 782-3987

Indiana Department of Health
1330 W Michigan St, PO Box 1964
Indianapolis, IN 46206-1964
317 383-6400   Fax 317 383-6779

Iowa Department of Public Health
Lucas State Office Bldg, Des Moines, IA 50319
515 281-5605   Fax 515 281-4958

Kansas Department of Health and Environment
Division Health, Landon State Office Bldg
900 SW Jackson St, Topeka, KS 66612-1290
913 296-1086   Fax 913 296-1231

Kentucky Human Resources Cabinet
Health Services Department
275 E Main St, Frankfort, KY 40621
502 564-3970   Fax 502 564-6533

Louisiana Department of Health and Hospitals
Public Health Services Office
PO Box 3214, New Orleans, LA 70177
504 342-8094   Fax 504 342-8098

Maine Department of Human Services
Health Bureau
State House, Sta 11, Augusta, ME 04333
207 287-3201   Fax 207 287-3005

Maryland Department of Health and Mental Hygiene
Public Health Services Office
201 W Preston St, 5th Fl, Baltimore, MD 21201
410 225-6525   Fax 410 225-6489

Massachusetts Executive Office of Health and
Human Services
Public Health Department
150 Tremont St, Boston, MA 02111
617 727-0201   Fax 617 727-2559

Michigan Department of Public Health
3423 N Logan, PO Box 30195, Lansing, MI 48909
517 335-8024   Fax 517 335-9476

Minnesota Department of Health
717 Delaware St SE, PO Box 9441
Minneapolis, MN 55440
612 623-5460   Fax 612 623-5794

Mississippi Department of Public Health
PO Box 1700, Jackson, MS 39215-1700
601 960-7634   Fax 601 960-7948

Missouri Department of Public Health
PO Box 570, Jefferson City, MO 65102
314 751-6001   Fax 314 751-6010

Montana Department of Health and
Environmental Sciences
Health Services Division
PO Box 2009D1, Cogswell Bldg, Room C-108
Helena, MT 59620
406 444-4473

Nebraska Department of Health
301 Centennial Mall S, 3rd Fl
PO Box 95007, Lincoln, NE 68509
402 471-2133   Fax 402 471-0383

Nevada Department of Human Resources
Health Division
505 E King St, Rm 201, Carson City, NV 89710
702 687-4740

New Hampshire Department of Health and
Human Services
Public Health Services Division
6 Hazen Dr, Concord, NH 03301
603 271-4501   Fax 603 271-3745

New Jersey Department of Health
John Fitch Plaza, CN 360, Trenton, NJ 08625-0360
609 292-7837   Fax 609 984-5474

New Mexico Department of Health
Public Health Division
1190 St Francis Dr, PO Box 26110
Santa Fe, NM 87502-6110
505 827-2389   Fax 505 827-2329

New York State Department of Health
Corning Tower, Empire State Plaza
Albany, NY 12237-0001
518 474-2011   Fax 518 474-5450

North Carolina Department of Environment,
Health, and Natural Resources
Health Director's Office
PO Box 27687, Raleigh, NC 27611-7687
919 715-4125   Fax 909 715-3060

North Dakota Department of Health and
Consolidated Laboratories
600 E Boulevard Ave, Bismarck, ND 58505
701 328-2373   Fax 701 328-4727

Ohio Department of Public Health
246 N High St, Columbus, OH 43215
614 466-2253   Fax 614 644-0085

Oklahoma Department of Public Health
1000 NE 10th St, Oklahoma City, OK 73117-1299
405 271-4200   Fax 405 271-7339

Oregon Department of Human Resources
Health Division
PO Box 14450, Portland, OR 97214-0450
503 731-4078

Pennsylvania Department of Health
PO Box 90, Harrisburg, PA 17108
717 787-6436   Fax 717 787-0191

Puerto Rico Department of Public Health
PO Box 70184, San Juan, PR 00936
809 766-2210

Rhode Island Department of Health
3 Capitol Hill, Providence, RI 02908-5097
401 277-2231   Fax 401 277-2210

South Carolina Department of Health and
Environmental Control
Health Services Office
J. Marion Sims & R. J. Aycock Bldg
2600 Bull St, Columbia, SC 29201
803 734-3900   Fax 803 737-3946

South Dakota Department of Health
445 E Capitol, Pierre, SD 57501-3185
605 773-3361   Fax 605 773-5683

Tennessee Department of Health
Health Services Bureau
312 8th Ave N, 12th Fl, Nashville, TN 37247-4501
615 741-7305   Fax 615 741-2491

Texas Department of Health
1100 W 49th St, Austin, TX 78756-3199
512 458-7375   Fax 512 458-7477

Utah Department of Health
PO Box 142802, Salt Lake City, UT 84114-2802
801 538-6111   Fax 801 538-6694

Vermont Agency of Human Services
Health Department
PO Box 70, Burlington, VT 05402
802 863-7280   Fax 802 863-7425

Virgin Islands Department of Health
Office of the Governor, Kogens Glade
St Thomas, VI 00802
809 776-8311

Virginia Office of Health and Human Resources
Health Department
1500 E Main St, PO Box 2448
Richmond, VA 23218
804 786-3561   Fax 804 786-4616

Washington Department of Health
PO Box 45890, Olympia, WA 98504-7890
360 753-5871   Fax 360 586-7424

West Virginia Department of Health and
Human Resources
Public Health Bureau, State Capitol Complex
Bldg 3, Room 518, Charleston, WV 25305-7890
304 558-2971   Fax 304 558-1035

Wisconsin Department of Health and Social Services
Health Division
1 W Wilson St, PO Box 7850, Madison, WI 53707-7850
608 266-1511   Fax 608 267-2832

Wyoming Department of Health
Public Health Division
4th Fl, Hathaway Bldg, Cheyenne, WY 82002-0710
307 777-6186   Fax 307 777-5402

Pulmonary

American Association of Cardiovascular and
Pulmonary Rehabilitation
7611 Elmwood Ave, Ste 201, Middleton, WI 53562
608 831-6989   Fax 608 831-5122
E-mail: aacvpr@mang.com

American College of Chest Physicians
3300 Dundee Rd, Northbrook, IL 60062-2348
800 343-ACCP   847 498-1400   Fax 847 498-5460

Board Certification in Pulmonary Disease:
American Board of Internal Medicine
3624 Market St, Philadelphia, PA 19104
800 441-2246   215 243-1500   Fax 215 382-4702

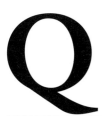

Quality

Quality qualms

Linda Prager
AM News Feb 24, 1997 p 7

Americans are anxious about the quality of US health care, recent polls show. Many feel quality has been sacrificed in the name of cost reduction.

	Agree Completely	Agree Somewhat	Disagree Somewhat	Disagree Completely
There are serious problems with the quality of health care	40%	35%	16%	7%
Quality care is often compromised by insurance companies to save money	49	25	15	6
Hospitals have cut corners to save money	47	33	10	6
Quality health care is almost unaffordable for the average person	57	22	14	5
The federal government can can play an important role in making health care better	43	26	11	18

Source: National Coalition on Health Care, 1997.

Editorial

Managed Care: a work in progress
[editorial excerpt]

Paul Ellwood, Jr, MD, George Lundberg, MD
JAMA 1996 Oct 2; 276(13): 1083-1086.

Editorials represent the opinions of the authors and The Journal and not those of the American Medical Association.

The health care system is coming out of the closet. Professional black boxes and undocumented claims of superior individual credentials and results are no longer enough! Organizational transparency and readily available objective evidence of health improvement is in!

Getting there will require the application of the following principles.

Principles of Accountability to the Public for Health Quality:
• The quality measures must be powerful enough to provide direction to the new American health system. Plans and providers will seek to achieve the results on which they are measured and for which they are accountable. If the measures are sound and the public understands and values them, they will become the central tool of health care reform and redesign.
• The measures must anticipate the behavioral changes they induce. If one plan or system proves to be exceptional at treating AIDS or diabetes, it will attract the sickest people in the community, and that's good! We should want the most competent and committed organizations to care for those most in need. But we should pay them for the additional responsibility and costs they incur. Quality measures and payment systems must be risk adjusted in order to shape the kind of health system we want. Despite its importance, there is no well-funded coordinated effort to devise risk adjustors and to reward health plans that serve the sickest patients well.
• Patient opinions should come first. Our patients pay us, receive our services, and have faith in our skill. In the market environment, they increasingly judge us. In the last 20 years, the science of measuring health outcomes and patient satisfaction has made enormous progress.[1,2] Although not without limits, many self-report measures are more reliable and rigorous than traditional clinical measures. The new measures of quality should emphasize consumers' perceptions of their own health function and well-being. At the same time, they should provide the level of feedback to providers that allows them to continuously improve medical practice.
• It's time for outcomes accountability. Managed care organizations are structured to facilitate accountability.

Q We finally have the measures and the structures in place to assess whether different practices or systems perform better. And we have an audience in purchasers and patients that is craving that information. As organizations become responsible for outcomes, we will see a growing link between the maturing disciplines of health services research and the clinical practices embraced by health systems.[3] Already many large health plans have created sophisticated research centers to help infuse their practices with evidence-based strategies, and they are building large observational series to continuously refine the care they provide.

The influence of health plans on the measures chosen should be minimized. Health plans are one important device for organizing and financing medical services, but there are others—some not invented yet. The standards for assessing performance must be based on the patient's experience of health and illness, independent of the particular structure or philosophy of the care providers. With billions of competitive dollars at stake, no plan can be objective about how it should be judged. The measures used to assess quality should not be constrained by the self-interest of the provider or financing organizations. We should not ignore the practical experience of health plans that have learned a great deal about measuring and managing quality, and we should remain sensitive to unnecessary burden or cost. But our health system is accountable to the public, and the public must decide what level of reporting or burden is appropriate.

The first phase of the health maintenance strategy was a bold and successful experiment that focused on and produced lower-cost health care. Now we are ready for the next phase that will measure and produce better-quality health care. And, surely, from the enormous savings that have been made through this revolution, we also will be able to find an incremental way to provide access to basic health care for all of our people.[4]

References

1. Ellwood PM. The Shattuck Lecture outcomes management: a technology of patient experience. *N Engl J Med.* 1988;318: 1549-1556.

2. Ware HE Jr, Bayliss MS, Rodgers WH, Kosinski M, Tarlov AR. Differences in 4-year outcomes for elderly and poor, chronically ill patients treated in HMO and fee-for-service systems: results from the Medical Outcomes Study. *JAMA.* 1996;276:1039-1047.

3. Yelin HE, Criswell LA, Feigenbaum G. Health care utilization and outcomes among persons with rheumatoid arthritis in fee-for-service and prepaid group practice settings. *JAMA.* 1996;276:1048-1053

4. Davis K. Incremental coverage of the uninsured. *JAMA.* 1996;276:831-832.

NCQA courts doctors with practicing physicians panel

Linda O. Prager
AM News Oct 28, 1996 p 7

Eager to tap the expertise of physicians in the field and quell complaints from the profession, the National Committee for Quality Assurance recently formed its Practicing Physicians Advisory Council.

The health plan accreditor had been under fire from medical leaders who complained that the organization's policies were not physician-friendly. A chief bone of contention: duplicative office reviews that physicians with multiple managed care contracts have faced as the plans work to comply with NCQA standards.

NCQA officials see the new panel as a tool to highlight potential problems as policies are formed and revise them as necessary.

"Many NCQA activities have very tangible effects on practicing physicians," says spokesman Barry Scholl. "But one of the gaps in our organization had been that there was no mechanism to get regular insight into that impact. There was no mode of direct communication."

The 19-member panel held its first meeting late last month and plans to meet quarterly. The next meeting will be held in December. The accreditor sought nominations from a wide range of physician groups earlier this year before assembling the panel.

The advisory council will be called on to help NCQA identify areas within managed care in which opportunities for quality improvement exist, provide input on NCQA activities, and educate providers about the accreditor's work.

Although physicians have long been members of NCQA's board, many had wanted more. Members of the AMA's House of Delegates had called for a physician-designated seat on the board, a structure similar to that of the Joint Commission on Healthcare Organizations.

NCQA officials and physician leaders had emphasized that the Joint Commission was originally formed and is still largely governed by provider groups. NCQA, in contrast, is a private organization with no slotted board seats.

AMA Chair-elect Thomas R. Reardon, MD, sits on the NCQA board, but not as an official representative of organized medicine.

Dr. Reardon applauded the creation of the new practicing physicians council. "This is an opportunity to spur communication in both directions," he said. "NCQA never realized how much its standards for managed care would affect practicing physicians. This committee will create a method by which concerns can be taken to NCQA and hopefully some consensus on some of the more contentious issues will be reached."

Resources

American College of Medical Quality
9005 Congressional Ct, Potomac, MD 20854
301 365-3570   Fax 301 365-3202

American Health Quality Association
(formerly the American Peer Review Association)
1140 Connecticut Ave NE, Ste 1050
Washington, DC 20036
202 331-5790   Fax 202 331-9334
E-mail: ahqa@ahqa.org

Joint Commission on Accreditation of
Healthcare Organizations
1 Renaissance Blvd
Oakbrook Terrace, IL 60181
630 916-5600   Fax 630 792-5001
Web address: http://www.jacho.org

National Committee for Quality Assurance
2000 L St NW, Ste 500, Washington, DC 20036
202 955-3500 Fax 202 955-3599
Web address: http://www.NCQA.org

Foundation for Accountability: FAACT
220 NW Second Ave, Ste 725, Portland, OR 97209
503 223-2228   Fax 503 223-4336
E-mail: info@facct.org

Quality Assurance

Quality Assurance Coordinator. Interprets and implements quality assurance standards in hospital to ensure quality care to patients. Reviews quality assurance standards, studies existing hospital policies and procedures, and interviews hospital personnel and patients to evaluate effectiveness of quality assurance program. Writes quality assurance policies and procedures. Reviews and evaluates patients' medical records, applying quality assurance criteria. Selects specific topics for review, such as problem procedures, drugs, high volume cases, high-risk cases, or other factors. Compiles statistical data and writes narrative reports summarizing quality assurance findings. May review patient records, applying utilization review criteria, to determine need for admission and continued stay in hospital. May oversee personnel engaged in quality assurance review of medical records. (DOT-1991)

Agency for Health Care Policy and Research materials

The Agency for Health Care Policy and Research (AHCPR) has issued a two-volume report discussing how to translate their clinical practice guidelines into medical review criteria, performance measures, and standards of quality to measure and evaluate the degree to which guideline recommendations are being implemented. Copies are available free of charge by calling the AHCPR at 800 358-9295.

Resource

American Board of Quality Assurance and
Utilization Review Physicians
4890 W Kennedy Blvd, Ste 260, Tampa, FL 33609
813 286-4411   Fax 813 286-4387

Quality Improvement

Six ways to improve your practice

Howard Larkin
AM News May 13, 1996 p 30

Continuous quality improvement has been proven time and again to improve health care outcomes while lowering costs. But it takes more than mere knowledge of statistical process control to succeed. It also takes a change in practice culture, says Ernie Rutherford, MD.

What that means is a change in the way people think about and do their jobs, says Dr. Rutherford, who led an effort that drastically reduced mortality rates and costs at five renal dialysis centers in northern Louisiana. Even more important, it means a change in how physicians and staff relate to one another and to patients.

Dr. Rutherford has codified into six principles what he learned from the transformation of his practice:

Keep the focus on the patient and listen to what the patient says. This also entails educating patients about their conditions and treatments to improve patient compliance. As a result, many problems are prevented before they become life-threatening or require expensive hospitalization.

Integrate into daily practice a computer-based patient record that is easily accessible yet maintains patient confidentiality. Computer records are the only practical way to maintain and manipulate the mass of data needed to do comprehensive statistical analysis.

Manage integration and change at the grassroots level. Change is always stressful for an organization. Staff must be taught not just a new static system but how to change, for continuous quality improvement means procedures will constantly change.

Integrate continuous quality improvement into the daily practice and collection of data. Quality measurement is not something that can be layered on top of existing procedures. It is and must be a process that standardizes, measures, and changes the procedures themselves. As such, it becomes an integral part of daily practice.

Implement the principles of the scientific methods of measurement to the medical review process. CQI is nothing more than a systematic application of the scientific method to daily practice. Practice algorithms are developed based on best available knowledge. Their outcomes are measured and changes are made. When those changes yield better results, they are incorporated into the algorithm, which always has the status of the best working hypothesis and therefore always can be improved.

Create a learning organization that fosters constant interaction between health care providers and patients, including the education of patients about their conditions and treatments. A learning organization is one in which all members, from physician to maintenance technician, are free to teach and learn from each other. Barriers among departments and classes of professionals must be lowered for this to occur.

Questionable Doctors

Public Citizen Health Research Group
2000 P St NW, 6th Fl, Washington, DC 20036
202 833-3000

R

Radiologic Technology

History

In 1944, X-ray technology, the predecessor of radiologic technology, joined the health professions of occupational therapy, clinical laboratory sciences, and medical records as the fourth health occupation to establish standards of education and qualifications for accreditation. The first *Essentials of an Acceptable School for X-Ray Technicians* were the product of negotiation between the American Society of X-Ray Technicians, now the American Society of Radiologic Technologists (ASRT), and the Council on Medical Education and Hospitals of the American Medical Association (AMA). During this time, X-ray technology was limited to diagnostic imaging using radiation produced by the simple and, certainly by today's standards, primitive equipment. Very little radiation therapy was performed—the X-ray technician "did it all." Radiation therapy technology, the treating of malignant diseases with radiation, was recognized as a separate discipline from radiography in 1964. The ASRT and the American College of Radiology (ACR) adopted the first set of dedicated radiation therapy technology *Essentials* in 1968. In 1994, the discipline became known as radiation therapy, and practitioners as radiation therapists.

In 1969, the ASRT and the ACR established the Joint Review Committee on Education in Radiologic Technology (JRCERT) within the structure for allied health educational accreditation provided by the AMA Council on Medical Education (AMA CME).

The AMA CME delegated responsibility for allied health educational accreditation to a newly formed Committee on Allied Health Education and Accreditation (CAHEA) in 1976. In 1992, the Association of Educators in Radiological Sciences joined the ASRT and ACR as a participating organization in the JRCERT. That same year, the AMA announced that it had elected to dissolve CAHEA as of June 1994. In January 1994, the United States Department of Education recognized the JRCERT as the national accrediting agency for radiography and radiation therapy educational programs.

Known as *Essentials* since 1944, educational standards continually evolve. In 1997, a totally new document, *Standards for an Accredited Program in Radiologic Sciences*, was implemented. The *Standards* define the requirements to achieve and maintain programmatic accreditation.

The *Standards* measure a program's compliance in areas of mission and goals, integrity, effectiveness and outcomes, curriculum, academic practices, human and learning resources, physical safety, student services, fiscal responsibility, and student outcomes. Accreditation ensures that a program operates in substantial compliance with these *Standards*.

Radiation Therapist

Occupational description

Radiation therapists deliver radiation to patients for therapeutic purposes. Radiation therapists provide for appropriate patient care and safety; apply problem-solving and critical thinking skills in the administration of prescribed treatment protocols, tumor localization, and dosimetry; and maintain pertinent records. Radiation therapists are particularly concerned with the principles of radiation protection for the patient, themselves, and others while performing these responsibilities.

Job description

Professional competence requires that radiation therapists apply knowledge of anatomy and physiology, oncologic pathology, radiation biology, radiation oncology techniques, treatment planning procedures, and dosimetry in the performance of their duties. They must also communicate effectively with patients, health professionals, and the public.

The radiation therapist accepts responsibility for administering a radiation oncologist (physician)–prescribed course of radiation therapy, observing the patient during treatment, and maintaining pertinent records of treatment. Radiation therapists also evaluate and assess treatment delivery components, evaluate and assess the daily physiologic and psychological responsiveness of the patient, and promote total quality care for patients undergoing radiation therapy. Additional duties may include tumor localization, dosimetry, patient follow-up, and patient education. Radiation therapists must display competence, compassion, and concern in meeting the special needs of the oncology patient.

Employment characteristics

Radiation therapists are employed in health care facilities, including cancer centers and private offices; they are also employed in settings where their responsibilities focus on education, management, research, and sales. Salaries and benefits vary with experience and employment location, but are generally competitive with other health specialties. (AHRP-1997)

Radiographer

Occupational description

Radiographers use imaging equipment to provide patient services as prescribed by physicians. When providing patient services, radiographers continually strive to provide quality patient care and are particularly concerned with limiting radiation exposure to patients, themselves, and others. Radiographers utilize problem-solving and

R

critical thinking skills to perform medical imaging procedures by adapting variable technical parameters of the procedure to the condition of the patient and by initiating life support procedures as necessary during medical emergencies.

Job description
Professional competence requires that radiographers apply knowledge of anatomy, physiology, positioning, radiographic technique, and radiation biology and protection in the performance of their responsibilities. They must be able to communicate effectively with patients, other health professionals, and the public. Additional duties may include evaluating radiologic equipment, conducting a radiographic quality assurance program, providing patient education, and managing a medical imaging department. The radiographer must display compassion, competence, and concern in meeting the special needs of the patient.

Employment characteristics
Radiographers are employed in health care facilities—including specialized imaging centers, urgent care clinics, and private physicians' offices—and as educators or imaging department administrators. Salaries and benefits are generally competitive with other health professions, and vary according to experience and employment location. (AHRP-1997)

Resources
AMA Allied Health Department
312 553-9355

American Society of Radiologic Technologists
15000 Central Ave SE, Albuquerque, NM 87123-3909
505 298-4500   Fax 505 298-5063

American Registry of Radiologic Technologists
1255 Northland Dr, Mendota Heights, MN 55120
612 687-0048

Joint Review Committee on Education in
Radiologic Technology
20 N Wacker Dr, Ste 900, Chicago, IL 60606-2901
312 704-5300   Fax 312 704-5304

Radiology

Radiologist. Diagnoses and treats diseases of human body, using X ray and radioactive substances. Examines internal structures and functions of organ systems, making diagnoses after correlation of X-ray findings with other examinations and tests. Treats benign and malignant internal and external growths by exposure to radiation from X ray, high-energy sources, and natural and man-made radioisotopes directed at or implanted in affected areas of body. Administers radiopaque substances by injection, orally, or as enemas to render internal structures and organs visible on X-ray films or fluoroscopic screens. May specialize in diagnostic radiology or radiation oncology. May diagnose and treat diseases of human body, using radioactive substances, and be certified in nuclear radiology or nuclear medicine. (DOT-1991)

Resources
American Board of Radiology
5255 E Williams Ct, Ste 6800, Tucson, AZ 85711-7401
520 790-2900   Fax 520 790-3200

American College of Radiology
1891 Preston White Dr, Reston, VA 22091
800 ACR-LINE   703 648-8989   Fax 708 648-9176

American Roentgen Ray Society
c/o Paul R. Fullagar
1891 Preston White Dr, Reston, VA 22091
800 438-2777   703 648-8992   Fax 703 264-8863

American Society for Therapeutic Radiology and Oncology
1891 Preston White Dr, Reston, VA 22091
800 962-7876   703 716-7588   Fax 703 476-8167

Radiological Society of North America
2021 Spring St, Ste 600, Oak Brook, IL 60521
630 571-2670   Fax 630 571-7837
Web address: http://www.rsna.org/

Rare Disorders

This list, prepared by the Consortium on Rare Diseases, is intended as a starting point for individuals or groups seeking information on rare diseases or disorders, and the types of information they may be able to provide.

Biotechnology Industry Organization
1625 K St NW, Ste 1100, Washington, DC 20006
800 255-3304   202 857-0244   Fax 202 857-0237
(current funded research, and drug and product
information)

Alliance of Genetic Support Groups
4301 Connecticut Ave NW, Ste 404
Washington, DC 20008
800 336-GENE
E-mail: alliance@capaccess.org
(general disease information, voluntary and patient
organizations)

Coalition for Heritable Disorders of Connective Tissue
c/o National Marfan Foundation
382 Main St, Port Washington, NY 11050
800 862-7326   516 883-5712
(voluntary and patient organizations)

General Clinical Research Centers
Rare Disorder Network
AA 3223 MCN

Vanderbilt University Medical Center
Nashville, TN 37232-2195
800 428-6626   615 343-6499   Fax 615 343-8649
E-mail: david.robertson@mcmail.anderbilt.edu
(clinical trial subjects, current funded research, patient
care)

Biotechnology Industry Organization
1625 K St NW, Ste 1100, Washington, DC 20006
800 255-3304   202 857-0244   Fax 202 857-0237
(professional inquiries only; current funded research,
drug and product information)

March of Dimes Birth Defects Foundation
1275 Mamaroneck Ave, White Plains, NY 10605
914 428-7100   Fax 914 428-8203
(general disease information)

Metabolic Information Network
PO Box 670847, Dallas, TX 75367-0847
800 945-2188   214-696-2188
(prevalence data, clinical trial subjects, patient care)

National Center for Education in
Maternal and Child Health
2000 15th St N, Ste 701, Arlington, VA 22201-2617
703 524-7802   Fax 703 524-9335
E-mail: ncemch01@gumedlib.dml.georgetown.edu
(voluntary and patient organizations)

National Information Center for Orphan Drugs &
Rare Diseases
PO Box 1133, Washington, DC 20013-1133
800 336-4797
(voluntary and patient organizations, drug and product
information)

National Organization for Rare Disorders
PO Box 8923, New Fairfield, CT 06812-1783
800 999-NORD 203 746-6518   Fax 203 746-6481
E-mail: orphan@nordrdb.com
Web address: http://www.pcnet.com/~orphan
(general disease information, prevalence data, research
funding sources, clinical trial subjects, current research
results, travel assistance, voluntary and patient
organizations)

Office of Orphan Products Development, FDA
5600 Fishers Ln (HF 35), Rockville, MD 20857
301 443-4903
(prevalence data, research funding sources)

Pharmaceutical Manufacturers Association
Commission on Drugs for Rare Diseases
1100 15th St NW, Washington, DC 20005
202 835-3550   Fax 202 835-3429
(research funding sources, drug and product information)

World Life Foundation
PO Box 571, Bedford, TX 76095
800 289-5433 817 282-1405
(travel assistance)

Reference Criteria for Short Stay Hospital Review
Order from NTIS (US Department of Commerce)
5285 Port Royal Rd, Springfield, VA 22161
703 487-4650
Order #PB81-179889

References

The following is excerpted from *American Medical
Association Manual of Style*, 9th ed.

References serve two primary purposes—documentation
and acknowledgment. Authors may cite a reference to
support their own arguments or lay the foundation for
their theses; in this case, the emphasis is on documentation. They may also cite a reference as a source of information or to credit other authors; in this case, the emphasis is on acknowledgment.

References are a critical element of a manuscript and, as
such, the reference list demands close scrutiny by authors, editors, peer reviewers, copy editors, and proof-
readers. Authors bear primary responsibility for all reference citations. Editors and peer reviewers should examine
manuscripts for completeness, accuracy, and relevance of
documentation and references. Copy editors and proof-
readers are responsible for assessing the completeness of
references and for ensuring that references are presented
in proper style and format.

Much has been written about problems with bibliographic inaccuracies[4] (eg, the first author's name is misspelled, the journal name is incorrect, the year of publication or the volume or page numbers are incorrect). Such
errors make it difficult for the interested reader to retrieve the documents cited. An even more serious problem is inappropriate citation (eg, a speculative commentary is cited in a way that implies proved causality; an
article about an association between diet and heart disease in men is cited as if it represents data on the association in all adults). Not only is accuracy critical for the
integrity of the individual document, but because authors
may sometimes rely on secondary rather than primary
sources, an inaccurate citation in a document's reference
list may be replicated in subsequent articles whose authors do not consult the primary source. Authors should
always consult the primary source and should never cite a
reference that they themselves have not read.[5-8] (See also
2.12.21, Abstracts and Other Material Taken From
Another Source, and 2.12.48, Secondary Citations and
Quotations [Including Press Releases].)

**2.12.1 Reference Style and the Uniform Require-
ments.** For greater uniformity in technical requirements
for manuscripts submitted to their journals, the International Committee of Medical Journal Editors, meeting in
1978 in Vancouver, British Columbia, developed the
*Uniform Requirements for Manuscripts Submitted to
Biomedical Journals.*[1] Suggested formats for bibliographic style, developed for uniformity by the US National Library of Medicine (NLM), are included in that
document, which has been revised and updated several
times. Editors of approximately 500 journals have agreed
to receive manuscripts prepared in accordance with this
uniform style. Although *Uniform Requirements* is intended to aid authors in the preparation of their manuscripts for publication, not to dictate publication style to
journal editors, many journals have drawn on them for
elements of their publication style. References that adhere exactly to the *Uniform Requirements* will be acceptable without challenge in manuscripts submitted for
publication to AMA journals, and any necessary changes
will be made by AMA copy editors.

The reference style followed by AMA journals is also
based on recommendations of the NLM described in the
*National Library of Medicine Recommended Formats for
Bibliographic Citation.*[9] Both the *Uniform Requirements*
and AMA style represent modifications of the NLM style
but follow the general principles outlined in the NLM
document. Whatever reference style is followed, consistency throughout the document and throughout the
publication (journal, book) is critical.

Each reference is divided by periods into the following
bibliographic groups (listed in order):
• Author(s)
• Title
• Edition
• Imprint group (place and name of publisher, date of
  publication, volume number, issue number, inclusive
  page numbers)
• Physical description (physical construction or form)
• Series statement
• Supplementary notes (identifiers of the uniqueness of
  the reference or material necessary for added clarity)

R

The period serves as a field delimiter, making each bibliographic group distinct and establishing a sequence of bibliographic elements in a reference. The items within a bibliographic group are referred to as bibliographic elements. Bibliographic elements may be separated by the following punctuation marks:

A semicolon: if the elements are different or if there are multiple occurrences of logically related elements within a group; also, before volume identification data.

A comma: if the items are subelements of a bibliographic element or a set of closely related elements.

A colon: before the publisher's name, between the title and the subtitle, and after a connective phrase (eg, In, Taken from, Located at, Accompanied by, Available from).

2.12.2 Reference List. Reference to information that is retrievable is appropriately made in the reference list. This includes but is not limited to (1) articles published or accepted for publication in scholarly or mass circulation print or electronic journals, magazines, or newspapers, (2) books that have been published or accepted for publication, (3) papers presented at professional meetings, (4) abstracts, (5) theses, (6) CD-ROMs, films, videotapes, (7) package inserts or a manufacturer's documentation, (8) monographs, (9) official reports, (10) databases, (11) legal cases, and (12) patents.

References should be listed in numerical order at the end of the manuscript (except as specified in 2.12.3, References Given in Text, and 2.12.5, Numbering). Each reference is a separate entry.

References to material not yet accepted for publication or to personal communications (oral, written, and electronic) are not acceptable as listed references and instead should be included parenthetically in the text (see 2.12.3, References Given in Text; 2.12.46, Electronic Citations; and 2.12.47, Unpublished Material).

2.12.3 References Given in Text. Parenthetical citation in the text of references that meet the criteria for inclusion in a reference list should be restricted to those features that do not use reference lists, such as news articles or obituaries. Note that in the text (1) author(s) may not be named, (2) the title may not be given, (3) the name of the journal is abbreviated only when enclosed in parentheses, and (4) inclusive page numbers are given.

The findings were reported recently by Kessler et al (*Arch Gen Psychiatry.* 1995;52:1048-1060).

The results were reported recently by Kessler et al in the *Archives of General Psychiatry* (1995;52:1048-1060).

The *JAMA* article (1995;274:1591-1598) on the frequent failure of physicians to heed dying patients' wishes was picked up by *Time* (December 4, 1995:76) and *Newsweek* (December 4, 1995:74-75) as well as many major newspapers (eg, *Chicago Tribune.* December 3, 1995;1:19).

2.12.4 Minimum Acceptable Data for Print References. To be acceptable, a reference to print journals or books must include certain minimum data, as follows:

Journals: Author(s). Article title. Journal Name. Year; volume: inclusive page numbers.

Books: Author(s). Book Title. Place of publication: publisher; year: inclusive pages.

Enough information to identify and retrieve the material should be provided. More complete data (see 2.12.12, References to Journals, Complete Data, and 2.12.28, References to Books, Complete Data) should be used when available. (For detailed information on references to material available in electronic form and unpublished material, see 2.12.46, Electronic Citations, and 2.12.47, Unpublished Material.)

2.12.5 Numbering. References should be numbered consecutively by means of arabic numerals in the order in which they are cited in the text. Unnumbered references, in the form of a selected reading list, are rarely used in AMA journals. If they are, these references would appear alphabetically in a list separate from the specifically cited reference list.

2.12.6 Citation. Each reference should be cited in the text, tables, or figures in consecutive numerical order by means of superscript arabic numerals. It is acceptable for a reference to be cited only in a table or a figure legend and not in the text if it is in sequence with references cited in the text. For example, if Table 2 contains reference 13, which does not appear in the text, this is acceptable as long as the last reference cited (for the first time) before text citation of Table 2 is reference 12.

Use arabic superscript numerals outside periods and commas, inside colons and semicolons. When more than two references are cited at a given place in the manuscript, use hyphens to join the first and last numbers of a closed series; use commas without space to separate other parts of a multiple citation.

As reported previously,[1,3-8,19]

The derived data were as follows[3,4]:

Avoid placing a superscript reference citation immediately after a number or an abbreviated unit of measure to avoid any confusion between the superscript reference citation and an exponent.

Avoid: The two largest studies to date included 26[2] and 18[3] patients.

Better: The two largest studies to date included 26 patients[2] and 18 patients.[3]

Avoid: The largest lesion found in the first study was 10 cm.[2]

Better: The largest lesion found in the first study[2] was 10 cm.

When a multiple citation involves more than 23 characters (including spaces and punctuation), use an asterisk in the text and give the citation in a footnote at the bottom of the page (see example below). Note that reference numerals in such a footnote are set full size and on the line rather than as superscripts. Also note that the spacing is different from that in superscript reference citations.

As reported previously,*

*References 3, 5, 7, 9, 11, 13, 21, 24-29, 31.

If the author wishes to cite different page numbers from a single reference source at different places in the text, the page numbers are included in the superscript citation and the source appears only once in the list of references. Note that the superscript may include more than one page number, citation of more than one reference, or both, and that all spaces are closed up.

These patients showed no sign of protective sphincteric adduction.[3(p21),9]

Westman[5(pp3,5),9] reported 8 cases in which vomiting occurred.

In listed references, do not use *ibid* or *op cit.*

2.12.7 Authors. Use the author's surname followed by initials without periods. In listed references, the names of all authors should be given unless there are more than six, in which case the names of the first three authors are used, followed by "et al."

Note spacing and punctuation. Do not use *and* between names. Roman numerals and abbreviations for Junior (Jr) and Senior (Sr) follow author's initials.

Note: The NLM guidelines recommend listing the first 10 authors and, if more than 10, the first 10 and et al. For space considerations, and because et al means and others (ie, more than one—a problem in citing an article with 11 authors and listing the first 10 followed by et al), we have elected to depart from the NLM guidelines on this point.

One author: Doe JF.

Two authors: Doe JF, Roe JP III.

Six authors: Doe JF, Roe JP III, Coe RT Jr, Loe JT Sr, Poe EA, van Voe AE.

More than six authors: Doe JF, Roe JP III, Coe RT Jr, et al.

One author for a group: Doe JF, for the Laser ROP Study Group

One author and a group: Doe JF, and the Laser ROP Study Group

More than six authors for a group: Doe JF, Roe JP III, Coe RT Jr, et al, for the Laser ROP Study Group

More than six authors and a group: Doe JF, Roe JP III, Coe RT Jr, et al, and the Laser ROP Study Group

When mentioned in the text, only surnames of authors are used. For a two-author reference, list both surnames; for references with more than two authors or authors and a group, include the first author's surname followed by et al, and associates, and coworkers, or and colleagues.

Doe[7] reported on the survey.

Doe and Roe[8] reported on the survey.

Doe et al[9] reported on the survey.

Note: Do not use the possessive form et al's; rephrase the sentence.

The data of Doe et al[9] support our findings.

2.12.8 Prefixes and Particles. Surnames that contain prefixes or particles (eg, von, de, La, van) are spelled and capitalized according to the preference of the persons named.

1. van Gylswyk NO, Roche CI.

2. Van Rosevelt RF, Bakker JC, Sinclair DM, Damen J, Van Mourik JA.

3. Al-Faquih SR.

4. Kang S, Kim KJ, Wong T-Y, et al.

2.12.9 Titles. In titles of articles, books, parts of books, and other material, retain the spelling, abbreviations, and style for numbers used in the original. Note, however, that all numbers are spelled out at the beginning of a title

(although exceptions are made for years). See below for capitalization and typeface style.

Articles and Parts of Books: In English-language titles, capitalize only (1) the first letter of the first word, (2) proper names, and (3) abbreviations that are ordinarily capitalized (eg, DNA, EEG, VDRL). Do not enclose article and book chapter titles in quotation marks. However, if a book, book chapter, or article title contains quotation marks in the original, retain them as double quotation marks (unless both double and single quotation marks are used).

Journals, Books, Government Bulletins, Documents, and Pamphlets: Capitalize the first letter of each major word in titles and subtitles. Do not capitalize articles, prepositions of three or fewer letters, coordinating conjunctions (and, or, for, nor, but), or the *to* in infinitives. Do capitalize a two-letter verb, such as *Is.*

Capitalization: For journal article titles, follow the capitalization in *Index Medicus.* For books, pamphlets, reports, government documents, and parts of books, retain the capitalization used in the original or consult the author or publisher. *Note:* In non–English-language titles, capitalization does not necessarily follow the same rules. For example, in German titles (both articles and books), all nouns and only nouns are capitalized; in French, Spanish, and Italian book titles, capitalize only the first word, proper names, and abbreviations that are capitalized in English.

Names of Organisms: In all titles, follow AMA style for capitalization of scientific names of organisms and use of italics. Use roman type for genus and species names in book titles.

2.12.10 Non–English-Language Titles. Non–English-language titles may be given as they originally appeared, without translation:

1. Hachulla E, Hatron PY, Robert Y, Devulder B. Artèrite digitale, thrombose et syndrome hyperèosinophilique: une complication exceptionnelle. *Rev Med Interne.* 1995;16:434-436.

2. Aranete MRG, Mascola L, Eller A, et al. Transmissao de HIV atraves de inseminacao artificial de doador. *JAMAILGO.* 1995;3:1956-1972. Originally published, in English, in: *JAMA.* 1995;273:854-858.

If non–English-language titles are translated into English, bracketed indication of the original language should follow the title:

3. Salmon RJ, Vilcoq JR. Breast cancer after preventive subcutaneous mammectomy [in French]. *Presse Med.* 1995;24:1167-1168.

If both the non–English-language title and the translation are provided, both may be given, as shown below, with the non–English-language title given first, followed by the English translation, in brackets:

4. Kolmos HJ. Antibiotika i almen praksis [Antibiotics in general practice]. *Ugeskr Laeger.* 1996;158:258-260.

Non–English-language titles should be verified from the original when possible. Consult a dictionary in the appropriate language for accent marks, spelling, and other particulars.

Reference to the primary source is always preferable, but if the non–English-language article is not readily available or not accessible, the translated version is acceptable. The citation should always be to the version consulted.

Such words as *tome* (volume), *fascicolo* (part), *Seite* (page), *Teil* (part), Auflage (edition), *Abteilung* (section or part), *Band* (volume), *Heft* (number), *Beiheft* (supplement), and *Lieferung* (part or number) should be translated into English.

2.12.11 Subtitles. Style for subtitles follows that for titles (see 2.12.9, Titles) with regard to spelling, abbreviations, numbers, capitalization, and use of italics, except that for journal articles the subtitle begins with a lowercase letter. A colon and space separate title and subtitle. If the subtitle is numbered, as is common when articles in a series have the same title but different—numbered—subtitles, use a comma after the title, followed by a roman numeral immediately preceding the colon.

1. Guyatt GH, Sackett DL, Sinclair JC, Hayward R, Cook DJ, Cook RJ, for the Evidence-Based Medicine Working Group. Users' guides to the medical literature, IX: a method for grading health care recommendations. *JAMA.* 1995;274:1800-1804.

References to journals

2.12.12 Complete Data. A complete journal reference includes the following:
- Authors' surnames and initials
- Title of article and subtitle if any
- Abbreviated name of journal
- Year
- Volume number
- Part or supplement number, when pertinent, and issue month or number when pagination is not consecutive throughout a volume
- Inclusive page numbers

2.12.13 Names of Journals. Abbreviate and italicize names of journals. Use initial capital letters. Abbreviate according to the listing in the current *Index Medicus.*[10] Include parenthetical designation of a city if it is included in the abbreviations given in *List of Journals Indexed in Index Medicus*[10]; for example, *Acta Anat (Basel), J Physiol (Lond).*

In journal titles listed in *Index Medicus,* information enclosed in brackets should be retained without brackets, eg, *J Comp Physiol A* for *J Comp Physiol [A].*

If the name of a journal has changed since that used at the time the reference was published, retain the name used during the time of publication but use the currently recommended NLM abbreviations for the words involved. For example, the journal formerly called *Transactions of the Ophthalmological Societies of the United Kingdom* is now called *Eye.* If a citation was from the older-named journal, do not change the journal name to Eye, but do use the current style of abbreviating the former title: *Trans Ophthalmol Soc U K.*

2.12.14 Page Numbers and Dates. Do not omit digits from inclusive page numbers. The year, followed by a semicolon, the volume number, a colon, the initial page number, a hyphen, the final page number, and a period are set without spaces.

1. Davis JT, Allen HD, Powers JD, Cohen DM. Population requirements for capitation planning in pediatric cardiac surgery. *Arch Pediatr Adolesc Med.* 1996;150:257-259.

2.12.15 Discontinuous Pagination. For an article with discontinuous pagination, the cited parts of which appear in the same issue, follow this example:

1. Altman LK. Medical errors bring calls for change. *New York Times.* July 18, 1995:C1, C10.

2.12.16 Journals Without Volume Numbers. In references to journals that have no volume numbers or that have volume numbers but paginate each issue beginning with page 1, use one of the following styles:

1. Timmerman MG. Medical problems of adolescent female athletes. *Wis Med J.* June 1996:351-354.

2. Hardy AM. Incidence and impact of selected infectious diseases in childhood. *Vital Health Stat 10.* 1991;No. 180:5.

3. Hastings C. Differences in professional practice model outcomes: the impact of practice setting. *Crit Care Nurs Q.* November 1995;18:75-86

2.12.17 Parts of an Issue. If an issue has two or more parts, the part cited should be indicated in accordance with the following example:

1. Newman KM, Johnson CL, Jean-Claude J, Li H, Ramey WG, Tilson MD. Cytokines which activate proteolysis are increased in abdominal aortic aneurysms. *Circulation.* 1994;90(pt 2):224-227.

2.12.18 Issue Number. Do not include the issue number or month except in the case of a special issue (see 2.12.19, Special or Theme Issue) or when pagination is not consecutive throughout the volume (ie, when each issue begins with page 1). In the latter case, the month or the date of the issue is preferable to the issue number.

1. Taulbee P. Maryland Quality Project puts new focus on processes of care. *Rep Med Guideline Outcomes Res.* June 1994;5:10-11.

2.12.19 Special or Theme Issue. The *NLM Recommended Formats*[7] defines a special or theme issue as follows: "Special issues are frequently published to present the papers from conferences.... They may also be published to commemorate a specific event or to bring together papers on a specific subject." AMA journals refer to these as theme issues. References to all or part of a special or theme issue of a journal should be cited as follows:

1. Marais AD, Firth JC, Batemon M, Jones J, Mountney J, Marten C. Atorvastatin is a powerful and safe agent for lowering plasma cholesterol concentrations in heterozygous familial hypercholesterolaemia. *Atherosclerosis.* 1994;109(special issue):316. Abstract 226.

2. Winker MA, Flanagin A, guest eds. Emerging and reemerging global microbial threats. *JAMA.* 1996;275(theme issue):163-256.

Special or theme issues may be published as supplements (see also 2.12.20, Supplements). In this case, the following form is used:

3. Warrell DA, Molyneux ME, Beales PF, eds. Severe and complicated malaria. *Trans R Soc Trop Med Hyg.* 1990;84(suppl 2):1-65. Theme issue.

2.12.20 Supplements. The following example illustrates the basic format:

1. Lagios MD. Evaluation of surrogate endpoint biomarkers for ductal carcinoma in situ. *J Cell Biochem.* 1994;19(suppl):186-188.

If pagination is not consecutive with that of the volume, use the following form; there may be several supplements to a volume, each referred to by month.

2. Novick LF, Glebatis DM, Striacof RL, MacCubbins PA, Lessner L, Berns DS. New York State HIV Seroprevalence Project, II: Newborn Seroprevalence Study: methods and results. *Am J Public Health.* May 1991;81(suppl):15-21.

If the supplement is numbered, use the following form; pagination in each supplement is independent of that in others.

3. Schmidt D. Behavioural abnormalities and retention rates of antiilepilepsy drugs during long-term treatment of epilepsy: a clinical perspective. *Acta Neurol Scand.* 1995;92(suppl 162): 7-10.

When numbered supplements have several parts, each with independent pagination, use the following form:

4. Sofferman RA. The recovery potential of the optic nerve. *Laryngoscope.* 1995;105(suppl 72, pt 3):1-38.

The following example shows the pagination that may be found in a supplementary issue:

5. Ball P. Bacterial resistance to fluoroquinolones: lessons to be learned. *Infection.* 1994;22(suppl 2):S140-S147.

Other variations, akin to supplements, use a form similar to that for supplements. Below is an example of a supplement (*Recommendations and Reports*) published June 17, 1994; there is an issue of the *Morbidity and Mortality Weekly Report* (weekly) with that date as well.

6. Centers for Disease Control and Prevention. Compendium of animal rabies control, 1994. *MMWR Morb Mortal Wkly Rep.* 1994;43(RR-10):1-9.

2.12.21 Abstracts and Other Material Taken From Another Source. Several types of published abstracts may be cited: (1) an abstract of a complete article taken from another publication, as in the Abstracts section of *JAMA,* (2) a published abstract of a paper before presentation at a conference, and (3) a rewritten abstract of a published article with an appended commentary. (For examples of abstracts presented at meetings, published or unpublished, see 2.12.39, Serial Publications, and 2.12.47, Unpublished Material.)

Ideally, reference to any of these types of abstracts should be permitted only when the original article is not readily available (eg, non–English-language articles or papers presented at meetings but not yet published). If an abstract is published in the society proceedings section of a journal, the name of the society before which the paper was read need not be included.

Abstract of a complete article taken from another publication:

1. Falco NA, Upton J. Infantile digital fibromas [abstract]. *J Hand Surg Am.* 1995;20:1014-1020. Taken from: *JAMA.* 1996;275:1462h.

2. Salmon RJ, Vilcoq JR. Breast cancer after preventive subcutaneous mammectomy [in French; English abstract]. *Presse Med.* 1995;24:1167-1168. Taken from: *JAMA.* 1996;274:1896h.

Published abstract of a paper to be presented at a conference:

3. Schwartz RH, O'Donnell R, Mann L, Baugh J. Adolescents who smoke cigarettes: criteria for addiction, health concerns, and readiness to quit [abstract]. *AJDC.* 1993;147:417. Abstract 3.

Note that if an abstract number is given, it appears in the final field.

Rewritten abstract of a published article with an appended commentary:

4. Long-term clomiphene therapy may increase the risk of ovarian cancer [abstract]. *Arch J Club/Womens Health.* October 1995:43. Abstract of: Rossing MA, Daling JR, Weiss NS, Moore DE, Self SG. Ovarian tumors in a cohort of infertile women. *N Engl J Med.* 1994;331:771-776.

2.12.22 Special Department, Feature, or Column of a Journal. When reference is made to material from a special department, feature, or column of a journal, the department should be identified only in the following cases:

The cited material has no byline or signature. (*Note:* This is preferable to citing Anonymous, unless Anonymous or something similar was actually used.)

1. Health effects of sanctions on Iraq [editorial]. *Lancet.* 1995;346:1439-1440.

2. Case records of the Massachusetts General Hospital: weekly clinicopathological exercises. *N Engl J Med.* 1995;333:1625-1630. Case 38-1995.

The column or department name (1) might help the reader identify the nature of the article and (2) is not apparent from the title itself. *Note:* In these cases, the inclusion of the department or column name is optional and should be used as needed, at the editor's discretion.

3. Voelker R. Hypnosis for diagnosis [Quick Uptakes]. *JAMA.* 1996;275:272.

4. Seifer SD, Grumbach K. Migrating docs: studying physician practice location [letter]. *JAMA.* 1995;274:1914.

Note: Identification of other special departments, features, or columns may not require additional notation (eg, book or journal reviews, cover stories) as their identity will be apparent from the citation itself:

5. Schreiner GE, reviewer. *Ann Intern Med.* 1995;123:975-976. Review of: Kissick WL. Medicine's Dilemmas: Infinite Needs Versus Finite Resources.

6. Bowden VM, Long MJ, reviewers. JAMA. 1995;273:1395. Review of: Cohen GD, ed. *American Journal of Geriatric Psychiatry.*

7. Southgate MT. The Cover (Felix Nussbaum, Carnival Group). *JAMA.* 1993;269:477.

2.12.23 Other Material Without Named Author(s). Reference may be made to material that has no named author or is prepared by a committee or other group. The following forms are used:

1. National Institute of Neurological Disorders and Stroke rt-PA Stroke Study Group. Tissue plasminogen activator for acute ischemic stroke. *N Engl J Med.* 1995;333:1581-1587.

2. NIH Consensus Development Panel on Cochlear Implants in Adults and Children. Cochlear implants in adults and children. *JAMA.* 1995;274:1955-1961.

2.12.24 Discussants. If reference citation in the text names a discussant specifically rather than the author(s), eg, as noted by Allo,[1] the following form is used (see also 2.12.48, Secondary Citations and Quotations [Including Press Releases]).

1. Allo MD. In discussion of: McKindley DS, Fabian TC, Boucher BA, Croce MA, Proctor KG. Antibiotic pharmacokinetics following fluid resuscitation from traumatic shock. *Arch Surg.* 1995;130:1321-1329.

2.12.25 Corrections. If the reference citation is to an article with a published correction, provide both the information about the article and the information about the published correction, if available, as follows.

1. Nelson HD, Nevitt MC, Scott JC, Stone KL, Cummings SR, for the Study of Osteoporotic Fractures Research Group. Smoking, alcohol, and neuromuscular and physical function of older women [published correction appears in *JAMA.* 1996;275:446]. *JAMA.* 1994;272:1825-1831.

2.12.26. If the reference citation is to an article that has since been retracted, or to the retraction notice itself, use the appropriate example below, as adapted from *Uniform Requirements.*[1] *Uniform Requirements* notes, "Ideally, the first author should be the same in the retraction as in the article, although under certain circumstances the editor may accept retractions by other responsible people."

Article containing retraction:

1. Garey CE, Schwarzman AL, Rise ML, Seyfried TN. Ceruloplasmin gene defect associated with epilepsy in EL mice [retraction of Garey CE, Schwarzman AL, Rise ML, Seyfried TN. In: *Nat Genet.* 1994;6:426-431]. *Nat Genet.* 1995;11:104.

Article retracted:

2. Liou GI, Wang M, Matragoon S. Precocious IRBP gene expression during mouse development [retracted in: *Invest Ophthalmol Vis Sci.* 1994;35:3127]. *Invest Ophthalmol Vis Sci.* 1994;35:1083-1088.

2.12.27 Duplicate Publication. The following form is suggested for citation of a notice of duplicate publication.

1. Shadey IM. Notice of duplicate publication: Prevalence of measles in day-care centers [Duplicate publication of Shadey IM. Measles in children attending day care: an epidemiological assessment. *J New Results.* 1994;32:150-154.]. *JAMA.* 1994;270:2004-2008.

References to books

2.12.28 Complete Data. A complete reference to a book includes the following:
- Authors' surnames and first and middle initials
- Chapter title (when cited)
- Surname and first and middle initials of book authors or editors (or translator, if any)
- Title of book and subtitle, if any
- Volume number and volume title, when there is more than one volume
- Edition number (do not indicate first edition)
- Place of publication
- Name of publisher
- Year of copyright
- Page numbers, when specific pages are cited

2.12.29 Reference to an Entire Book. When referring to an entire book, rather than pages or a specific section, use the following form (see also 2.12.7, Authors).

1. Sherlock S, Dooley J. *Diseases of the Liver and Biliary System.* 9th ed. Oxford, England: Blackwell Scientific Publications; 1993.

2. LaFollette MC. *Stealing Into Print: Fraud, Plagiarism, and Misconduct in Scientific Publishing.* Berkeley: University of California Press; 1992.

3. Sutcliffe A, ed. *The New York Public Library Writer's Guide to Style and Usage.* New York, NY: HarperCollins Publishers Inc; 1994.

2.12.30 Reference to a Chapter in a Book. When citing a chapter of a book, capitalize as for a journal title (see 2.12.9, Titles); do not use quotation marks. Inclusive page numbers of the chapter should be given (see also 2.12.36, Page Numbers or Chapter Number).

1. Nahas GG, Goldfrank LR. Marijuana. In: Goldfrank LR, Flomenbaum NE, Lewin NA, Weisman RS, Howland MA, Hoffman RS, eds. *Goldfrank's Toxicologic Emergencies.* 5th ed. Norwalk, Conn: Appleton & Lange; 1994:889-898.

2. Cole BR. Cystinosis and cystinuria. In: Jacobson HR, Striker GE, Klahr S, eds. *The Principles and Practice of Nephrology.* Philadelphia, Pa: BC Decker Inc; 1991:396-403.

3. Huth EJ. Revising prose structure and style. In: *How to Write and Publish Papers in the Medical Sciences.* 2nd ed. Baltimore, Md: Williams & Wilkins; 1990:109-136.

4. Haddy FJ, Buckalew VM. Endogenous digitalis-like factors in hypertension. In: Laragh HJ, Brenner MB, eds. *Hypertension: Pathophysiology, Diagnosis, and Management.* New York, NY: Raven Press; 1995:1055-1067.

2.12.31 Editors and Translators. Names of editors, translators, translator-editors, or executive and section editors are given in accordance with the following forms:

1. Plato. *The Laws.* Taylor EA, trans-ed. London, England: JM Dent & Sons Ltd; 1934:104-105. [Plato is the author; Taylor is the translator-editor.]

2. Gwei-Djen L, Needham J. Diseases of antiquity in China. In: Kiple KF, ed; Graham RR, exec ed. *The Cambridge World History of Human Disease.* New York, NY: Cambridge University Press; 1993:345-354.

[Gwei-Djen and Needham are the authors of a chapter in a book edited by Kiple, for which Graham was the executive editor.]

3. Bloom FE. Neurotransmission and the central nervous system. In: Gilman AG, consulting ed; Hardman JG, Limbird LE, eds-in-chief; Molinoff PB, Roddon RW, eds. *Gilman's The Pharmacological Basis of Therapeutics.* 9th ed. New York, NY: McGraw-Hill Book Co; 1996:267-293.

[Bloom is the author of a chapter in a book edited by Molinoff and Roddon, for which Gilman was the consulting editor and Hardman and Limbird were the editors-in-chief.]

4. Jacobson MS, ed. *Pediatric Atherosclerosis Prevention: Identification and Treatment of the Child With High Cholesterol.* Chur, Switzerland: Harwood Academic Publishers; 1991. Lanzkowsky P, ed. Monographs in Clinical Pediatrics.

5. Goligorsky MS, ed. *Acute Renal Failure: New Concepts and Therapeutic Strategies.* New York, NY: Churchill Livingstone; 1995. Stein JH, ed. Contemporary Issues in Nephrology; No. 30.

6. Warner R, ed. *Alternatives to the Hospital for Acute Psychiatric Treatment.* Washington, DC: American Psychiatric Press; 1995. Clinical Practice Series; No. 32.

No authors are named in the three examples above. Each book has an editor and is part of a series; in examples 4 and 5, the series also has an editor. *Note:* The name of the series, as well as the series editor, if any, is given in the final field. If the book has a number within the series, the number is also given in the final field.

2.12.32 Volume Number. Use arabic numerals for volume number if the work cited includes more than one volume.

If the volumes have no separate titles, merely numbers, the number should be given after the general title.

1. Bithell TC. Hereditary coagulation disorders. In: Lee GR, Bithell TC, Foerster J, Athens JW, Lukens JN, eds. *Wintrobe's Clinical Hematology.* Vol 2. 9th ed. Philadelphia, Pa: Lea & Febiger; 1993:1422-1472.

2. Widiger TA, Frances AJ, Pincus HA, Ross R, First MB, Davis WW. *DSM-IV Sourcebook.* Vol 2. Washington, DC: American Psychiatric Press; 1996.

If the volumes have separate titles, the title of the volume referred to should be given first, with the title of the overall series of which the volume is a part given in the final field, along with the name of the general editor and the volume number, if applicable.

3. Creager MA, ed. *Vascular Disease.* St Louis, Mo: Mosby; 1996. Braunwald E, ed. *Atlas of Heart Disease;* vol 7.

In the example above, Creager is the editor of *Vascular Disease,* which is volume 7 in the series *Atlas of Heart Disease.* Braunwald is the editor of the entire series.

When a book title includes a volume number, use the title as it was published. Three examples are given below. *Note:* The volume number does not need to be repeated in its customary place after the year if it is included in the book's title.

4. Rous SN. *1995 Urology Annual Volume 9.* New York, NY: WW Norton & Co; 1995.

5. Lewin B. Gene numbers: repetition and redundancy. In: *Genes V.* New York, NY: Oxford University Press; 1994:703-731.

6. Hames BD, Higgins SJ, eds. *Gene Probes 1.* New York, NY: Oxford University Press; 1995. Rickwood D, Hames BD, eds. The Molecular Approach Series.

2.12.33 Edition Number. Use arabic numerals to indicate an edition, but do not indicate a first edition. If a subsequent edition is cited, the number should be given. Abbreviate "New revised edition" as "New rev ed"; "Revised edition" as "Rev ed"; "American edition" as "American ed"; and "British edition" as "British ed."

1. Frolich ED. Pathophysiology of systemic arterial hypertension. In: Schlant RC, Alexander RW, eds. *Hurst's The Heart: Arteries and Veins.* 8th ed. New York, NY: McGraw-Hill Book Co; 1994:1391-1401.

2. Baker PC, Keck CK, Mott FL, Quinlan SV. *NYLS Child Handbook: A Guide to the 1986-90 National Longitudinal Survey of Youth and Child Data.* Rev ed. Columbus: Ohio State University; 1993.

2.12.34 Place of Publication. Use the name of the city in which the publishing firm was located at the time of publication. Follow AMA style in the use of state names. Do not list the state name if it is part of the publisher's name. If more than one location appears, use the one that appears first in the edition you consulted. A colon separates the place of publication and the name of the publisher.

1. Perkins AC. Nuclear Medicine: *Science and Safety.* London, England: John Libbey; 1995.

2. Chalmers I, Altman DG. *Systematic Reviews.* London, England: BMJ Publishing Group; 1995.

3. Scioscia AL. Reproductive genetics. In: Moore TR, Reiter RC, Rebar RW, Baker VV, eds. *Gynecology & Obstetrics: A Longitudinal Approach.* New York, NY: Churchill Livingstone; 1993:55-77.

4. Dougherty CJ. *Back to Reform: Values, Markets, and the Health Care System.* New York, NY: Oxford University Press; 1996.

5. Parkes MB. *Pause and Effect: An Introduction to the History of Punctuation in the West.* Berkeley: University of California Press; 1993.

2.12.35 Publishers. The full name of the publisher (publisher's imprint, as shown on the title page) should be given, abbreviated in accordance with AMA style but without punctuation. Even if the name of a publishing firm has changed, use the name that was given on the published work.

Consult the latest *Books in Print*[11] to verify names of publishers.

2.12.36 Page Numbers or Chapter Number. Use arabic numerals, unless the pages referred to use roman pagination (eg, the preliminary pages of a book).

1. Litt IE. Special health problems during adolescence. In: Nelson WE, senior ed; Behrman RE, Kliegman RM, Arvin AM, eds. *Nelson Textbook of Pediatrics.* 15th ed. Philadelphia, Pa: WB Saunders Co; 1996:541-560.

2. Grossman J. Preface. In: *The Chicago Manual of Style.* 14th ed. Chicago, Ill: University of Chicago Press; 1993:vii-xi.

If a book uses separate pagination within each chapter, follow the style used in the book.

3. Trunkel AR, Croul SE. Subacute and chronic meningitides. In: Bleck TP, ed. *Central Nervous System and Eye Infections.* Philadelphia, Pa: Current Medicine; 1995:2.1-2.27. Mandell GL, ed. *Atlas of Infectious Diseases;* vol 3.

Inclusive page numbers are preferred. The chapter number may be used instead if the author does not provide the inclusive page numbers.

4. Shils ME. Magnesium. In: Shils ME, Young VR, eds. *Modern Nutrition in Health and Disease.* 7th ed. Philadelphia, Pa: Lea & Febiger; 1988:chap 6.

Special materials

2.12.37 Newspapers. References to newspapers should include the following, in the order indicated: (1) name of author (if given), (2) title of article, (3) name of newspaper, (4) date of newspaper, (5) section (if applicable), and (6) pages. Note that newspaper titles are not abbreviated.

1. Gianelli DM. AMA launching ethics institute for research, outreach projects. *American Medical News.* November 4, 1996:1, 75.

2. Steinmetz G. Kafka is a symbol of Prague today; also, he's a T-shirt. *Wall Street Journal.* October 10, 1996:A1, A6.

3. Auerbach S. Tomorrow's MDs unready for managed care? Studies say that medical schools' training methods are behind the times. *Washington Post.* September 17, 1996;Health section:11.

4. Travis D. Advertising our dishonor: my industry should be ashamed of itself for pushing cigarettes on kids. *Washington Post.* September 8, 1996:C3.

5. Grady D. So, smoking causes cancer: this is news? *New York Times.* October 27, 1996;sect 4:3.

2.12.38 Government Bulletins. References to bulletins published by departments or agencies of the US government should include the following information, in the order indicated: (1) name of author (if given); (2) title of bulletin; (3) place of publication; (4) name of issuing bureau, agency, department, or other governmental division (note that in this position, Department should be abbreviated Dept; also note that Government Printing Office should be used only if the name of the issuing bureau, agency, or department cannot be obtained); (5) date of publication; (6) page numbers, if specified; (7) publication number, if any; and (8) series number, if given.

1. US Bureau of the Census. *Statistical Abstract of the United States: 1993.* 113th ed. Washington, DC: US Bureau of the Census; 1993.

2. US General Accounting Office. *Trauma Care: Life-saving Systems Threatened by Unreimbursed Costs and Other Factors.* Washington, DC: US General Accounting Office; 1991. Publication HRD 91-57.

3. Clinical Practice Guideline Number 5: *Depression in Primary Care, 2: Treatment of Major Depression.* Rockville, Md: US Dept of Health and Human Services, Agency for Health Care Policy and Research; 1993. AHCPR publication 93-0551.

4. Food and Drug Administration. *Jin Bu Huan Herbal Tablets.* Rockville, Md: National Press Office; April 15, 1994. Talk Paper T94-22.

2.12.39 Serial Publications. If a monograph or report is part of a series, include the name of the series and, if applicable, the number of the publication.

1. Steahr TE, Roberts T. *Microbial Foodborne Disease: Hospitalizations, Medical Costs and Potential Demand for Safer Food.* Storrs: Food Marketing Policy Center, University of Connecticut; 1993. Private Strategies, Public Policies and Food System Performance Working Paper Series, No. 32.

2. Hardy AM. *AIDS Knowledge and Attitudes for Oct-Dec 1990: Provisional Data From the National Health Interview Survey.* Hyattsville, Md: National Center for Health Statistics; 1991. Advance Data From Vital and Health Statistics, No. 204.

3. Miller JE, Korenman S. *Poverty, Nutritional Status, Growth and Cognitive Development of Children in the United States.* Princeton, NJ: Princeton University Office of Population Research; 1993. Working Paper 93-5.

2.12.40 Theses and Dissertations. Titles of theses and dissertations are given in italics. References to theses should include the location of the university (or other institution), its name, and year of completion of the thesis. If the thesis has been published, it should be treated as any other book reference (see References to Books, Complete Data, 2.12.28).

1. Knoll EG. *Mental Evolution and the Science of Language: Darwin, Müller, and Romanes on the Development of the Human Mind* [dissertation]. Chicago, Ill: Committee on the Conceptual Foundations of Science, University of Chicago; 1987.

2. King L. *Modern Literary Apparitions and Their Mind-Altering Effects* [master's thesis]. Evanston, Ill: Northwestern University; 1994.

2.12.41 Special Collections. References to material available only in special collections of a library take this form:

1. Hunter J. An account of the dissection of morbid bodies: a monograph or lecture. 1757;No. 32:30-32. Located at: Library of the Royal College of Surgeons, London, England.

2.12.42 Package Inserts. Package inserts may be cited as follows:

1. Lamasil [package insert]. East Hanover, NJ: Sandoz Pharmaceuticals Corp; 1993.

2.12.43 Patents. Patent citations take the following form:

1. Furukawa Y, Kishimoto S, Nishikawa K, inventors; Takeda Chemical Industries Ltd, assignee. Hypotensive imidazole derivatives. US patent 4340598. July 20, 1982.

2.12.44 Audiotapes, Videotapes. Occasionally, references may include citation of audiotapes or videotapes. The form for such references is as follows:

1. *The Right to Die . . . The Choice Is Yours* [videotape]. New York, NY: Society for the Right to Die; 1987.

2. *Obsessive-compulsive Disorder: Pharmacotherapy and Psychotherapy* [videotape]. Washington, DC: American Psychiatric Press; 1995. Alger I, ed; Treatment of Psychiatric Disorders Video Series.

3. Cohen LB, Basuk PM, Waye JD. *Video Guide to Flexible Sigmoidoscopy* [videotape]. New York, NY: Igaku-Shoin Medical Publishers; 1995.

2.12.45 Transcript of Television or Radio Broadcast. Citation of transcripts of television or radio broadcasts take the following form:

1. Lundberg GD. The medical profession in the 1990s [transcript]. American Medical Television. September 15, 1993.

2. An American dilemma [transcript]. *60 Minutes.* CBS television. January 14, 1996.

2.12.46 Electronic Citations. The *NLM Recommended Formats*[9] document includes guidelines for many types of electronic citations, examples of which are given below. As electronic forms of documents proliferate and the number of citations to them increases, additional guidelines will likely be required. Already, specific guidelines on these forms of citations are appearing.[12-14] The recommendations in this section combine those in *NLM's Recommended Formats*[9] and those at the Li/Crane Web site.[14] When citing an electronic document that also exists in print form, you should cite the version you consulted. Annotation of an additional version of the same publication might also be helpful.[15]

Software: To cite software, use the following form. Note that when the computer program is mentioned only in passing and is not the subject of the report, the software used does not need to be added to the reference list. However, in these cases, the manufacturer of the software, and the manufacturer's location, should be included in parentheses in the text.

1. Epi Info [computer program]. Version 6. Atlanta, Ga: Centers for Disease Control and Prevention; 1994.

Software Manual: If it is not the software but the software manual or guide that is being cited, use the following form, which follows that for citation of a book (see References to Books, Complete Data, 2.12.28).

1. Dean AG, Dean JA, Coulombier D, et al. *Epi Info, Version 6: A Word-Processing, Database, and Statistics Program for Public Health on IBM-Compatible Microcomputers.* Atlanta, Ga: Centers for Disease Control and Prevention; 1994.

2. Dixon WJ, Brown MB, Engelman L, Jennrich RI, eds. *BMDP Statistical Software Manual.* Los Angeles: University of California Press; 1990.

Online Journals: References to articles cited in online journals may take one of the two following forms:

Journals without volume and page information: For online journals that do not use the typical year, volume, and page format of print journal citations, a document number, preceded by a date of publication, may be used.

1. Harrison CL, Schmidt PQ, Jones JD. Aspirin compared with acetaminophen for relief of headache. *Online J Curr Clin Trials* [serial online]. January 2, 1992;doc 1.

Journals with volume and page information: Citations to online journals that do use year, volume, and page formats take a form similar to that of citations to print journals. Note that the inclusion of date accessed (consulted) is appropriate and especially important when articles in online journals that allow changes to be made in the article after its publication are cited.

1. Friedman SA. Preeclampsia: a review of the role of prostaglandins. *Obstet Gynecol* [serial online]. January 1988;71(1):22-37. Available from: BRS Information Technologies, McLean, Va. Accessed December 15, 1990.

CD-ROMs: When citing a book or monograph in a CD-ROM format, use the following form:

1. *The Oxford English Dictionary* [book on CD-ROM]. 2nd ed. New York, NY: Oxford University Press; 1992.

2. *The American Heritage Dictionary: Reference Tool for Windows* [book on CD-ROM]. Cambridge, Mass: SoftKey International Inc; 1995. Based on: *American Heritage Dictionary of the English Language,* Third Edition. Boston, Mass: Houghton Mifflin Co; 1992.

3. *AMA Drug Evaluations Annual 1993* [book on CD-ROM]. Jackson, Wyo: Teton Data Systems; 1993. Based on: Sugden R, ed. *AMA Drug Evaluations Annual 1993.* Chicago, Ill: American Medical Association; 1993. STAT!-Ref Medical Reference Library.

4. *Williams Obstetrics* [book on CD-ROM]. Jackson, Wyo: Teton Data Systems; 1993. Based on: Cunningham FG, MacDonald PC, Grant NF, Leveno KJ, G-strap LC III. *Williams Obstetrics.* 19th ed. East Norwalk, Conn: Appleton & Lange; 1993. STAT!-Ref Medical Reference Library.

Citation of a journal article on CD-ROM takes the following form:

5. Gershon ES. Antisocial behavior. *Arch Gen Psychiatry* [serial on CD-ROM]. 1995;52:900-901.

Databases: When citing a database, use the following form:

1. CANCERNET-PDQ [database online]. Bethesda, Md: National Cancer Institute; 1996. Updated March 29, 1996.

World Wide Web Site: Citations to material on a home page or Web site take the following form:

1. Rosenthal S, Chen R, Hadler S. The safety of acellular pertussis vaccine vs whole-cell pertussis vaccine [abstract]. *Arch Pediatr Adolesc Med* [serial online]. 1996;150:457-460. Available at: http://www.amailassn.org/sci-pubs/journals/archive/ajdc/vol_150/no_5/abstract/htm. Accessed November 10, 1996.

2. Gostin L. Drug use and HIV/AIDS [JAMA HIV/AIDS Web site]. June 1, 1996. Available at: http://www.amailassn.org/special/hiv/ethics. Accessed July 19, 1996.

3. LaPorte RE, Marier E, Akazawa S, Sauer F, et al. The death of biomedical journals. *BMJ* [serial online]. 1995;310:1387-1390. Available at: http://www.bmj.com/bmj/archive/6991ed2.htm. Accessed March 17, 1997.

4. Food and Drug Administration home page. Available at: http://vm.cfsan.fda.gov/;aplrd/sodium.txt. Accessed October 1, 1995.

5. Health on the Net Foundation. Health on the Net code of conduct (HONcode) for medical and health web sites. Available at: http://www.hon.ch/Conduct.html. Accessed September 5, 1996.

6. Health Care Financing Administration. 1996 statistics at a glance. Available at: http://www.hcfa.gov/stats/stath-i.htm. Accessed December 2, 1996.

E-mail: References to e-mail messages, as to other forms of personal communication (see also 2.12.47, Unpublished Material), should be listed parenthetically in the text and should include (1) the name of the person who sent the message, (2) the sender's e-mail address, and (3) the date the message was sent. An example of an e-mail citation, appearing in running text, appears below:

Unlike e-mail addresses, URLs [uniform resource locators] may be case-sensitive (J. M. Kramer, K. Kramer [jmkramer@umich.edu], e-mail, March 6, 1996).

2.12.47 Unpublished Material. References to unpublished material may include articles or abstracts that have been presented at a society meeting but not published and material accepted for publication but not published. If, during the course of the publication process, these materials are published or accepted for publication, and if the author is familiar with the later version, the most up-to-date bibliographic information should be included.

Items presented at a meeting but not published: These oral presentations take the following form:

1. Eisenberg J. Market forces and physician workforce reform: why they may not work. Paper presented at: Annual Meeting of the Association of American Medical Colleges; October 28, 1995; Washington, DC.

2. Coyle J. Glutamate, oxidative stress and schizophrenia. Paper presented at: International Congress on Schizophrenia Research; April 10, 1995; Hot Springs, Va.

3. Donegan J. Anesthesia for patients with ischemic cerebrovascular disease. Refresher course lectures presented at: American Society of Anesthesiologists; October 17-21, 1981; New Orleans, La.

Note that once these presentations do become published, they take the form of reference to a book, journal, or other medium in which they are ultimately published, as in the example below (see 2.12.28, References to Books, Complete Data):

4. Slama K, ed. *Tobacco and Health: Proceedings of the Ninth World Conference on Tobacco and Health, Paris, France, 10-14 October 1994.* New York, NY: Plenum Press; 1995.

Material accepted for publication but not published: Formats suggested for both journal articles and books, accepted for publication but not yet published, are shown below:

5. Klassen TP, Watters LK, Feldman ME, Sutcliffe T, Rowe PC. The efficacy of nebulized budesonide in dexamethasone-treated outpatients with croup. *Pediatrics*. In press.

6. Akil H, Morano MI. The biology of stress: from periphery to brain. In: Watson SJ, ed. *Biology of Schizophrenia and Affective Disease*. Washington, DC: American Psychiatric Press. In press.

7. Mrak RE. Ultrastructural diagnosis of tumors of the nervous system. In: Garcia JH, ed. *Diagnostic Neuropathology. Vol 4*. New York, NY: Oxford University Press. In press.

Note: Some publications require that authors demonstrate proof that acceptance for publication has been granted.[9,16] Some publishers also prefer the term *forthcoming* to *in press* because they feel that the latter is not appropriate for electronic citations,[9,16] in which case online designation would also be used, as shown in 2.12.46, Electronic Citations.

In the list of references, do not include material that has been submitted for publication but has not yet been accepted. This material, with its date, should be noted in the text as unpublished data, as follows:

These findings have recently been corroborated (H. E. Marman, MD, unpublished data, January 1996).

Similar findings have been noted by Roberts[6] and H. E.Marman, MD (unpublished data, 1996).

Numerous studies[12-20] (also H. E. Marman, MD, unpublished data, 1996) have described similar findings.

If the unpublished data referred to are those of the author, indicate this as follows:

Other data (H.E.M., unpublished data, 1996)....

Do not include personal communications in the list of references. The following forms may be used in the text:

In a conversation with H. E. Marman, MD (August 1996)....

According to a letter from H. E. Marman, MD, in August 1996....

Similar findings have been noted by Roberts[6] and by H. E. Marman, MD (written communication, August 1996).

According to the manufacturer (H. R. Smith, oral communication, May 1996), the drug became available in Japan in January 1995.

Note that the author should give the date of the communication and indicate whether it was in an oral or written form. Highest academic degrees should also be given. On occasion, the affiliation of the person might also be included to better establish the relevance and authority of the citation.

See also 2.12.46, Electronic Citations, E-mail.

Some journals now require that the author obtain written permission from the person whose unpublished data or personal communication is thus cited.[1,16]

2.12.48 Secondary Citations and Quotations (Including Press Releases). Reference may be made to one author's citation of, or quotation from, another's work. Distinguish between citation and quotation (ie, between work mentioned and words actually quoted). In the text, the name of the original author, rather than the secondary source, should be mentioned. (See also 2.12.24, Discussants.) As with citation of an abstract of an article rather than citation of the original document (see 2.12.21, Abstracts and Other Material Taken From Another Source), citation of the original document is

preferred unless it is not readily available. Only items actually consulted should be listed. The forms for listed references are as follows:

1. Gordis E. Relapse and craving: a commentary. *Alcohol Alert*. 1989;6:3. Cited by: Mason BJ, Kocsis JH, Ritvo EC, Cutler RB. A double-blind, placebo-controlled trial of desipramine for primary alcohol dependence stratified on the presence or absence of major depression. *JAMA*. 1996;275:761-767.

Occasionally, though rarely, a more complex citation history is required.

2. Wang YX, Jin X, Jiang HF, et al. Studies on the percutaneous absorption of four radioactive labeled pesticides. *Acta Acad Med Primae Shanghai*. 1981;8:370. Cited by: Bartelt N, Hubbell JP. *Percutaneous Absorption of Topically Applied 14C-Permethrin in Volunteers: Final Medical Report*. Research Triangle Park, NC: Burroughs Wellcome Co/Fairfield American Corp; 1989:378-410. Publication 86182. Cited by: Permethrin (Permanone Tick Repellent): *Risk Characterization Document* (Revised). Sacramento: Dept of Pesticide Regulation, California Environmental Protection Agency; 1994.

3. Leary WE. Quoted by: Smoking Control Advocacy Resource Center (SCARC) Action Alert. Issue: *Study Correlates Advertising With Increased Youth Consumption*. Washington, DC: Advocacy Institute; March 15, 1994.

4. Cigarette smoking among American teens rises again in 1995 [press release]. Ann Arbor: University of Michigan Survey Research Center; December 15, 1995.

2.12.49 Classical References. Classical references may deviate from the usual forms in some details. In many instances, the facts of publication are irrelevant and may be omitted. Date of publication should be given when available and pertinent.

1. Shakespeare W. *A Midsummer Night's Dream*. Act 2, scene 3, line 24.

2. Donne J. *Second Anniversary*. Verse 243.

For classical references, *The Chicago Manual of Style*[17] may be used as a guide.

3. Aristotle. *Metaphysics*. 3. 2.966[b] 5-8.

In biblical references, do not abbreviate the names of books. The version may be included parenthetically if the information is provided. References to the Bible are usually included in the text.

The story begins in Genesis 3:1.

Paul admonished against succumbing to temptation (I Corinthians 10:6-13).

Occasionally they may appear as listed references at the end of the article.

4. I Corinthians 10:6-13 (RSV).

2.12.50 Legal References. A specific style variation is used for references to legal citations. Because the system of citation used is quite complex, with numerous variations for different types of sources and among various jurisdictions, only a brief outline can be presented here. For more details, consult *The Bluebook: A Uniform System of Citation*.

Method of citation: A legal reference may be included in full in the text or in the reference list, or partially in the text and partially in the reference list.

In a leading decision on informed consent (*Cobbs v Grant*, 502 P2d 1 [Cal 1972]), the California Supreme Court stated . . . .

In a leading decision on informed consent,[1] the California Supreme Court stated. . . .

In the case of *Cobbs v Grant* (502 P2d 1 [Cal 1972]). . . .

In the case of *Cobbs v Grant*[1] . . . .

Citation of cases: The citation of a case (ie, a court opinion) generally includes, in the following order:

The name of the case in italics (only the names of the first party on each side are used, never with et al, and only the last names of individuals).

The volume number, name, and series number (if any) of the case reporter in which it is published.

The page in the volume on which the case begins and, if applicable, the specific page or pages on which is discussed the point for which the case is being cited.

In parentheses, the name of the court that rendered the opinion (unless the court is identified by the name of the reporter) and the year of the decision. If the opinion is published in more than one reporter, the citations to each reporter (known as parallel citations) are separated by commas. Note that v, 2d, and 3d are standard usage in legal citations.

1. *Canterbury v Spence,* 464 F2d 772,775 (DC Cir 1972).

This case is published in volume 464 of the *Federal Reporter,* second series. The case begins on page 772, and the specific point for which it was cited is on page 775. The case was decided by the US Court of Appeals, District of Columbia Circuit, in 1972.

The proper reporter to cite depends on the court that wrote the opinion. Table T.1 of *The Bluebook* contains a complete list of all current and former state and federal jurisdictions.

US Supreme Court: Cite to *US Reports* (abbreviated as US). If the case is too recent to be published there, cite to *Supreme Court Reporter* (SCt), *US Reports, Lawyer's Edition* (LEd), or *US Law Week* (USLW)—in that order. Do not include parallel citation.

US Court of Appeals (formerly known as Circuit Courts of Appeals): Cite to *Federal Reporter,* original or second series (F or F2d). These intermediate appellate-level courts hear appeals from US district courts, federal administrative agencies, and other federal trial-level courts. Individual US Courts of Appeals, known as circuits, are referred to by number (1st Cir, 2d Cir, etc) except for the District of Columbia Circuit (DC Cir) and the Federal Circuit (Fed Cir), which hears appeals from the US Claims Court and from various customs and patent cases. Citations to the *Federal Reporter* must include the circuit designation in parentheses with the year of the decision.

2. *Wilcox v United States,* 387 F2d 60 (5th Cir 1967).

US District Court and claims courts: Cite to *Federal Supplement* (F Supp). (There is only the original series so far.) These trial-level courts are not as prolific as the appellate courts; their function is to hear the original cases rather than review them. There are more than 100 of these courts, which are referred to by geographical designations that must be included in the citation (eg, the Northern District of Illinois [ND Ill], the Central District of California [CD Cal], but District of New Jersey [D NJ], as New Jersey has only one district).

3. *Sierra Club v Froehlke,* 359 F Supp 1289 (SD Tex 1973).

State courts: Cite to the appropriate official (ie, state-sanctioned and state-financed) reporter (if any) and the appropriate regional reporter. Most states have separate official reporters for their highest and intermediate appellate courts (eg, *Illinois Reports* and *Illinois Appellate Court Reports*), but the regional reporters include cases from both levels. Official reporters are always listed first, although an increasing number of states are no longer publishing them. The regional reporters are the *Atlantic Reporter* (A or A2d), *North Eastern Reporter* (NE or NE2d), *South Eastern Reporter* (SE or SE2d), *Southern Reporter* (So or So2d), *North Western Reporter* (NW or NW2d), *South Western Reporter* (SW or SW2d), and *Pacific Reporter* (P or P2d). If only the regional reporter citation is given, the name of the court must appear in parentheses with the year of the decision. If the opinion is from the highest court of a state (usually but not always known as the supreme court), the abbreviated state name is sufficient (except for Ohio St). The full name of the court is abbreviated (eg, Ill App, NJ Super Ct App Div, NY App Div). A third, also unofficial, reporter is published for a few states; citations solely to these reporters must include the court name (eg, *California Reporter* [Cal Rptr], *New York Supplement* [NYS or NYS2d]).

4. *People v Carpenter,* 28 Ill2d 116, 190 NE2d 738 (1963).

5. *Webb v Stone,* 445 SW2d 842 (Ky 1969).

When a case has been reviewed or otherwise dealt with by a higher court, the subsequent history of the case should be given in the citation. If the year is the same for both opinions, include it only at the end of the citation. The phrases indicating the subsequent history are set off by commas, italicized, and abbreviated (eg, *aff'd* [affirmed by the higher court], *rev'd* [reversed], *vacated* [made legally void, annulled], *appeal dismissed, cert denied* [application for a writ of certiorari, ie, a request that a court hear an appeal, has been denied]).

6. *Glazer v Glazer,* 374 F2d 390 (5th Cir), cert denied, 389 US 831 (1967).

This opinion was written by the US Court of Appeals for the Fifth Circuit in 1967. In the same year, the US Supreme Court was asked to review the case in an application for a writ of certiorari but denied the request. This particular subsequent history is important because it indicates that the case has been taken to the highest court available and thus strengthens the case's value as precedent for future legal decisions.

Citation of statutes: Once a bill is enacted into law by the US Congress, it is integrated into the US Code (USC). Citations of statutes include the official name of the act, the title number (similar to a chapter number), the abbreviation of the code cited, the section number (designated by §), and the date of the code edition cited.

7. Comprehensive Environmental Response, Compensation, and Liability Act, 42 USC 9601-9675 (1988).

The above example cites sections 9601-9675 of title 42 of the US Code.

If a federal statute has not yet been codified, cite to Statutes at Large (abbreviated Stat, preceded by a volume number, and followed by a page number), if available, and the Public Law number of the statute.

8. Pub L No. 93-627, 88 Stat 2126.

The name of the statute may be added if it provides clarification.

9. Labor Management Relations (Taft-Hartley) Act 301(a), 29USC 185a (1988).

Citation forms for state statutes vary considerably. Table T.1 in *The Bluebook* lists examples for each state.

10. Ill Rev Stat ch 38, 2

This is section 2 of chapter 38 of Illinois Revised Statutes.

11. Fla Stat 202.

This is section 202 of Florida Statutes.

12. Mich Comp Laws 145.

This is section 145 of Michigan Comp-ed Laws.

13. Wash Rev Code 45.

This is section 45 of Revised Code of Washington.

14. Cal Corp Code 300.

This is section 300 of California Corporations Code.

Citation of federal administrative regulations: Federal regulations are published in the *Federal Register* and then codified in the Code of Federal Regulations.

15. 55 *Federal Register* 36612 (1990) (codified at 26 CFR 52).

If a rule or regulation is known by its name, the name should be given.

16. Medicare, Medicaid and CLIA programs: regulations implementing the Clinical Laboratory Improvement Amendments of 1988 (CLIA), 57 *Federal Register* 7002 (1992).

Regulations promulgated by the Internal Revenue Service retain their unique format. Temporary regulations must be denoted as such.

17. Treas Reg 1.72 (1963).

18. Temp Treas Reg 1.338 (1985).

Citation forms for state administrative regulations are especially diverse. Again, Table T.1 in *The Bluebook* lists the appropriate form for each state.

Citation of congressional hearings: Include the full title of the hearing, the subcommittee (if any) and committee names, the number and session of the Congress, the date, and a short description if desired.

19. *Hearings Before the Consumer Subcommittee of the Senate Committee on Commerce,* 90th Cong, 1st Sess (1965) (testimony of William Stewart, MD, surgeon general).

20. *Discrimination on the Basis of Pregnancy, 1977: Hearings on S995 Before the Subcommittee on Labor of the Senate Committee on Human Resources,* 95th Cong, 1st Sess (1977) (statement of Ethel Walsh, vice-chairman, EEOC).

Citations to services: Many legal materials, including some reports of cases and some administrative materials, are published by commercial services (eg, Commerce Clearing House), often in looseleaf format. These services attempt to provide a comprehensive overview of rapidly changing areas of the law (eg, tax law, labor law, securities regulation) and are updated frequently, sometimes weekly. The citation should include the volume number

of the service, its abbreviated title, the publisher's name (also abbreviated), the paragraph or section or page number, and the date.

21. 7 Sec Reg Guide (P-H) 2333 (1984).

The above example cites volume 7, paragraph 2333, of the *Securities Regulation Guide,* published by Prentice-Hall in 1984.

22. 54 Ins L Rep (CCH) 137 (1979).

This is volume 54, page 137, of *Insurance Law Reports,* published by Commerce Clearing House in 1979.

23. 4 OSH Rep (BNA) 750 (1980).

This is volume 4, page 750, of the *Occupational Safety and Health Reporter,* published by the Bureau of National Affairs in 1980.

Acknowledgment
Principal author: Cheryl Iverson.

References
1. International Committee of Medical Journal Editors. Uniform requirements for manuscripts submitted to biomedical journals. *JAMA.* 1993;269:2282-2286.

2. JAMA instructions for authors. *JAMA.* 1997;277:74-82.

3. Haynes RB, Mulrow CD, Huth EJ, Altman DG, Gardner MJ. More informative abstracts revisited. *Ann Intern Med.* 1990;113:69-76.

4. Yankauer A. The accuracy of medical journal references. *CBE Views.* April 1990;13:38-42.

5. Broadus RN. An investigation of the validity of bibliographic citations. *J Am Soc Information Sci.* 1983;34:132-135.

6. Evans JT, Nadjari HI, Burchell SA. Quotational and reference accuracy in surgical journals: a continuing peer review problem. *JAMA.* 1990;263:1353-1354.

7. Shenoy BV. Peer review [letter]. *JAMA.* 1990;264:3142.

8. Schofield EK. Accuracy of references [letter]. *CBE Views.* June 1990;13:68.

9. Patrias K. *National Library of Medicine Recommended Formats for Bibliographic Citation.* Bethesda, Md: National Library of Medicine, Reference Service; 1991.

10. *List of Journals Indexed in Index Medicus: 1996.* Washington, DC: National Library of Medicine; 1996. NIH publication 96-267.

11. *Books in Print: 1995-96.* New Providence, NJ: RR Bowker; 1995:1-9.

12. Williams MA. Citing electronic information. *CBE Views.* 1995;18:60.

13. Guernsey L. Cyberspace citations: scholars debate how best to cite research conducted on the Internet. *Chron Higher Educ.* January 12, 1996:A18, 20-21.

14. Li X, Crane N. Electronic Styles: *An Expanded Guide to Citing Electronic Information.* Westport, Conn: Meckler Publishers. In press. Examples available at: http://www.uvm.edu/xli/reference/estyles.html.

15. Ivey KC. Citing Internet souces. *Editorial Eye.* August 1996:10.

16. Council of Biology Editors Style Manual Committee. *Scientific Style and Format: The CBE Manual for Authors, Editors, and Publishers.* 6th ed. New York, NY: Cambridge University Press; 1994.

17. *The Chicago Manual of Style.* 14th ed. Chicago, Ill: University of Chicago Press; 1993.

18. *The Bluebook: A Uniform System of Citation.* 15th ed. Cambridge, Mass: The Harvard Law Review Association; 1991.

Additional readings and general references
Council of Biology Editors Style Manual Committee. *Scientific Style and Format: The CBE Manual for Authors, Editors, and Publishers.* 6th ed. New York, NY: Cambridge University Press; 1994.

Hall GM, ed. *How to Write a Paper.* London, England: BMJ Publishing Group; 1994.

Huth EJ. *How to Write and Publish Papers in the Medical Sciences.* 2nd ed. Baltimore, Md: Williams & Wilkins; 1990. (MAN-1997)

Referrals, Medical Facilities

AMA Policy

Conflicts of interest. Physician ownership of medical facilities (H.140.961) CEJA Rep C, I-91; Reaffirmed: Sub Res 4, I-92. (Section)

(*g*) Physicians must disclose their investment interest to their patients when making a referral. Patients must be given a list of effective alternative facilities if any such facilities become reasonably available, informed that they have the option to use one of the alternative facilities, and assured that they will not be treated differently by the physician if they do not choose the physician-owned facility. These disclosure requirements also apply to physician investors who directly provide care or services for their patients in facilities outside their office practice.

Introduction to Stark I

In 1991, the Health Care Financing Administration (HCFA) published regulations for the Ethics in Patient Referrals Act. This Act was called "Stark I" because of its author, US Representative Fortney "Pete" Stark (D Calif). Stark's Act prohibited physician referrals of Medicare patients to clinical laboratories where the physicians had ongoing financial involvement. The financial involvement or relationship was defined as "any ownership or investment interest (including both equity and debt) or any compensation arrangement."

Overview

Stark I was enacted through the consolidated Omnibus Budget Reconciliation Act of 1990, and published in late 1991. Limited in its scope, the primary objective of this law is the prevention of physician referrals to clinical laboratories in which they have financial relationships. Many practicing physicians operating private laboratories as an adjunct to their medical practice experienced financial repercussions from this law. However, subsequent "Stark" legislation rendered widespread financial consequences on practicing physicians.

Introduction to Stark II

The Consolidated Omnibus Budget Reconciliation Act of 1993 authorized an extension of the initial provisions of Stark I. As of January 1, 1995, Stark II prohibited physicians and physician family members with financial relationship to an organization from referring a patient to that organization for clinical laboratory services and to any of 10 additional "designated health services." Distinguishing itself from Stark I, Stark II restricted referrals of Medicaid patients in addition to Medicare patients.

Overview

With Stark II becoming effective January 1, 1995, the primary objective of this law was to preclude physicians from the Medicare and Medicaid referrals noted above. Primarily, this was for referrals to clinical laboratories and the other "designated health services." These were designed to be preclusions from organizations with whom physicians maintain financial relationships. Such "designated health services" are following:

1. Physical therapy.
2. Occupational therapy.
3. Radiology or other diagnostic.
4. Radiation therapy.
5. Durable medical equipment (DME).
6. Parenteral and enteral nutrients, equipment, and supplies.
7. Prosthetics, orthotics, and prosthetic devices.
8. Home health care.
9. Outpatient prescription drugs.
10. Inpatient and outpatient hospital care.

Together a comprehensive list, number 10 alone—inpatient and outpatient hospital services—brings immense implications for the operations of physicians and to the valuation of physician practices.

Introduction to Stark III

Now, Stark III legislation is under way. This is a broad and sweeping bill aiming at extending the current referral bands to all patients, whatever payor. Further, this legislation anticipates including all ancillary services. With the shift of the United States Congress to a Republican majority in 1995, Congress has reduced, or placed on extended hold, the Stark III legislation.

Summary

Stark legislation has caused sweeping changes in health care and, in addition, uncertainty and questions of the legality of certain transactions. Overall, the Stark legislation attempts to prohibit any provider transactions that are illegal referrals of patients by the physician. The true objectives of all Stark legislation are curbing physician referral practices based on perceived conflicts of interest, and preventing overutilization of identified medical services.

Due to the complicated nature of this legislation and its implications, health care entities contemplating buying, selling, or contracting should consult qualified legal counsel and experienced valuation experts quickly. This should preclude costly misunderstandings about the legality of certain business practices and their bearing on valuation. (AVMP-1996)

Referrals, Physician

What you can't—or shouldn't—do to get referrals

Ryan Ver Berkmoes
AM News Oct 23, 1993 p 48

Boosting your referrals calls not just for sharp business acumen, but sensitivity and tact as well. Just as a hot-pink door would be a major no-no in certain suburban subdivisions, so would behavior in the hospital that goes against accepted norms.

And some referral-boosting efforts might even violate federal law.

As you plan your referral strategy, keep in mind what the law and local norms dictate. In some communities, a comprehensive marketing package of brochures, Rolodex cards, and the like would be considered quite proper, in others it would be much too showy.

And in addition to examining how your efforts will be seen by others, take into account as well any hospital or local medical society regulations.

In some hospitals, entertaining the emergency department staff would be seen as at least proper, if not generous. In others, the gesture would run afoul of conflict-of-interest doctrines, and may raise the ire of other physicians who consider it a form of kickback.

And speaking of kickbacks, keep in mind that it's illegal to offer or accept any kind of consideration for referral of Medicare or Medicaid patients.

While an occasional cup of coffee or dinner might be OK, attorneys warn that any kind of gift, particularly any routine gift, could be construed as a violation under the broad language of the federal kickback ban. You may want to check with legal counsel if you're uncertain about what you're doing, or limit gifts to physicians who refer only private-pay patients.

Regulations aside, the bottom line is to have a referrals strategy that earns the respect and admiration of your colleagues—not their ire.

Public:
Contact county medical society.

Rehabilitation

American Academy of Physical Medicine and Rehabilitation
1 IBM Plaza, 25th Fl, Chicago, IL 60611-3604
312 464-9700   Fax 312 464-0227
Web address: http://www.aapmr.org

American Board of Physical Medicine and Rehabilitation
21 First St SW, Ste 674, Rochester, MN 55902
507 282-1776   Fax 507 282-9242

American Congress of Rehabilitation Medicine
4700 W Lake St, Glenview, IL 60025-1485
847 375-4725
E-mail: acrm@amctec.com

National Rehabilitation Information Center
8455 Colesville Rd, Ste 935
Silver Spring, MD 20910-3319
800 346-2742   301 588-9284   Fax 301 587-1967

Rehabilitation Counselor

History of profession

Initially, rehabilitation professionals were recruited from a variety of human service disciplines, including public health nursing, social work, and school counseling. Although educational programs began to appear in the 1940s, it was not until the availability of federal funding for rehabilitation counseling programs in 1954 that the profession began to grow and establish its own identity.

Historically, rehabilitation counselors primarily served working-age adults with disabilities. Today, the need for rehabilitation counseling services extends to children and the elderly. Rehabilitation counselors may also provide general and specialized counseling to people with disabilities in public human service programs and private practice settings.

Accreditation history

In 1969, a group of rehabilitation professionals met to discuss the need for accreditation of rehabilitation counselor education (RCE) programs. After 2 years of planning, the Council on Rehabilitation Education (CORE) was formed in 1971 and incorporated in 1972. Five professional rehabilitation organizations were represented by CORE:

- American Rehabilitation Association (ARA), formerly the International Association of Rehabilitation Facilities.
- American Rehabilitation Counseling Association (ARCA).
- Council of State Administrators of Vocational Rehabilitation (CSAVR).
- National Council on Rehabilitation Education (NCRE), formerly the Council on Rehabilitation Educators.
- National Rehabilitation Counseling Association (NRCA).

Today, these five organizations—except ARA, which has been replaced by the National Council of State Agencies of the Blind (NCSAB)—comprise CORE and as such represent the professional and organizational constituencies concerned with the training, evaluation, and employment of rehabilitation counselors. CORE accredits approximately 80 university- and college-based rehabilitation counselor educational programs at the master's degree level. Accreditation serves to promote the effective delivery of rehabiltation services to people with disabilities by stimulating and fostering continual review and improvement of master's degree rehabilitation counselor educational programs.

Occupational description

Working directly with an individual with a disability, the rehabilitation counselor determines and coordinates services to assist people with disabilities in moving from psychological and economic dependence to independence.

Job description

Rehabilitation counselors assist people with physical, mental, emotional, or social disabilities to become or remain self-sufficient, productive citizens. Disabilities may result from birth defects, illness and disease, work-related injuries, automobile accidents, the stresses of war, work, and daily life, and the aging process. Rehabilitation counselors help individuals with disabilities deal with societal and personal problems, plan careers, and find and keep satisfying jobs. They may also work with individuals, professional organizations, and advocacy groups to address the environmental and social barriers that create obstacles for people with disabilities. The rehabilitation counselor builds bridges between the often isolated world of people with disabilities and their families, communities, and work environments.

Other responsibilities for the rehabilitation counselor include:
- Evaluating an individual's potential for independent living and employment and arranging for medical and psychological care and vocational assessment, training, and job placement.
- Evaluating medical and psychological reports and conferring with physicians and psychologists about the types of work individuals can perform.
- Working with employers to identify and/or modify job responsibilities to accommodate individuals with disabilities.

The rehabilitation counselor draws on knowledge from several fields, including psychology, medicine, psychiatry, sociology, social work, education, and law. Their specialized knowledge of disabilities and environmental factors that interact with disabilities, as well as specific knowledge and skills, differentiate rehabilitation counselors from other types of counselors.

Employment outlook
Rehabilitation counselors serve a large portion of the US population. An estimated 43 million Americans have physical, mental, or psychological disabilities that restrict their activities and prevent them from obtaining or maintaining jobs.

Consequently, the employment outlook for the profession is excellent: Based on national employment outlook studies and regional and state surveys, hundreds of rehabilitation counselor positions are expected to be available throughout the 1990s and into the next century for qualified masters-level professionals. Recent studies show that RCE programs are not graduating sufficient numbers of qualified students to meet current and anticipated marketplace needs.

Recently the roles and responsibilities of rehabilitation counselors have expanded, further increasing the attractiveness of a career in the profession. Rehabilitation counselors, for example, have begun to determine, coordinate, and arrange for rehabilitation and transition services for children within school systems. In addition, rehabilitation counselors are providing geriatric rehabilitation services to older persons with health problems, and workers injured on the job are increasingly receiving rehabilitation services through private rehabilitation counseling companies and employers' disability management and employment assistance programs.

Many former teachers, attorneys, nurses, physical therapists, occupational therapists, clergy, and businesspeople have found second careers as rehabilitation counselors.

Employment characteristics
Most rehabilitation counselors work in state or federal rehabilitation agencies. Because all state rehabilitation agencies follow the same general procedures, a rehabilitation counselor has geographical mobility and can find employment throughout the United States and its territories. Other potential employers include comprehensive rehabilitation centers, universities and academic settings, insurance companies, substance abuse rehabilitation centers, correctional facilities, halfway houses, and independent living centers. Reflecting this wide range of job opportunities, rehabilitation counselors are often employed in positions with different job titles, such as counselor, job placement specialist, substance abuse counselor, probation and parole officer, mental health counselor, marriage and family counselor, and independent living specialist.

According to the NCRE, the average starting salary for rehabilitation counselors in the public sector is more than $23,000 and can range between $16,000 and $32,000; the salary ranges in the private sector are considerably higher. The average overall salary is estimated at more than $30,000. (AHRP-1997)

Resources
American Rehabilitation Counseling Association (ARCA)
5999 Stevenson Ave, Alexandria, VA 22304
703 620-4404

Commission on Rehabilitation Counselor Certification (CRCC)
1835 Rohlwing Rd, Ste E, Rolling Meadows, IL 60008
847 394-2104

Council on Rehabilitation Education (CORE)
1835 Rohlwing Rd, Ste E, Rolling Meadows, IL 60008
847 394-1785   Fax 847 394-2108

National Association of Rehabilitation Professionals in the Private Sector (NARPPS)
PO Box 697, Brookline, MA 02146
617 566-4432

National Council on Rehabilitation Education (NCRE)
c/o Dr Garth Eldredge
Department of Special Education and Rehabilitation
Utah State University, Logan, UT 84322-2870
801 797-3241

National Rehabilitation Counseling Association (NRCA)
8807 Sudley Rd #102, Manassas, VA 22110-4719
703 361-2077

Research
The Albert Lasker awards
Jane Kenamore, AMA Archives, 1997

Established in 1945, The Albert Lasker awards recognize achievement in basic medical research, clinical medical research, and public service. Considered by many to be among the most significant prizes in the field of medicine, the Lasker awards have recognized approximately 300 individuals, 56 of whom have gone on to become Nobel Laureates.

Lasker award recipients are selected annually by a jury of 20 individuals. Appointed by the Albert and Mary Lasker Foundation, the jurors are themselves leaders in the medical profession, many having received Lasker or Nobel prizes before their appointments to the jury. Over the past 52 years, the Lasker awards have commemorated such medical milestones as the discovery of penicillin as a cure for syphilis (1946), development of polio vaccines (1954), development of the birth control pill (1960), development of the heart-lung machine making open heart surgery possible (1968), design of a total hip joint replacement (1974), research on the retrovirus that causes AIDS (1986), and investigation revealing that DNA is the chemical substance of heredity (1994). Individuals cited by the Foundation include such well-known physicians and scientists as George Papanicolaou, MD (1950), Jonas Salk, MD (1956), Paul Dudley White, MD (1953), Albert Sabin, MD (1965), and Michael E. DeBakey, MD (1963), among many others. Public Service recipients have included Eunice Kennedy Shriver (1966), Anne Landers (1985), and Lyndon Baines Johnson (1965).

Albert Lasker, after whom the award is named, was born in Germany in 1880 and raised in Galveston, Texas. After working for a short time for newspapers in Galveston and Dallas, Lasker moved to Chicago, where he accepted a position for $10/week in the advertising firm of Lord and Thomas. Within 10 years, Lasker owned the company. Amassing a sizable fortune in advertising, Lasker displayed an interest in medical research as early as 1922, when he contributed $50,000 to the Cancer Institute. Six years later, he contributed over $1 million to the University of Chicago for a study of degenerative diseases.

Lasker married Mary Woodward Reinhardt in 1940, his first wife having died in 1936 and his second marriage having ended in divorce. In 1942, the Laskers established the Albert and Mary Lasker Foundation; and 2 years later, Mary Lasker conceived the first Albert Lasker Medical Research Award, as a birthday gift to her husband. Envisioning the award as an annual prize to produce a cure for cancer, Mary Lasker wrote in her birthday note: "I hope the person who discovers the cure will be the 10th recipient of the Albert Lasker Medical Research Award."

After Lasker died in 1952, Mary Lasker remained a leader in the support of medical research until her own death at the age of 92 in 1993. The Mary Woodward Lasker Charitable Trust has been created from her estate, and it is expected that the Lasker Foundation will use the funds to establish new programs to advance medical research.

References

Albert and Mary Lasker Foundation. *The Albert Lasker Medical Research Awards* [program]. New York, NY: Albert and Mary Lasker Foundation; 1996.

Lasker Saga Recounted. *Galveston News,* June 26, 1960, p 4-B.

Resources

Albert and Mary Lasker Foundation
865 First Ave, New York, NY 10017
212 753-8222   Fax 212 832-8514
Web address: http://www.laskerfoundation.com.

Piccirelli A, ed. *Research Centers Directory.* 17th ed. 2 vols. Detroit, Mich: Gale Research; 1993. ISBN 0-8103-7617-2 (set)

Computer Retrieval of Information on Scientific Projects (CRISP)
Research Documentation Section
Information Systems Branch
Division of Research Grants
Westwood Bldg, Room 148, 5333 Westbard Ave
Bethesda, MD 20895
301 496-7543

National Research Council, Office of Public Affairs
2101 Constitution NW, Washington, DC 20418
202 334-2000
Web address: http://www.nas.edu

Research, Ethics

AMA Policy

Support of biomedical research: (H.460.998) BOT Rep S, A-74; Reaffirmed; CLRPD Rep C, A-89.

The AMA endorses and supports the following 10 principles considered essential if continuing support and recognition of biomedical research vital to the delivery of quality medical care is to be a national goal: (1) The support of biomedical research is the responsibility of both government and private resources. (2) The National Institutes of Health must be budgeted so that they can exert effective administrative and scientific leadership in the biomedical research enterprise. (3) An appropriate balance must be struck between support of project grants and of contracts. (4) Federal appropriations to promote research in specifically designated disease categories should be limited and made cautiously. (5) Funds should be specifically appropriated to train personnel in biomedical research. (6) Grants should be awarded under the peer review system. (7) The roles of the private sector and of government in supporting biomedical research are complementary. (8) Although the AMA supports the principle of committed federal support of biomedical research, the Association will not necessarily endorse all specific legislative and regulatory action that affects biomedical research. (9) To implement the objectives of section 8, the board will establish mechanisms for continuing study, review, and evaluation of all aspects of federal support of biomedical research. (10) The AMA will accept responsibility for informing the public on the relevance of basic and clinical research to the delivery of quality medical care.

Helsinki Report
(Recommendations regarding biomedical research involving humans)

World Medical Association Handbook of Declarations
World Medical Association
(Association Medicale Mondiale—AMM)
28, Avenue des Alpes,
F-01210 Ferney-Voltaire, France
To call from the United States, dial the following numbers: 011-33-50-40-7575
Fax 011-33-50-40-5937

Residents

Report finds abuse of NY resident rules; hospitals say no [excerpt]

Leigh Page
AM News Jan 16, 1995 pp 5-7

Ground-breaking state regulations on residents' working conditions are being widely violated in New York City hospitals, a new study suggests.

The report, by the city's Office of the Public Advocate, was released as former residents were being tried in the case that led to the creation of the work rules—the 1984 death of a patient at a prestigious Manhattan hospital.

Broader lessons?

New York is the only state that regulates residents' work conditions. But what happened there—especially in New York City—may have important ramifications for the rest of the nation. The city's hospitals have all the problems of residency programs elsewhere, only on a larger, more urgent scale.

Critics of US residency training say it exposes trainees to exploitation, arguing that they can be a cheap form of labor for cash-strapped hospitals that can't afford to hire attending physicians. And since residents must complete training for board certification, they are not likely to protest poor working conditions, critics allege.

New York City residents are especially exploited, they say. City hospitals, beset by constant financial problems, serve large indigent populations, often in dangerous neighborhoods where most doctors won't practice. Virtually every community hosptial in the city runs several training programs, with residents doing work that in the suburbs would be performed by highly paid, fully trained physicians.

As a result, New York City has the largest contingent of residents in the nation. Some 12,000 residents train in the city, amounting to an estimated 160 residents per 100,000 population, four times the national average. Only Washington, DC, has a higher concentration.

Critics say a system that overworks unsupervised trainees can have tragic consequences for patients. The city study, for example, alleged that two people died, apparently because of mistakes made by unsupervised residents.

In one case, an ob-gyn resident performing an unsupervised delivery allegedly overlooked evidence of fetal distress, leading to the newborn's death 11 hours later, the report said. In the other case cited, a 10-year old boy "died in agony" after a medical resident reportedly ignored pleas by the boy's mother that he needed "a simple, yet life-saving operation."

A grim warning of what such mistakes can lead to was playing out in a Manhattan courtroom when the study was released. Four physicians at New York Hospital are fighting a malpractice suit alleging that errors by unsupervised residents led to the death of patient Libby Zion when she was admitted to the hospital 10 years ago.

The suit, filed in state court, names three former residents and one supervising physician at the time of Zion's death. The defendants deny any wrong-doing.

Intern. Historically "intern" was used to designate individuals in the first post-MD year of hospital training; less commonly it designated individuals in the first year of any residency program. Since 1975 the *Graduate Medical Education Directory* and the Accreditation Council for Graduate Medical Education (ACGME) have not used the term, instead referring to individuals in their first year of training as residents.

Resident. An individual at any level of graduate medical education in a program accredited by the ACGME. Trainees in subspecialty programs are specifically included.

Fellow. A term used by some hospitals and in some specialties to designated trainees in subspecialty GME programs. *The Graduate Medical Education Directory* and the ACGME use "resident" to designate all GME trainees in ACGME-accredited programs. (GME-1996)

JAMA Issue of Note: Medical Education

JAMA's Medical Education issue appears annually the fourth week of September

Resources

National Association of Residents and Interns
292 Madison Ave, New York, NY 10017
800 221-2168   212 949-5900   Fax 212 949-5910

National Resident Matching Program
2450 N St NW, Ste 201, Washington, DC 20037-1141
202 828-0676
Web address: http://www.aamc.org

Respiratory Therapy

History

In 1957, a resolution to develop schools of inhalation therapy was introduced to the American Medical Association (AMA) House of Delegates by the Medical Society of New York. Following approval, the resolution was referred to the Council on Medical Education (CME) and subsequently resulted in the proposed report titled *Standards (Essentials) for an Approved School of Inhalation Therapy Technicians*. The proposed *Standards* were tested during the next few years, after which they were recommended for adoption by the CME and formally approved by the AMA House of Delegates in December 1962. The *Standards* were revised in 1967 and included the requirements of an 18-month program.

In 1970, the Board of Schools was reorganized and incorporated as the Joint Review Committee for Inhalation Therapy Education. In 1972, the American Thoracic Society became another sponsor of the Joint Review Committee. In 1972, the *Standards* underwent a third revision, and additional *Standards* were developed for a shorter educational program for training individuals to function as technicians. The *Standards* were approved by the sponsors of the Board of Schools for Inhalation Therapy, the American Society of Anesthesiologists, the American College of Chest Physicians, the American Association of Inhalation Therapy, and the AMA CME, and were adopted by the AMA House of Delegates in June 1972. In 1977, the review committee's name was changed to the Joint Review Committee for Respiratory Therapy Education (JRCRTE).

In 1986, *Standards* for both the respiratory therapy technician and the respiratory therapist were consolidated and the revision was adopted by the sponsors of the JRCRTE and by the AMA.

Respiratory Therapist

Occupational description
The respiratory therapist applies scientific knowledge and theory to practical clinical problems of respiratory care. The respiratory therapist is qualified to assume primary responsibility for all respiratory care modalities, including the supervision of respiratory therapy technician functions. The respiratory therapist may be required to exercise considerable independent clinical judgment, under the supervision of a physician, in the respiratory care of patients.

Job description
In fulfillment of the therapist role, the respiratory therapist may:
- Review, collect, and recommend obtaining additional data. The therapist evaluates all data to determine the appropriateness of the prescribed respiratory care and participates in the development of the respiratory care plan.
- Select, assemble, and check all equipment used in providing respiratory care.
- Initiate and conduct therapeutic procedures, and modify prescribed therapeutic procedures to achieve one or more specific objectives.
- Maintain patient records and communicate relevant information to other members of the health care team.
- Assist the physician in performing special procedures in a clinical laboratory, procedure room, or operating room.

Employment characteristics
Respiratory therapy personnel are employed in hospitals, nursing care facilities, clinics, physicians' offices, companies providing emergency oxygen services, and municipal organizations.

According to 1996 data from the American Association for Respiratory Care, a respiratory therapist, on average, earns $32,926. (AHRP-1997)

Respiratory Therapy Technician

Occupational description
The respiratory therapy technician administers general respiratory care. Technicians may assume clinical responsibility for specified respiratory care modalities involving the application of well-defined therapeutic techniques under the supervision of a respiratory therapist and a physician.

Job description
In fulfillment of the technician role, the respiratory therapy technician may:
- Review clinical data, history, and respiratory therapy orders.
- Collect clinical data by interview and examination of the patient. This includes collecting portions of the data by inspection, palpation, percussion, and auscultation of the patient.
- Recommend and/or perform and review additional bedside procedures, X rays, and laboratory tests.
- Evaluate data to determine the appropriateness of the prescribed respiratory care.
- Assemble and maintain equipment used in respiratory care.
- Ensure cleanliness and sterility by the selection and/or performance of appropriate disinfecting techniques and monitor their effectiveness.
- Initiate, conduct, and modify prescribed therapeutic procedures.

Employment characteristics
Respiratory therapy personnel are employed in hospitals, nursing care facilities, clinics, doctors' offices, companies providing emergency oxygen services, and municipal organizations.

According to 1996 data from the American Association for Respiratory Care, a respiratory therapy technician, on average, earns $26,707. (AHRP-1997)

Resources
AMA Allied Health Department
312 553-9355

American Association for Respiratory Care
11030 Ables Ln, Dallas, TX 75229-4593
214 243-2272   Fax 214 484-2720
E-mail: aarc@spaceworks.com

Joint Review Committee for Respiratory
Therapy Education
1701 W Euless Blvd, Ste 300, Euless, TX 76040
800 874-5615   817 283-2835   Fax 817 354-8519

National Board for Respiratory Care
8310 Nieman Rd, Lenexa, KS 66214
913 599-4200   Fax 913 541-0156

Retinitis Pigmentosa
RP Foundation Fighting Blindness
1401 Mt Royal Ave, 4th Fl
Baltimore, MD 21217-4245
800 638-2300   410 225-9400   Fax 410 225-3936

Retirement
Selecting a corporate retirement plan

Retirement plans that meet certain Internal Revenue Service requirements (ie, qualified plans) offer significant tax advantages to physicians. Briefly, the major advantages are:

1. Amounts contributed by the professional corporation (or to the noncorporate entity in which the physician practices) to a qualified retirement plan are immediately deductible from the income of the corporation or other entity.

2. Physicians do not have to pay current income tax on these contributions to the plan at the time they are made. Rather, physicians will not be taxed on those benefits until they are actually distributed to them.

3. Earnings and capital gains made by investments of the plan's funds are not subject to state or federal income taxes when received, but only after they're distributed to the physician. That means the yearly earnings of the plan compound tax-free, and therefore increase at a much greater rate than if they were subject to taxes.

4. Certain distributions from a qualified plan can be taxed in advantageous ways:

a. If the physician receives a lump-sum distribution of the benefits under the plan after age 59½, the distribution can be subject to 5-year averaging if it meets certain requirements. Under 5-year averaging, the amount received is taxed in the year it is received, but it is taxed at rates that would have been applicable if it had been received over a 5-year period.

b. Individuals who are over 50 by January 1, 1986, may elect 10-year averaging under the rate schedule in effect in 1986, and in some cases may elect capital gains treatment for a portion of the distribution.

c. In order to qualify for 5-year averaging, 10-year averaging, or capital gains treatment, however, the distribution must be received on account of certain specified events, and must meet several complex conditions.

d. Certain distributions from qualified plans may be rolled over into an individual retirement account (IRA), and will not be taxed until they are withdrawn from the IRA. The rollover must occur no later than 60 days after the distribution is received, and this deadline cannot be extended for any reason.

A physician receiving a distribution from a plan should always seek the advice of a tax attorney or an accountant who is familiar with the physician's individual financial situation.

5. The first $5000 of a lump-sum death benefit from a qualified retirement plan can pass to a beneficiary free of income tax.

There are basically two types of qualified plans: defined-contribution plans and defined-benefit plans. Some plans, such as target-benefit plans, combine features of both type of plans.

Defined-contribution plans

Under this type of plan, contributions are made in an amount equal to a fixed percentage of each employee's salary or other compensation (hence the term *defined-contribution*). The employee's share of the contribution will be placed in his or her "account" in the plan, and that account will be adjusted from time to time by the employee's share of the plan's earnings, gains, and losses. The plan doesn't say anything about how much the employee will receive in benefits when he or she retires. The employee will simply get a pension (or lump-sum distribution) equal in value to the amount held in his or her account at the time of retirement.

Defined-contribution plans come in two basic forms: profit-sharing and money-purchasing pension plans. The former is usually based on corporate profits, although it is now possible to make a contribution even in the absence of profits. The latter is usually a straight percentage of the employee's annual compensation. These two forms are very similar, but the distinctions can be important for financial and tax-planning purposes. Money-purchase pension plans require a fixed contribution every year, no matter what. On the other hand, a profit-sharing plan is much more flexible, since the corporation isn't required to make a contribution every year, and even when it does it can change from year to year. The primary advantage of a money-purchase plan is that the contribution can

often go as high as 25% of a participant's compensation—but not more than $30,000 (1995 figure) per participant. However, the maximum contribution that can be made to a profit-sharing plan is generally 15% of compensation.

A professional corporation or a noncorporate entity should, in most cases, start out with a profit-sharing plan, since at first the practice's financial picture will be unclear, and this type is most flexible. Later, if retirement-plan contributions greater than 15% of employee compensation are desired, then a money-purchase pension plan can be adopted either instead of or in addition to the profit-sharing plan to make aggregate contributions of up to 25% of compensation. Contributions cannot be based on more than $150,000 (1995 figure) in compensation for any one employee. Therefore, a contribution level of at least 20% is necessary to make the maximum $30,000 contribution on behalf of any participant.

Defined-benefit plans

A defined-benefit plan is one in which the amount of benefit that the employee will receive upon retirement is guaranteed to be a certain amount—usually a specified percentage of the employee's compensation at the time of retirement. The contributions required to achieve that benefit level, however, can vary from year to year. In a defined-benefit plan, an actuary must figure, from the participant's age and other factors, how much must be contributed every year.

The most important feature of a defined-benefit plan is that the employer must contribute every year whatever sum is necessary to fund the plan adequately, which makes the plan very inflexible for financial-planning purposes. These plans are also complicated and often misunderstood by physicians and other corporate employees. However, for some physicians, defined-benefit plans may be an option worth exploring.

The primary advantage of a defined-benefit plan is that older physicians who have not previously maintained plans can often make larger contributions than are permissible in a defined-contribution plan. If an older physician has employees who are substantially younger than he or she is, that contribution can often be obtained at a substantially lower cost for covering the staff than would be the case in a defined-contribution plan.

Where several physicians are participating in the same plan, a defined-benefit plan will tend to favor the older participants, since the majority of contributions will be used to pay for benefits to the older physician participants. This may be an advantage if the group wishes to make substantially larger contributions on behalf of the older physicians than are made on behalf of the younger physicians. However, if younger physicians also wish to have substantial contributions made for them, a defined-benefit plan may, depending on their exact ages and certain other factors, actually reduce the maximum retirement-plan contributions that can be made on their behalf.

Target-benefit plans

A target-benefit plan has some features of a defined-benefit plan and some features of a defined-contribution plan. Its formula is structured as though it were a defined-benefit plan, and a contribution amount, based on

R that formula, is determined actuarially. Thus, older participants will generally receive larger contributions than younger ones. However, the formula used is only a "target" formula, and the targeted benefit is not guaranteed. Once the contribution amount is calculated, that amount is allocated to the participant's account as it would be in any other defined-contribution plan, and the participant's ultimate benefit from the plan is based on his or her account balance at the time of retirement. Target-benefit plans have become much more popular in recent years because of the increasing limitations on defined-benefit plans. (PRO-1989 with 1995 revision)

Resources

American Medical Association
Senior Physicians Services
515 N State Street, Chicago, IL 60610
312 464-2460

American Association of Retired Persons
601 E St NW, Washington, DC 20049
202 434-2277   Fax 202 434-2320
Web address: http://www.aarp.org

Review Courses

Note: These programs are not affiliated with the AMA, and their appearance in this directory does not constitute an endorsement or an approval by the AMA.

ArcVentures, Inc Educational Services
820 W Jackson Blvd, Chicago, IL 60607
312 258-5290

Sites available:
Chicago: 312 258-5290
New Jersey: 201 712-0897
Miami: 305 530-1930
Los Angeles: 213 258-5290

Postgraduate Medical Review Education, Inc
PO Box 414174, Miami Beach, FL 33141
800 433-3539

Stanley H. Kaplan
810 Seventh Ave, New York, NY 10019
800 527-8378 212 492-5810

Reye's Syndrome

Reye's Syndrome is a rare disorder characterized by brain and liver damage following an upper respiratory tract infection, chickenpox, or influenza. Reye's Syndrome is almost entirely confined to children under age 15.

Causes
Evidence suggests that Reye's Syndrome is often (but not invariably) related to taking aspirin for a viral infection. Physicians recommend that children be given acetaminophen instead of aspirin for viral infections or fever of unknown origin.

Symptoms and signs
Reye's Syndrome develops as the child is recovering from the infection, starting with uncontrollable vomiting, often with lethargy, memory loss, disorientation, or delirium. Swelling of the brain may cause seizures, deepening coma, disturbances in heart rhythm, and cessation of breathing. Jaundice indicates severe liver involvement. (ENC-1989)

Resource
National Reye's Syndrome Foundation
426 N Lewis, Box 829, Bryan, OH 43506
800 233-7393 (outside OH)   800 231-7399 (in OH)
419 636-2679   Fax 419 636-3366
E-mail: reyessyn@bright.net

Rheumatism

American College of Rheumatology
60 Executive Park S, Ste 150, Atlanta, GA 30329
404 633-3777   Fax 404 633-1870
Web address: http://www.rheumatology.org/~acr

Board Certification:
American Board of Internal Medicine
3624 Market St, Philadelphia, PA 19104
800 441-2246 215 243-1500   Fax 215 382-4702

Rhinology

American Rhinologic Society
Long Island College Hospital
Otolaryngology Department, c/o Frank Lucente
Brooklyn, NY 11201
718 780-1281   Fax 718 270-3924

American Laryngological, Rhinological and Otological Society
10 S Broadway, Ste 1401, St Louis, MO 63102
314 621-6550   Fax 314 621-6688

Runaway Hotlines

Missing Child Hotline
800 843-5678 9 am-Midnight

National Center for Missing and Exploited Children
2101 Wilson Blvd, Ste 550, Arlington, VA 22201
800 843-5678   703 235-3900   Fax 703 235-4067

Runaway Hotline
800 231-6946

Rural Health

Poetry and Medicine

Outliers

Tony Garland, MD
JAMA 1997 Feb 26; 277(8): 608h

Sadly, a scarcity of rural physicians is likely to be a continuing feature of medicine in the USA, even in the face of a physician surplus[1]

Facultative anaerobes,
We
Metabolize irony
In
The frequently airless
Outer reaches.

Obligate opportunists,
We
Recognize irony
As
The bioavailable form of
Truth here.

Scattergraphic outliers,
We
Realize irony
Has
Not been shown to
Sustain life.

Yet,
We dig in.

The agar yields.

Reference

1. Schroeder SA. Physician shortages in rural America. *Lancet.* 1995;345:1002.

A Piece of My Mind

Daddy

William H. Hunter, MD
JAMA 1984 May 4; 251(17): 2184

Back in 1953 I had just begun my practice in the small town of Clemson at the foot of the Blue Ridge Mountains in South Carolina. In the beginning I spent a lot of time reading medical journals and waiting for the local people to find out I was in town.

One August evening near dusk, my wife, Jane, and I were sitting in the swing when two farmers approached the porch and asked: "You the new doctor?" I nodded.

"Well, Doc, Daddy's down and sick and the doctor we called isn't treating him right."

"What's the matter?"

"This here doctor wants to put Daddy in a hospital."

I asked what he'd been treating him for.

"He hadn't been treating him for nothin'. Last time Daddy had a doctor was in '33, when he fell out of the loft and broke his leg."

"Well, what did the doctor say was the matter?" I asked.

"He said Daddy was havin' a heart attack, and damned if he was gonna treat him at home. He wanted to take him down to the hospital in Anderson, Doc. That's 20 miles away. Are you comin' to see him or we just gonna stand here and talk?"

So, after going by my office and getting my new ECG machine that had never been used on a sick patient, I followed their truck up through the rolling hills toward the foot of the mountains.

This was the most beautiful country in the world, covered with small and middle-sized farms inhabited by very independent people. They'd come from Celtic stock and had been there since they drove out the Cherokee in 1781 (after the Indians came out for King George). They were fiercely loyal to each other, shared a common dislike for revenuers, voted Republican in a Democratic state, and yet were the most hospitable people I'd ever met. Pickens County, South Carolina, had produced more Congressional Medal of Honor recipients than any other in the United States, and while there's no record, they probably had more court-martialings as well.

"Daddy," whom I was going to see, turned out to be the patriarch of this part of the country. When we arrived, there were about 50 people standing around under the white oaks. Daddy raised himself from his bed, gasping a bit. He gave me a look that said: "Is this the best those boys could do? Guess I'll just have to put up with him."

He was 76 years old. The ECG confirmed a myocardial infarction with numerous PVCs, and there were wet rales in both lung bases. I was six weeks out of what I thought was a good internship in one of the best teaching hospitals in the Carolinas, but I wasn't prepared for this. My looks must have betrayed me (Celtic types read a lot into looks), because Daddy gasped: "Doc, I was born in this house, lived here all my life, and I'm gonna die in this house. You just do the best you can."

I sent for an oxygen tank and sent Jane to the hospital for heparin. I used mercuhydrin intravenously and sat by his bed poking nitroglycerin into him and injecting Demerol until about 1 am, when he was finally free of pain and his lungs began to clear. I went back out on the porch for some fresh air and saw more than 100 people had gathered under the trees. When I left at sunrise, many of them were still there.

I'm sure, deep down, that Daddy's recovery had more to do with his tough constitution, but I got the credit. There's never been a want of patients in my practice since then. And from that time, I was always invited to their family reunions, where the preacher would sit on one side of Daddy and I sat on the other.

Resources

National Rural Health Association
1 W Armour Blvd, Ste 301, Kansas City, MO 64111
816 756-3140   Fax 816 756-3144

National Health Service Corps Headquarters
(recruiting physicians for rural areas)
5600 Fishers Ln, Rockville, MD 20857
301 443-2900

Rural Information Center Health Services (RICHS)
National Agricultural Library
Beltsville, MD 20705
800 633-7701   301 344-2547
Web address: http://www.nal.usda.gov/ric/richs

Safety

AMA Policy

Injury Prevention (H-10.982) Res 410, A-92; Reaffirmed by BOT Rep 19 - I-94, Reaffirmed by BOT Rep 34, A-95, Modified and Reaffirmed by BOT Rep 52, I-95

The AMA (1) supports the CDC's efforts to (*a*) conduct research, (*b*) develop a national program of surveillance and focused interventions to prevent injuries, and (*c*) evaluate the effectiveness of interventions, implementation strategies, and injury prevention programs; (2) supports a Public Health Service public information campaign to inform the public and its policymakers of the injury problem and the potential for effective intervention; (3) supports the development of a National Center for Injury Control at the CDC; and (4) encourages state and local medical societies to support, in conjunction with state and local health departments, efforts to make injury control a priority, and advise the leadership of the United States Congress of this unqualified support; and the AMA remains open to working with all interested parties in efforts to deal with and lessen the effects of violence in our society.

Mountain bike injuries mount

Rebecca Voelker
JAMA 1997 Mar 26; 277(2): 951

It's good exercise and a thrilling sport. But mountain bike riders suffered 23,409 injuries in 1994, 7% of which warranted admission to a hospital.

During the American Academy of Orthopaedic Surgeons meeting last month in San Francisco, Calif., Mary Bos, MD, of the Institute for Bone and Joint Disorders in Phoenix, Ariz., reported that half the injuries were to bikers' upper extremities, particularly the shoulder and rib areas. About 22% of the injuries were to the face and head. Knee injuries were less common, occurring in about 7% of those injured.

About one fourth of the injured bikers sustained a fracture, and another one fourth had lacerations. Other common injuries were contusions, strains, sprains, and dislocations.

Mountain bikers should take note of the findings. The US Consumer Product Safety Commission has reported that in 1995 mountain biking injuries more than doubled, to 48,604. According to the National Sporting Goods Association, about 16.2 million people participate in mountain biking, which became an Olympic event last year.

JAMA Article of Note: Helmets and preventing motorcycle and bicycle-related injuries.

JAMA 1994 Nov 16; 272(19): 1535-1538

Resources
American Academy of Pediatrics
141 Northwest Point Blvd
Elk Grove Village, IL 60009-0927
847 228-5005   Fax 847 228-5097
E-mail:kidsdoc@aap.org
Web address: http://www.aap.org/dogl/dogl.html
(injury prevention program)

CareAmerica
6300 Canoga Ave, Woodland Hills, CA 91367
818 228-2567   Fax 818 228-5128

Center for Safety in the Arts
5 Beekman St, New York, NY 10038
212 227-6220   Fax 212 233-3846

National Center for Injury Prevention and Control
Centers for Disease Control and Prevention
4770 Buford Hwy NE, Atlanta, GA 30341-3724
404 488-4690
Web address: http://www.cdc.gov

National Child Safety Council
4065 Page Ave, PO Box 1368, Jackson, MI 49204
517 764-6070   Fax 517 764-3068

National Safety Council
1121 Spring Lake Dr, Itasca, IL 60143-3201
630 285-1121   Fax 630 285-1315
Web address: http://www.nsc.org

Safety, Automobile

A Piece of My Mind

Accomplices

Douglas S. Diekema
JAMA 1991 Feb 13; 265(6): 802

The news coverage began with scenes of the tragedy, eerily illuminated by the flashing lights of emergency vehicles and the glow of floodlights that could not overcome the deeper shadows. A man, on top of the smashed vehicle, was trying to force his way into the wreckage.

Although disturbed by the scenes of the automobile accident, I was haunted most by a brief home video that immediately followed. Because it was shown on the 10 o'clock news by all the major television stations, I saw the home movie three times. I recognized two of its stars

S from the previous night, although I had known them only as dead bodies. My eyes fixed on the pretty young mother, smiling as her husband hammed in front of the camera. The scene shifted to a cheery bedroom, where the same man, the father, tickled his 6-week-old son. He made no effort to hide his pride in this recent addition to their young family. His wife sat quietly to the side until he playfully pulled her in front of the camera.

Each news program followed these images with a brief narrative of the tragedy—three people killed when their car was struck head-on by another vehicle whose driver was drunk. Each newscaster commented on the evils of drunk driving. But none seemed aware of the knowledge I held. None seemed to realize there had been accomplices.

I had difficulty clearing my mind as I picked up the telephone and tried to understand—at 1 o'clock that morning—what the emergency room clerk was telling me. Slowly, some of her words began to penetrate. I was wanted downstairs. Fire rescue was 6 minutes away with two victims of a motor vehicle accident. Neither had a pulse. Neither was breathing. One was a baby. No other information was available. Could I please hurry. My nightmare.

Stumbling down the stairs, I began to review resuscitation medications and dosages. What size endotracheal tube would I need for the child? Anxiety greeted me in the faces of our small emergency room team. We don't see many babies with traumatic injuries.

I had 2 minutes to gather a few supplies, find an endotracheal tube I hoped would be small enough, and prepare myself for the worst. As I reached over to confirm that an intraosseous needle lay nearby, the emergency room entrance burst open. A frightened EMT ran through the door carrying a limp blue baby. He slid the small body onto a cart and backed away, apparently relieved to be done with his part. The rest of us slipped into the rhythm of resuscitation: intubation, intraosseous line, large volumes of fluid, several rounds of drugs. Most of it is a blur to me now. As we waited for some response to the medications, the nurse to my left suggested I feel the head. Her eyes locked on mine as I touched the soft skin of this small child's head and felt the crushed skull. Holding back a rush of tears, I nodded. We had nothing more to offer.

My colleague had declared the father dead even before we ended our efforts. Word arrived that the mother, the driver, had died at the university hospital across town. The driver of the other car had a few bruises and cuts but would be fine. His intoxicated state had not prevented him from putting on his seat belt.

As I sat in the television's glow, tears of anger joined those of sadness. My frustration with the victims unnerved me. One small detail, provided us by the sheriff soon after our failed resuscitation attempt, greatly magnified this tragedy. He had found the infant's car seat 70 feet from the smashed vehicle. Obviously it had not been secured, nor had it carried the baby. Rescue workers had discovered the infant while removing his father from the car. The child had apparently been riding on his father's lap as the family returned from a visit with Grandpa and Grandma. Neither parent had been restrained. The baby had been crushed between his father and the passenger side of the dashboard.

The young family I had watched on television, so alive with joy and love, could have done nothing about the fact that a drunk driver would cross their path on that cold December evening. But the truth was that they had failed to protect themselves and their baby from the encounter they couldn't prevent. It grieved me that they had been accomplices.

Resources

Association for the Advancement
of Automotive Medicine
22340 Des Plaines Ave, Ste 106
Des Plaines, IL 60018
847 390-8927   847 390-9962
E-mail: AAAMI@aol.com

Auto Safety Hotline
800 424-9393   202 426-0123 (in DC)

National Highway Traffic Safety Administration
HTS-10, US Department of Transportation
400 7th St SW, Rm 5130, Washington, DC 20590
202 426-9294

Safety, Patient

Hippocrates said: "'First do no harm"—but what happens when mistakes do occur?

Wendy Sue Morphew

The US health care system has the best-trained physicians, nurses, and providers and the most resources in the world. It is considered the safest health system in the world. Yet among the millions of medical interactions that take place annually, a very small number of frightening medical errors do occur. We've all read about them: the amputation of the "wrong" leg; a catheter being mistaken for a feeding tube; an accidental dose of chemotherapy administered by one of the nation's leading cancer treatment hospitals. Just how can such things happen?

It's easy to settle for simple answers. "The physician was negligent, or the hospital was careless, or the insurance company put corporate profits ahead of patient welfare." It would be comforting if mistakes like these could be attributed to "bad doctors" or careless providers because then all we'd have to do is eliminate the "bad" ones and the problem of medical errors would be solved. In truth, however, the names of some fine, wonderfully skilled and caring physicians can sometimes be connected to a tragic mistake. Those who investigate medical injuries say that when they do happen, it's because a breakdown in the health care system allows a human error to occur. Until we stop asking "Who's to blame?" and start focusing on reducing the likelihood of a good professional making a mistake, we will not succeed in preventing the few errors that mar our wonderful health care safety records.

To address these infrequent anomalies, the American Medical Association created this past September the AMA's National Patient Safety Foundation. The Foundation will fund research into ways to make health care delivery systems safer, will encourage health care providers to discuss their experiences with errors—so that physicians and hospitals can learn from each other still better ways to prevent mistakes—and will educate patients about steps that they can take to help ensure their safety.

"Any error that injures a patient will always be one error too many," said Dr Nancy W. Dickey, chair of the AMA's Board of Trustees. According to Dr Dickey, the Foundation hopes to ensure that patient safety remains a top priority as health care continues to move through rapid changes. The American Medical Association is convinced that the Foundation can reduce the rate of medical error and patient injuries.

Finding solutions

Look no further than anesthesiology. Not so long ago, anesthesiology had one of the highest death rates of any medical specialty. Nobody knew why. It was simply assumed that anesthesia involved extremely high-risk procedures and that a certain number of patients would have negative reactions to the drugs administered. Then a group of anesthesiologists decided to see if they could improve anesthesia safety and were amazed at what they found. Though many physicians believed previously that drugs or the patient's diseases were to blame for an anesthesia death, the researchers found that human error was also a factor. The Anesthesia Patient Safety Foundation was formed to analyze what factors made human error more likely. Researchers focused on the "process" of error—its causes, the circumstances that surround it, and its association with specific procedures. They found patterns to predict where errors were likely to occur and they were able to recommend changes to lessen the chance of a mistake occurring. Anesthesia equipment was redesigned, and better monitoring systems were put in place. This all-volunteer effort by dedicated doctors met with great success. In only 10 years' time, there was a 20-fold drop in the anesthesiology mortality rate. From June of 1985 to June of 1990, over the course of 392,000 anesthesia procedures, there was only one accident.

The AMA's Patient Safety Foundation will build on such accomplishments, working with safety experts, not only from medicine but from all high-risk fields, including the airline industry and our national space program.

Yes, physicians are held to the highest standards of accountability. As patients, we accept nothing less than perfect medical outcomes. So when an error does occur, the first reaction is to assign personal blame—to find the "bad actor." Society's remedies have also been focused on assessing personal blame. The emphasis is on discipline and deterrence. This approach has led to more and more lawsuits, but it hasn't stopped those relatively few errors from continuing to occur. Medical lawsuits are not like product liability suits where large awards against a manufacturer can influence the next manufacturer to be more careful. When a McDonald's gets sued for serving scalding hot coffee, other McDonald's can respond by lowering the temperature of the coffee they serve. A lawsuit against a physician, on the other hand, is not going to influence the next physician never to make a mistake. There is no incentive that can ensure human perfection. "The way to prevent errors is not lawsuits," says Dr Dickey, "but system analysis and improvement. That's exactly what the National Patient Safety Foundation is going to do."

Once we understand that medicine ca.. begin the task of reducing risk to as close to z.. possible. Studying the problems, sharing the lessons, .. managing the risks are parts of the solution. We may have the best and safest health care system in the world, but there is room for improvement, and Americans can continue to look to the AMA to take the lead and make those improvements happen. "We owe it to our patients," says Dr Dickey, "and we won't quit until we get there."

JAMA Article of Note: The safety effects of child-resistant packaging for oral prescription drugs

JAMA 1996 June 5;275(21): 1661-1665

Resources

Anesthesia Patient Safety Foundation
1400 Locust St, 9 Ermire, Pittsburgh, PA 15219
Web address: http://gasnet.med.yale.edu/apsf

Institute for Safe Medication Practices
300 W Street Rd, Warminster, PA 18974
215 956-9181   Fax 215 956-9266
Web address: http://www.ismp.org

National Patient Safety Foundation
515 N State St, Chicago, IL 60610
Fax 312 464-4154
E-mail: npsf@ama-assn.org
Web address: http://www.ama-assn.org/med-sci/main.htm

Safety, Product

The Consumer Product Safety Commission protects the public against unreasonable risks of injury from consumer products; assists consumers in evaluating the comparative safety of consumer products; develops uniform safety standards for consumer products and minimizes conflicting state and local regulations; and promotes research and investigation into the causes and prevention of product-related deaths, illnesses, and injuries. (USG-1996)

Consumer Product Safety Commission
4330 E West Hwy, Bethesda, MD 20814
800 638-2772   301 504-0100
Hearing impaired teletypewriter 800 638-8270
Web address: http://www.cpsc.gov

Sample Criteria

Sample Criteria for Procedure Review: Screening Criteria to Assist PSROS
(#PB81-179871)
Reference Criteria for Short-Stay Hospital Review
(#PB81-179889)

Order either from:
National Technical Information Serivce (NTIS)
US Department of Commerce
5285 Port Royal Rd, Springfield, VA 22161
703 487-4650
E-mail: orders@ntis.fedworld.gov
Web address:http://www.ntis.gov

S

Sarcoidosis

Sarcoidosis Family Aid and Research Foundation
760 Clinton Ave, Newark, NJ 07108
800 223-6429

School Health

American School Health Association
7263 State Rte 43, PO Box 708, Kent, OH 44240
216 678-1601   Fax 216 678-4526

Science

American Association for the Advancement of Science
1333 H St NW, Washington, DC 20005
202 326-6400   202 289-4021

National Science Foundation
4201 Wilson Blvd, Arlington, VA 22230
800 628-1487   703 306-1070   Fax 703 306-0157
E-mail: info@nsf.gov
Web address: http://www.nsf.gov

Scleroderma

United Scleroderma Foundation, Inc
PO Box 399, Watsonville, CA 95077-0399
800 722-HOPE (outside CA)   408 728-2202 (in CA)
Fax 408 728-3328

Scoliosis

National Scoliosis Foundation
5 Cabol Pl, Staughton, MA 020172-4624
800 673-6922   617 341-6333   Fax 617 341-8333
E-mail: scoliosis@aol.com

The Scoliosis Association
PO Box 811705, Boca Raton, FL 33481-1705
800 800-0669   407 994-4435   Fax 407 368-8518

Scuba

Handicapped Scuba Association
7172 W Stanford Ave, Littleton, CO 80123
714 498-6128   805 648-6740   Fax 714 498-6128
E-mail: 1034243535@compuserve.com

Divers Alert Network (DAN)
3101 Tower Blvd, Ste 1300, Durham, NC 27707
800 446-2671   919 684-2948   Fax 919 490-6630
E-mail: shust001@mc.duck.edu

Second Opinion (for Patients)

Department of Health and Human Services
800 638-6833   800 492-6603 (Maryland)

For free brochure, write:
Surgery Department
Department of Health and Human Services
Washington, DC 20201

Self-help

AMA examines roles of self-help groups

Hannah L. Hedrick, PhD [Adapted]
The AMA Reporter, Feb 1992

For the past decade, the American Medical Association has been in the vanguard of associations willing to examine the benefits of self-help groups and has increasingly recognized them as one of many established helping methods. AMA policies, publications, and activities have supported the study of self-help in educational programs and have increased the number of professional researchers and writers who understand groups and their role in the health care system.

At the corporate level, the AMA Employee Assistance Program refers employees, as appropriate, to self-help groups. The AMA has also sponsored support groups for smoking cessation, nutrition and weight loss, expectant mothers, and the Persian Gulf conflict. These autonomous grassroots self-help groups, which operate without professional control and without a great deal of professional involvement, reflect the maturing of a movement that came of age during the 1980s.

Throughout that decade, the *Journal of the American Medical Association* and *American Medical News* were among the varied publications—including *Chicago Medicine, Good Housekeeping, New Woman,* the *New York Times, The New Yorker, Newsweek, Population Reports, Psychology Today, The Wall Street Journal, The Washington Post* and *World Medical News*—that featured articles on the benefits of self-help groups.

Phil Donahue, Ann Landers, Oprah Winfrey, and other media figures refer frequently to the benefits provided by peer support groups in dealing with a multitude of problems. Almost all of the national and local docudramas on the "disease of the week," depicting people affected by AIDS, Alzheimer disease, cancer, child abuse, domestic violence, mental illness, etc, involve and promote a successful self-help group.

Self-help groups typically exhibit the following characteristics and benefits:

Common problem: Members immediately identify with one another.

Mutual aid helper therapy: Members benefit as much from giving help as from receiving it.

Network for support: Members provide a network of emotional and social support through regular and special gatherings, telephone calls, newsletters, visits, and computers.

Shared information: Through the group process and written material, members capture and share their successful techniques for coping.

Low cost: Expenses are shared through collections at meetings, minimal membership dues, or fund-raising projects.

Unconditional acceptance: Members are usually encouraged to share their personal situations in a nonjudgmental, caring environment.

"Prosumer" concept: Self-help group members frequently acquire a special ability to help, based on their development as both consumers and professionals ("prosumers") in the area of their problem.

Increasing support in AMA policies

Examination of and support for the self-help group movement has not been happenstance. An early blueprint for action vis-a-vis the contributions of self-help groups to public health appeared in the AMA report of *The Health Policy Agenda for the American People* (271 pages; 1987). The report emanated from a 5-year collaborative effort involving 172 health-related, business, government, and consumer groups; the project was coordinated and largely financed by the AMA. Dissemination of information about self-help groups and regional coordination of self-help efforts was cited in conjunction with reducing disease and injury and promoting healthy behaviors. The report advised self-help groups to "make their presence known in the community through coalitions to develop and distribute regional directories" and establish clearinghouses "as a means of integrating these efforts at the state level."

This important policy was among the AMA contributions to the self-help movement reported by the AMA vice president for Medical Education, Carlos J. M. Martini, MD, at the 1989 Symposium on the Impact of Life Threatening Conditions: "Self-help Groups and Health Care Providers in Partnership," which was cosponsored and cochaired by the AMA. Dr Martini summarized the many self-help group activities coordinated or supported by AMA staff at the national level, including:

- featuring self-help programs and open meetings at the National Leadership Conference, the National Conference for Impaired Professionals, and other meetings;
- initiating and participating in the 1978 Surgeon General's Workshop on Self-help and Public Health;
- using AMA publications to promote the involvement of health and human service providers in self-help groups; and
- providing leadership to the National Council on Self-help and Public Health.

Resources

American Self-help Clearinghouse
NW Covenant Medical Center
25 Pocono Rd, Denville, NJ 07834-2995
973 625-7101

National Self-help Clearinghouse
25 W 43rd, Rm 620, New York, NY 10036-7406
212 354-8525   Fax 212 642-1956

Self-help Centers, Statewide

Arizona (East Valley area)
Rainy Day People
Box 472, Scottsdale, AZ 85252
602 231-0868

Arkansas (Northeast area)
Arkansas Self-help Center
PO Box 9028, Jonesboro, AR 72403
501 932-5555

California
California (Sacramento)
Mental Health Associates
8912 Volunteer Ln, #210, Sacramento, CA 95826
916 368-3100

California (Davis)
Mental Health Association
PO Box 447, Davis, CA 95617
916 756-8181

Connecticut
Self-help Mutual Support Network
389 Whitney Ave, New Haven, CT 06511
203 789-7645

Illinois (Champaign County)
Family Services Center
405 S State St, Champaign, IL 61820
217 352-0099

Iowa
Iowa Pilot Parents Center
33 N 12th St, PO Box 1151, Fort Dodge, IA 50501
800 383-4777 (IA only)   515 576-5870

Kansas
Self-help Network
Wichita State University
1845 Fairmount, Box 34, Wichita, KS 67260-0034
800 445-0116 (KS only)   316 978-3843

Massachusetts
Clearinghouse of Mutual Help Groups
Massachusetts Cooperative Extension
University of Massachusetts
113 Skinner Hall, Amherst, MA 01003
413 545-4800

Michigan
Self-help Clearinghouse
106 W Allegan, Ste 210, Lansing, MI 48933-1706
800 752-5858 (MI only)   517 484-7373

Minnesota
First Call for Help
166 E 4th St, #310, St Paul, MN 55101
612 224-1133

Nebraska
Self-help Information Services
1601 Euclid Ave, Lincoln, NE 68502
402 476-9668

New Hampshire
800 852-3388 (NH only)

New Jersey
New Jersey Self-help Clearinghouse
Pocono Rd, Denville, NJ 07834
800 367-6274 (NJ only)   973 625-7101

New York (Westchester Cty)
Self-help Clearinghouse
456 North St, White Plains, NY 10605
914 949-0788, ext 237

S

New York City
American Self-help Center
NW Covenant Medical Center
25 Pocono Rd, Denville, NJ 07834-2995
973 625-7101

National Self-help Center
Graduate School & University
Center CUNY
25 W 43rd St, Rm 620, New York, NY 10036
212 354-8525

North Carolina
Support Works
1018 East Blvd, Ste 5, Charlotte, NC 28203-5779
704 331-9500

Ohio (Dayton area)
Family Services
184 Salem, Dayton, OH 45406
937 225-3004

Ohio (Toledo area)
Harbor Behavioral Healthcare
4334 Secor Ave, Toledo, OH 43623
419 475-4449

Oregon (Portland area)
United Way
Attn: NW Regional Self-help Clearinghouse
619 SW 11th Ave, Ste 300, Portland, OR 97205
503 222-5555

Pennsylvania (Pittsburgh area)
Self-help Network
1323 Forbes Ave, Ste 200, Pittsburgh, PA 15219
412 261-5363

Pennsylvania (Scranton area)
Voluntary Action Center
538 Spruce St, Ste 420, Scranton, PA 18503-1816
717 961-1234

South Carolina (Midlands area)
803 791-9227
Message advising they will call back.

Tennessee (Memphis area)
Mental Health Association
2400 Poplar St, Ste 410, Memphis, TN 38112
901 323-0633

Texas
Mental Health Association
8401 Shoal Creek Blvd, Austin, TX 78757-7597
512 454-3706   Fax 512 454-3725

Selling a Medical Practice

Sample letter to notify patients of practice transfer

[Date]

Dear Patients (personalize if computer database system permits):

This letter is to inform you that I am leaving active practice on _____, 19____. I write this letter with mixed emotions because caring for you and all of my patients has been a great source of satisfaction and pleasure. I have made the decision because _____

_____ .

Since my concern for you is that you continue to receive the same kind of personal medical care that I have tried to provide you over the years, I am very pleased to announce that Dr. _____ will be taking over my practice. [Insert effective data if appropriate.]

Doctor _____ comes to the practice with excellent credentials. [He/she] is a graduate of _____ medical school and received [his/her] residency training in _____ at _____. We share the same philosophies about the practice of medicine and it is reassuring to me to leave my practice in the hands of such a competent physician.

I am also happy to inform you that [office manager, medical assistant, nurse] will continue in the office. When you wish to make appointments just call the same telephone number _____ and speak with_____

_____ .

I believe you will find Doctor _____ to be not only well trained but very compassionate and attentive to your needs.

You do not have an obligation to accept Dr. _____ as your physician. If you wish, you may request that your records be transferred to another physician. If so, we will need an authorization form from you. If you elect to be treated by Dr _____, you can authorize the release of your records to [him/her] from my files on your next visit to our office.

Let me take this opportunity to thank you for your many years of loyalty and friendship. It has been a pleasure to serve as your personal physician. My [wife/husband], _____, and I extend our best wishes to you for your future health and happiness.

Sincerely,

_____ , MD

(BUY-1990)

Sex Education Report

Guidelines for comprehensive sexuality education:
National Guidelines Task Force
c/o Sex Information and Education Council of the US (SIECUS)
130 W 42nd St, Ste 350, New York, NY 10036
212 819-9770   Fax 212 819-9776

Sexual Assault

AMA Press Release

June 1996

AMA report card on violence: Sexual assault

Subject includes: Sexual assaults, date, acquaintance, spousal rape, stranger rape

Grade: D–

Summary of status: Sexual assault remains the most dramatically underreported crime, with an estimated two thirds of attacks unreported. And while it is said to be our nation's most expensive crime, outstripping even murder, it is still not considered a priority problem in our society.

The relatively small group of dedicated individuals who are working diligently to put this problem on society's radar screen and to assist and advocate for victims deserve an A+—hands-down. Further, in November 1995, the American Medical Association declared sexual assault a "silent violent epidemic" and launched a public awareness campaign encouraging patients not to be afraid to talk to their doctors. In addition, the AMA sent guidelines to physicians to help them better identify and treat victims of sexual assault. Even so, society as a whole is making no progress on this issue.

Incidence and reporting
Accurate estimates of the incidence of sexual assault are nearly impossible to obtain, primarily because the crime remains grossly underreported. According to the most recent National Crime Victimization Survey (NCVS), released in April 1996, an estimated 430,000 sexual assaults occurred in victims over the age of 12 in the United States in 1994. This constitutes no statistically significant change from the previous year. The NCVS reports that only 36% of rapes, 20% of attempted rapes, and 41% of other sexual assaults are reported to police.

Most victims of sexual assault are under age 24. Unfortunately, many who experience attacks meeting the legal definition of rape do not label their experience as such, illustrating continued confusion among legal definitions, medical terminology, and lay usage of terms relating to sexual assault.

Societal attitudes
Negative societal attitudes and social myths about rape are still prevalent. In a 1995 survey of 1965 eighth and ninth graders: Eleven percent agreed that if a girl says "no" to sex she usually means "yes"; half said that being raped was sometimes the victim's fault; and 40% agreed that girls who wear sexy clothes are "asking to be raped."

Reporting is severely impeded by victims' feelings of embarrassment, fear of further injury, and anxiety about court procedures that too often scrutinize and judge the victim's behavior and history. Male rape victims worry that their sexuality will come into question. "In rape cases, unlike any other crime, it is the victim who is put on trial," said Ronet Bachman, PhD, author of the Justice Department's 1995 Violence Against Women Report.

The legal system
In recent years, some progress has been made in reforming rape laws, particularly in the area of victims' rights. However, many states still lag far behind, and harassment of victims by the system persists. "We need to go back to the table and stress that strong, victim-centered approaches must be developed to assure victims are not neglected or abused while making their way through the system," said Patricia Giggans, chair of the California Coalition on Sexual Assault and executive director of the nation's oldest rape crisis center.

Apprehension and conviction of rapists are still too rare. Experts say that the justice system is not successfully deterring this crime because would-be offenders view the likelihood of being caught and punished as highly improbable.

When offenders are apprehended one question must be answered—"Was the sex consensual?" While the means to show concrete evidence to answer this question exists, it is not being used by the courts.

Colposcopy research has established that rape victims suffer internal injuries that are not apparent in women who engage in consensual sex. This is a major breakthrough in documenting injuries sustained in sexual assaults, which will prove invaluable in helping prosecutors prove victimization. But the results are still unpublished and there are no plans to conduct the corroborating research needed to establish the findings as a national standard. Funding for rape-related research is scarce. "If you're not working on research related to cholesterol, you don't get any money," said Dr Laura Slaughter, former medical director of the San Luis Obispo Sexual Assault Reaction Team (SART). "We have to put our money where our mouth is."

Medicine
Although there is universal agreement that a national standard for handling sexual assault is needed, no significant progress has been made toward establishing one. However, in the interim, individual groups like the American Medical Association have developed and distributed their own procedural and educational protocols to assist health care professionals in better identifying, treating, and referring victims of sexual assault. These protocols are particularly important because medical personnel, who are a first point of contact for victims, often don't receive formal training in this area.

Often victims are cared for in busy emergency departments, where they may wait behind life-threatening cases as their emotional trauma escalates and physical evidence erodes. They also are rarely seen for follow-up care. "We need to stop treating victims like they're dead, sending them home and never following up," said Dr Slaughter. "If you break your arm you get better follow-up."

It is clear that more extensive coordination is needed between the medical, legal, and social service communities to ensure that victims' needs are fully met. This goal is being accomplished through multidisciplinary sexual assault reaction teams (SART). Unfortunately, these teams exists in only a handful of states.

Social service
Over the past 25 years, a good national network of crisis intervention centers, hotlines, support groups, and other services has developed that meet victim needs in varying degrees. Still, services are out of reach for victims in rural areas and are of no use to the hundreds of thousands of victims who do not seek help.

"In 25 years, we have not solved this problem," said Giggans. "Women are not safer than they were 25 years ago, but if they can plug into this system, at least they can get though the process and begin healing."

Traditionally it has been a challenge to find funding for antirape programs and, to date, the focus has been on intervention. Experts feel that a greater commitment must be made to prevention and education. "It takes a long time to educate and change attitudes, and you have to change attitudes before you can change behaviors," said Giggans. "There is not enough of a mobilization in

S our society to get everyone to buy into changing attitudes."

The Violence Against Women Act (VAWA), which was passed as part of the 1994 Crime Bill, "constitutes a giant leap forward," according to Pam McMahon, PhD, Centers for Disease Control and Prevention. The funds were slow in coming, but in May were formally approved and made available to states for the development of prevention programs.

Conclusion

Until our society is willing to make a firm commitment to making the eradication of sexual assault a priority, we cannot hope for much progress. As a society, we must begin to talk openly about this very private crime and to forge a unified educational movement for prospective victims and offenders. It is only with education that we can begin to change negative attitudes and behaviors, squelch ridiculous myths, bring victims out of the shadows, and see that justice is served.

The AMA will continue its crusade to educate the public and the medical profession about this "silent violent epidemic" and will continue to urge victims to talk to their doctors.

Facts about sexual assault

Incidence

- Sexual assault continues to represent the most rapidly growing violent crime in America.[1]
- Over 700,000 women are sexually assaulted each year.[2]
- It is estimated that fewer than 50% of rapes are reported.[1]
- Approximately 20% of sexual assaults against women are perpetrated by assailants unknown to the victim. The remainder are committed by friends, acquaintances, intimates, and family members. Acquaintance rape is particularly common among adolescent victims.[3]
- Male victims represent 5% of reported sexual assaults.[4]
- Among female rape victims, 61% are under age 18.[2,4]
- At least 20% of adult women, 15% of college women, and 12% of adolescent women have experienced some form of sexual abuse or assault during their lifetimes.[5]

Societal attitudes

A survey of 6159 college students enrolled at 32 institutions in the United States[5] found:

- Fifty-four percent of the women surveyed had been the victims of some form of sexual abuse; more than one in four college-aged women had been the victim of rape or attempted rape.
- Fifty-seven percent of the assaults occurred on dates.
- Seventy-three percent of the assailants and 55% of the victims had used alcohol or other drugs prior to the assault.
- Twenty-five percent of the men surveyed admitted some degree of sexually aggressive behavior.
- Forty-two percent of the victims told no one.

In a survey of high school students, 56% of the girls and 76% of the boys believed forced sex was acceptable under some circumstances.[6]

A survey of 11- to 14-year-olds[6] found:

- Fifty-one percent of the boys and 41% of the girls said forced sex was acceptable if the boy "spent a lot of money" on the girl.

- Thirty-one percent of the boys and 32% of the girls said it was acceptable for a man to rape a woman with past sexual experience.
- Eighty-seven percent of boys and 79% of girls said sexual assault was acceptable if the man and the woman were married.
- Sixty-five percent of the boys and 47% of the girls said it was acceptable for a boy to rape a girl if they had been dating for more than 6 months.

In a survey of male college students:

- Thirty-five percent anonymously admitted that, under certain circumstances, they would commit rape if they believed they could get away with it.
- One in 12 admitted to committing acts that met the legal definitions of rape, and 84% of men who committed rape did not label it as rape.[7,8]

In another survey of college males[9]:

- Forty-three percent of college-aged men admitted to using coercive behavior to have sex, including ignoring a woman's protest, using physical aggression, and forcing intercourse.
- Fifteen percent acknowledged they had committed acquaintance rape.
- Eleven percent acknowledged using physical restraints to force a woman to have sex.

Women with a history of rape or attempted rape during adolescence were almost twice as likely to experience a sexual assault during college, and were three times as likely to be victimized by a husband.[10] Sexual assault is reported by 33% to 46% of women who are being physically assaulted by their husbands.[11]

References

1. Dupre AR, Hampton HL, Morrison H, Meeks GR. Sexual assault. *Obstet Gynecol Surv.* 1993;48:640-648.

2. *Rape in America: A Report to the Nation.* Arlington, Va: National Victim Center and Crime Victims Research and Treatment Center; 1992:1-16.

3. Heise LL. Reproductive freedom and violence against women: where are the intersections? *J Law Med Ethics.* 1993;21(2):206-216.

4. American Academy of Pediatrics, Committee on Adolescence. Sexual assault and the adolescent. *Pediatrics.* 1994;94(5):761-765.

5. Koss MP. Hidden rape: sexual aggression and victimization in a national sample of students in higher education. In: Burgess AW, ed. *Rape and Sexual Assault.* New York, NY: Garland Publishing; 1988;2:3-25.

6. White JW, Humphrey JA. Young people's attitudes toward acquaintance rape. In: Parrot A, ed. *Acquaintance Rape: The Hidden Crime.* New York, NY: John Wiley and Sons Inc; 1991.

7. Koss MP, Dinero TE, Seibel CA. Stranger and acquaintance rape: are there differences in the victim's experience? *Psychol Women Q.* 1988;12:1-24.

8. Malamuth NM. Rape proclivity among males. *J Soc Issues.* 1981;37:138-157.

9. Rapaport KR, Posey CD. Sexually coercive college males. In: Parrot A, ed. *Acquaintance Rape: The Hidden Crime.* New York, NY: John Wiley and Sons Inc; 1991.

10. Ellis, Atkeson, Calhoun, 1982: Gidycz, Coble, Latham, Layman, 1993; Guthrie, Notgrass, 1992.

11. Frieze IH, Browne A. Violence in marriage. In: Ohlin L, Tonry M, eds. *Family Violence: Crime and Justice, A Review of Research.* Chicago, Ill: University of Chicago Press; 1989:163-218.

Strategies for the treatment and prevention of sexual assault

Contact the American Medical Association
Department of Mental Health
312 464-5563

Web address: http://www.ama-assn.org/public/releases/assault/sa-guide.htm

Resources

Stop Prison Rape (SPR)
PO Box 2713, Manhattanville Station
New York, NY 10027-8817
212 663-5562

National Resource Center on Child Sexual Abuse
2204 Whitezburg Dr, Ste 200
Huntsville, AL 35801
800 543-7006   205 534-6868 (direct contact with information specialist)

National Organization of Victim Assistance (NOVA)
1757 Park Rd NW, Washington, DC 20010
800 879-6682 202 232 6682

National Coalition on Sexual Assault (NCASA)
912 N 2nd St, Harrisburg, PA 17102
717 232-7460

National Resource Center Against Domestic Violence
800 537-2238

National Clearinghouse on Marital and Date Rape
510 524-1582 (fee-based telephone service)

National Victims Center
800 FYI-CALL 703 276-2880

Rape, Abuse & Incest National Network (RAIN)
Contact: Scott Berkowitz
635B Pennsylvania Ave SE, Washington, DC 20003
800 656-HOPE (national referral to local service)
202 544-1034   Fax 202 544-1401
E-mail: rainnmail@aol.com
Web address: http://www.rain.org

Department of Health and Human Services (HHS)
Council on Sexual Violence
Contact: Virginia Cox, Assistant to the Secretary
202 690-8157
American Bar Association recommends for legal assistance: Call the local bar association and request the lawyer referral service.

Sexual Issues in the Practice of Medicine

Sex and the physician

Harold I. Lief, MD

Dealing with sexual problems of patients is an important part of medical practice and should be a significant concern of almost all physicians who are comfortable about inquiring into the sexual lives of their patients, and when they take the initiative by asking appropriate questions, sexual problems are discovered in 15% to 50% of patients, depending upon the type of practice.[1] Although sexual problems are rarely if ever fatal, many thousands of people are deeply troubled, anxious, and depressed because of them. Marital disruption, even divorce, commonly results from untreated sexual problems.

Not all sexual problems confronting the physician are the usual sexual dysfunction, such as premature ejaculation and impotence in men or orgasmic dysfunction in women. Conflicts over sexual behavior, such as frequency, oral sex, and coital positions, are even more common and sometimes more troublesome.[2] Sexual concerns resulting from illness and from medical procedures, such as hysterectomy, mastectomy, and colostomy, also require counseling. Physical disorders may bring about sexual dysfunction; diabetes is the most common of these, but there are many others that may adversely affect sexual function. Medications, such as those used to treat hypertension, often cause sexual dysfunction.[3]

Unlike most other subjects in medical practice, sexuality often creates intense feelings in physicians. Because sex is a private and intimate subject, physicians are likely to be uncomfortable when taking a sexual history until they become experienced in treating patients with sexual problems.

Tendencies to regard sexual behavior as good or bad, important or unimportant—in short, values—are significant considerations. Probably more than in any other dimension of practice, values and ethics have to be taken into account—the physician's as well as the patient's. The physician must recognize that he or she has sexual values or preferences and that these may differ from those of the patient.

In dealing with sexual problems, the physician has a splendid opportunity to practice preventive as well as therapeutic medicine. By assisting a young patient to overcome sexual anxieties and inhibitions, he or she helps prepare that person for satisfactory relationships throughout life, perhaps eventually for marriage. By counseling a married couple, enabling them to obtain greater mutuality and sexual pleasure, the physician reduces marital discord and may even prevent divorce and its emotional and physical sequelae for the couple and their children.

Marital unhappiness, separation, and divorce have been implicated as causative factors in a variety of illnesses, especially depression, which, in turn, often contributes to many diseases. Somers quotes a report of the National Institute of Mental Health: "The single most powerful predictor of stress-related physical as well as emotional illness is marital disruption."[4] Helping patients with sexual problems is more than enriching, important as that is: It is good medical care because, by reducing one of the most common sources of human suffering, it helps prevent illness, the uprooting of families, and the resultant social disorganization.

Most sexual problems brought to the attention of physicians, especially to family physicians, are those of couples. Some of these problems are primary causes of marital dysfunction. Most are consequences of other kinds of marital discord and, in turn, perpetuate and increase marital unhappiness. It seems reasonable, then, to make sex counseling and marriage counseling a "package" in the training of physicians and the delivery of medical care. Training in sex and marriage counseling is a logic requisite for primary care physicians—those practicing

S internal medicine, family medicine, and obstetrics/gynecology. It is logical even in pediatrics, for it helps the practitioner to recognize the connections between the parents' relationship and a child's sexual problems. An example of such a connection is the covertly seductive father of a teenage daughter, abetted by a sexually repressed wife, who interferes with the separation that is necessary for a girl in her early adolescence to transfer attachment from her father to male peers.

Sex counseling and couple counseling are not the only ways the physician can practice preventive medicine. Early intervention can occur in many other sexually related clinical situations, such as unwanted teenage pregnancies, premarital counseling, family-planning services during pregnancy, postpartum care, and family-life education for teenagers and young adults. The pediatrician and obstetrician, dealing with children and adolescents or with young parents, have excellent opportunities to practice effective preventive medicine.

Physician's attitudes

There is general agreement that the physician's capacity to help his or her patient is a result of three primary factors: attitudes, skill, and knowledge (sometimes called the ASK formula). Attitudes can inhibit or enhance the acquisition of skills and even of knowledge from physician to patient. In few other aspects of medical practice are attitudes more important than in caring for patients with sexual problems.

Physicians have been socialized as boys and men or as girls and women before they become medical students. Sexual feelings, beliefs, and values stemming from a particular religious, ethnic, and social-class background are often intense and firmly held; therefore, physicians cannot learn about sex in the same relatively dispassionate way that they can study the Krebs cycle. In all of us, an interplay between our beliefs or ideas about sexual functions and dysfunctions on the one hand, and our values or preferences on the other, determines what our attitudes will be.

If a future physician grows up believing that masturbation is sinful, for example, he or she will retain the value judgment in practice that it is bad; thus the physician might react strongly and negatively to a patient's discussion of masturbation. If the physician believes that masturbation is normal for unmarried males and females but abnormal and bad in marriage, that judgment would influence the discussion of masturbation with a married partner.

Society impresses on its members many sexual values, some of them so gradually and covertly that they are absorbed and accepted without awareness. In addition, every person has life experiences that subtly leave marks largely outside his or her conscious recognition. The physician who is unaware of his or her own moral values may unwittingly impose them on the patient. On the other hand, some physicians who are fully aware of their values also try to impose them on patients.

A physician who cannot countenance premarital intercourse under any circumstance is clearly a poor choice for a single girl seeking contraceptive help. The physician who, because of strong religious beliefs, unconsciously regards out-of-wedlock pregnancy as justified punishment for premarital coitus may find it impossible to prescribe a contraceptive even for a girl who has already had an out-of-wedlock pregnancy. It is thus that physicians may project their own values onto the clinical situation.

Similarly, personal attitudes may be held toward such sexual behaviors as oral-genital and anal-genital intercourse, extramarital sex, homosexual practices, sexual expression among the elderly, and group sex. Even the idea that women may enjoy and actively pursue sex was strange to many gynecologists until the 1960s.[5] If a physician believes that women are essentially passive and submissive and should be paced by the husband's sexual interests, his or her attitude toward a woman who reports that she took the initiative sexually and that she actively enjoys it probably affects the way the physician deals with her.

Every physician who wishes to be a competent sex counselor must try to discern patients' values and to become more aware of his or her own. It doesn't matter whether the physician's values are more conservative or liberal than the patient's. The patient may become threatened and respond with shame or anger if the physician attempts to change the patient's value abruptly. A good physician-patient relationship depends on the clarification of values and of possible conflicts between those of the patient and the physician.

Ethical issues and concerns in sex counseling

Ethical issues in sex counseling in many ways are like those in other aspects of medical care—professional competence, responsible care, informed consent, and confidentiality. However, the intimate nature of sexual function, the self-esteem affected by it, and the strong emotions associated with it intensify the significance of such issues. There are also unique aspects of sex counseling (eg, the enhanced possibility of erotic feelings arising in the patient or the physician, the way in which the patient's and/or physician's erotic feelings are managed) that make accompanying ethical issues an even more important consideration for the physician than they are in medical care in general.

Imposing standards. Although the general rule is not to impose sexual standards on patients, the patient's values must be the most significant factors in sexual inhibitions or symptoms. An inhibited couple's puritanical ideas may have kept their sexual pleasure minimal; their values and those of the physician are the keys to successful therapy. Some attitude change toward greater tolerance and permissiveness often occurs, as the physician tries to modify an archaic conscience and rigid standards of behavior. When it happens, it happens slowly, often as a by-product of treatment, rather than by value confrontation and imposition. Occasionally, however, explicit reference to the differences in values of patient and physician is necessary.

In many sex counseling situations, the physician must take a permission-giving role, eg, permission to a couple to experiment with new behaviors so that they can expand and enrich their sexual experiences. However, the physician must be sensitive to the patients' values and extremely careful not to jeopardize their trust in him or her by demanding that they behave in ways that are inimical to their values. The correct timing of interventions is most important; decisions about how and when to offer recommendations should be made on the basis of sensitivity and experience.

Value conflicts between sexual partners are common. The physician's neutrality by no means precludes his or her making these conflicts as explicit as possible in an attempt to reach a satisfactory resolution.

Competence. The physician must judge whether he or she has the competence to undertake therapy in a given situation. Certainly, it is unethical to promise to deliver more than is possible; even the most skillful practitioners have their share of failures. A physician's competence increases with experience in an ongoing process; yet physicians have to be reasonably certain that they are not only willing to help, but that their skills are equal to the clinical task. The levels of competence—diagnostician, educator, counselor, and skilled therapist—are discussed in Chapter 8 and guidelines are given for judging one's own level.[6]

Exploitation. Exploitation may be financial or sexual. Financial exploitation occurs when the physician continues to treat beyond his or her level of competence or uses inappropriate therapy merely to retain the patient. Financial exploitation is possible in any clinical situation. Sexual exploitation is more of a possibility in sex counseling than in other forms of counseling or psychotherapy. Patients with sex problems are particularly vulnerable to seduction, and sometimes they themselves use seduction as a magical means of reassurance about being worthwhile, of gaining power over a person perceived as more dominating, or of overcoming inhibitions of sexual desire, excitement, or orgasm. The physician who actively or passively engages in erotic contacts with a patient is violating the patient's trust, and there is a very strong likelihood that the patient will be psychically damaged, if not by the contact then by the termination of an illusory love relationship with the therapist. The few authors who claim that sex between patient and therapist is helpful to the patient are unconvincing.[7,8]

There is a "gray area" in which affectionate touching, hugging, even kissing—the "laying on of hands" in a parental way—may be misinterpreted by the patient as erotic. Malpractice suits have been based on such misconceptions. Without duly restraining his or her warmth and affection, the physician must be cautious about the degree and the manner in which he or she displays affection for a patient.

Special therapeutic techniques. Special techniques, such as the sexological examination and the use of surrogate partners, raise ethical issues. Both techniques are controversial. The physician without special training should not carry out theses procedures, but he or she should know about them and the pitfalls that are involved. Very few sex therapists actually watch their patients during sexual encounters; that procedure, too, is highly questionable, and the physician is advised not to refer to therapists who use it. It is not only ethically controversial, but it involves invasion of privacy and has potential legal complications.

Recommending sexually explicit books or films is ethical, provided the physician has first determined what the patient's attitudes toward such material are, and provided the physician does not impose his or her values in an authoritarian way.

Confidentiality and informed consent. Confidentiality and informed consent raise ethical issues as they do in other aspects of medicine, but feelings about violation may be more intense. Many patients would not want others to know about their reason for seeking help or that they are even undergoing sex therapy. The charged feelings that most people have make it mandatory that the physician explain in detail the procedures and methods he or she intends to use.

There is a full discussion of the ethical issues in sex therapy and research in the publications on sex ethics by Masters et al.[9,10]

Sexual health care is requested by many patients and needed by many more who are too embarrassed to ask for it. A sensitive, thoughtful, caring physician can be of enormous help to such patients. Sexual problems cannot be ignored. Even the physician who is disinterested or uncomfortable with this part of medical care must be willing to listen, to inquire, and to refer tactfully and competently. The interested physician who gradually acquires greater competence as a sex counselor will derive a great deal of satisfaction from his or her efforts—usually short term and often effective. Helping patients with sexual problems can, in fact, be one of the most gratifying aspects of practice.

References

1. Burnap DW, Golden JS. Sexual problems in medical practice. *J Med Educ.* 1967;42:673-680.

2. Frank E, et al. Frequency of sexual dysfunction in 'normal' couples. *N Engl J Med.* 1978;299:111-115.

3. Reichgott MJ. Problems of sexual function in patients with hypertension. *Cardiovasc Med.* 1979;3:149-156.

4. Somers AR. Marital status, health, and use of health services. *JAMA.* 1979;241:1818-1822.

5. Scully D, Bart P. A funny thing happened on the way to the orifice: women in gynecology text books. *Am J Sociol.* 1973;78:1045-1050.

6. Lief H. Sex education in medicine: retrospect and prospect. In: Rosenweig N, Pearsall FP, eds. *Sex Education for the Health Professional.* New York, NY: Grune & Stratton; 1978.

7. McCartney J. Overt transference. *J Sex Res.* 1966;2:227-237.

8. Shepard M. *The Love Treatment: Sexual Intimacy Between Patients and Psychotherapist.* New York, NY:PH Wyden; 1971.

9. Masters WH, et al. *Ethical Issues in Sex Therapy and Research,* Vol 1. Boston, Mass: Little, Brown & Co; 1977.

10. Masters WH, et al. *Ethical Issues in Sex Therapy and Research.* Vol 2. Boston, Mass: Little, Brown & Co; 1977.

(SMP-1981)

Office procedures

Robert C. Long, MD

Leaders in the field of human sexuality commonly express the opinion that primary care physicians (family physicians, obstetrician-gynecologists and internists) should provide care to those couples who are experiencing sexual problems—even though these physicians, with infrequent exceptions, have had no specialized education in psychiatry, psychology, behavioral therapy, or counseling beyond medical school. What is the justification for

S this belief which, on its face, does not seem to make much sense?

Physician-patient relationship

Primary care physicians establish long-term relationships with many of their patients; these relationships may extend to two to three decades or even longer. No other health care practitioners are in such a unique position to intervene to prevent a self-perpetuating cycle of sexual anxiety. These physicians see patients at every stage of life and each encounter furnishes an opportunity to provide appropriate information on the varieties of normal sexual development and behavior. The opportunities to serve as a resource person, to practice preventive medicine, to maintain health, to treat illness, and to counsel patients during times of stress are numerous. They occur daily.

In times of physical and emotional illness, most patients turn first to their family physician. Although most physicians perform creditably in response to their patients' health care needs, in the field of human sexuality they have failed. No physician, for example, would ignore mitral valve insufficiency or stenosis discovered on physical examination. He or she would either carry out appropriate diagnostic studies and therapy or refer the patient to an appropriate specialist. At the same time, however, this same otherwise competent physician ignores a specific sexual complaint. How can this behavior be explained?

There are several reasons. Many physicians separate sexual anxiety and dysfunction from the patient's general health status. This separation of sexual disease from other kinds of disease and activity is deeply rooted in our culture. Sex as a cause of illness has largely been ignored in medical education and practice. For example, most physicians, especially those in primary care, are familiar with the concept of psychosomatic medicine. Daily they encounter patients with somatic complaints whose origins lie in emotional stress. Yet all too infrequently do they recognize that how the patient feels about himself or herself as a sexual person and how he or she relates to others sexually provide a very common source of psychosomatic symptomatology. Fatigue, pelvic pain, mild depression, low back pain, headache, urinary tract symptoms, hyperacidity with or without ulcer formation, and dyspareunia are commonly found in patients who lead sexual lives that they consider unsatisfactory.

Another reason for inattention to sexual problems by physicians is that many of them have never become comfortable with themselves as sexual persons. In this respect, they differ not a whit from the general population. Until recently it was believed that the study of anatomy, physiology, and pathology prepared a physician to deal with the sexual problems of others. This belief and the cultural tradition that sex is a taboo subject effectively blocked the teaching of human sexuality in medical schools until a decade or so ago. Lief reported that in 1961 only three of 82 medical schools offered courses in human sexuality[1]; today many of the 126 medical schools offer programs in this subject. This augurs well for the future, not only because of the availability of larger numbers of trained personnel, but also because primary care physicians will have a more solid academic background for treating sexual problems.

The point of all this is that most physicians are reared to believe that sex is evil, dirty, or harmful. Consequently, the changing of attitudes that results in feeling comfortable about sex, and dealing comfortably with it in relation to ourselves and others, has to be a learned experience. A physician's inability to deal comfortably with sexual questions can have a devastating effect upon patients. Physician embarrassment blocks communication and further investigation, and the patient's belief that nothing helpful can be done is often reinforced.

Another reason given by primary care physicians for eschewing investigation of their patient's sexuality is a feeling of incompetence with the subject. In addition, many are fearful of doing harm. These reasons are legitimate but, for most physicians, the lack of competence can be rather easily overcome through participation in such continuing medical education courses as sexual attitude restructuring (SAR) and office management of sexual dysfunctions.

It is essential not only that physicians be comfortable with themselves as sexual persons, but also that they learn to keep their personal, ethical, and moral value system away from the counseling table. This is often difficult, but it is important to recognize that each individual has his or her own moral-ethical value system that must be respected by the physician. The physician's role is to serve as a resource person in a comfortable, nonjudgmental way, to establish an accurate diagnosis, and to work with couples in the development of therapeutic strategies that have emerged from the work of Masters and Johnson, Kaplan, and others.

Management

Management encompasses four dimensions: time, adjunctive aids, record keeping, and insurance.

Time. Time is said to be an important barrier to the inclusion of a marital-sexual history as part of the routine investigation of a person's health care status by primary care physicians. Although this may be true, I know of no data to substantiate the conclusion. I also believe that there is a general misconception concerning the amount of time needed to investigate sexual problems with patients.

The incorporation of a marital-sexual history as a routine part of the physical examination takes only a brief period of time. The determination of whether the sexual problem is primarily marital or primarily sexual takes a bit longer but should not present a real problem to those physicians who have made a commitment to the sexual health of their patients. Much can be accomplished even in a busy practice. The physician can spend 5 to 10 minutes to determine whether the problem is primarily marital or sexual. The differentiation is not difficult. For those patients whose problems are primarily marital, referral to a marriage counselor can be made. For those who describe a good marital relationship but for whom sex has never met the couple's expectations in terms of pleasure, intimacy, and response, a choice then arises. The physician can counsel the patient or refer the patient to appropriate resources within the community, ie, health professionals, most of whom are not physicians, who are qualified sex therapists. It is essential, therefore, that physicians know the resources available within the community.

If the physician who engages in sex counseling or therapy undertakes specialized training based on the work of Masters and Johnson, Chaplain, and others, special time must be allotted in his or her practice. There are probably as many models as there are individuals engaged in this therapy. As a solo gynecologist, I have evolved the following useful and practical model over a period of several years. The first 4 days of the week are engaged in the practice of general gynecology. The fifth day is devoted entirely to counseling couples whom I have carefully screened. The couples come directly from my practice or have been referred by other physicians.

Therapy in my office is confined to the diagnosis and treatment of the dysfunctions of the sexual response system: general sexual dysfunction (eg, frigidity, lack of lubrication), anorgasmia and vaginismus in the female; premature ejaculation, retarded ejaculation, and erectile incompetence in the male. Mental problems and deviant sexual behavior, eg, fetishism, voyeurism, are referred. However, as a primary care physician, I often serve as a bridge in the referral of patients to other health professionals engaged in therapy in which I am not competent. This often requires two or three sessions. However, it has been my experience that after several sessions couples will accept referral more readily. Patients whom I treat are seen once a week or once every 2 weeks depending upon need and progress. The initial interview lasts 1 hour. Subsequent sessions last 25 to 40 minutes and charges are based on time.

Adjunctive aids. Several aids are available to the primary care physician who has made a commitment to include an inquiry into the sexual health of his or her patient. For example, a preprinted form[2] can be given to the patient to complete prior to seeing the physician. This particular form consists of 49 questions that appear on separate cards and that the patient responds to with yes or no answers. The questions begin very generally (eg, the existence of allergies, past serious illness or accident, immunizations, weight) and cover most of the organ systems. Those questions that concern marriage and sex appear near the bottom of the list: marital problems, husband's attitudes, pregnancy, vaginal discharges, menstrual periods, problems about sex, questions about sex or birth control, and a final question indicating whether the patient wishes to talk about a problem privately. My patients and I have found this very useful. They understand that discussion of almost any subject is acceptable and encouraged, although most patients will deny that they have serious marital sexual problems. The physician receives much general information without spending a good deal of effort and time.

Another valuable aid in obtaining information and conserving time is a detailed questionnaire that evaluates sexual performance.

Audiovisual material also can be helpful. For example, I can describe sensate focus, the sine qua non of Masters and Johnson therapy, but illustrating this with three 10-minute audiovisual cassettes is much more effective.[3] The same applies to the "stop and go" or "stimulate squeeze" exercises and to the employment of masturbation in cases of anorgasmia. Although I do not believe that audiovisual materials are essential to carry out sex therapy, they do serve to demonstrate and clarify, and they provide more time for dialogue in the exploration of other aspects of a problem. Such materials also increase my effectiveness and shorten therapy. The cassettes and the projector never leave my office and are used for no other purpose. I am not present in the room during the showing of the films, but there is a brief discussion about their contents immediately following.

Record keeping. When personnel are interviewed for employment, they are apprised of the nature of the practice and the absolute necessity for confidentiality. No separate list of sex therapy patients is kept. That is, there is no cross filing. Employees are forbidden to extract charts from the files except for office visits, telephone calls, insurance purposes, or other matters of absolute necessity. The objective is not to highlight the sexual aspect of my practice, but rather to regard it as an integral part no different than any other aspect. However, because of possible stigma, another precaution is taken. When a patient transfers from my practice to another physician's practice and later we receive a signed release form pertaining to her records, the patient is contacted and asked specifically whether record transfer is to include information regarding sexual, marital sexual functioning, and counseling. Those patients who instruct me to forward all material are then requested to sign a statement releasing this material.

Insurance. All patients are billed in accordance with fee-for-service based upon time. Sex therapy by physicians may be reimbursed by third-party payers if a *DSM-III* diagnosis, such as anxiety, generalized disorder state, or depressive neurosis, can be made with respect to one of the spouses.

References

1. Lief HL. Sex education of medical students and doctors. *Pac Med Surg.* 1965;72:52-58.

2. Data Sheets, Series 4000. Medical Practice Systems, Inc; 1970.

3. EDCOA Productions, Inc, 310 Cedar Ln, Teaneck, NJ 07666.

(SMP-1981)

Sexually Transmitted Diseases

STDs a 'hidden epidemic.' US rate highest in the Western world; knowledge, awareness lag

Deborah L. Shelton
AM News Dec 9, 1996 p 1

The nation is experiencing a "hidden epidemic" of sexually transmitted diseases (STDs), and physicians are key to combating it, an Institute of Medicine panel said in a major new report.

STDs are called a hidden problem because many are asymptomatic and many people, including care providers, are reluctant to talk about them.

The United States has the world's highest rates of STDs. Five of the 10 most common diseases reported to the Centers for Disease Control and Prevention in 1995 were sexually transmitted.

Yet awareness and knowledge about STDs are low, and there is no national strategy to address this, said the

S

S report, "The Hidden Epidemic: Confronting Sexually Transmitted Diseases."

The IOM panel said HIV was not included in the report because it is now the most recognized STD, and HIV-prevention efforts are relatively well funded. Such is not the case with other STDs, however.

12 million new cases a year

More than 25 infectious organisms are transmitted sexually. And about 12 million new STD cases a year are reported to the CDC, with about a quarter occurring among adolescents.

Prevention efforts have been hampered on many levels, however, by the "biological characteristics of STDs, societal problems, unbalanced media messages, lack of awareness, fragmentation of STD-related services, inadequate training of health care professionals, inadequate health insurance coverage and access to services, and insufficient investment in STD prevention," the report said.

Between 1973 and 1992, more than 150,000 US women died as a result of STDs or related complications. Women are biologically more susceptible to certain STDs and more likely to have asymptomatic infections that result in delayed diagnosis and treatment.

Quality of care varies

The report noted a wide variation in the quality, scope, accessibility, and availability of services provided by publicly funded clinics, some of which "do not provide high-quality services."

The public sector spends only $1 to prevent STDs for every $43 spent on treatment and other costs. Private health plans were faulted for doing an inadequate job of reimbursing care and integrating treatment and prevention of STDs into the mainstream of primary care.

The IOM panel recommended establishing a national campaign to promote healthy sexual behavior. At the heart of the initiative is the promotion of open discussion between care providers and their patients. That's especially needed when working with adolescents, who have the highest rates of STDs but who often go untreated. The consequences of an untreated STD include infertility and cervical and other cancers, and sometimes aren't known for years.

The national campaign would include promotion of school-based sex education and age-appropriate STD services, including access to condoms. The report noted that the average age at which American women first engage in sexual intercourse is about 16.

According to the report, teens are more likely to engage in unprotected sex and other high-risk sexual behaviors, are more susceptible to cervical infections, and often lack access to adequate health services. About a quarter of adolescents are uninsured.

The Institute of Medicine proposes a national, long-term campaign to promote healthy sexual behaviors by making the public and health professionals more knowledgeable about sexually transmitted diseases. The recommendations include:

- Increased funding for prevention.
- Improved surveillance systems and monitoring of prevention programs.
- Innovative services for adolescents and underserved populations.
- More complete health care coverage of STD-related services for members and their sexual partners.
- Raising of the skill level of health professionals in sexual health issues.
- Better integration of STD-related services into primary care.

Resources

American Social Health Association
PO Box 13827, Research Triangle Park, NC 27709
919 361-8400   Fax 919 361-8425
Web address: http://sunsite.unc.edu/ASHA

National VD Hotline
American Social Health Association
800 227-8922 (CA 800 982-5883)

SIECUS (Sex Information and Education
Council of the US)
130 W 42nd, Ste 350, New York, NY 10036
212 819-9770   Fax 212 819-9776

Sick Building Syndrome

Sick building syndrome is a collection of symptoms sometimes reported by people who work in modern office buildings. The symptoms include loss of energy, headaches, and dry, itching eyes, nose, and throat.

The cause of the syndrome is unknown, although it has been attributed to air conditioning, fluorescent lighting, loss of natural ventilation and light, and psychological factors, especially frustration at being unable to control physical conditions (such as temperature and ventilation) in the working environment. Some authorities believe that many outbreaks of sick building syndrome may be pseudoepidemics (conditions without physical causes that are thought to be a form of hysteria). (ENC-1989)

Resource

National Safe Workplace Institute
3008 Bishops Ridge, Monroe, NC 28110
704 289-6061   Fax 704 289-6766

Sickle Cell Anemia

Center for Sickle Cell Disease
Howard University
2121 Georgia Ave NW, Washington, DC 20059
202 636-7930   Fax 202 806-4517

Sickle Cell Disease Association of America
200 Corporate Pointe, Ste 495
Culver City, CA 90230-7633
800 421-8453 310 216-6363   Fax 310 215-3722

Sjogren's Syndrome

Sjogren's Syndrome Foundation, Inc
333 N Broadway, Ste 200, Jericho, NY 11753
800 475-6473   516 933-6365   Fax 516 933-6368
Web address: http://www.w2.com/ss.html

Sleep

American Sleep Disorders Association
1610 14th St NW, Ste 300, Rochester, MN 55901
507 287-6006   Fax 507 287-6008
Web address: http://www.cloud9.net/~thorpy

Smoking

AMA Policy

Dangers of passive smoking to children (505.975)
Amended Res 417, A-93

The AMA calls on corporate headquarters of fast food franchisers to require that one of the standards of operation of such franchises be a no-smoking policy for such restaurants; and endorses the passage of laws, ordinances, and regulations that prohibit smoking in fast food restaurants and other entertainment and food outlets which target children in their marketing efforts, in view of the long-term health effects and severe impact on future health care costs in the United States.

AMA guidelines: Make it a habit

AM News Feb 7, 1994 p 22

Starting a stop-smoking program in your practice can be as easy as A-B-C. In fact, forget B and C, and follow the AMA's five A's:

Ask—Determine smoking status of every patient.

Advise—Urge all smokers to stop.

Assist—Provide motivational and self-help materials, set a "quit date" and tailor a plan for each patient.

Arrange—Set follow-up visits to encourage success and prevent relapse.

Anticipate—Be ready with a prevention strategy for adolescent nonsmokers.

JAMA Theme Issue: Smoking

JAMA 1996 Oct 9; 276(14)

Over the past decade, several issues have discussed the perils and controversies revolving around smoking (for example, see also February 23, 1994; December 11, 1991; September 26, 1990). This issue looks at macular degeneration and smoking.

Magazines without tobacco advertising

JAMA 1994 Feb 23; 271(8): 571-576

Since its first list appeared (*JAMA* 1989 Sept 8; 262[10] 1290-1291, 1295), many titles have come and gone, but the list is still substantial. Credit for the idea of having only "smoke-free magazines" in physicians' reception rooms goes to Doctors Ought to Care (DOC), a group of physicians devoted to educating people about the causes of preventable illness. Publication of such a list in *JAMA* follows a resolution adopted by the American Medical Association's House of Delegates in 1987. The list below has been updated with address changes since the last publication of the list.

Accent on Living
PO Box 700, Bloomington, IL 61701-0700

Adirondack Life
PO Box 97, Jay, NY 12941

Air & Space
370 L'Enfant Promenade SW
Washington, DC 20024-2518

Alaska
808 E St, Anchorage, AK 99501

American Baby
249 W 17th, New York, NY 10011

American Health
28 W 23rd St, New York, NY 10010

American Heritage
60 Fifth Ave, New York, NY 10011

American History Illustrated
PO Box 822, Harrisburg, PA 17105

American Philatelist
PO Box 8000, State College, PA 16803

American Square Dance
PO Box 488, Huron, OH 44839

American Woman
1700 Broadway, New York, NY 10019

American Woodworker
33 E Minor St, Emmaus, PA 18098

Americas
1889 F St NW, Washington, DC 20006

Animal Kingdom
185th St & Southern Blvd, Bronx, NY 10460

Antique Automobile
501 W Governor Rd, PO Box 317, Hershey, PA 17033

Antiques
PO Box 10547, Des Moines, IA 50347

Archaeology
135 William St, New York, NY 10038

Arizona Highways
2039 W Lewis Ave, Phoenix, AZ 85009

Arthritis Today
1314 Spring St NW, Atlanta, GA 30309

Artist's Magazine
1507 Dana Ave, Cincinnati, OH 45207

ArtNews
PO Box 11680, Boulder, CO 80323

Art & Antiques
3 E 54th St, New York, NY 10022

Astronomy
PO Box 1612, Waukesha, WI 53187

Audubon
950 3rd Ave, New York, NY 10022

Aviation Week & Space Technology
1221 Ave of the Americas, New York, NY 10020

Backpacker
33 E Minor St, Emmaus, PA 18098

Basketball America
PO Box 2982, Durham, NC 27715

S

Bicycling
33 E Minor St, Emmaus, PA 18098

Bird Watcher's Digest
PO Box 110, Marietta, OH 45750

Black Elegance
475 Park Ave S, New York, NY 10016

Boating
PO Box 51055, Boulder, CO 80323

Business Start-Ups
2392 Morse Ave, PO Box 57050, Irvine, CA 92714

Business Week
1221 Ave of the Americas, New York, NY 10020

Byte
1 Phoenix Mill Lane, Peterborough, NH 03458

Canoe & Kayak
PO Box 3146, Kirkland, WA 98083

Cars & Parts
911 Vandermark Rd, Sidney, OH 45365

Cash Saver
PO Box 16958, North Hollywood, CA 91615

Cat Fancy
PO Box 6050, Mission Viejo, CA 92690

Child
110 Fifth Ave, New York, NY 10017

Common Cause Magazine
2030 M St NW, Washington, DC 20036

Complete Woman
875 N Michigan Ave, Chicago, IL 60611-1901

Consumer Reports
101 Truman Ave, Yonkers, NY 10703-1057

Consumer's Research
800 Maryland Ave NE, Washington, DC 20002

Cooking Light
2100 Lakeshore Dr, Birmingham, AL 35209

Country Home
1716 Locust St, Des Moines, IA 50309-3023

Country Journal
6405 Flank Dr, Harrisburg, PA 17112

Crafts
PO Box 1790, Peoria, IL 61656

Craftworks for the Home
70 Sparta Ave, Sparta, NJ 07871

Crosstrainer
63 Grand, River Edge, NJ 07661

Cruising World
PO Box 3029, Harlan, IA 51593

Cyclist
20916 Higgins Court, Torrance, CA 90501

Dance Magazine
33 W 60th St, New York, NY 10023-7990

Diabetes Forecast
1660 Duke St, Alexandria, VA 22314

Dive Travel
PO Box 2992, Boulder, CO 80329

Dog Fancy
PO Box 6050, Mission Viejo, CA 92690

Dog World
29 N Wacker Dr, Chicago, IL 60606

Down Beat
102 N Haven Rd, Elmhurst, IL 60126

Down East Magazine
PO Box 679, Camden, ME 04843

Earth
PO Box 1612, Waukesha, WI 53187

The Economist
PO Box 58510, Boulder, CO 80321

Elks Magazine
425 W Diversey Pkwy, Chicago, IL 60614

Entrepreneur
PO Box 57050, Irvine, CO 92619-7050

Exceptional Children
1920 Association Dr, Reston, VA 22091

Exceptional Parent
120 State St, Hackensack, NJ 07601-5421

The Family Handyman
7900 International Dr, Minneapolis, MN 55425

Fine Cooking
63 S Main St, Newtown, CT 06470

Fine Gardening
63 S Main St, Newtown, CT 06470

Fine Homebuilding
63 S Main St, Newtown, CT 06470

Fine Woodworking
63 S Main St, Newtown, CT 06470

Fishing Facts
1901 Bell Ave, Des Moines, IA 50315

Florida Sportsman
5901 SW 74th St, Miami, FL 33143

Flower & Garden
700 W 47th St, Ste 310, Kansas City, MO 64112

Folk Art
Museum of American Folk Art
61 W 62nd St, New York, NY 10023

Flying
500 W Putnam Ave, Greenwich, CT 06830

Flying Models
PO Box 700, Newton, NJ 07860

Freshwater & Marine Aquarium
PO Box 487, Sierra Madre, CA 91204

The Futurist
7910 Woodmont Ave, Ste 450, MD 20814

Golf Illustrated
3 Park Ave, New York, NY 10016

Good Housekeeping
959 Eighth Ave, New York, NY 10019

Good Old Days
306 E Parr Rd, Berne, IN 46711

Guideposts
39 Seminary Hill Rd, Carmel, NY 10512

Guitar World
1115 Broadway, 8th Fl, New York, NY 10010

Hadassah Magazine
50 W 58th St, New York, NY 10019

Harvard Business Review
60 Harvard Way, Boston, MA 02163

Harvard Lampoon
44 Bow St, Cambridge, MA 02138

Harvard Medical School Health Letter
79 Garden St, Cambridge, MA 02138

Harvard Women's Health Watch
PO Box 420234, Palm Coast, FL 32142

Health News & Review
27 Pine St, New Canaan, CT 06840

Historic Preservation
1785 Massachusetts Ave, Washington, DC 20036

Home
PO Box 53969, Boulder, CO 80323

Home Office Computing
411 Lafayette St, 4th Fl, New York, NY 10003

Horn Book Magazine
11 Beacon St, Boston, MA 02108

Horse Illustrated
PO Box 6050, Mission Viejo, CA 92690

Horticulture
98 N Washington St, Boston, MA 02114

Income Opportunities
1500 Broadway, New York, NY 10036-4015

Instructor
555 Broadway, New York, NY 10012

International Travel News
2120 28th St, Sacramento, CA 95818

Isaac Asimov's Science Fiction
380 Lexington Ave, New York, NY 10017

Itinerary
PO Box 1084, Bayonne, NJ 07002-1084

Journal of Irreproducible Results
350 E Sauk Trail, South Chicago Heights, IL 60411

Kaleidoscope
326 Locust St, Akron, OH 44302

The Lion
300 22nd St, Oak Brook, IL 60521

Longevity
277 Park Ave, New York, NY 10172

Macworld
501 Second St, San Francisco, CA 94107

MAD
485 Madison Ave, New York, NY 10022

Maine Fish & Wildlife
284 State St, Ste 41, Augusta, ME 04333

Maine Life
250 Center St, Auburn, ME 04210

Mature Outlook
1716 Locust, Des Moines, IA 50309-3023

Mayo Clinic Health Letter
Mayo Clinic, Rochester, MN 55905

Men's Fitness
21100 Erwin St, Woodland Hills, CA 91367

Men's Health
33 E Minor St, Emmaus, PA 18098

Men's Workout
1115 Broadway, New York, NY 10160

Midwest Living
1716 Locust St, Des Moines, IA 50309-3023

Model Railroader
21027 Crosswroads Circle, PO Box 1612
Waukesha, WI 53186

Modern Drummer Magazine
12 Old Bridge Rd, Cedar Grove, NJ 07009

Modern Maturity
3200 E Carson St, Lakewood, CA 90712

Mondo 2000
PO Box 10171, Berkeley, CA 94709

Montana Magazine
PO Box 5630, Helena, MT 59604

Mother Jones
731 Market St, Ste 600, San Francisco, CA 94103-2021

Motorboating & Sailing
250 W 55th St, 4th Fl, New York, NY 10019

Ms.
230 Park Ave, New York, NY 10069

Muscle & Fitness
21100 Erwin St, Woodland Hills, CA 91367

Nation
72 Fifth Ave, New York, NY 10011

National Gardening
180 Flynn Ave, Burlington, VT 05401

National Geographic
1145 17th St NW, Washington, DC 20036

National Parks
1776 Massachusetts Ave NW, Washington, DC 20036

National Wildlife
8925 Leesburg Pike, Vienna, VA 22184

Natural History
Central Park West at 79th St, New York, NY 10024

New Mexico Magazine
PO Box 12002, Sante Fe, NM 87504

The New Yorker
20 W 43rd St, New York, NY 10036

North American Review
University of Northern Iowa, Cedar Falls, IA 50614-0516

Nutrition Action Healthletter
1501 16th St NW, Washington, DC 20036

Old House Journal
2 Main St, Gloucester, MA 01930-5725

Opera Magazine
PO Box 816, Madison Square Station
New York, NY 10159

Organic Gardening
35 E Minor St, Emmaus, PA 18098

Out West
10522 Brunswick Rd, Grass Valley, CA 95945

Parenting Magazine
301 Howard St, San Francisco, CA 94105

S

Parents
685 Third Ave, New York, NY 10017

PC Magazine
1 Park Ave, New York, NY 10016

PC World
501 2nd St, 5th Fl, San Francisco, CA 94107

Personal Computing
PO Box 2492, Boulder, CO 80322

Petersen's Hunting
6420 Wilshire Blvd, Los Angeles, CA 90048-5515

Petersen's Photographic Magazine
6420 Wilshire Blvd, Los Angeles, CA 90048-5515

Popular Communications
76 N Broadway, Hicksville, NY 11801

Popular Photography
1633 Broadway, New York, NY 10019

Prevention
33 E Minor St, Emmaus, PA 18098

Railfan & Railroad
PO Box 700, Newton, NJ 07860

Reader's Digest
Pleasantville, NY 10570

Runner's World
33 E Minor St, Emmaus, PA 18098

Salt, Inc
PO Box 1400, Kennebunkport, ME 04046

Satellite Orbit
8330 Boone Blvd, Vienna, VA 22182

Saturday Evening Post
1100 Waterway Blvd, Indianapolis, IN 46202

Science
1200 New York Ave NW, Washington, DC 20005

Science News
1719 N St NW, Washington, DC 20036

Scientific American
415 Madison Ave, New York, NY 10017

Sea Frontiers
400 SE 2nd Ave, 4th Fl, Miami, FL 33131

Shape
21100 Erwin St, Woodland Hills, CA 91367

Sierra
85 2nd St, San Francisco, CA 94105

Single Parent
401 N Michigan Ave, Chicago, IL 60611

Sixteen Magazine
233 Park Ave S, New York, NY 10003

Skiing
2 Park Ave, New York, NY 10016

Ski Magazine
PO Box 52013, Boulder, CO 80321

Skin Diver Magazine
6420 Wilshire Blvd, Los Angeles, CA 90048-5515

Smithsonian
900 Jefferson Dr, Washington, DC 20560

Society
Rutgers University, New Brunswick, NJ 08903

Southern Accents
2100 Lakeshore Dr, Birmingham, AL 35209

Southern Living
2100 Lakeshore Dr, Birmingham, AL 35209

Sports Afield
250 W 55th Ave, New York, NY 10019

Sunset
80 Willow Rd, Menlo Park, CA 94025

Texas Highways
PO Box 141009, Austin, TX 78714-1009

The Texas Observer
307 W 7th St, Austin, TX 78701

Theatre Crafts
135 Fifth Ave, New York, NY 10010

Threads
63 S Main St, Newtown, CT 06470

Traditional Home
1716 Locust St, Des Moines, IA 50309-3023

Travel & Leisure
1120 Ave of the Americas, New York, NY 10036

Travel Holiday
19 W 22nd St, 10th Fl, New York, NY 10010-5204

Twins
6740 Antioch, Merriam, KS 66204-1261

University of California, Berkeley Wellness Letter
PO Box 420148, Palm Coast, FL 32142

Vegetarian Times
PO Box 570, Oak Park, IL 60303

Venture
Christian Service Brigade
PO Box 150, Wheaton, IL 60189

Veranda
455 E Paces Ferry Rd, Atlanta, GA 30305

Vermont Life
61 Elm St, Montpelier, VT 05602

Vermont Magazine
PO Box 389, Bristol, VT 05443

Vibrant Life
55 W Oak Ridge Dr, Hagerstown, MD 21740

Walking Magazine
9-11 Harcourt St, Boston, MA 02116

The Washington Monthly
1611 Connecticut Ave NW, 4th Fl
Washington, DC 20009

Weight Watchers Magazine
360 Lexington Ave, New York, NY 10017

West Coast Review of Books
5265 Fountain, Upper Terrace 6, Los Angeles, CA 90029

Western Outdoors
PO Box 2027, New Port Beach, CA 92659-1027

Westways
2601 S Figueroa, Los Angeles, CA 90007

Wildlife Conservation
New York Zoological Society
2300 Southern Blvd, Bronx, NY 10460

Women's Sports & Fitness
2025 Pearl St, Boulder, CO 80302

Wood
6060 Spine Rd, PO Box 55049
Boulder, CO 80323

The Woodworkers' Journal
517 Litchfield Rd, PO Box 1629
New Millford, CT 06776

Workbasket
700 W 47th St, Ste 310, Kansas City, MO 64112

Workbench
700 W 47th St, Ste 310, Kansas City, MO 64112

Worth
PO Box 55424, Boulder, CO 80323

Writer's Digest
1507 Dana Ave, Cincinnati, OH 45207

Yachting
PO Box 52277, Boulder, CO 80323

Your Money
5705 N Lincoln Ave, Chicago, IL 60659

Zoogoer
National Zoological Park, Washington, DC 20008

For Children and Teenagers

Big Bopper
3500 W Olive Ave, Burbank, CA 91505

Black Beat
355 Lexington Ave, New York, NY 10017

Boy's Life
1325 Walnut Hill Lane, PO Box 152079
Irving, TX 75015-2079

Cricket
315 5th St, Peru, IL 61354

Highlights for Children
803 Church St, Honesdale, PA 18431

Humpty Dumpty
PO Box 567, Indianapolis, IN 46206

Jack and Jill
PO Box 567, Indianapolis, IN 46206

Kid City
1 Lincoln Plaza, New York, NY 10023

Ladybug
315 5th St, Peru, IL 61354

Ranger Rick
8925 Leesburg Pike, Vienna, VA 22184-0001

Right On!
233 Park Ave S, 6th Fl, New York, NY 10003

Sesame Street
1 Lincoln Plaza, New York, NY 10022

Seventeen
850 Third Ave, New York, NY 10022

Teen
6420 Wilshire Blvd, Los Angeles, CA 90048-5515

3-2-1 Contact
1 Lincoln Plaza, New York, NY 10023

YM
685 Third Ave, New York, NY 10017

Resource
Office on Smoking and Health
Technical Information Center
5600 Fishers Ln, Park Bldg, Room 1-16
Rockville, MD 20857
301 443-1690

Snake Bite

To locate antivenom:
Arizona Poison and Drug Information Center Center
602 626-6016

Contact local zoo for exotic snakes.

Social Health

American Social Health Association
PO Box 13827, Research Triangle Park, NC 27709
919 361-8400   Fax 919 361-8425
Web address: http://sunsite.unc.edu/ASHA

Socioeconomic Characteristics of Medical Practice

Gonzalez ML. *Socioeconomic Characteristics of Medical Practice.* Chicago, Ill: American Medical Association; 1997 Annual; 177 pp
ISBN 0-89970-865-X OP192697

Spanish

Interamerican College of Physicians & Surgeons
915 Broadway, Ste 1510, New York, NY 10010
212 777-3642   Fax 212 505-7984

(Spanish-speaking physicians, list of)

Special Purpose Examination (SPEX)

Exam administered by individual state licensing boards:

Federation of State Medical Boards of the US
6000 Western Pl, Ste 707, Fort Worth, TX 76107
817 735-8445   Fax 817 738-6629

Specialists, Board Certified

AMA Policy

Patient Access to Specialty Care in Managed Care Systems (H-165.908) CMS Rep I-93-5

Amended by Res 707, I-96

(1) That the AMA take all appropriate action to require all health plans or sponsors of such plans that restrict a patient's choice of physicians or hospitals to offer, at the time of enrollment and at least for a continuous one-month period annually thereafter, an optional "point-of-service-type" feature so that patients who choose such plans may elect to self-refer to physicians outside of the plan at additional cost to themselves. (CMS Rep 5, A-95; Reaffirmed by CMS Rep 5, I-95; Reaffirmed by Ref Cmt G, A-96; Reaffirmed by Rules & Credentials Cmt, A-96; Reaffirmed by Sub Res 706, I-96)

(2) urges managed care plans to provide patients, on an ongoing basis, with the right to select a new primary physician from the panel of physicians contracting with that managed care plan, and appeal to the plan when the patient is dissatisfied with his/her present primary physician; (CMS Rep I-93-5)

(3) encourages medical specialty societies, through the Specialty and Service Society, the Practice Parameters Partnership, and other appropriate channels, to conduct further research to define the circumstances better when patient self-referrals to specialists of their choice are appropriate and cost-effective; (CMS Rep I-93-5)

(4) opposes any governmental incentives or mandates that would favor managed care, the gatekeeper concept, and restrictions upon patient self-referral in the absence of any research to demonstrate conclusively the cost-effectiveness of such a system; (CMS Rep I-93-5)

(5) will study the impact on access to specialty care if the government mandates the use of "gatekeepers" in health system reform, and the AMA will take appropriate action based on the results of its study and

(6) encourages all components of organized medicine to minimize the use of the term "gatekeeper" when making any reference to primary care physicians or to their role.

A Piece of My Mind

An omission rectified

Spence Meighan, MD
JAMA 1994 Aug 24/31; 272(8): 586

Recently I referred to some colleagues as "a bunch of doctors." Immediately it became apparent that bunch was an entirely inappropriate descriptive term for a group of such eminent professional people. Realizing my error, I tried to identify a more upscale term than bunch and discovered that we lack a collective noun for our profession. Lions have a *pride*; geese, a *gaggle*; and larks, an *exaltation*. But for physicians, all is silent.

On the spot I took it upon myself to rectify this deficiency in our heritage and come up with a word to describe a group of physicians. To my consternation I found my talents were unequal to the task. I started with a *band,* moved to *orchestra,* then to *family.* A *perversity* (suggested by my spouse), *safari,* and *praestigium* crossed my mind but were quickly rejected. The advent of managed care made me think of *bundle, package,* or even *contract.* But none of these nouns came close to doing us justice.

Ultimately, I came to the conclusion that we are so specialized that no single collective noun can represent the rich diversity of talent that graces our distinguished profession; each specialty must be afforded its own noun. The following list represents a starting point. Additions and refinements will follow in due course.

A *stash* of addictionists.
A *hive* of allergists.
A *block* of anesthesiologists.
A *murmur* of cardiologists.
A *rash* of dermatologists.
A *crush* of emergency physicians.
A *surge* of endocrinologists.

A *plague* of epidemiologists.
A *practicum* of family physicians.
A *bolus* of gastroenterologists.
A *marsupialization* of general surgeons (in small groups, a *knot*).
A *pool* of geneticists.
A *wrinkle* of geriatricians.
A *smear* of gynecologists.
A *clot* of hematologists.
A *system* of immunologists.
An *outbreak* of infectious disease specialists.
A *deliberation* of internists.
A *sample* of nephrologists.
A *network* of neurologists (in small groups, a *nucleus*).
A *drill* of neurosurgeons.
A *nest* of obstetricians.
A *field* of ophthalmologists.
A *mass* of oncologists.
A *union* of orthopedic surgeons (in small groups, a *brace*).
A *drum* of otolaryngologists.
A *twinge* of pain managers.
A *cross-section* of pathologists.
A *giggle* of pediatricians.
An *artifice* of plastic surgeons.
A *Fleet* of proctologists.
A *complex* of psychiatrists (when confidentiality must be preserved, a *thingamajig*).
An *inspiration* of pulmonologists.
A *series* of radiologists.
A *hobble* of rheumatologists.
A *conjugation* of sexologists.
A *scrimmage* of sports medicine physicians.
A *puddle* of urologists (in small groups, a *dribble*).

Although I may be accused of transcending my legitimate boundaries, I felt I should offer my newly honed skills to some other professions with which we work. I propose the following:
A *proliferation* of administrators.
A *cavity* of dentists.
An *uprising* of nurses.
A *dose* of pharmacists.
A *collection* of phlebotomists.
A *repetition* of physical therapists.
A *standing* of podiatrists.
A *quandary* of psychologists.
A *utopia* of social workers.
A *stampede* of veterinarians.

All of these collective nouns are offered as suggestions as to a place to begin the process of final selection—a responsibility that will require the approval of a *congress of body politics.*

But, it *is* a beginning.

Jim Kronenberg, Oregon Medical Association, aided and abetted in this craziness.

ABMS Compendium of Certified Medical Specialists available, annually revised, from:
American Board of Medical Specialties
1007 Church St, Ste 404, Evanston, IL 60201-5913
847 491-9091   Fax 847 328-3596

S

Directory of Medical Specialists
Marquis Who's Who, Macmillan Directory Division
3002 Glenview Rd, Wilmette, IL 60091
800 621-9669 (outside IL) 847 441-2387

Resource
Council of Medical Specialty Societies
51-A Sherwood Terrace, Lake Bluff, IL 60044
847 295-3456 Fax 847 295-3759
E-mail:76324.2156@compuserve.com

Specialty Boards

Medical practice: specialization [excerpt]

Lester S. King

Shortly after the middle of the 19th century, specialization in medicine increased greatly. It formed part of the vast expansion of knowledge and the improvement in patient care that characterized the era. However, there also developed many internal strains whose study provides an excellent approach to medical practice and the sociology of medicine.

Central to the story of specialization is the consultant, who could help the general practitioner with a difficult case. In the 17th and 18th centuries, in Great Britain, the physician, who held an MD degree, would act as consultant for the apothecary who did not have university training.[1] In the United States, even though the distinction of physician and apothecary did not obtain, the consultation always had a prominent part in medical practice: By virtue of training and expertise, the consultant was qualified to give advice. When called in consultation he could unearth new evidence, or reinterpret the data already amassed, to reach a diagnosis or evaluate treatment. He was an expert who gave an opinion and made recommendations but did not ordinarily take over the conduct of the case.

In the larger cities, especially among medical school faculty, a consultation practice was a much sought goal, one that might accrue almost automatically to the professor of medicine. Such an honor, however, had to be earned, for such men had to be better trained and more knowledgeable than their colleagues. They generally had a long apprenticeship in pathology, and spent a great deal of time in teaching, as well as in keeping up with current developments. The paradigm of consultant was, perhaps, William Osler. In the smaller and nonacademic communities a consultant would have a less exalted status. He would be a fellow practitioner who engaged in regular medical practice in the community. While not necessarily better trained than his colleagues, he would have acquired a reputation in some particular area and his opinion would be received with respect.

In its annual meetings the American Medical Association recognized a trend toward specialization. The presentation of papers took place in sections, where men with special interests could meet to promote those interests. By 1859 six such sections were recognized for the annual meeting: (1) anatomy and physiology; (2) chemistry and materia medica; (3) practical medicine and obstetrics; (4) surgery; (5) meteorology, medical topography, and epidemic diseases; and (6) medical jurisprudence and hygiene. The first two groups comprehended what we now call the basic sciences; group three, significantly enough, combined general medicine and obstetrics; surgery, in group four, remained by itself. Infectious diseases were bracketed with environmental data, an interesting sidelight on the prebacteriologic era.[2]

Gradually the number of sections increased. When the AMA decided to sponsor the International Congress of Medicine, to be held in Washington, DC, in 1887, the original plans called for 18 separate sections at which papers might be presented. The purely clinical sections embraced the following areas: medicine, surgery, obstetrics, gynecology, ophthalmology, otology, dermatology and syphilis, nervous diseases and psychiatry, laryngology, and diseases of children. These subjects had thus received formal recognition as approved specialties.[3]

The AMA, which served primarily the general practitioner, crystallized its position in 1869.[4] Specialism was certainly advantageous for the science of medicine, but opinions differed regarding "its benefits to the profession." There was objection that the specialties "operate unfairly toward the general practitioner, in implying that he is incompetent to properly treat certain classes of disease, and narrowing his field of practice." The report went on, "It is natural that in any changes from old-beaten paths, there should be some temporary confusion, but...as soon as the relations between special and general practice become better adjusted...great advantages will accrue, even to the general practitioner."

The AMA formally adopted the view that specialties were a proper field of practice, that specialists should obey the same rules of professional "etiquette" as general practitioners, and that "it shall not be proper for specialists publicly to advertise themselves as such, or to assume any title not specially granted by a regular chartered college."[5]

The AMA had officially accepted specialism as a major movement in medicine but was relatively powerless to smooth out the conflicts between the specialists and the general practitioners. The dissensions between the two groups could not be settled by official ukase and surfaced progressively over the next 40 years. In the medical literature during that time the specialties at first showed a defensive posture. Later the general practitioners were on the defensive. In 1874 an editorial pointed out that the previous 15 years had witnessed bitter opposition "against the cultivation of specialties" but these nevertheless had proved themselves "indispensable to progress in medicine." The great problem was how to find the proper distinction between "general and special practice" to achieve the best interests of medicine and the greatest good of the patients.

The general practitioner was expected to treat the simpler affections and should be "competent" to judge between mild and serious conditions. As soon as special skill was required, the case should be "gracefully resigned" to the specialist. Since this, the writer admitted, "is not the general custom," he offered a highly simplistic remedy. In medical schools the teachers should emphasize "the symptoms which should always demand the resignation of the case to the expert." The practitioner should be aware of his limitations. No practitioner "who has the best interests of his patient at heart" can ignore the claims of the experts. To do so is to "sacrifice the dearest

S of all professional obligations to the paltry and mean consideration of a few extra dollars in his own purse." This mixture of high moral principle and concrete economic consideration was a fairly constant ingredient of the entire controversy.

In 1906 a general practitioner, John L. Hildreth, in a well-balanced presentation published in the *Boston Medical Surgery Journal,* illustrated some of the issues troublesome at that time.

The people at large were showing an increasing demand for specialists, and often might bypass the family doctor and go directly to a specialist. The complaints against the specialists are delicately phrased and qualified, but when we analyze the rather long paper we find two main areas of discontent. The one involves status, and the other the monetary aspects of practice.

Frankly expressed is the practitioner's fear of losing the patient. The writer also feared that the specialist would disparage what had already been done for the patient. There existed, as well, a widespread feeling that the specialist was prompted by pecuniary considerations. The general practitioner "spends all his time looking after $3 ailments," while the specialist collects $5 and $10 a visit, or performs surgical operations for which he makes a substantial charge.

There was strong emphasis on the "commercialism" that the author saw as invading medicine and especially affecting specialists. He admitted, however, that the doctor "who deprives himself of many of the pleasures of life that he may minister to suffering humanity, should be properly remunerated so that he may have the ordinary comforts of life." We must realize that the physician—certainly the general practitioner—was not at that time really well-to-do, and that the problem of making a living loomed large in the first part of the 20th century.

Between 1866 and 1906 the same problems and complaints, variously phrased, recurred again and again. The literature shows quite a repetitive character. The general practitioner feared that he might lose patients, along with status. In the medical literature defense took the form partly of counterattack against the specialists, partly of recommendations toward self-improvement.

Counterattack was directed against the shortcomings of specialists. The general practitioner derived satisfaction from pointing to individual instances of bad practice. Specialists were criticized for inadequate training, rendering them prone to ignore whatever fell outside their own field of interest. There resulted diagnostic errors that no experienced general practitioner would make.

The fault was attributed chiefly to insufficient experience in general practice—premature specialism. One practitioner in 1887 noted the "rattlebrained person who, having tried general practice for a year or so and miserable failed, immediately takes up some sub-department of medicine...and becomes a specialist."[6] Of course, the better and more vocal specialists agreed that physicians who wanted to specialize should have extensive experience in general practice before limiting themselves to a particular field.

The specialists were also subjected to the charges of money-grubbing and commercialism. An important complaint declared that they were always able to find something to operate on. Such charges were directed particularly at gynecologists. "The older men are more conservative, but the younger men are making their reputation and are doing at the expense of the general practitioner."[7] While the gynecologists were commonly the subject of attack, specialists in eye, ear, nose, and throat came off fairly well.

Despite the various charges, specialism was firmly established. The real problem was, how far would the process of subdivision go, and what effect would this have on the general practitioner—problems still oppressive today. With the growth of specialism general practitioners expressed a very real fear that they would sink to the level of mere referral centers, shunting patients to this or that specialist. One physician told of a woman who came to him, saying she did not want to consult him but wanted the name of "the best man in Pittsburgh on livers."[8] Patients would bypass their family doctor and go to some specialist they thought would be appropriate for their self-diagnosed condition.

Leaders in the profession might decry the overspecialization and brand it as absurd. F. C. Shattuck[9] said scornfully, in 1897, "We have an Association of Orificial Surgeons in this country. A few years ago a recent graduate asked me, apparently seriously, to give the name of a specialist in rheumatism. We can afford to laugh at these things." Later he declared, sarcastically, in discussing specialism, "Why not a chair in medical schools for the diseases of old age as well as for the diseases of children?"[10] Yet specialism did progress inexorably until the "absurdities" of 1900 have turned into the flourishing specialties of rheumatology and gerontology.

By way of a more positive approach, some generalists encouraged their fellow practitioners to have greater confidence in themselves. The general practitioners could assimilate the great progress that specialism had made and thus treat their patients more intelligently. Postgraduate courses would help so that the general practitioner could do for himself what formerly went to specialists. One practitioner declared[11] that the graduate from "any good hospital" should be able to perform creditably "such operations as tracheotomy, thoracentesis, and amygdalotomy, repair the recently lacerated perineum, attend to simple and many compound fractures, do minor gynecological work," as well as the work of the family physician, "and still leave enough for the specialist." A little self-confidence will often enable one to do as good work in such cases as the specialists, and at the same time advance his own professional and financial interests.

Another practitioner voiced his complaints against the "crazes" that derived from the work of specialists, particularly in gynecology. He encouraged his colleagues by saying, "The specialist is beginning to acknowledge his dependence of the practicing physician...The humble general practitioner is the real 'Ironsides' of the army of medical science."[12]

The struggle between specialists and general practitioners was merely one aspect of a much wider conflict, involving an elite group that claimed special knowledge and ability and expected corresponding rewards. These claims had to be hammered out on the anvil of experience—did in fact the special knowledge yield better results commensurate with the increased cost? Furthermore, were any advantages vitiated by compensatory drawbacks? In one or another form these conflicts had afflicted the medical profession for hundreds of years.

Medical practice had always involved competition for patients. The growth of specialism in the last third of the 19th century rendered the process more acute than ever. The struggle, however, was taking place in a constantly shifting environment. The entire culture was in flux, and the relation of physicians to each other and to their patients had to undergo severe and constant readjustments as the cultural and economic environment changed.

Bibliographic notes

1. King LS. The British background for American medicine. *JAMA*. 1982;248:217-220; Medical education: the early phases, ibid, pp 731-734.

2. *Trans AMA*. 1859;12:639.

3. *JAMA* 1884;3:671; see also: King LS. The AMA gets a new code of ethics. *JAMA*. 1983;249:1338-1342.

4. Report of the Committee on Specialties, and on the propriety of specialists advertising. *Trans AMA*. 1869;20:111-113.

5. *Trans AMA*. 1869;20:28.

6. The relations of general practice to specialism. *Med Rec*. 1874;9:597-598.

7. A particularly important source of opinion is the extensive discussion that followed several papers on specialism. The discussion is much more revealing than the actual papers and is found in *Bull Am Acad Med* 1899;4:186-199. The present reference is on page 195.

8. Ibid, p 191.

9. Shattuck FC. Specialism, the laboratory, and practical medicine. *Boston Med Surg J*. 1897;136:613-617.

10. Quoted in editorial: Specialism in medicine. *Boston Med Surg J*. 1900;143:379-380.

11. Gordon OA. Specialists and general practitioners. *NY Med J*. 1896;63:601.

12. Hutchinson W. Some of the disadvantages of specialism. *Med Rec*. 1895;48:518-519.

(AGE-1984)

Resources

American Board of Medical Specialties
1007 Church St, Ste 404, Evanston, IL 60201-5913
847 491-9091   Fax 847 328-3596
Web address: http://www.certifieddocs.org
(to verify board certification)

Council of Medical Specialty Societies
51-A Sherwood Terrace, Lake Bluff, IL 60044
847 295-3456   Fax 847 295-3759
E-mail:76324.2156@compuserve.com

Specialty boards

American Board of Allergy and Immunology
University City Science Ctr, 3624 Market St
Philadelphia, PA 19104
215 349-9466   Fax 215 222-8669
Includes the subspecialty of Diagnostic Laboratory Immunology

American Board of Anesthesiology
4101 Lake Boone Trail, Ste 510
Raleigh, NC 27607-7506
919 881-2570   Fax 919 881-2575
Includes the subspecialties of Critical Care Medicine and Pain Management

American Board of Colon and Rectal Surgery
20600 Eureka Rd, Ste 713, Taylor, MI 48180
313 282-9400   Fax 313 282-9402
E-mail: admnABCRS@aol.com

American Board of Dermatology
Henry Ford Hospital, 1 Ford Pl, Detroit, MI 48202-3450
313 874-1088   Fax 313 872-3221
Includes the subspecialties of Dermapathology, Dermatological Immunology, and Diagnostic Laboratory Immunology

American Board of Emergency Medicine
3000 Coolidge Rd, East Lansing, MI 48823-6319
517 332-4800   Fax 517 332-2234
Includes the subspecialty of Pediatric Emergency Medicine

American Board of Family Practice
2228 Young Dr, Lexington, KY 40505
606 269-5626   Fax 606 266-9699
Includes the subspecialties of Geriatric Medicine and Sports Medicine

American Board of Internal Medicine
University City Science Ctr, 3624 Market St
Philadelphia, PA 19104
800 441-2246 215 243-1500   Fax 215 382-4702
Includes the subspecialties of Cardiac Electrophysiology, Cardiovascular Disease, Critical Care Medicine, Diagnostic Laboratory Immunology, Endocrinology and Metabolism, Gastroenterology, Geriatric Medicine, Hematology, Infectious Disease, Medical Oncology, Nephrology, Pulmonary Disease, and Rheumatology

American Board of Neurological Surgery
6550 Fannin St, #2139, Houston, TX 77030-2722
713 790-6015
Includes the subspecialty of Critical Care Medicine

American Board of Nuclear Medicine
900 Veteran Ave, Rm 12-200
Los Angeles, CA 90024-1786
310 825-6787   Fax 310 825-9433
Includes the subspecialties of Nuclear Radiology and Radioisotopic Pathology

American Board of Obstetrics and Gynecology
2915 Vine St, Dallas, TX 78204-1069
214 871-1619   Fax 214 871-1943
Includes the subspecialties of Critical Care Medicine, Gynecologic Oncology, Maternal and Fetal Oncology, and Reproductive Endocrinology

American Board of Ophthalmology
111 Presidential Blvd, Ste 241
Bala Cynwyd, PA 19004
215 664-1175

American Board of Orthopaedic Surgery
400 Silver Cedar Ct, Chapel Hill, NC 27514
919 929-7103   Fax 919 942-8988
Includes the subspecialty of Hand Surgery

S

American Board of Otolaryngology
2211 Norfolk, Ste 800, Houston, TX 77098-4044
713 528-6200

American Board of Pathology
5401 W Kennedy Blvd, PO Box 25915
Tampa, FL 33622
813 286-2444   Fax 813 289-5279
Includes certification in Anatomic and Clinical Pathology as well as the subspecialties of Blood Banking Transfusion Medicine, Chemical Pathology, Cytopathology, Dermatopathology, Forensic Pathology, Hematology, Immunopathology, Medical Microbiology, Neuropathology, Pediatric Pathology, and Radioisotopic Pathology

American Board of Pediatrics
111 Silver Cedar Ct, Chapel Hill, NC 27514
919 929-0461   Fax 919 929-9255
Includes the subspecialties of Adolescent Medicine, Diagnostic Laboratory Immunology, Neonatal-Perinatal Medicine, Pediatric Cardiology, Pediatric Critical Care, Pediatric Emergency Medicine, Pediatric Endocrinology, Pediatric Gastroenterology, Pediatric Hematology-Oncology, Pediatric Infectious Disease, Pediatric Nephrology, Pediatric Pulmonary Disease, and Pediatric Sports Medicine

See also:
American Board of Pathology—Pediatric Pathology
American Board of Surgery—Pediatric Surgery

American Board of Physical Medicine and Rehabilitation
Ste 674, Norwest Center
21 First St SW, Rochester, MN 55902
507 282-1776   Fax 507 282-9242

American Board of Plastic Surgery
7 Penn Center, Ste 400
1635 Market St, Philadelphia, PA 19103
215 587-9322
Includes the subspecialty of Hand Surgery

American Board of Preventive Medicine
9950 W Lawrence Ave, Ste 106
Schiller Park, IL 60176
847 671-1750   Fax 847 691-1751
Includes certification in Aerospace Medicine, Occupational Medicine, Public Health and Preventive Medicine, as well as the subspecialty of Undersea Medicine

American Board of Psychiatry and Neurology
500 Lake Cook Rd, Ste 335, Deerfield, IL 60015
847 945-7900   Fax 847 564-6180
E-mail: amerotho@aol.com
Includes certification in Psychiatry and Neurology, as well as the subspecialties of Child and Adolescent Psychiatry, Geriatric Psychiatry, and Clinical Neurophysiology

American Board of Radiology
5255 Williams Cir, Ste 6800, Tucson, AZ 85711-7401
520 790-2900   Fax 520 790-3200
Includes certification in Diagnostic Radiology, Radiation Oncology, Radiological Physics, and Radiology as well as the subspecialty of Nuclear Radiology

American Board of Surgery
1617 John F. Kennedy Blvd, Ste 860
Philadelphia, PA 19103
215 568-4000   Fax 215 563-5718
Includes the subspecialties of General Vascular Surgery, Pediatric Surgery, Surgical Critical Care, and Surgery of the Hand

American Board of Thoracic Surgery
1 Rotary Center, Ste 803, Evanston, IL 60201
847 475-1520   Fax 847 475-6240

American Board of Urology
31700 Telegraph Rd, Ste 150
Birmingham, MI 48025
810 646-9720

Speech

Speech Pathologist. Alternate titles: speech clinician; speech therapist. Specializes in diagnosis and treatment of speech and language problems, and engages in scientific study of human communication. Diagnoses and evaluates speech and language skills as related to educational, medical, social, and psychological factors. Plans, directs, or conducts habilitative and rehabilitative treatment programs to restore communicative efficiency of individuals with communication problems of organic and nonorganic etiology. Provides counseling and guidance and language development therapy to handicapped individuals. Reviews individual files to obtain background information prior to evaluation to determine appropriate tests and to ensure that adequate information is available. Administers, scores, and interprets specialized hearing and speech tests. Develops and implements individualized plans for assigned clients to meet individual needs, interests, and abilities. Evaluates and monitors individuals, using audiovisual performance to modify, change, or write new programs. Maintains records as required by law, establishment's policy, and administrative regulations. Attends meetings and conferences and participates in other activities to promote professional growth. Instructs individuals to monitor their own speech and provides ways to practice new skills. May act as consultant to educational, medical, and other professional groups. May conduct research to develop diagnostic and remedial techniques. May serve as consultant to classroom teachers to incorporate speech and language development activities into daily schedule. May teach manual sign language to student incapable of speaking. May instruct staff in use of special equipment designed to serve handicapped. See Audiologist in Chapter A of this book for one who specializes in diagnosis of, and provision of rehabilitative services for, auditory problems. (DOT-1991)

Resource

American Speech-Language-Hearing Association
10801 Rockville Pike, Rockville, MD 20852
301 897-5700   Fax 301 897-7348
800 638-TALK (referrals to speech-language pathologists)
E-mail: irc@asha.org

Sperm Bank

American Society for Reproductive Medicine
1209 Montgomery Hwy, Birmingham, AL 35216-2809
205 978-5000   Fax 205 978-5005

Cryo Laboratory Facility
100 E Ohio St, Chicago, IL 60611
312 751-2632

Spinal Cord Injury

American Spinal Injury Association
250 E Superior, Rm 1436, Chicago, IL 60611
312 908-3425   Fax 312 503-0869

National Spinal Cord Injury Association
545 Concord Ave, Ste 29, Cambridge, MA 02138-1122
800 926-9629   617 441-8500   Fax 617 441-3449
E-mail: nscia@aol

Spinal Cord Injury Care Center
Northwestern Memorial Hospital
Rehabilitation Institute
312 908-6000

Learning Resource Center: 312 908-2859
Spinal Cord Injury Hotline:
800 526-3456   800 638-1733 (MD only)

Spinal Cord Society
Wendell Rd, Fergus Falls, MN 56537
218 739-5252   Fax 218 739-5262

Sports Medicine

JAMA Issue of Note: Sports medicine

JAMA 1996; July 17: 276(3)

This issue takes a look at different clinical issues involved in sports. Articles include an NIH consensus development panel on physical activity and cardiovascular health, performance-enhancing drugs, the legacy of Olympic sport, and sudden death in young athletes.

Resources

American College of Sports Medicine
PO Box 1440, 1 Virginia Ave
Indianapolis, IN 46206-1440
317 637-9200   Fax 317 634-7817

American Orthopaedic Society for Sports Medicine
6300 N River Rd, Ste 200, Rosemont, IL 60018
847 292-4900   Fax 847 292-4905

Board Certification:
American Board of Family Practice
2228 Young Dr, Lexington, KY 40505
606 269-5626   Fax 606 266-9699

Sports injuries hotline:
Women's Sports Foundation
Eisenhower Park, East Meadow, NY 11554
800 227-3988   516 542-4700   Fax 516 542-4716

State Medical Societies

More state societies try HMOs. Groups learn start-up secrets for health plans; some report success

Julie A. Jacob
AM News Feb 3, 1997 pp 1, 16-17

Following the theory that if you can't beat 'em, join 'em, state medical societies across the country are setting up their own managed care plans.

Results are mixed. Some fail to raise enough money to get off the ground, while others are giving bigger HMOs a dose of competition.

In Florida, plans for a physician-owned HMO fell through last month when Doctors Health Plan fell far short of raising the $20 million it needed to launch operations.

But in other states—including Louisiana, California, Kansas, and Colorado—doctor-owned managed care plans are off to a strong start.

Success takes a combination of staunch member support, good timing, thorough planning, niche marketing, and professional management, say executives who run these plans.

Although medical society–sponsored plans use similar cost-control policies as conventional managed care arrangements, physicians say their plans are superior because they offer broad provider networks, less red tape, peer-established utilization guidelines, and low administrative costs.

But some HMO industry executives say that medical society–sponsored health plans aren't selective enough in the make-up of their physician panels to ensure good quality of care. While large commercial HMOs tend to restrict their plans to a tight network of board-certified physicians, medical society HMOs generally are more open and admit all licensed physicians who meet their credentialing criteria.

Waiting too long to jump into the managed care market caused Doctors' Health Plan in Florida to sputter before it ever enrolled its first patient.

The idea sounded promising. A 1994 survey by the Florida Medical Association showed that more than 1300 physicians supported the idea. Both the state medical society and the Florida Osteopathic Medical Association endorsed the concept of forming a doctor-owned plan.

The plan needed $20 million to get up and running, says Jack McAbee, a vice president with FMA's insurance subsidiary who was tapped to head the new corporation. Physicians could invest anywhere from $500 to $50,000 in the venture. But response was sluggish. By the time the stock offering closed at the end of 1996, only 350 doctors had purchased a total of $2.4 million in shares.

McAbee blames the plan's failure on the quick growth of managed care in Florida. HMOs, which already commanded 23% of the market in 1994, spread like wildfire during the next 2 years.

Doctors deciding whether to invest in the medical society's plan probably wondered "if it would really

S change much because they would still have to deal with the other HMOs," speculates McAbee.

Bayou success

But in Louisiana, a doctor-owned health plan looks promising.

Within six months of the initial stock offering last spring, the Louisiana State Medical Society's corporation, called MD HealthShares, had raised $12 million by selling 2000 shares at $6000 apiece. A key difference allowing Louisiana to succeed where Florida did not is the state's low managed care penetration, now just 10%. That figure is projected to jump to 50% in the next five years, says Rene Abadie, MD HealthShares' director of provider relations.

The state medical society had to act quickly to take advantage of that "window of opportunity" before it slammed shut, says Abadie.

Before launching its health plan, the medical society conducted a feasibility study that examined physician and employer attitudes toward doctor-owned health plans and the financial and legal issues involved in launching one.

Results were encouraging, so the group appointed an ad hoc physician committee to serve as the board of directors and moved immediately to set up the corporation.

Last month, the corporation began marketing a PPO and direct-access HMO under the name Patient's Choice. It hopes to enroll 2400 members by the end of 1997, says Abadie.

The health plans emphasize their wide array of doctors and hospitals, says Melanie Firmin, MD, vice president of MD HealthShares. Unlike other HMOs that contract with only a few facilities, "we want every facility that wants to reasonably negotiate with us," she says.

Small-business niche

Although a glut of health plans foiled the formation of a doctor-owned HMO in Florida, the California Medical Association used niche marketing to get its doctor-owned plan off the ground in a mature managed care market.

Within months of its initial stock offering in April 1995, California Advantage had sold 6000 shares at $1000 per share, meeting its target of a $6 million start-up fund.

California Advantage kept start-up costs low by incorporating as an insurer, not an HMO, which requires less capital and has fewer legal restrictions, says CEO John Gray.

California Advantage offers an exclusive provider organization, which is similar to an HMO but is governed differently; a point-of-service plan; and a PPO.

The CMA-sponsored health plan has 7450 physician-owners and provider contracts with 27,000 physicians, 350 hospitals, and 3800 pharmacies.

It got a boost from a 1992 law that offered health insurance at cheaper rates to businesses with fewer than 50 employees. Small businesses can choose from among 22 health plans. Among the point-of-service plans offered, California Advantage's one was the most popular, chosen by 56% of the program's participants.

Although only 5000 people have joined California Advantage so far, the insurer's goal is to capture 10% of the market, or 3.3 million enrollees, within 10 years, says Gray.

CMA members are beginning to see their investment pay off, says Jack C. Lewin, MD, the group's executive vice president. "Most of them are getting patients now who are enrolled in California Advantage and they are realizing that it is beginning to work."

Starting small

Starting small also has proved a winning strategy for the Kansas Medical Society's physician-owned insurer, Heartland Health. The health plan currently focuses on rural areas and small towns, although it intends to expand into Kansas City and compete head-on with larger HMOs, says Jimmie Gleason, MD, a Heartland board member.

Like California Advantage, Heartland is incorporated as an insurer and offers PPO and point-of-service products, as well as workers' compensation. It also owns an HMO subsidiary, which serves the Medicaid managed care market.

About two thirds of Kansas doctors, some 2100 physicians, own Heartland stock at $2000 a share. Heartland has 8000 enrollees and a network of 90 hospitals. Dr. Gleason predicts that, based on current rates, the plan will have 35,000 members by year's end.

The difference between Heartland and its large competitors is physician involvement, says Dr. Gleason. "We want to change health care, not just pay for it. Physicians are really in the trenches of what works and what doesn't."

Teaming up with others

Not all medical society health plans are going it alone, however.

The Colorado Medical Society created a nonprofit corporation called Colorado Physicians Network, which teamed up with Rocky Mountain HMO, a Boulder-based nonprofit HMO. Patients enrolled in the HMO are treated by doctors who participate in the medical group's network.

The doctors' network chose Rocky Mountain HMO because of its reputation for respecting physicians, says president David Martz, MD. And forming an alliance with the third-largest HMO in Colorado enabled the network to tap into a base of 90,000 subscribers.

Doctors who participate in the arrangement hope it's a step toward greater physician participation in managed care.

"We see this as an example of physicians stepping forward to influence the delivery of health care and the way it should be," says Dr. Martz.

But not every medical society is leaping into the managed care business.

For the past few years, the Idaho Medical Association has rejected the idea of a society-sponsored health plan after concluding that the state's population was too sparse and member support too shaky. Managed care penetration is only 5%, and Idaho physicians prefer to retain more local control, says Robert K. Seehusen, IDA's executive director.

Even though Florida's plans for a doctor-owned HMO fizzled, McAbee says it was worth finding out whether the idea could succeed.

"The main thing is that the effort had to be tried. We're disappointed, but that doesn't mean that something else might not happen in the future."

Resources

Medical Association of the State of Alabama
195 Jackson St, Montgomery, AL 36102-1900
205 263-6441   205 269-5200
Web address: http://www.maslink.org/

Alaska State Medical Association
4107 Laurel St, Anchorage, AK 99508
907 562-2662   Fax 907 561-2063

Arizona Medical Association
810 W Bethany Home Rd, Phoenix, AZ 85013
602 246-8901   Fax 602 242-6283

Arkansas Medical Society
PO Box 5776, 10 Corporate Hill Dr, Ste 300
Little Rock, AR 72215-5776
501 224-8967   Fax 501 224-6489

California Medical Association
221 Main St, PO Box 7690
San Francisco, CA 94120-7690
415 541-0900   Fax 415 882-5116
Web address: http://www.cmanet.org/

Colorado Medical Society
7800 E Dorado Place, Englewood, CO 80111-2306
303 779-5455   Fax 303 771-8657
Web address: http://www.cms.org/

Connecticut State Medical Society
160 St Ronan St, New Haven, CT 06511
203 865-0587   Fax 203 865-4997

Medical Society of Delaware
1925 Lovering Ave, Wilmington, DE 19806
302 658-7596   Fax 302 658-9669
Web address: http://www.medsocdel.org/

Medical Society of the District of Columbia
2215 M St NW, Washington, DC 20037
202 466-1800   Fax 202 452-1542

Florida Medical Association
760 Riverside Ave, PO Box 2411
Jacksonville, FL 32203
904 356-1571   Fax 904 353-1247
Web address: http://www.medone.org/

Medical Association of Georgia
938 Peachtree St NE, Atlanta, GA 30309
404 876-7535   Fax 404 874-8651

Guam Medical Society
850 Governor Camacho Rd, Tamuning, GU 96911
671 646-5801

Hawaii Medical Association
1360 S Beretania St, Honolulu, HI 96814
808 536-7702   Fax 808 528-2376

Idaho Medical Association
PO Box 2668, 305 W Jefferson, Boise, ID 83701
208 344-7888   Fax 208 344-7903

Illinois State Medical Society
20 N Michigan Ave, Ste 700, Chicago, IL 60602
312 782-1654   Fax 312 782-2023
Web address: http://www.isms.org/

Indiana State Medical Association
322 Canal Walk, Indianapolis, IN 46202
317 261-2060   Fax 317 261-2076
Web address: http://www.ismanet.org/

Iowa Medical Society
1001 Grand Ave, West Des Moines, IA 50265
515 223-1401   Fax 515 223-8420
Web address: http://www.iowamedicalsociety.org/

Kansas Medical Society
623 SW 10th Ave, Topeka, KS 66612-1627
800 332-0156 913 235-2383   Fax 913 235-5114
Web address: http://www.inlandnet/~smeddoc/
kms.html

Kentucky Medical Association
301 N Hurstbourne Ln, Ste 200
Louisville, KY 40222-8512
502 426-6200   Fax 502 426-6877

Louisiana State Medical Society
3501 N Causeway Blvd, Ste 800
Metairie, LA 70002-3673
504 832-9815   Fax 504 833-7685
Web address: http://www.lsms.org/

Maine Medical Association
PO Box 190, Manchester, ME 04351
207 622-3374   Fax 207 622-3332
Web address: http://www.mainmed.com

Medical and Chirurgical Faculty of the
State of Maryland
1211 Cathedral St, Baltimore, MD 21201
410 539-0872   Fax 410 547-0915

Massachusetts Medical Society
1440 Main St, Waltham, MA 02154-1649
617 893-4610   Fax 617 893-3481
Web address: http://www.masssmed.org/

Michigan State Medical Society
120 W Saginaw, East Lansing, MI 48823
517 337-1351   Fax 517 337-2490
Web address: http://www.voyager.net/msms

Minnesota Medical Association
2221 University Ave SE, Ste 400
Minneapolis, MN 55414
612 378-1875   Fax 612 378-3875
Web address: http://www.mnmed.org/

Mississippi State Medical Association
735 Riverside Dr, Jackson, MS 39202
601 354-5433   Fax 601 352-4834
Web address: http://www.msmed.org/

Missouri State Medical Association
PO Box 1028, 113 Madison St
Jefferson City, MO 65102
314 636-5151   Fax 314 636-8552
Web address: http://www.msma.org

Montana Medical Association
2021 11th Ave, Ste 1, Helena, MT 59601
406 443-4000   Fax 406 443-4042

Nebraska Medical Association
233 S 13th St, Ste 1512, Lincoln, NE 68508-2091
402 474-4472   Fax 402 474-2198

Nevada State Medical Association
3660 Baker Ln, #101, Reno, NV 89509
702 825-6788   Fax 702 825-3202

New Hampshire Medical Society
7 N State St, Concord, NH 03301-4018
603 224-1909   Fax 603 226-2432
Web address: http://www.mednexus.com/nhms/
index.html

Medical Society of New Jersey
2 Princess Rd, Lawrenceville, NJ 08648
609 896-1766   Fax 609 896-1368

New Mexico Medical Society
7770 Jefferson NE, Ste 400
Albuquerque, NM 87109
505 828-0237   Fax 505 828-0336
Web address: http://www.nmms.org/nmms/

Medical Society of the State of New York
420 Lakeville Rd, Lake Success, NY 11042-5404
516 488-6100   Fax 516 488-1267
Web address: http://www.mssys.org/

North Carolina Medical Society
222 N Person St, PO Box 27167, Raleigh, NC 27167
919 833-3836   Fax 919 833-2023

North Dakota Medical Association
PO Box 1198, Bismarck, ND 58501-1198
701 223-9475   Fax 701 223-9476

Ohio State Medical Association
1500 Lake Shore Dr, Columbus, OH 43204-3824
614 486-2401   Fax 614 486-3130

Oklahoma State Medical Association
601 NW Expressway, Oklahoma City, OK 73118
405 843-9571   Fax 405 842-1834
Web address: http://www.osmaonline.org/

Oregon Medical Association
5210 SW Corbett Ave, Portland, OR 97201
503 226-1555   Fax 503 241-7148

Pennsylvania Medical Society
777 E Park Dr, PO Box 8820
Harrisburg, PA 17105-8820
717 558-7750   Fax 717 558-7830
Web address: http://www.pamedsoc.org/

Puerto Rico Medical Association
PO Box 9387, Santurce, PR 00908
809 721-6969   Fax 809 722-1191

Rhode Island Medical Society
106 Francis St, Providence, RI 02903
401 331-3207   Fax 401 751-8050

South Carolina Medical Association
PO Box 11188, Columbia, SC 29211
803 798-6207   Fax 803 772-6783

South Dakota State Medical Association
1323 S Minnesota Ave, Sioux Falls, SD 57105
605 336-1965   Fax 605 336-0270
Web address: http://www.usd.edu/med/sdsma/

Tennessee Medical Association
2301 21st Ave S, PO 120909
Nashville, TN 37212-0909
615 385-2100   Fax 615 383-5918
Web address: http://www.medwire.org/

Texas Medical Association
401 W 15th St, Austin, TX 78701-1680
512 370-1300   Fax 512 370-1633
Web address: http://www.texmed.org/

Utah Medical Association
540 E 500 South, Salt Lake City, UT 84102
801 355-7477   Fax 801 531-0381
Web address: http://www.xmission.com/~utahmed/
webfiles/umahome.htm

Vermont State Medical Society
136 Main St, Box 1457, Montpelier, VT 05601
802 223-7898   Fax 802 223-1201

Medical Society of Virginia
4205 Dover Rd, Richmond, VA 23221-3267
804 353-2721   Fax 804 355-6189
Web address: http://www.msv.org/

Virgin Islands Medical Society
PO Box 5986, St Croix, VI 00823
809 778-5305

Washington State Medical Association
2033 Sixth Ave, Ste 1100, Seattle, WA 98121
206 441-9762   Fax 206 441-5863

West Virginia State Medical Association
PO Box 4106, Charleston, WV 25364
304 925-0342   Fax 304 925-0345
Web address: http://www.wvsma.com

State Medical Society of Wisconsin
PO Box 1109, Madison, WI 53701
608 257-6781   Fax 608 283-5401
Web address: http://www.wismed.com/

Wyoming Medical Society
PO Drawer 4009, Cheyenne, WY 82003
307 635-2424   Fax 307 635-1973

Statistics, Health-related

The following essay presents some examples of health policy issues for which physicians will likely encounter data and statistics in their medical practices. Selected examples include hospital mortality data; variations in utilization of health care services; and utilization review, quality assurance, and peer review.

Since the importance of these issues will likely increase in the coming years, it is essential that physicians understand the appropriate role of statistics in their evaluations. This is particularly true in those instances (eg, release of hospital mortality data) where physicians may be called on by patients to explain the clinical meaning of published data.

Hospital mortality data

The Health Care Financing Administration (HCFA), which administers the Medicare program, releases selected statistical information on the performance of those hospitals that participate in the Medicare program.

The information released includes, for each hospital, the number of Medicare beneficiaries treated and the percentage of beneficiaries who died within 30 days of admission. This information is compared with an estimate of the number of deaths that would be expected at the same hospital (calculated through a regression analysis) if that hospital's experience conformed to the national experience with patients of similar age, sex, incidence of complicating diseases, and prior hospitalization. HCFA has taken the position that a comparison of data drawn from the individual hospital with the estimate drawn from the population as a whole will give consumers useful information about the quality of care provided by individual hospitals.

Release of such data can, of course, have important implications. As such, it is essential that any information not be misleading to the public. However, there is at least one fundamental flaw in the design of this plan that may foster the proliferation of misleading statistics: In essence, the HCFA plan invites reviewers of these data to compare noncomparable populations.

The population that is subject to comparison consists of Medicare beneficiaries with a specific diagnosis in a hospital. Given the approach used by HCFA, the population to which comparisons will be made may differ from this population in several important ways. These include the following:

1. *Race*. In drawing an estimate from the overall population, HCFA has ignored race as a factor that could influence the outcome of specific procedures. Thus, a hospital that, because of location, has a preponderance of patients who are of one race may be compared with a hospital population that serves several races.

2. *Medicare status*. While each hospital's data are drawn from Medicare patients alone, the national population of citizens over the age of 65 includes people who are not on Medicare. Medicare covers those with prior social security coverage and their dependents. It does not include those who did not work, or who did not work in a covered occupation, such as federal employees without other jobs. In addition, while Medicare does cover some individuals under age 65, such as those with end-stage renal disease, these individuals are not comparable to members of the population as a whole who are in the same age group.

3. *Severity of illness*. No measure of the severity of illness is included in the estimate drawn from the national population. As a result, a hospital that may selectively receive patients whose condition is more critical, or that receives more terminally ill patients, will inevitably show mortality rates higher than those estimated.

Because of these deficiencies, questions have been raised about whether the methods being used by HCFA can produce valid predictions of mortality rates for specific hospitals. It has further been questioned as to whether it is appropriate to imply that differences between a hospital's mortality rate and an estimated national mortality rate are due solely to the quality of care provided by the hospital. The number of factors that could influence such an outcome (ie, the mortality experience) is simply too great to permit inferences to be drawn about any one factor.

The limitations of the data, of course, center on outliers—cases where the actual mortality rate falls outside the range of predicted mortality rates. These data lead one to believe that there may be a quality problem whenever the actual mortality rate is above the upper end of the range of predicted mortality rate.

The key question that must be addressed is the reasons that any such outlier might occur. An example is the diagnostic category "HS-severe acute heart disease." The actual rate shown of 48% is above that predicted, 28% to 35%. This outlier could occur for several reasons:

1. The normal random error that is expected in any statistical model. Some observations always lie above the regression line.

2. The exclusion of important explanatory variables from the predictive model (eg, severity of illness, race, Medicare status of the hospital).

3. An actual quality problem in this diagnostic category in this hospital.

The problem is that there is no easy way for the public to discern which of the reasons is the correct one. Accordingly, it is essential that physicians understand, and be able to inform their patients, what can be legitimately inferred from these data.

Geographic variations in the utilization of health care services

A substantial and growing body of research has identified significant differences from one geographic area to another in the utilization of health care services. For example, in the past, tonsillectomies have been found to vary from 151 per 10,000 population in one area to as few as 13 per 10,000 in another. Hysterectomies have been found to be performed on 70% of women in one locality compared to 30% in another.

A key issue raised by these data is whether these differences in utilization can be explained by demographic or epidemiologic factors. (In other words, are these populations comparable?) Are there a greater number of elderly in one area than in another, for example? Is it possible that individuals requiring certain types of treatment are being referred from one geographic area into another? Statistical research indicates that often such area-to-area differences cannot be explained solely in terms of demographic or epidemiologic differences. Any number of other factors (eg, variations in patient needs, differences in medical practice styles) may be important.

Another issue raised by such variations is whether certain health care services are being provided unnecessarily in some areas of the country. Simply because in one area there is a relatively high incidence of a specific procedure, it cannot be assumed that the procedure is being performed unnecessarily. It is equally possible that in an area with a relatively low rate of a given procedure, the procedure may not be performed often enough. Too little provision of medical services is as undesirable as too much.

Utilization review, quality assurance, and peer review

The application of statistical concepts to medical practice data is a major component of utilization assurance processes. There is likely to be increasing use of such statistical applications in these areas, due to the greater amount of medical care data being generated by payment systems, and due to the increasingly sophisticated techniques for evaluating and comparing such data.

Nearly all medical review programs make u[...] statistical principles. For example, it is [...] mon for reviewing bodies to exa[...]

S

specific hospitals or physicians who exhibit practice patterns that significantly deviate from the median level of care provided for a particular diagnosis. Such analysis can lead to the identification of utilization "outliers," ie, hospitals or physicians who provide significantly more or less services to a particular kind of patient compared to other hospitals or physicians. The same analysis can be applied to mortality rates and other data that may be regarded as indicators of possible quality problems.

While definitive judgments concerning appropriate utilization and quality of care typically must await the review of the medical chart by a physician, a key component of review programs is the development of screening criteria that can be applied to all, or a sample, of cases as an administratively efficient means of detecting possible utilization or quality problems. Those flagged as possible problems can then be referred for further medical review to determine if a problem in fact exists. (MMP-1987)

Resources

Accidents:
National Safety Council
1121 Spring Lake Dr, Itasca, IL 60143-3201
630 285-1121   Fax 630 285-1315
Web address: http://www.nsc.org

Diseases:
National Center for Health Statistics
6525 Belcrest Rd, Rm 1140, Hyattsville, MD 20782
301 436-7016
Web address: http://www.cdc.gov

Hospital Procedures:
Healthcare Knowledge Resource
3853 Research Park, PO Box 303
Ann Arbor, MI 48106-0303
313 930-7830

Hospital Statistics:
Health Statistics Group
American Hospital Association
1 N Franklin, Chicago, IL 60606
Statistics Center 312 422-3000   Fax 312 422-4796

Pharmaceuticals:
American Pharmaceutical Association
Academy of Pharmacy Practice and Management
c/o Susan C. Winckler
2215 Constitution Ave NW, Washington, DC 20037
800 237-APHA   202 628-4410   Fax 202 783-2351

St　istics, Physicians

*　earch:*
　for Health Policy Research
　2

*　ation:*
　lph L, Seidman, B.
　ristics and Distribution in the US.
　n Medical Association; 1997-1998.
　0-89970-893-5 OP390297

Stress

Preventing burnout among health care professionals

To recognize and reduce the cultural and individual factors that promote burnout in caring professionals, doctors must respond as a profession, as specialists or institutional groups, and as individuals, giving specific attention to the factors causing burnout. The warning signs are emotional exhaustion, denial of the need for self-care (eg, adequate rest, recreation, nutrition, friendship, humor, quiet time, and space), and clinical detachment. Personal and professional partners who wish to help the individual to "recharge" could respond when they recognize dependence upon short-term "corrective" aids such as overeating, overworking, blaming, out-of-control outbursts, and overuse of alcohol or self-prescribed psychoactive substances. Physicians are often lonely and suffer alone needlessly. It is necessary to develop a system that offers choices for the early correction of burnout behavior. This system could offer "flex-time" schedules, flexible contracts, mini-sabbaticals, night-shift backup, funding for "tune-ups" (counseling or retreats), process interventions ("debriefings" after catastrophes or patient deaths), and support groups. (DRS 9-1994)

Stroke

Poetry and Medicine

the stroke in 111a

Richard Donze, DO, MPH
JAMA 1995 Oct 11; 274(14): 1094e

is somebody's uncle
who was part of
safe warm week-over friday night
visits, making chuckling kitchen din
over coffee and coffee cake
while nephew half-watched half-dreamed
77 sunset strip
on the living room floor

is somebody's father
who watched his daughter's
first birthday through the
gray square of an old
super-eight, blinding everyone
with the floodlight rack he
balanced in one hand while
motioning with the other to
move the cake closer
closer to the baby

is somebody's husband
who took his wife to
atlantic city after the war
and charted a sunny future
in sand finger doodles
when hope bubbled like lava
out of the victory volcano

is getting orders to "go"
so he goes with
loose gown flapping like
motorcade flags and
leads a paretic parade of
trailing tethering tubing
to the bathroom
pulling out balloon-and-all foley
felling i.v. pole
falling
into a tube-spill puddle that
spreads red from sliced-scalp-drip as

the family walks in
nephew daughter wife who will
crash vision against memory
like cymbals and
cover their ears

Damage to part of the brain caused by interruption to its blood supply or leakage of blood outside of vessel walls is a stroke. Sensation, movement, or function controlled by the damaged area is impaired. Strokes are fatal in about one third of cases and are a leading cause of death in developed countries. (ENC-1989)

Resources

National Institute of Neurological Disorders and Stroke
9000 Rockville Pike, Bethesda, MD 20892
301 496-5751

National Stroke Association
96 Inverness Dr E, Ste I, Englewood, CO 80112-5112
800 STROKE   303 649-9299   Fax 303 649-1328

The Stroke Foundation
898 Park Ave, New York, NY 10021
212 734-3461

Stuttering

National Center for Stuttering
200 E 33rd St, New York, NY 10016
800 221-2483 9 am-5 pm EST
800 221-2483   212 532-1460

Stuttering Resource Foundation
123 Oxford, New Rochelle, NY 10804
800 232-4773

Sudden Infant Death Syndrome

American Sudden Infant Death Syndrome Institute
6065 Roswell Rd, Ste 876, Atlanta, GA 30328
800 232-SIDS   404 843-1030   Fax 404 843-0577

SIDS Alliance
1314 Bedford Ave, Ste 210
Baltimore, MD 21208
800 221-SIDS (800 221-7437)   410 653-8226
Fax 410 653-8709   410 964-8000

National SIDS Resource Center
8201 Greensboro, Ste 600, McLean, VA 22102
703 821-8955   Fax 703 821-2098

Suicide

Poetry and Medicine

Overdose

L. Jeffry Price, MD
JAMA 1992 Mar 11; 267(10): 1304

Your life was neatly packaged
when you came to us,
all hopes and farewells
written in two looseleaf testaments.
You had taken the whole amount
and cast yourself on
the quiet barbiturate flood.
The hospital linen you
willed a winding sheet
and floated so much
at peace, I thought yours
the dreaming face of God,
uncreased by human care.
We kept you tethered
with IV line
and respirator tubing
throughout that long dream.
After a week, you lay
aground on the mattress,
your face awake and twisted
by the world again.
I wished for you
a modicum of peace,
short of that one
in which all souls cast
their perfect reflection.

Resources

American Association of Suicidology
2459 S Ash, Denver, CO 80222
303 692-0985

Survivors of Suicide
(for family and friends of the deceased)
Send stamped self-addressed envelope to:
3251 N 78th St, Milwaukee, WI 53222

Suicide, Physicians

A Piece of My Mind

The smell of gardenias

Charles A. Koller
JAMA 1994 May 4; 271(17): 1366

Rounds were finished, labs checked, and orders written. I had done everything I could for my patients, and for the moment, things seemed calm. Now at 2 o'clock in the afternoon, the thought of lunch passed quickly through my mind, but as quickly, left. Instead I went back to a special patient's room.

Upon entering her room, I was immediately captivated by the smell of gardenias. The fragrance rose from eight or 10 huge blossoms floating in a large, flat bowl on the bed stand near the patient's bed. My patient, an attractive middle-aged woman, was lying still in her perfectly made hospital bed. Her eyes were closed, sleeplike, revealing no sign of tension or stress. Her hair was stylishly

Short, several shades of gray darker now as it grew back after her recent radiation therapy. She had quietly lapsed into a coma the night before. An emergency evaluation, the works, done in the middle of the night, had confirmed that her condition was hopeless. The fight was over.

I had come back this afternoon to comfort her ever-caring family and to begin my personal process of mourning for a special patient. However, I stood there distracted by the gardenias, their fragrance holding me sway for several seconds. Her husband, almost always at her side, told me that he had gone home after our morning rounds and picked the gardenia blossoms from a bush in their yard. His face also seemed totally free of anxiety. Thus, the atmosphere in the room was entirely different from the one I had anticipated for a patient who would never again open her eyes or talk to anyone.

This family and I had come a long way together since our first formal meeting only a few weeks before. Their deep affection for each other had immediately formed a beautiful and sturdy image in my mind. This woman loved life, lived with joy and intensity until the end, and with her husband and family bravely faced the inevitable.

However, the arbitrary and capricious vagaries that govern life or death in leukemia patients were different for this patient. One could make the case that this patient was a delayed victim of the same self-inflicted gunshot wound to the head that, with no explanation, took the life of my partner. He was her physician. He had crafted her remission induction. He had constantly encouraged her to comply with her maintenance program despite a natural reluctance on her part to take therapy when she felt well and had no objective evidence of disease. Her relapse occurred while therapy was interrupted in the aftermath of her physician's death. She had suspended maintenance herself when she had detected the opportunity.

Why did he do it? I was unable to answer. There was no note, no warning. The mortality of her physician had exposed a weakness in her that would soon result in her own death. I had not heard the horrible shot, but I was watching its reverberation.

Surgery

Poetry and Medicine

Flowers after surgery

Katharine Weber
JAMA 1997 Apr 23/30; 277(16): 1263

Orchids, a calla lily
(they bloom again, mother),
sweetly tousled baskets (though two are identical,
like airplane salad).
Eleven sweetheart roses—
Loving gestures start to smother;
they make this invalid feel invalid.

(Silly, this need of another flower,
but where's the twelfth?
Filched? Or a sly florist's stealth?)
Drugs steal time in this hospital bower.

While I wander lonely as a cloud,
the last delivery crowds the sill:
a funereal bucket two feet high
spills delphinia, ranunculi
(obscenely tumorous homunculi)—
Pedunculated, the doctor said, but benign.
(A half-dozen, all mine.)
Did I mention the tuberous begonia?
Begone. Removed.

I am moved again
by friends, by knowledge that I didn't die—
At times, when on my couch I lie
in vacant or in pensive mood
I think of blooms and solitude
and know for sure with friends like these,
who really needs anemones?

Surgeon. Performs surgery to correct deformities, repair injuries, prevent diseases, and improve function in patients. Examines patient to verify necessity of operation, estimate possible risk to patient, and determine best operational procedure. Previews reports of patient's general physical condition, reactions to medications, and medical history. Examines instruments, equipment, and surgical setup to ensure that antiseptic and aseptic methods have been followed. Performs operations, using variety of surgical instruments and employing established surgical techniques appropriate for specific procedures. May specialize in particular type of operation, as on nervous system, and be designated neurosurgeon. May specialize in repair, restoration, or improvement of lost, injured, defective, or misshapen body parts and be designated plastic surgeon. May specialize in correction or prevention of skeletal abnormalities, utilizing surgical, medical, and physical methodologies, and be designated orthopedic surgeon. (DOT-1991)

Resources
American Board of Surgery
1617 John F. Kennedy Blvd, Ste 860
Philadelphia, PA 19103
215 568-4000   Fax 215 563-5718

American College of Surgeons
55 E Erie St, Chicago, IL 60611
312 664-4050   Fax 312 440-7014
E-mail: postmaster@facs.org

International College of Surgeons
1516 N Lake Shore Dr, Chicago, IL 60610
312 642-3555   Fax 312 787-1624
E-mail: exa@aol.com

National Second Opinion Program
800 638-6833 (MD 800 492-6603)

Surgical Technologist

History
The profession of surgical technology was developed during World War II when there was a critical need for assistance in performing surgical procedures and a shortage of qualified personnel to meet that need. Individuals were educated specifically to assist in surgical procedures and to function in the operative theater.

The Association of Surgical Technologists (AST) was organized in July 1969, with an advisory board of representatives from the American College of Surgeons (ACS), the Association of Operating Room Nurses (AORN), the American Hospital Association (AHA), and the American Medical Association (AMA).

In December 1972, the AMA's Council on Medical Education (CME) adopted the recommended educational standards for this field, and the Accreditation Review Committee on Education in Surgical Technology (ARC-ST) was formed. The ARC-ST is jointly sponsored by the AST, ACS, and AHA, in collaboration with the AMA.

The accreditation policies and processes of the ARC-ST comply with the standards for nationally recognized agencies established by the US Department of Education and the Commission on Recognition of Postsecondary Accreditation.

Occupational description
Surgical technologists are allied health professionals who are an integral part of the team of medical practitioners providing surgical care to patients in a variety of settings.

Job description
Surgical technologists prepare the operating room by selecting and opening sterile supplies. Preoperative duties also include assembling, adjusting, and checking nonsterile equipment to ensure that it is in proper working order. Common duties include operating sterilizers, lights, suction machines, electrosurgical units, and diagnostic equipment.

When patients arrive in the surgical suite, surgical technologists assist in preparing them for surgery by providing physical and emotional support, checking charts, and observing vital signs. They have been educated to properly position the patient on the operating table, assist in connecting and applying surgical equipment and/or monitoring devices, and prepare the incision site. Surgical technologists have primary responsibility for maintaining the sterile field, being constantly vigilant that all members of the team adhere to aseptic technique.

They most often function as the sterile member of the surgical team who passes instruments, sutures, and sponges during surgery. After "scrubbing," they don gown and gloves and prepare the sterile setup for the appropriate procedure. After other members of the sterile team have scrubbed, they assist them with gowning and gloving and with the application of sterile drapes that isolate the operative site.

In order that surgery may proceed smoothly, surgical technologists anticipate the needs of surgeons, passing instruments and providing sterile items in an efficient manner. They share with the circulator the responsibility for accounting for sponges, needles, and instruments before, during, and after surgery.

Surgical technologists may hold retractors or instruments, sponge or suction the operative site, or cut suture materials as directed by the surgeon. They connect drains and tubing and receive and prepare specimens for subsequent pathologic analysis. They are responsible for preparing and applying sterile dressings following the procedure and may assist in the application of nonsterile dressings, including plaster or synthetic casting materials.

After surgery, they prepare the operating room for the next patient.

Surgical technologists are most often members of the sterile team but may function in the nonsterile role of circulator. The circulator is not gowned and gloved during the surgical procedure but is available to respond to the needs of the individual providing anesthesia, keep a written account of the surgical procedure, and participate jointly with the scrubbed person in counting sponges, needles, and instruments before, during, and after surgery. In operating rooms where local anesthetics are administered, they meet the needs of the conscious patient.

Certified surgical technologists with additional specialized education or training may also act in the role of the surgical first assistant. The surgical first assistant provides aid in exposure, hemostasis, and other technical functions under the surgeon's direction that will help the surgeon carry out a safe operation with optimal results for the patient.

Surgical technologists also may provide staffing in postoperative recovery rooms where patients' responses are carefully monitored in the critical phases following general anesthesia.

Employment characteristics
A majority of surgical technologists work in hospitals, principally in the surgical suite and also in emergency rooms and other settings that call for knowledge of, and ability in, maintaining asepsis, such as materials management and central service. A number work in a wide variety of settings and arrangements, including outpatient surgicenters, private employment by physicians, or as self-employed technologists.

Those who work in hospital and other institutional settings are usually expected to work rotating shifts or to accommodate on-call assignments to ensure adequate staffing for emergency surgical procedures during evening, night, weekend, and holiday hours. Otherwise, surgical technologists follow a standard hospital workday.

According to a recent study conducted by the US Bureau of Labor Statistics, the forecast for employment opportunities for surgical technologists is one of rapid growth. Demand for technologists varies among communities and geographic regions. Prospective students are advised to assess the market for graduates within the region in which they would like to work before matriculating in an educational program. Such information is likely to be available through local employment offices, local accredited programs, and hospital councils or hospitals.

Salaries vary depending on the experience and education of the individual, the economy of a given region, the responsibilities of the position, and the working hours.

According to the AST, salaries for certified surgical technologists average $22,786 per year. (AHRP-1997)

Resources
AMA Allied Health Department
312 553-9355

Association of Surgical Technologists
7108-C S Alton Way, Englewood, CO 80112-2106
303 694-9130   Fax 303 694-9169

Surrogate Motherhood/Parents

Center for Surrogate Parenting
8383 Wilshire Blvd, Ste 750D
Beverly Hills, CA 90211
213 655-1974   Fax 213 852-1310

Systematized Nomenclature of Medicine (SNOMED)

College of American Pathologists
325 Waukegan Rd, Northfield, IL 60093-2750
800 323-4040   847 446-8800   Fax 847 446-8807

Teaching Hospitals

Council on Teaching Hospitals
2450 N St NW, Washington, DC 20037-1127
202 828-0490   Fax 202 828-4792

Technology Assessment

The life and death of the Congressional Office of Technology Assessment

Clyde J. Behney
Technology News Jan/Feb 1996 pp 1-2, 6-8

On September 30, 1995, the Office of Technology Assessment (OTA) terminated its research operations, shut its doors, and began a 4-month process of distributing its furniture and computers, archiving its records, and looking for homes for its electronic and paper publications. The agency had been abolished by the 104th Congress. OTA could now add to its list of "firsts" the fact that it was the first total casualty of the changes sweeping Congress.

OTA was created by the US Congress in 1972, in reaction to societal and congressional concerns about some highly visible advances in science and technology (such as the supersonic transport, emerging biomedical technologies including genetic engineering, fear of environmental degradation) and an increased recognition of the importance of science and technology in legislative decisions. In addition, it was created to respond to Congress's dramatic and growing science and technology "knowledge deficit" when compared to the executive branch. OTA was one of the four research support agencies of the Congress, and the only one with a focus on science and technology. Twenty-three years and 750 studies later, OTA was abolished by a very different Congress than the one that had established it.

What was OTA?

The Office of Technology Assessment was established by the Technology Assessment Act of 1972. Its mission was to help Congress deal with policy issues affected by the complexities of science and technology, from biotechnology to fusion energy, from telecommunications to space launch capabilities. OTA's staff of 200 represented every major field of science and technology.

OTA was designed to operate in an expert, objective, and nonpartisan fashion, governed by a 12-member Technology Assessment Board composed of six senators and six representatives, equally divided by party.

OTA undertook assessments at the request of any congressional committee chairman or ranking minority member. In practice, most assessments were requested by both the chairman and the ranking minority member of a committee, and a great many were supported by more than one committee. The Board made the final decision on whether OTA could proceed with all reports, to be sure that OTA followed the appropriate research and review process, prior to their release.

Most of OTA's work concentrated on in-depth assessment that took one to two years to complete, but a variety of mechanisms—interim reports, shorter efforts, briefings, testimony, umbrella projects (same overall topic but consisting of a series of shorter, more focused reports)—were used increasingly, especially in the health area, to respond to more immediate needs of congressional committees. OTA's studies were guided by advisory panels of outside experts and stakeholders, who served as advisors but did not control the studies. All studies underwent extensive, open peer review.

In short, "Congress's own think-tank" functioned as a unique information resource in the intersection between national policy and science and technology.

OTA's contributions

The medical and health care–related body of work produced over a period of about 20 years by OTA was primarily the result of studies by its Health Program, but also of studies by its Biological Application Program and its Environment Program. OTA's accomplishments stem not so much from the sheer number of studies—the agency was far too small for that to have been the case—but rather from: 1) studies in contentious or controversial areas that others either wouldn't do or couldn't do with credibility (such as unconventional cancer treatments or the costs of and returns to pharmaceutical research and development); and 2) studies that demonstrated the feasibility of certain analytical approaches and the importance of evaluation, of knowing what works.

The earliest contributions of OTA in the health area were its studies on the process of and need for assessment of clinical effects and costs. The result was a series of studies in the late 1970s and the early 1980s: Development of Medical Technology: Opportunities for Assessment (1976); Assessing the Efficacy and Safety of Medical Technology (1978); Policy Implications of the Computed Tomography (CT) Scanner (1978); The Implications of Cost Effectiveness Analysis of Medical Technologies (1980); and Strategies for Medical Technology Assessment (1982). These reports, I believe, were influential in demonstrating the dramatic lack of valid information about the effectiveness and safety of many medical technologies and, for the latter two, in legitimizing the comparison of effects with costs. We tend to forget how hostile the climate of the late 1970s and early 1980s was with regard to the use of cost-effectiveness analysis as an aid to health care decision-making. This strand of

T analysis was revisited in a lesser fashion occasionally, with the most notable being the recent OTA report, *Identifying Health Technologies that Work: Searching for Evidence*.

OTA also is well known for its specific studies of prevention, particularly its cost-effectiveness analyses on pneumococcal vaccine, influenza vaccine, mammography screening, and a series of cost-effectiveness studies of preventive technologies. OTA examined screening for cervical cancer, colorectal cancer, glaucoma, osteoporosis, prostate cancer, and hypercholesterolemia. In addition, prenatal care and postnatal screening were examined. Several of the computer models developed by OTA represented significant contributions to the state of the art and have been in high demand by other researchers.

A good example of OTA's being able to conduct a study in a controversial area is the report on the cost of pharmaceutical research and development and the financial return to the companies on that investment. The preparation of that report was an enormous methodological challenge with the inevitable backdrop of interest group controversy, attacks on the study results and process, and high visibility. Several of the, if not unique then certainly rare, elements of OTA's world are illustrated by that example. First, the results and the analysis must withstand methodological scrutiny. Second, the process of the study had to both be and be perceived as open, fair, and rigorous. If these conditions were met, then the members of OTA's congressional board would be willing to defend OTA and insulate it from undue pressure. Great intellectual freedom was balanced by the need to produce good work in an open fashion.

One of the areas that received the most media attention was OTA's estimates of the human and economic costs of smoking. In an earlier Background Paper and more recently in formal testimony, OTA calculated the billions of dollars spent on the direct and indirect consequences of smoking cigarettes. These estimates received great attention, even though other estimates were available; OTA's status as a congressional agency and its independence from any community with a stake in the debate lent greater weight to the figures.

Other areas in which OTA's studies seem to have had significant impact are aging and long-term care (especially regarding dementias), disability technology (OTA's studies have had a substantial and lasting effect on how the disability policy/technology system was viewed and approached), the biotechnology industry (OTA's earlier studies are credited by many observers with countering the misinformed fears that many members of Congress once held about biotechnology, thus diminishing the chances of restrictive legislation), and biomedical ethics.

Many other OTA studies have had an impact in the broadly defined areas of public health such as global climate, clean air, or other environmental concerns. OTA did much work for the Congress in areas such as environmental modeling for the Clean Air Act reauthorization deliberations, or studies around issues of global warming and climate change. It also produced an excellent series of reports on nuclear weapons dismantling and disposal or storage of nuclear weapons materials and on the effects of Soviet nuclear contamination in the Arctic. It examined Superfund, ATSDR, dioxin, and Agent Orange, and in a landmark study, technologies for determining cancer risks. Of significance, the agency and its contractors—Doll and Peto—called into serious question the conventional wisdom that a huge percentage of cancers are caused by the environment.

The decision to abolish OTA

The beginning of FY95 found management and staff of the Office of Technology Assessment involved in adjusting to and continuing the implementation of a major reorganization that was initiated in fiscal year 1994. In addition, the analytical agenda of the agency was a full and challenging one. Due to the elections of November 1994, OTA staff were beginning the process of ascertaining the research needs of the new Republican chairpersons and planning the year's research agenda in ways that could accommodate new requests from them. Thus, OTA in early fall of 1994 had a double focus: the conduct of a wide range of important research and the continuing challenge of guiding a newly reorganized agency.

This focus was blurred in December 1994, when the Senate Republican Caucus voted in favor of the elimination of OTA, and shifted entirely in the ensuing months, as further legislative actions moved closer and closer to a formal decision for elimination. For 10 months there was a nearly palpable sense of uncertainty. It was a period of extreme ups and downs, with the "ups" being a sense that the agency would continue to exist in some form but with the loss of a substantial proportion (from 20% to 50%) of its resources and, especially, staff. The "downs" were periods when OTA's termination seemed the most likely outcome.

Both the House and the Senate Appropriations Subcommittees on the Legislative Branch included the elimination of OTA in the bills they reported to the floor of their respective bodies. On the House floor, an amendment to restore OTA at a reduced funding level was approved, aided by the votes of numerous Republicans, including the chairs of many full committees and subcommittees. OTA lost narrowly on the Senate floor. In conference, the house conferees acceded to the Senate position, a vote to reverse that failed by one vote, and OTA's fate was sealed.

OTA was given an appropriation sufficient to conduct agency close-out activities and authority to continue 17 staff members from October 1995 to about January 1996 for that purpose.

Among these activities were steps to ensure that OTA's documents, in electronic form, remain available in the future. OTA's World Wide Web site, for example, is being "mirrored" at the National Academy of Sciences, the Government Printing Office (GPO), and about five other sites, primarily universities. In addition, OTA has prepared a set of five CD-ROMs containing, in searchable format, all 750 of its publications. This set will be available through the GPO.

The initial arguments against OTA (eg, that we were not doing quality work, that we only work for Democrats, that our work was not used) were dropped from the debate as overwhelming evidence of their lack of substance was offered. In the end, one substantive and one political argument remained. The substantive argument was that we were a luxury, since many other sources of information existed for Congress. Some Republican members argued, for example, that when OTA was founded there was much less information and fewer studies available than now exist, so that the country is awash in information, and thus we are unnecessary. The reverse of this argument, that in a sea of information, OTA's type of analysis becomes more, not less valuable, seems to be a stronger one. Thus, many observers were left with the opinion that the major reason for OTA's demise was that Congress needed to have a symbol of its willingness to cut its own budget by eliminating an entire agency from the legislative branch. The bottom line is that only the members involved know for sure.

Implications of OTA's death

Numerous organizations and individuals will ponder the "Why" and the "What It Means" of OTA's death (eg, the Milbank Memorial Fund is planning such an activity), and it may take some time and perspective for successful answers. There are a few preliminary ideas that make it seem clear that Congress and the country will be without an organization that has quite the same role. (The National Academy of Sciences, especially the Institute of Medicine, probably comes closest.)

Second, the agency will be missed in specific cases and not in the aggregate lessening of analysis, as the agency was too small for a substantial effect of the latter type. In the specific cases for which the loss of OTA is significant, it will probably not be because there is too little information in an area but because there is a great deal. That great deal of information, though, will be primarily or entirely from organizations (including the executive branch) with a stake in decisions, and the information often will be contradictory, unclear, not valid, or of suspicious validity. On top of this, it will probably be the case that Congress is unable to sort out that mass of information by itself.

Perhaps more importantly, is the loss of OTA an isolated incident or an example of a broader trend? That is, was the elimination of OTA a symbol of Congress's showing that frugality can start at home? Or was it, along with AHCPR's troubles, a symbol of a deeper lack of appreciation for the knowledge-producing and evaluating organization?

Article of Note: Technology assessment in medicine.

Arch Intern Med 1992 Jan; 152 (1):46-50

Abstract: The rapid proliferation of health care technology and the increasing concern about cost containment are major converging forces in today's health care system. These forces argue persuasively for the rigorous evaluation of the safety and effectiveness of technologies and for the use of such evaluative information as the foundation of both clinical decision making and public policy formulation. Thus, technology assessment is an essential tool in improving the quality of health care delivered and in maximizing the efficiency of the health care system. The American Medical Association historically has been dedicated to the provision of sound scientific information to enhance the appropriate utilization of health care technology. This objective remains the primary goal of the American Medical Association's activities in technology assessment. Additionally, with the ascendancy of nonphysician segments of the health care community in making policies that affect the availability of technology, the American Medical Association's assessment programs must represent physicians' views and concerns cogently in public policy debates (eg, coverage). The Council on Scientific Affairs and the Council on Medical Service examined the area of technology assessment and its influence on the payment for and the utilization of health care technology. The councils made specific recommendations to ensure that the American Medical Association maintains the sophisticated capabilities and sufficient capacity to meet the needs of physicians and patients alike in today's complex health care environment.

Resources

American Medical Association Diagnostic and Therapeutic Technology Assessment (DATTA) Program. For a list of DATTA Reports, see the AMA section.

US Department of Health and Human Services Agency for Health Care Policy and Research Wilco Bldg, Ste 309 6000 Executive Blvd, Rockville MD 20852 800 358-9295 410 381-3150 Publications clearinghouse: 800 358-9295 E-mail: info@ahcpr.gov Web address: http://www.ahcpr.gov

AHCPR InstantFax makes brief technology assessment and practice guideline materials available via fax-on-demand. This service operates 24 hours a day, 7 days a week. A fax machine with a telephone headset is needed to access the system. Dial the system through a fax handset and request a contents list by pressing #1. 301 594-2800

Telemedicine

AMA Policy

The Promotion of Quality Telemedicine
(H-160.937) CME/CMS Rep, I-96

1. The AMA adopts the following principles for the supervision of nonphysician providers and technicians when telemedicine is used:

   a. The physician is responsible for, and retains the authority for, the safety and quality of services provided to patients by nonphysician providers through telemedicine.

   b. Physician supervision (eg, regarding protocols, conferencing, and medical record review) is required when nonphysician providers or technicians deliver services via telemedicine in all settings and circumstances.

   c. Physicians should visit the sites where patients receive services from nonphysician providers or technicians through telemedicine, and must be knowledgeable regarding the competence and qualifications of the nonphysician providers utilized.

   d. The supervising physician should have the capability to immediately contact nonphysician providers or technicians delivering, as well as patients receiving, services via telemedicine in any setting.

   e. Nonphysician providers who deliver services via telemedicine should do so according to the applicable nonphysician practice acts in the state where the patient receives such services.

T

f. The extent of supervision provided by the physician should conform to the applicable medical practice act in the state where the patient receives services.

g. Mechanisms for the regular reporting, recording, and supervision of patient care delivered through telemedicine must be arranged and maintained between the supervising physician, nonphysician providers, and technicians.

h. The physician is responsible for providing and updating patient care protocols for all levels of telemedicine involving nonphysician providers or technicians.

2. The AMA urges those who design or utilize telemedicine systems to make prudent and reasonable use of those technologies necessary to apply current or future confidentiality and privacy principles and requirements to telemedicine interactions.

3. The AMA emphasizes to physicians their responsibility to ensure that their legal and ethical requirements with respect to patient confidentiality and data integrity are not compromised by the use of any particular telemedicine modality.

4. The AMA advocates that continuing medical education conducted using telemedicine adhere to the standards of the AMA's Physician Recognition Award and the *Essentials and Standards of the Accreditation Council for Continuing Medical Education.*

Today's licensure law, tomorrow's telemedicine: a snapshot

Curtis Rooney, Dennis Wentz

Most practitioners of interstate telemedicine are concerned about individual state licensure law, or they should be. Many physicians ask, Is it necessary to obtain a license in another state when telemedicine consultations are performed? Others have begun to ask the more philosophical question; that is, what type of medical license should be required of physicians who provide services by means of telemedicine? The issue of medical licensure and the practice of telemedicine may prompt lively debate in Washington and in the states in the near future.

Background

At present, each state has primary responsibility for regulating the health, safety, and welfare of its citizens. The various Medical Practice Acts, as developed by the states, govern physician licensure law. The laws of each state are unique, but they share many provisions. What the impending debate will determine is whether the present system is deemed adequate to meet the challenges of 21st century medicine or whether a change is required.

The following are alternative approaches to physician licensure law:

National licensure: Either complete nationalization or creation of a federal minimum standard or "floor" that states would implement.

Mutual recognition of licensure: State-based licensure that relies on the principles of reciprocity to allow for licensing in another jurisdiction upon "notice" of intent to practice in another state.

Full licensure: Requiring a full and unrestricted license in any state in which the practitioner provides medical services by means of telemedicine.

Limited licensure: A modified type of state licensure that requires a secondary "limited" license for telemedicine services in the second state, in addition to a primary full and unrestricted license in the primary state.

Extended jurisdiction licensure: A state-based approach that would allow state medical boards to assert their jurisdiction into another state where their own licensed physician is engaged in the practice of medicine.

Creating or clarifying consultation exceptions: Creation or clarification of state "consultation exceptions" from the definition of the "practice of medicine" that reduce additional licensure requirements on physicians for telemedicine services if the physician is consulting at the request of a fully licensed physician.

Licensure options

National Licensure. A national licensure system could take two forms. For example, a national licensure approach to telemedicine was recently proposed as an amendment to the Communications Act of 1995 (HR 1555) by then Representative, now Senator Ron Wyden (D-Ore) that would have preempted state law in cases in which a physician was conducting a consultation using telecommunications. The American Medical Association (AMA) and the Federation of State Licensing Boards (FSMB) opposed this amendment vigorously, citing the lack of any evidence demonstrating the need for such a system. Both the AMA and the FSMB expressed the belief that enforcement of standards should be a state issue, left to the individual licensing boards. The specter of a new federal bureaucracy that would govern medical licensure without local input and flexibility was viewed harshly by most of organized medicine. The Wyden amendment was withdrawn.

The other approach to national licensure would be for Congress to develop a set of minimum criteria for states to implement. These rules would be implemented by the states as a floor to which the state could enact additional conditions and requirements that were not inconsistent with the federal law. Although this concept has not been formally proposed, some members of Congress have recently expressed their interest in developing such a measure. Whether national licensure takes the form of federal standards or a nationalized program, proponents of this general approach have vowed to continue to advance this issue onto the congressional agenda in the future.

Mutual Recognition of Licensure. One alternative to national licensure is for states mutually to recognize the licenses of other states. For example, under this system a physician licensed in one state would give "notice" to the relevant medical board of another state of his or her intent to practice in that state. The licensing board would have 1 month to act on the registration. The board could not reject an applicant on the grounds that the primary qualifications were not sufficient under its medical practice act. In short, a physician's current registration in one jurisdiction would be qualification to practices of reciprocity; some maintain that this system of mutual recognition of licensure is similar to licensure by endorsement but is less burdensome to physicians.

Proponents of this approach to licensure argue that it would maintain elements of state control while allowing for a more seamless administrative and disciplinary system. Although this system is conducive to standardization, opponents argue that it would result in a lowest common denominator effect whereby the jurisdiction with the least requirements would become the de facto jurisdiction of choice. Opponents also assert that this system is insensitive to local needs, variations, and control. Although it is used in both Australia and the European community, a movement toward this type of approach does not appear to have taken a firm hold in the United States.

Full Licensure. Under a full licensure approach, state law would require physicians to obtain a full and unrestricted license in any state in which a physician provides medical services. There appears to be growing sentiment in some states for requiring out-of-state physicians to obtain a full and unrestricted license. This movement appears particularly strong among physicians concerned about the potential effects of telemedicine on traditional patterns of referrals and the challenges posed by managed care. Many states have opted for full and unrestricted licensure, a position also adopted by some medical specialty societies, such as the American College of Radiology, and more recently by the California Medical Association.

A number of states have already enacted into law (either by legislation or regulation) a full and unrestricted physician licensure requirement. To date the states of Kansas, South Dakota, Texas, Florida, Nevada, and Massachusetts have put a full licensure requirement into place. Although it is expected that a number of other states will follow suit, opponents of this approach have suggested that the Interstate Commerce Commission (ICC) could step in to declare these practices a "barrier" to interstate commerce and trade in federal court. Opponents also cite these state statutes as greater reason for a national licensure law to be enacted by Congress. Although a challenge by the ICC against these state laws remains possible, the practical success of such a challenge is unclear given the current plans by the Republican majority in Congress to eliminate this federal agency. The greater challenge to these full and unrestricted medical licensure requirements appears to be from action taken on Capitol Hill.

Limited Licensure. A modified type of state licensure approach would require a secondary or "limited" license for telemedicine services in addition to a primary full and unrestricted license. For example, as the ostensible result of the introduction and withdrawal of the Wyden amendment, the FSMB recently issued a limited licensure proposal entitled "An Act to Regulate the Practice of Telemedicine to Medicine by Other Means Across State Lines." The FSMB released its proposal model legislation on November 8, 1995, and held an open hearing on the subject on January 17, 1996. The proposal would require a physician who maintains a full and unrestricted license in one state to obtain a "limited license" from the state in which he or she intends to practice telemedicine. Although the AMA has expressed reservations regarding specific items contained in the FSMB proposal, it has vowed to continue to work with the FSMB to perfect its

details and assist in the development of this state-based approach.

Extended Jurisdiction Licensure. Another state-based approach would be to allow the medical board of one state to assert its jurisdiction in another state where a licensed physician from the first state is engaged in the practice of medicine. This could be accomplished through enactment of a so-called long-arm type of statute that would allow a medical board to reach into another state and obtain "jurisdiction" over the physician licensed in the first state.

Although this approach would potentially lend strength to a more efficient disciplinary and administrative system of licensure due to the fact that only one state would have jurisdiction over the physician, it may also be weighted down by its state-by-state nature. In addition, conflicts could develop in situations in which a state extends the jurisdictions of its medical board into states that maintain a full licensure requirement without a consultation exception. In such cases, the visiting physician could be deemed to be engaged in the "unauthorized practice of medicine" by the visited state even though in the physician's state local law provides that it has jurisdiction over the physician conducting the telemedicine consultation.

Clarifying or Extending Consultation Exceptions
Currently, a substantial number of states have what are termed "consultation exceptions" (ie, an exception from the definition of the "practice of medicine" under the state Medical Practice Act). Such exceptions typically allow out-of-state physicians to enter the state at the request of a locally licensed physician for the purpose of consultation. This creates another alternative to the current licensure system.

States that do not now maintain such exceptions could enact legislation in which a licensed physician would have no additional or specific licensure requirement placed on him or her for telemedicine services if the physician is consulting at the request of a fully licensed physician in that state. For example, the state of Alaska has taken the approach of exempting from licensure requirements those physicians who are called in for a consultation by a physician licensed in the state, and the services provided are limited to that consultation. Some of the states that maintain these statutory exemptions, however, also prohibit an out-of-state physician from opening an office, receiving calls, or making appointments in the state.

Conclusion
It is worth noting that Newton's third law of physics often appears to apply to politics—that is, for every action, there is an equal and opposite reaction. For every state that enacts a full licensure requirement, it is likely that Congress will propose a national licensure law, just as the Wyden amendment caused a reaction on the state level. It is too early to tell where the debate regarding medical licensure law will end, but it is clear that the action and reaction have begun. (LIC-1996)

Resource
American Telemedicine Association
901 15th St NW, Ste 230, Washington, DC 20005-2301
202 408-1400

T Therapeutic Recreation Specialist

Occupational description
Practiced in clinical, residential, and community settings, the therapeutic recreation profession uses treatment, education, and recreation services to help people with illnesses, disabilities, and other conditions develop and use leisure activities to enhance health, independence, and well-being.

Job description
The day-to-day work experience of therapeutic recreation specialists can vary dramatically, depending upon the setting and clients they serve. All therapeutic recreation specialists, however, conduct assessments of physical, mental, emotional, and social functioning to determine the client's needs, interests, and abilities. The therapeutic recreation specialist works with the client, family, and others to design and implement an individualized treatment, education, or program plan.

Professional therapeutic recreation services are divided into three specific "service areas," which represent a comprehensive continuum approach based upon individual needs:

Therapy is intended to improve functional skills for individuals with disabilities who require treatment or remediation of functional skills as a prerequisite to their involvement in meaningful leisure experiences.

Leisure education provides persons in clinical, residential, and community settings—including individuals with disabilities—opportunities to attain skills, knowledge, and attitudes of leisure involvement.

Recreation participation provides opportunities for voluntary involvement in recreation interests and activities. Specialized recreation participation programs are provided when assistance and/or adapted recreation equipment are needed or when appropriate community recreation opportunities are not available.

During a typical day, a therapeutic recreation specialist will be responsible for one or more group activities. These might include a stress management group, a high or low ropes course activity, a community outing, a family activity, an exercise group, or a leisure education group. The therapeutic recreation specialist might also meet with individual clients to conduct an assessment, develop a leisure discharge plan, or plan evening and weekend activities. Charting client progress and communicating with professionals in other disciplines and family members are also part of a typical day.

A therapeutic recreation specialist working in a community recreation agency also conducts assessments to determine client needs and interests and is responsible for adapting activities as needed and for providing adaptive equipment to enable individuals with disabilities or limitations to participate. In addition, the therapeutic recreation specialist provides in-service training for recreation staff who have individuals with disabilities in their programs to orient them to the needs of these individuals and to promote general sensitivity. The therapeutic recreation specialist will generally seek to integrate clients into existing recreation programs, activities, and classes when possible.

An important responsibility for a therapeutic recreation specialist in both community and clinical settings is to serve as an advocate on behalf of individuals with disabilities. This includes addressing such issues as limited transportation resources, inaccessible facilities, and legislation that affects people with disabilities or limitations. A therapeutic recreation specialist frequently serves on advisory committees and consults with outside agencies to ensure that resources and services are provided for people with disabilities.

One of the most attractive qualities of the therapeutic recreation profession is the opportunity for variety and diversity. The many changes in the health care delivery system have provided—and will continue to offer—an array of challenges and opportunities for continued growth in therapeutic recreation. And the opportunity to positively affect the quality of life of an individual with a disability or limitation is extremely rewarding.

Employment characteristics
In clinical settings, such as hospitals and rehabilitation centers, therapeutic recreation specialists treat and rehabilitate individuals with specific medical problems, usually in cooperation with physicians, nurses, psychologists, social workers, and physical and occupational therapists. In nursing homes, residential facilities, and community recreation departments, they use leisure activities—mostly group oriented—to improve general health and well-being, but may also treat medical problems.

Therapeutic recreation specialists assess patients, based on information from medical records, medical staff, family, and patients themselves. They then develop therapeutic activity programs consistent with patient needs and interests. For instance, a patient having trouble socializing may be helped to play games with others, or a client with right-side paralysis may be helped to use the left arm to throw a ball or swing a racket. Therapeutic recreation specialists observe and record patients' participation, reactions, and progress. These records are used by the medical staff and others to monitor progress, to justify changes or end treatment, and for billing.

Community-based therapeutic recreation specialists work in park and recreation departments, special education programs, or programs for older adults or people with disabilities. In these programs, therapeutic recreation specialists help clients develop leisure activities and provide them with opportunities for exercise, mental stimulation, creativity, and fun.

Therapeutic recreation specialists often lift and carry equipment as well as participate in activities. They generally work a 40-hour week, which may include some evenings, weekends, and holidays.

Therapeutic recreation specialists held about 32,000 jobs in 1990. Two fifths were in hospitals and one third were in nursing homes. Others were in community mental health centers, adult day care programs, correctional facilities, residential facilities, community programs for people with disabilities, and substance abuse centers. Some were self-employed, generally contracting with nursing homes or community agencies to develop and oversee programs.

According to a 1994 study of members of the National Therapeutic Recreation Society, the average salary of therapeutic recreation specialists was $31,472. In nursing homes, where therapeutic recreation specialists are often classified as activity directors, the average annual salary was $28,720 in 1994. Average annual earnings for therapeutic recreation specialists in the federal government were $30,559 in 1991.

Employment outlook

Employment of therapeutic recreation specialists is expected to grow faster than the average for all occupations through the year 2005 because of anticipated expansion in long-term care, physical and psychiatric rehabilitation, and services for people with disabilities.

Hospital-based adult day care and outpatient programs and units offering short-term mental health and alcohol or drug abuse services will provide a large number of jobs through the year 2005.

The rapidly growing number of older people is expected to spur job growth for activity directors in nursing homes, retirement communities, adult day care programs, and social service agencies. Continued growth is expected in community residential facilities, as well as day care programs for people with disabilities.

National certification is available through the National Council for Therapeutic Recreation Certification (NCTRC), which awards the title of Certified Therapeutic Recreation Specialist (CTRS).

Through registration, qualified individuals are listed on an official roster maintained by a governmental or non-governmental agency. Information regarding registration requirements may be obtained from state recreation and park associations. (AHRP -1997)

Resources

National Council for Therapeutic Recreation Certification
PO Box 479, Thiells, NY 10984-0479
914 947-4346   Fax 914 947-1634

National Recreation and Park Association (NRPA)
2775 S Quincy St, Ste 300, Arlington, VA 22206-2236
703 578-5570

National Therapeutic Recreation Society (NTRS)
2775 S Quincy St, Ste 300, Arlington, VA 22206-2236
703 820-4940
800 626-NRPA (for membership information and other services)
703 671-6772
E-mail: Info@NRPA.org
Web address: http://www.nrpa.org

Thermography

A technique in which temperature patterns on the surface of the skin are recorded in the form of an image. (ENC-1989)

Resource

American Academy of Thermology
2740 Chain Bridge Rd, Ste 122, Vienna, VA 22180-5303
703 938-6140   Fax 703 938-1482

Thoracic Medicine

American Thoracic Society
1740 Broadway, New York, NY 10019-4374
212 315-8778   Fax 212 315-6498

American Association for Thoracic Surgery
13 Elm St, PO Box 1565, Manchester, MA 01944
508 526-8330   Fax 508 526-4018

American Board of Thoracic Surgery
1 Rotary Center, Ste 803, Evanston, IL 60201
847 475-1520   Fax 847 475-6240

Society of Thoracic Surgeons
401 N Michigan Ave, Chicago, IL 60611-4235
312 644-6610   Fax 312 527-6635

Tinnitus

American Tinnitus Association
PO Box 5, Portland, OR 97207-0005
503 248-9985   Fax 503 248-0024
E-mail: Tinnitus@ata.org

Tissue Banks

American Association of Tissue Banks
1350 Beverly Rd, Ste 220-A, McLean, VA 22101
703 827-9582

Tobacco

Editorial

The Brown and Williamson documents: where do we go from here?

JAMA 1995 Jul 19; 274(3) p 256

Editorials represent the opinions of the authors and *The Journal* and not those of the American Medical Association.

There is a massive body of evidence, derived from many scientific disciplines, that tobacco is addictive and kills smokers. Up to half of those who continue to smoke cigarettes will die prematurely from diseases caused by smoking, half of these deaths occurring in middle age.[1] Peto et al[2] have calculated that of the 1.25 billion people now living in developed countries, 250 million will, if present tobacco consumption patterns are maintained, die from tobacco. With 3 million deaths worldwide each year currently due to tobacco use, the consequences of tobacco to the public health have been, and will continue to be, staggering, and the importance of bringing this hazard under control is correspondingly great.

It is against this background that *JAMA* publishes several highly unusual articles this week.

The documents

On May 12, 1994, Stanton A. Glantz, PhD, a professor of medicine in the Division of Cardiology at the University of California, San Francisco (UCSF), and a scholar interested in the field of tobacco and the public health, received from an unknown source, "Mr Butts," approximately 4000 pages of memoranda, reports, and letters, covering a 30-year period, from the Brown and Williamson Tobacco Corporation (B&W) and its parent company, the British American Tobacco Company (now

T BAT Industries).[3] In the subsequent months, Glantz received several thousand additional pages of documents from Congressman Henry Waxman's House Subcommittee on Health and the Environment and another few hundred pages of documents from the estate of the chief scientist of BAT. Glantz ultimately put all the documents into the library at UCSF.

This issue of the *Journal* is largely devoted to an analysis by Glantz and his colleagues of these three sets of documents.[4-8]

The documents show:
- that research conducted by tobacco companies into the deleterious health effects of tobacco was often more advanced and sophisticated than studies by the medical community;
- that executives at B&W knew early on that tobacco use was harmful and that nicotine was addictive and debated whether to make the research public;
- that the industry decided to conceal the truth from the public;
- that the industry hid their research from the courts by sending the data through their legal departments, their lawyers asserting that the results were immune to disclosure in litigation because they were the privileged product of the lawyer-client relationship;
- that despite their knowledge to the contrary, the industry's public position was (and continues to be) that the link between smoking and ill health was not proven, that they were dedicated to determining whether there was such a link and revealing this to the public, and that nicotine was not addictive.

We think that these documents and the analyses merit the careful attention of our readership because they provide massive, detailed, and damning evidence of the tactics of the tobacco industry. They show us how this industry has managed to spread confusion by suppressing, manipulating, and distorting the scientific record. They also make clear how the tobacco industry has been able to avoid paying a penny in damages and how it has managed to remain hugely profitable from the sale of a substance long known by scientists and physicians to be lethal. We hope that publication of the articles will encourage all our readers to become even more active in the campaign against tobacco.

The B&W documents Glantz first received are believed to be copies of documents themselves copied by a paralegal, Merrell Williams, who had once worked for one of B&W's outside counsel. Merrell Williams had, in 1993, turned the documents over to the attorney he had hired to make a claim for health damages against B&W. His ex-employers filed action against him in September 1993 to prohibit the use and dissemination of the B&W documents. In October 1993, B&W intervened as a plaintiff in the case, claiming that the documents were protected from disclosure to the public by the attorney-client privilege and the work product doctrine.[9]

The documents surfaced publicly on May 7, 1994, when Philip Hilts published the first of a series of articles in the *New York Times*,[10] and since then there have been reports in several national newspapers and on radio and television. In addition, Congressman Waxman made more documents public at hearings by the Subcommittee on Health and the Environment of the US House of Repre-

sentatives in the summer of 1994. Since that time, in litigation in the District of Columbia, West Virginia, Massachusetts, Kentucky, and Mississippi, B&W has attempted to subpoena reporters and seal the documents. They have been unsuccessful. Judge Harold H. Greene of the US District Court for the District of Columbia quashed subpoenas directed at Congressmen Henry Waxman and Ron Wyden, concluding that B&W's course of conduct was "patently crafted to harass those who would reveal facts concerning B&W's knowledge of the health hazards of tobacco."[11]

In the case of the documents in the UCSF library, B&W has not only tried to remove the documents but also sought to obtain the names of scholars who have used them, something the university has interpreted as a violation of the privacy rights of library patrons. In addition, the company hired private investigators to stake out the area in the UCSF library where the documents were kept, an action that had the effect of harassing and intimidating library personnel.[12] On May 25, 1995, Judge Stuart Pollak in the Superior Court of the State of California, without ruling on whether the documents were privileged, recognized that the documents were already in the public domain. The judge said that there was a strong public interest in permitting the information in the documents to remain available to the university and others. He noted that to grant B&W's application would have the effect of preventing the information from being used in the public dialogue bearing on public health, public law, and litigation. He denied B&W's application to take possession of all copies of the documents in the hands of the UCSF and its employees.[13] An appeal by B&W was unanimously rejected by the California Supreme Court on June 29, 1995. The documents, the authenticity of which is not in doubt, not least because of the actions B&W has taken to retrieve them, are therefore in the public domain because judges across the country say they should be.

Who are the authors?
The authors of the first five articles we publish in this issue of *JAMA* are people who have produced careful scholarship in the past, some of it published in *JAMA*.[14-16] They are academic researchers interested in national policy to reduce the toll from this devastating hazard to the nation's health.

The articles
These five articles provide a careful analysis of the documents. They detail the sharp disparities between the tobacco industries' private knowledge, developed by their own research during more than 30 years, and their public stance. The articles show that the effect of tobacco company tactics, long suspected, has been to obfuscate the conclusions of scientists, to confuse the public, and to assist greatly the tobacco industry in its successful efforts to influence the political process in its favor. The surgeon general's report of 1964 would have been far more decisive in its conclusions and recommendations had the evidence available to the executives of B&W been available to the surgeon general's committee. We can only speculate how many lives would have been saved and how much suffering would have been averted.

JAMA hired Mr Tim Graham, a veteran editor with the Alameda Newspaper Group, which includes the *Oakland Tribune*. He, after reading the documents, has, according to usual journalistic practice, tried to contact executives of B&W and other interested parties to get their reactions. We publish Graham's article[17] together with the written questions he sent B&W and B&W's statement in response. We also publish an interview by Andrew Skolnick with Mr Victor Crawford, a lobbyist for the Tobacco Institute in Maryland, who is now dying of cancer of the oropharynx.[18]

Why are we publishing the articles?
For many decades, the mission of the American Medical Association (AMA) has been to "promote the science and art of medicine and the betterment of public health." To remain silent about the B&W papers would be to deny our mission. Quite simply, we are publishing this research because it is the right thing to do.

Analysis of these papers suggests that we would have seen a very different picture of tobacco use today if the group knowing the most about the dangers of tobacco use, the industry, had been honest with its customers. The documents and the *JAMA* articles show us in a stark way that some of those who speak for the tobacco industry dissemble, distort, and deceive, despite the fact that the industry's own research is consistent with the scientific community's conclusion that continued use of their product will endanger the lives and health of the public at home and abroad. The industry continues to use the same tactics: even now, it is suing the government over the release of the Environmental Protection Agency report that has classified environmental tobacco smoke as a group A carcinogen.[19] It is spending vast amounts of money to overturn antismoking laws.[20]

These papers show us how little the tobacco industry is to be trusted when they speak on health issues and that the "evidence" they put before regulatory and legislative bodies at the national, state, and local level is highly suspect.

Where do we go from here?
The AMA maintains an unequivocal stance against tobacco.[21] The AMA reminds physicians, the public, and politicians that the damning evidence against tobacco makes opposition to its use a pressing, nonpartisan public health issue. If the industry uses political weapons, so shall we. The AMA will not relent in its opposition to tobacco use.

To accomplish this goal, the AMA recommends and will pursue the following steps:
- Further efforts should be made to educate physicians, the public, and policymakers about the consequences of tobacco use, the predatory nature of the tobacco industry, and ways individuals can break their addiction to tobacco.
- Medical schools and research institutions, as well as individual researchers, should refuse any funding from the tobacco industry and its subsidiaries to avoid giving them an appearance of credibility. The B&W documents affirm our belief that such tobacco industry entities as the Council for Tobacco Research, the Smokeless Tobacco Research Council, and the Center for Indoor Air Research are used by the tobacco industry to convince the public that there still is a controversy about whether tobacco has ill effects, to buy respectability, and to silence universities and researchers. We concur with the recommendation of a

subcommittee of the National Cancer Advisory Board that federal funding be withdrawn from cancer research organizations that accept tobacco industry support.[22]
- Politicians should not accept money from the tobacco industry but should direct their efforts to protection of the nonsmoking majority. Those who do accept money should be identified publicly.
- The federal Occupational Safety and Health Administration should move forward with its proposal to require smoke-free workplaces nationwide.
- Local communities should continue to control smoking in public.
- State legislatures should assume responsibility for ensuring smoke-free areas. Any preemptive tobacco laws should be repealed by public demand.
- Purchase of tobacco should be strictly limited to adults, with severe penalties for those who transgress. Underage use of tobacco should carry consequences for the user. All tobacco advertising should be eliminated, and a vigorous counteradvertising campaign should be instituted.
- The Justice Department should enforce the ban against indirect tobacco advertising such as televised sports events.
- Tobacco itself should be considered a drug delivery vehicle and placed under the oversight of the Food and Drug Administration, with appropriate regulation as for other life-threatening drugs.[23]
- State and federal excise taxes on tobacco products should be dramatically increased, both to help defray costs of tobacco-induced diseases and to deter young people from becoming addicted.
- The federal government should prevent the export of tobacco to other countries.
- The continued contribution to knowledge of the control of tobacco by the National Cancer Institute should be strongly supported.
- Physicians and the public should support legal action against the tobacco industry to recover billions of dollars in excess medical costs from tobacco-related diseases borne by Medicare, Medicaid, and the Department of Veterans Affairs.
- All avenues of individual and collective redress should be pursued through the judicial system.

In summary, the evidence is unequivocal—the US public has been duped by the tobacco industry. No right-thinking individual can ignore the evidence. We should all be outraged, and we should force the removal of this scourge from our nation and by so doing set an example for the world. We recognize the serious consequences of this ambition, but the health of our nation is more important than the profits of any single industry.

On behalf of the physicians of this country and the people they serve, the AMA pledges its best efforts to the eradication of tobacco-related disease. We solicit the support of the public and our government in this endeavor. It is a worthy cause.

James S. Todd, MD, Drummond Rennie, MD, Robert E. McAfee, MD, Lonnie R. Bristow, MD, Joseph T. Painter, MD, Thomas R. Reardon, MD, Daniel H. Johnson, Jr, MD, Richard F. Corlin, MD, Yank D. Coble, Jr, MD, Nancy W. Dickey, MD, Timothy T. Flaherty, MD, Palma E. Formica, MD, Michael S. Goldrich, MD, William E. Jacott, MD,

T Donald T. Lewers, MD, John C. Nelson, MD, MPH, P. John Seward, MD, Randolph D. Smoak, Jr, MD, Michael Suk, JD, MPH, Frank B. Walker, MD, Percy Wootton, MD, George D. Lundberg, MD

References

1. Doll R, Peto R, Wheatley K, Gray R, Sutherland I. Mortality in relation to smoking: 40 years' observations on male British doctors. *BMJ*. 1994;309:901-911.

2. Peto R, Lopez AD, Boreham J, Thun M, Heath C Jr. Mortality from tobacco in developed countries: indirect estimation from national statistics. *Lancet*. 1992;339:1268-1278.

3. Glantz SA. Declaration to the Superior Court of the State of California for the County of San Francisco, in *Brown and Williamson Tobacco Corporation v Regents of the University of California*. May 15, 1995.

4. Glantz SA, Barnes DE, Bero L, Hanauer P, Slade J. Looking through a keyhole at the tobacco industry: the Brown and Williamson documents. *JAMA*. 1995;274:219-224.

5. Bero L, Barnes DE, Hanauer P, Slade J, Glantz SA. Lawyer control of the tobacco industry's external research program: the Brown and Williamson documents. *JAMA*. 1995;274:241-247.

6. Barnes DE, Hanauer P, Slade J, Bero L, Glantz SA. Environmental tobacco smoke: the Brown and Williamson documents. *JAMA*. 1995;274:248-253.

7. Hanauer P, Slade J, Barnes DE, Bero L, Glantz SA. Lawyer control of internal scientific research to protect against products liability lawsuits: the Brown and Williamson documents. *JAMA*. 1995;274:234-240.

8. Slade J, Bero L, Hanauer P, Barnes DE, Glantz SA. Nicotine and addiction: the Brown and Williamson documents. *JAMA*. 1995;274:225-233.

9. *Castano v The American Tobacco Company, et al.* US District Court Eastern District of Louisiana.

10. Hilts PJ. Tobacco company was silent on hazards. *New York Times*. May 7, 1994:A1.

11. Greene HH, in *Maddox v Williams*, June 6, 1994. DC District Court. 855 F Supp 406, pp 414-415.

12. Balderson AJ. UCSF library has tobacco firm's documents under lock and key. *UCFS Newsbreak*. March 11-24, 1995;10(5):1.

13. Pollack S, in *Brown and Williamson v Regents of the University of California*. Superior Court of the State of California for the County of San Francisco. May 25, 1995.

14. Traynor M, Begay M, Glantz S. The tobacco industry strategy to prevent tobacco control. *JAMA*. 1993;270:479-488.

15. Glantz S, Begay M. Tobacco industry campaign contributions are affecting tobacco control policymaking in California. *JAMA*. 1994;272:1176-1182.

16. Glantz SA, Parmley WW. Passive smoking and heart disease: mechanisms and risk. *JAMA*. 1995;273:1047-1053.

17. Graham T. The Brown and Williamson documents: the company's response. *JAMA*. 1995;274:254-255.

18. Skolnick A. Cancer converts tobacco lobbyist: Victor L. Crawford goes on the record. *JAMA*. 1995;274:199.

19. *Respiratory Health Effects of Passive Smoking: Lung Cancer and Other Disorders*. Washington, DC: US Environmental Protection Agency; December 1992. EPA/600-90-006F.

20. Mallory M. Full-flavored, unfiltered statehouse shenanigans: Big Tobacco's big bucks can still turn antismoking laws around. *Business Week*. May 22, 1995:52.

21. Lundberg GD. In the AMA, policy follows science: a case history of tobacco. *JAMA*. 1985;253:3001-3003.

22. National Cancer Advisory Board, Subcommittee to Evaluate the National Cancer Program. *Cancer at a Crossroads: A Report to Congress for the Nation*. Washington, DC: National Cancer Institute; September 1994.

23. Lundberg GD. Tobacco: for consenting adults in private only. *JAMA*. 1986;255:1051-1053.

A turning point in tobacco suits: Liggett's cooperation triggers accountability

Stephanie Stapleton
AM News Apr 14, 1997 p 3

In 1996, the Liggett Group Inc., the smallest of the nation's big five cigarette companies, earned profits of less than $8 million—a fraction of the $6.8 billion accumulated by tobacco giant Philip Morris USA or the $611 million garnered by R.J. Reynolds/Nabisco.

But size does not determine impact, as the rest of the industry learned on March 20. That's when Liggett broke ranks with the others, signing away 25% of its annual pretax earnings for the next 25 years as part of a settlement agreement with 22 state attorneys general who are suing the tobacco industry to recover billions of dollars in Medicaid costs associated with treating smoking-related illnesses.

The payments will amount to a modest sum when divvied among all those with a claim. But from the perspective of public health and tobacco-control advocates, dollars are not the issue. The insider information to which they will now have access is the bottom line.

The Durham, N.C.-based Liggett Group agreed to cooperate with the state attorneys general in their ongoing lawsuits against the rest of the industry—Philip Morris, R.J. Reynolds, Brown & Williamson, and Lorillard—by making public its own proprietary information. The first state trial begins June 2 in Mississippi.

In-house marketing plans, nicotine content reports, and other files formerly subject to Liggett's attorney-client privilege and work-product protections will be turned over. Liggett also is offering up thousands of pages of records on industrywide activities.

Other elements of the settlement require Liggett to:
• Acknowledge that smoking causes health problems, that nicotine has been found to be addictive, and that the tobacco industry markets its products to children younger than 18.
• Promise not to challenge Food and Drug Administration regulations concerning the sale and distribution of cigarettes and smokeless tobacco products, agree to comply with many of these regulations before they officially take effect, and add a warning to cigarette packages that smoking is addictive.

In exchange, no further damages can be sought from Liggett in the state Medicaid cases, and the forfeited documents cannot be used against the company in other legal actions.

Eliminates the clutter

Although the long-term implications of the settlement are difficult to predict, it will be important for a number of reasons, said Thomas P. Houston, MD, the AMA's director of public health and environmental medicine.

In legal proceedings to date, the tobacco industry has produced reams of paper to bury potentially damaging documents "like a needle in a haystack," Dr. Houston said. He offered as an example the reports that Philip Morris turned over two warehouses full of paperwork—28 million pages—in response to a suit filed by the state of Minnesota.

The difference here, he said, is that Liggett will "cut out the chaff and go right to the kernel," not only supplying documents but directing the plaintiffs' lawyers to the key information.

Liggett's cooperation also entails identifying employees to provide expert testimony regarding its marketing strategies and nicotine manipulation—"spilling the secrets of the industry in court," Dr. Houston said.

At the very least, tobacco control advocates predict the airing of Liggett's laundry will trigger industrywide accountability.

"This will change juries' perception," said Robert Kline, an attorney with Northeastern University's Tobacco Products Liability Project, an organization that assists litigation efforts against the tobacco industry.

Cigarette companies have been successful, up to this point, with their contention that people make the decision to smoke, and if they get sick, it is a result of that choice, he added.

"Now, there's a sense that tobacco companies are not clean," Kline said, pointing to Liggett's admission that cigarette marketing targets young people—"hooking them in" with an addictive substance.

The most valuable prizes, however, are locked in a second set of documents, the release of which—at press time—was being contested by the other tobacco companies.

According to Dr. Houston, these papers include intra-industry communications and records, such as minutes from meetings of a group known as the committee of counsel—the legal representatives of the five tobacco companies—that formed a united front in planning anti-litigation strategies.

Industry: Liggett 'reckless'

Even before the settlement was announced, the four other tobacco companies went to court to argue that these materials are subject to attorney-client privilege and were granted a temporary restraining order to prevent them from being turned over.

"There is a right way and a wrong way to pursue discovery in litigation. The attorneys general are proposing to take an inappropriate route. We cannot allow them to proceed in an unchecked, reckless fashion to undermine long-settled principles that protect from disclosure materials covered by attorney-client privilege," asserted an industry statement.

Judges in the 22 states where suits are pending will now likely decide on a case-by-case basis whether this argument has merit.

In Florida, for example, a judge is reviewing these documents in preparation for an April 14 hearing to determine whether, as allowed by state law, public safety concerns override the confidentiality claim. Similar proceedings have begun in at least three other jurisdictions.

"If they are released, it will blow the lid off of other tobacco companies," Dr. Houston said.

Tobacco companies have publicly claimed all along that cigarettes are not addictive, not carcinogenic, and not marketed to kids, said Kathryn Kahler Vose, communications director for the National Center for Tobacco-Free Kids.

"These documents will show they have been lying," she said.

But big tobacco is holding fast to its position.

"Smoking is a personal choice, and so is quitting. These are choices made by countless numbers of individuals every day. Nothing said or agreed to by [Liggett Director] Bennett LeBow can change these facts," asserted a statement issued by Philip Morris in response to the settlement.

Liggett's motives in making this deal are said to stem from the company's circumstances as the weakest financial link in the tobacco chain—least able to absorb costs stemming from protracted litigation and most anxious to reduce its liability burden to become more attractive to buyout bids.

It is the second time the company has been willing to cut bait.

In March, 1996, Liggett agreed to similar but less expansive stipulations to end the so-called Castano class-action lawsuit filed on behalf of addicted smokers and to partially reimburse five state governments for Medicaid costs.

That settlement, which was viewed as a maneuver to facilitate a merger with R.J. Reynolds, became void last year when a federal appeals court threw out the case. Several smaller suits have since been filed, and the number of Medicaid-related suits has grown.

Tobacco-control advocates, however, have little concern over the why behind Liggett's actions, focusing instead on the payoff.

They say the disclosure comes at "a critical time in the tobacco wars," when smoking among young people is at a 17-year high. A Stanford University study released on the same day the settlement was announced found that teen smoking increased 30% from 1991 to 1995.

"The acknowledgment that the tobacco industry has been deceitful, distrusting, and continues to sacrifice lives for their bottom lines is long overdue," said AMA Secretary-treasurer Randolph Smoak, MD, adding that Liggett's admission that young people were targeted by advertising is another overriding factor.

And advocates say that in addition to the strength the deal adds to the Medicaid lawsuits, the settlement also

T will galvanize public support for FDA efforts to limit youth access to tobacco products—a regulation now facing a separate legal challenge.

JAMA Issue of Note: Tobacco: the Brown and Williamson documents

JAMA 1995, Jul 19: 274(3)

This issue, as highlighted in the editorial above, presents documentation and commentary related to the discovery of the research documents and support materials from the tobacco giant.

Tourette Syndrome

Tourette Syndrome Association
42-40 Bell Blvd, Bayside, NY 11361
800 237-0717 718 224-2999 Fax 718 279-9596

Transitional Year

Accreditation Council of Graduate Medical Education
Transitional Year Review Committee
515 N State St, Ste 2000, Chicago, IL 60610
312 464-4920 Fax 312 464-4098

Transplantation

The early days of transplantation

Thomas E. Starzl, MD
JAMA 1994 Dec 7; 272(21): 1705

Although the fantasy of performing tissue and limb transplantation can be traced to antiquity, not until this century was the possibility of engrafting vital organs broached. The attempt began with failed kidney xenograft trials in Europe,[1] followed by the first recorded attempt at a renal allograft in 1936 by the Russian physician Y. Y. Voronoy. The modern era of transplantation truly began in 1944, when Peter Medawar demonstrated that allograft rejection is an immunologic process.

In a burst of clinical interest between 1950 and 1952, French surgeons Rene Kuss, Charles Dubost, and Marceau Servelle independently described essentially the same pelvic renal transplantation operation that is standard today; in 1952 Louis Michon and Jean Hamburger reported the first live kidney donation (mother to son).[2]

Immunosuppression was not used for these recipients, nor for those of David Hume at the Peter Bent Brigham Hospital, Boston, Mass, who transplanted allografts subcutaneously in the thigh.[3] Consequently, the few kidneys that had functioned up to the end of 1954 were doomed to be rejected. In the 1930s E. C. Padgett and J. B. Brown had shown that genetic identity was essential to permit the permanent exchange of skin in monozygotic twins. In a bold application of this knowledge, a team led by Joseph Murray and John Merrill successfully transplanted an identical twin kidney on December 23, 1954.

On January 24, 1959, the same Boston team successfully transplanted a kidney between dizygotic twins.[4] The successful breaching of such a genetic barrier makes this the single most important case in the history of transplantation. The claim was enhanced a few months later when a similar case was reported by Jean Hamburger's team in Paris. The recipients, who received total-body irradiation for immunosuppression, survived 20 and 26 years, respectively, before dying of cancer. Using irradiation, Hamburger's group[5] and a second Paris team headed by Kuss[6] produced four additional long-surviving recipients between 1959 and 1962, this time with more distant donors—a non-twin sibling, a cousin, and in the two Kuss cases, nonrelatives.

While encouraging, these six cases were exceptions. Unable after 11 more attempts to duplicate his 1959 achievement, Murray took an alternative historical step. On April 5, 1962, he transplanted an unrelated renal allograft that functioned for 17 months.[7] This was the first human example of successful chemical immunosuppression using azathioprine.[8]

Expectations from Boston and Paris generated a worldwide ripple that did not spare me in Chicago, where I had been experimenting with canine liver transplantation. By the end of 1960, I concluded that liver transplantation could never be tried until consistent success in renal grafts was achieved. In 1961, I joined William Waddell, at the University of Colorado School of Medicine, to begin a kidney transplant program that would be a forerunner for our liver program.

Which method of immunosuppression to use for our first kidney recipients remained undecided. Although total-body irradiation was considered dangerous and relatively ineffective, the best results were being obtained by Hamburger and Kuss in France,[5,6] who sporadically gave adrenal corticosteroids to their irradiated patients or even—in one of Kuss' 1,960 patients—6-mercaptopurine, the drug from which azathioprine is derived.

Our contribution was to combine azathioprine with prednisone.[9] Rejection could be reversed with prednisone in most azathioprine-treated recipients and, in many, the immune barrier could be reduced without general immune deficiency. During the year after the repeatedly successful use of this drug combination became known, nearly 50 US kidney transplant programs were formed. These "double-drug cocktails" also justified the first liver transplant trials in Colorado, beginning on March 1, 1963. When these failed, liver replacement suffered its own protracted birth pangs. The "baby" was finally delivered in 1967, with several recipients surviving more than 1 year. This success was quickly followed by attempts at other organ transplants.

Although transplantation of the liver and heart was sporadically successful during the next dozen years, the results of these procedures were unpredictable. The introduction of cyclosporine in 1978[10] and its systematic combination with prednisone[11] was followed by a proliferation of liver, cardiac, pancreas, lung, and intestinal transplant programs—as well as increased use of cadaveric kidneys. The consequence, by the late 1980s, was a shortage of all cadaveric organs and a drift back to live donors.

When transplantation procedures finally became routine, the social ramifications thrust a range of unfamiliar problems on health care providers. Ironically, the scientific and medical problems of transplantation have resolved more ingeniously and definitively than derivative ones associated with the dissemination of the fruits of scientists' labor of love.

References

1. Groth CG. Landmarks in clinical renal transplantation. *Surg Gynecol Obstet*. 1972;134:323-328.

2. Starzl TE. France and the early history of organ transplantation. *Perspect Biol Med*. 1993;37:35-47.

3. Hume DM, Merrill JP, Miller BF, Thorn GW. Experiences with renal homotransplantation in the human: report of nine cases. *J Clin Invest*. 1955;34:327-382.

4. Murray JE, Merrill JP, Dammin GJ, et al. Study on transplantation immunity after total body irradiation: clinical and experimental investigation. *Surgery*. 1960;48:272-284.

5. Hamburger J, Vaysse J, Crosnier J, Auvert J, LaLanne CM, Hopper J Jr. Renal homotransplantation in man after radiation of the recipient: experience with six patients since 1959. *Am J Med*. 1962;32:854-871.

6. Kuss R, Legrain M, Mathe G, Nedey R, Camey M. Homologous human kidney transplantation: experience with six patients. *Postgrad Med J*. 1962;38:528-531.

7. Murray JE, Merrill JP, Harrison JH, Wilson RE, Dammin GJ. Prolonged survival of human-kidney homografts by immunosuppressive drug therapy. *N Engl J Med*. 1963;268:1315-1323.

8. Calne RY. Inhibition of the rejection of renal homografts in dogs with purine analogues. *Transplant Bull*. 1961;28:445.

9. Starzl TE, Marchioro TL, Waddell WR. The reversal of rejection in human renal homografts with subsequent development of homograft tolerance. *Surg Gynecol Obstet*. 1963;117:385-395.

10. Calne RY, Rolles K, White DJG, et al. Cyclosporine A initially as the only immunosuppressant in 34 recipients of cadaveric organs: 32 kidneys, two pancreases, and two livers. *Lancet*. 1979;2:1033-1036.

11. Starzl TE, Weil R III, Iwatsuki S, et al. The use of cyclosporine A and prednisone in cadaver kidney transplantation. *Surg Gynecol Obstet*. 1980;151:17-26.

Resource

American Society of Transplant Surgeons
716 Lee St, Des Plaines, IL 60016
847 824-5700   Fax 847 824-0394

Transplants, Liver (Experimental Status)

More transplants planned

AM News Oct 19, 1992 p 2

Pittsburgh—About 10 patients with life-threatening hepatitis B are being considered for a baboon-liver transplant, despite the September 6 death of the first man to undergo the surgery, medical officials say. The first baboon-liver recipient, a 35-year-old man whose identity was never revealed, died 10 weeks after his transplant at Presbyterian University Hospital. A hospital spokeswoman says the new candidates are undergoing medical evaluations and discussing the possible risks and benefits with doctors.

Resource

National Institutes of Health
301 496-5787

Trauma

American College of Emergency Physicians
PO Box 619911, Dallas, TX 75261-9911
214 550-0911   Fax 214 580-2816

American Trauma Society
8903 Presidential Pkwy, Ste 512
Upper Marlboro, MD 20772
800 556-7890   301 420-4189   Fax 301 420-0617

Travel, International—Health Aspects

Centers for Disease Control and Prevention
Center for Preventive Services, Atlanta, GA 30333
404 332-4559 404 639-2779

International Association for Medical Assistance to Travelers (IAMAT)
417 Center St, Lewiston, NY 14092
716 754-4883   Fax 519 836-3412
E-mail: amat@sentex.net

Mobility International
(aid to handicapped people when traveling)
228 Borough High St, London, SEI 1JX, England
71 4035688

Mobility International, USA
(North American affiliate of Mobility International)
PO Box 10767, Eugene, OR 97440
541 343-1284   Fax 541 343-6812
E-mail: miusa@igc.apc.org

Yellow Book of Health Information for International Travel
Publication #017-023-00187-6
Superintendent of Documents
US Government Printing Office
Washington, DC 20402
202 783-3238

Inoculations:
Contact local county health department.

Travelers and Immigrant Aid Societies, Statewide

National Organization of Travelers Aid Societies
512 C St NE, Washington, DC 20002
202 546-3120   Fax 202 546-1625

Alabama
Traveler Aid Society of Birmingham
3600 Eighth Ave S, Ste 110-West
Birmingham, AL 35222
205 322-5426

Family Guidance Center
925 Forest Ave, Montgomery, AL 36106
205 265-6669

Arizona
Travelers Aid of Tucson
40 West Veterans Blvd, Tucson, AZ 85713
602 622-8900

California
Compass Community Services
PO Box 420137, San Francisco, CA 94142-0137
909 984-2252

Travelers Aid Society of Alameda County
520 16th St, Oakland, CA 94612
510 444-6834

Travelers Aid Society of the Inland Empire
1131 W 6th St, Ste 240, Ontario, CA 91762-1117

Travelers Aid Society of Long Beach
947 E 4th St, Long Beach, CA 90802
310 432-3485

Travelers Aid Society of Los Angeles
1720 N Gower, Hollywood, CA 90028
213 468-2500

Travelers Aid Society of Orange County
9872 Chapman Ave, Garden Grove, CA 92641
714 530-2426

Travelers Aid Society of San Diego
1765 Fourth Ave, Ste 100, San Diego, CA 92101
619 232-7991

Colorado
Travelers Aid Services
1245 E Colfax Ave, Ste 408, Denver, CO 80218
303 832-8194

Connecticut
Travelers Aid Services of Hartford
Catholic Family Services
896 Asylum Ave, Hartford, CT 06105
203 522-2247   203 522-8241

Family Counseling of Greater New Haven
1 Long Wharf Dr, New Haven, CT 06511
203 495-7437

Delaware
Family & Children's Service of Delaware
2005 Baynard Blvd, Wilmington, DE 19802
302 658-5303

District of Columbia
Traveler's Aid Society of Washington DC
512 C St NE, Washington, DC 20002
202 546-3120

Florida
Travelers Aid Society
330 Magnolia Ave, Daytona Beach, FL 32114
904 252-4752

Community Service Council
PO Box 14428, Fort Lauderdale, FL 33302
305 524-8371   305 467-6333

Travelers Aid Society of Tampa
1005 N Marion St, Tampa, FL 33602-3404
813 273-5936

The Center for Family Services
2218 S Dixie Hwy
West Palm Beach, FL 33401
407 655-4483

Georgia
Travelers Aid of Metropolitan Atlanta
40 Pryor St SW, Ste 400, Atlanta, GA 30303
404 527-7400

Savannah United Ministries
PO Box 9621, Savannah, GA 31412
912 236-7423

Illinois
Travelers & Immigrants Aid
208 S LaSalle St, Ste 1818, Chicago, IL 60604
312 435-4500

Kentucky
Family and Children's Agency
PO Box 3784, Louisville, KY 40201-3784
502 583-1741

Louisiana
Travelers Aid Society of New Orleans
846 Baronne St, New Orleans, LA 70113
504 525-8726

Maryland
PATH: People Aiding Travelers and the Homeless
111 Park Ave, Baltimore, MD 21201
410 685-3569

Massachusetts
Travelers Aid Society of Boston
17 East St, Boston, MA 02111
617 542-7286

Michigan
Travelers Aid Society of Detroit
211 W Congress, 3rd Fl, Detroit, MI 48226
313 962-6740

Minnesota
Metropolitan Airport Foundation
MSP International Airport, Rm 350
Minneapolis, MN 55111
612 726-5235

Missouri
Mullanphy Travelers Aid
The Globe Bldg, 702 N Tucker Blvd
St Louis, MO 63101
314 241-5820

Nevada
HELP of Southern Nevada
953 E Sahara, Ste 23-B, Las Vegas, NV 89104
702 369-4357

New Jersey
Travelers Aid of New Jersey
Newark International Airport, Terminal B
Newark, NJ 07114
201 623-5052

New York
Homeless and Travelers Aid Society
200 Green St, Albany, NY 12202
518 463-2124

Child and Family Services Travelers Aid Division
The Ellicott Square Bldg
295 Main St, Rm 828, Buffalo, NY 14203
716 854-8661

Travelers Aid Services
2 Lafayette St, 3rd Fl, New York, NY 10007-1307
212 577-3806

Family Services of Greater Utica, Inc
401 Columbia St, Utica, NY 13502
315 735-2236

North Carolina
Community Link
500 Spratt St, Charlotte, NC 28206
704 334-7288

T

Family Services Center
401 Hillsborough St, Raleigh, NC 27603
919 821-0790

Family Services Travelers Aid
PO Box 944, Wilmington, NC 28402
919 392-7051

Family Services of Winston-Salem
610 Coliseum Dr, Winston-Salem, NC 27106-5393
910 722-8173

Ohio
Travelers Aid International of Cincinnati
707 Race St, Ste 300, Cincinnati, OH 45202
513 721-7660

Family Service Association
184 Salem, Rm 790, Dayton, OH 45406
513 222-9481

Oklahoma
Travelers Aid Society of Oklahoma
412 NW 5th St, Oklahoma City, OK 73102
405 232-5507

Pennsylvania
Travelers Aid Society of Philadelphia
311 S Juniper St, Ste 500-05
Philadelphia, PA 19107
215 546-0571

Travelers Aid Society of Pittsburgh
Greyhound Bus Terminal
11th and Liberty Ave, Pittsburgh, PA 15222
412 281-5466

Commission on Economic Opportunity
211-213 S Main St, Wilkes-Barre, PA 18701
717 826-0510

Puerto Rico
Travelers Aid of Puerto Rico
Luis Marin Airport Station, PO Box 38017
Carolina, PR 00937-1017
809 791-1034

Rhode Island
Travelers Aid Society of Rhode Island
177 Union St, Providence, RI 02903
401 521-2255

South Carolina
Family Services Center
1800 Main St, Columbia, SC 29201
803 733-5450

United Ministries
606 Pendleton St, Greenville, SC 29601
803 232-6463

Tennessee
Travelers Aid Society
46 N 3rd St, Ste 708, Memphis, TN 38103
901 525-5466

Nashville Union Mission Travelers Aid
129 7th Ave S, Nashville, TN 37203
615 780-9471

Texas
Travelers Aid American Red Cross
2700 Southwest Frwy, PO Box 397
Houston, TX 77001-0397
713 526-8300

Utah
Travelers Aid Society of Salt Lake City
210 Rio Grande, Salt Lake City, UT 84101
801 328-8996

Virginia
Travelers Aid Society of Virginia
503 E Main, Richmond, VA 23219
804 643-0279

Washington
Travelers Aid Society
909 4th Ave, Rm 630, Seattle, WA 98104
206 461-3888

Wisconsin
Community Advocates Travelers Aid
4906 W Fond du Lac Ave, Milwaukee, WI 53216
414 449-4777

Tropical Medicine

Obituary

Walter Reed, MD
JAMA 1902 Nov 29; 39(22): 1402

In the death of Dr. Walter Reed of the Army, which occurred November 23, scientific medicine has suffered a severe loss, and the profession has been bereft of a constant and enthusiastic student. Walter Reed was born in Virginia in 1857, was graduated from the Medical Department of the University of Virginia, Charlottesville, and from Bellevue Hospital Medical College, New York. He was appointed from Virginia to the Medical Department of the Army and was commissioned first-lieutenant and assistant surgeon, June 26, 1875; five years later he was made captain and assistant surgeon, and on December 4, 1893, was promoted to the position of major and surgeon. At the time of his death he was at the head of the list of majors of the Medical Department of the Army. He made special studies in bacteriology at the Johns Hopkins Hospital, Baltimore, then was assigned to duty as attending surgeon at St. Paul, and from there was selected by the Surgeon-General as bacteriologist in his office, and was on duty there from 1893 until the outbreak of the Spanish-American War. During that time he was a member of the board of medical officers to investigate and report on the prevalence of typhoid fever in home camps and the commission recommended the plan of collecting excreta in galvanized iron tanks, which was afterwards successfully carried out at the US General Hospital, Presidio, Cal, and was followed by cessation of the disease. His especial work was in the line of preventive medicine and military hygiene. His most notable services to the science of medicine were those connected with yellow fever. He was appointed president of the board the other members of which were Drs. Carroll and Agramonte of the Army, which met in Cuba for the study of yellow fever, and their discoveries in connection with the cause and prevention of this disease mark an epoch in medicine. Their reports have already been published in the Journal and show the highest degree of scientific accuracy combined with excellent discrimination. Dr. Reed was operated on for appendicitis on November 17, but did not rally from the operation, and died November 23.

Memorial to Major Walter Reed

JAMA 1903 Aug 15; 41(9): 1402

A meeting of the committees appointed by the American Medical Association and the American Association for the Advancement of Science has been called to meet at Bar Harbor, Me, August 15, to confer regarding the memorial in honor of the late Major Walter Reed, MD. There are other committees beside the ones above mentioned, and the object is to secure immediate, concerted action and unanimity of purpose. The chairman of the committee representing the American Medical Association is Dr. W. W. Keen, Philadelphia, and Dr. Daniel C. Gilman, Baltimore, is chairman of the committee representing the American Association for the Advancement of Science. It is to be hoped that the various committees will be heartily supported by those whom they represent, and that in the immediate future a memorial worthy of the man and his work will be dedicated to Major Reed.

Resource

American Society of Tropical Medicine and Hygiene
8000 Westpark Dr, Ste 130, McLean, VA 22102
703 790-1745

Tuberous Sclerosis

National Tuberous Sclerosis Association
8181 Professional Pl, Ste 110, Landover, MD 20785
800 225-6872   301 459-9888   Fax 301 459-0394
E-mail: ntsa@capcon.net

Twins

Center for Study of Multiple Birth
333 E Superior St, Ste 464, Chicago, IL 60611
312 266-9093

National Organization of Mothers of Twins Club
PO Box 23188, Albuquerque, NM 87192-1188
505 275-0955

Twinline
2131 University Ave, Ste 234, Berkeley, CA 94704
415 644-0861

Ultrasound

Ultrasound is a painless and safe imaging procedure that uses sound waves to create a picture on a video screen. Doctors use ultrasound during pregnancy to help determine the age of the fetus, its rate of growth, and its position in the uterus. They can also tell if there is more than one fetus or any visible birth defect, such as a missing limb. Ultrasound shows the position of the placenta and the amount of amniotic fluid. Most pregnant women in the United States have an ultrasound examination at least once during their pregnancy. During the last months of a pregnancy, it is sometimes possible to determine the sex of the fetus. However, ultrasound is not a precise method of determining the sex of a fetus and is never recommended for this reason alone.

Although ultrasound can identify a variety of fetal abnormalities, including structural defects such as missing limbs, it cannot detect minor structural abnormalities such as an extra finger or toe; genetic disorders such as cystic fibrosis, sickle cell anemia, or Tay-Sachs disease; or chromosome abnormalities such as Down syndrome. (WHG-1996)

Ultrasonography task force, Council on Scientific Affairs reports

The following are citations with abstracts of articles written by a special AMA task force.

The Future of ultrasonography. Report of the Ultrasonography Task Force, Council on Scientific Affairs, American Medical Association. *JAMA* 1991 Jul 17; 266(3): 406-409
Abstract: Future advances in ultrasonography will undoubtedly occur in three major areas: diagnostic capability, instrumentation, and clinical applications. In the area of diagnostic capability, spatial and contrast resolution offer excellent opportunities for improvement. Continued research into tissue characterization is worthwhile, even though efforts to date have been more frustrating than fulfilling. Blood flow studies and new contrast agents are among the more promising areas for future development. New techniques of signal detection, analysis, and display in Doppler imaging may overcome some present limitations, including those in color flow imaging.

Gynecologic sonography. Report of the Ultrasonography Task Force, Council on Scientific Affairs, American Medical Association. *JAMA* 1991 Jun 5; 265(21): 2851-2855
Abstract: Sonography, because it is nonionizing, is the preferred imaging modality for the female pelvis. Traditionally, transabdominal, transcystic studies were performed. However, development of transvaginal and transrectal transducers has led to enhanced imaging capabilities of the pelvis. These new technologies will likely improve our ability to understand gynecologic pathology. The clinical use of pelvic ultrasonography depends on a thorough understanding of normal anatomy and cyclical changes and on the relative limitations of the imaging modality in specifically characterizing pathologic processes. This article reviews the accepted role of pelvic sonography in gynecologic disease and provides a preview of some of the potential applications of recent advances in sonographic technology.

Doppler sonographic imaging of the vascular system. Report of the Ultrasonography Task Force, Council on Scientific Affairs, American Medical Association. *JAMA* 1991 May 8; 265(18): 2382-2387
Abstract: Ultrasonic vascular imaging has been used for more than 20 years to define vascular anatomy, pathologic changes in vessel size, and perivascular abnormalities. In the last decade, development of duplex Doppler technology has permitted the evaluation of both anatomic vascular features and physiologic blood flow parameters in a variety of locations. Doppler "color flow" imaging promises to expand these applications. In many instances, duplex Doppler technology has replaced more invasive angiographic procedures for evaluation of suspected vascular abnormalities. Improved ultrasound duplex technology, combined with the relatively inexpensive, rapid, noninvasive aspects of ultrasonography, has made it a valuable screening examination for suspected flow abnormalities.

Ultrasonic imaging of the abdomen. Report of the Ultrasonography task force, Council on Scientific Affairs, American Medical Association. *JAMA* 1991 Apr 3; 265(13): 1726-1731
Abstract: As new imaging modalities emerge and existing technologies improve, indications for a particular imaging method may change. This article examines current indications for abdominal and prostatic ultrasound examination and, where possible, compares ultrasound with other imaging techniques. This is not an attempt to list all possible ultrasound indications or examinations, but rather an attempt to serve as an aid to informed imaging selection based on current literature and equipment.

Medical diagnostic ultrasound instrumentation and clinical interpretation. Report of the Ultrasonography Task Force, Council on Scientific Affairs. *JAMA* 1991 Mar 6; 265(9): 1155-1159
Abstract: Over the past 20 years, there has been a dramatic increase in the use of ultrasonography as an imaging modality. The introduction of real-time ultrasonography and Doppler units for the measurement of blood flow in the 1970s, recent advances in transducer design, signal processing, and miniaturization of electronics,

along with the lack of radiation exposure, have been primarily responsible for the increased use of ultrasound. However, although ultrasonography can provide diagnostic information safely and easily, interpretation of the information requires an understanding of the physics behind ultrasound, how that physics is translated into ultrasound instrumentation, recognition of artifacts that are associated with the various types of ultrasonography, and identification of the artifacts in specific anatomic locations.

Resource

American Institute of Ultrasound in Medicine
14750 Sweetzer Ln, Ste 100
Laurel, MD 20707-5906
800 638-5352   301 498-4100   Fax 301 498-4450

Undersea Medicine

Undersea and Hyperbaric Medical Society, Inc
10531 Metropolitan Ave, Kensington, MD 20895
301 942-2980   Fax 301 942-7804
E-mail: uhms@radix.net

Board Certification:
American Board of Preventive Medicine
9950 W Lawrence Ave, Ste 106, Schiller Park, IL 60176
847 671-1750   Fax 847 671-1751

University Health Centers

Association of Academic Health Centers
1400 16th Street NW, Ste 720, Washington, DC 20036
202 265-9600   Fax 202 265-7514
E-mail: ahc@acadhlthctrf.org

American College Health Association
PO Box 28937, Baltimore, MD 21240-8937
410 859-1500   Fax 410 859-1510

Urinary Incontinence

Help for Incontinent People, Inc (HIP)
PO Box 544, Union, SC 29379
800 BLA-DDER   803 579-7900   Fax 803 579-7902

Simon Foundation for Continence
PO Box 815, Wilmette, IL 60091
800 23-SIMON 847 864-3913   Fax 847 864-9758

Urology

Urologist. Diagnoses and treats diseases and disorders of genitourinary organs and tract. Examines patient, using X-ray machine, fluoroscope, and other equipment to aid in determining nature and extent of disorder or injury. Treats patient, using diathermy machine, catheter, cystoscope, radium emanation tube, and similar equipment. Performs surgery, as indicated. Prescribes and administers urinary antiseptics to combat infection. (DOT-1991)

Resources

American Association of Clinical Urologists, Inc
c/o Encyclopedia of Associations
1120 N Charles St, Baltimore, MD 21201
301 539-7168

American Board of Urology
31700 Telegraph Rd, Ste 150, Birmingham, MI 48025
810 646-9720

American Urological Association
1120 N Charles St, Baltimore, MD 21201
410 727-1100   Fax 410 625-2390

Utilization Review

AMA Policy

Confidentiality and Utilization Review (H-320.986)
Res 64, A-87

(1) The AMA believes that: (*a*) in order to protect patient care and confidentiality, physicians should use judicious restraint when discussing any patient's care over the telephone; and (*b*) physicians who receive patient permission for a case discussion by telephone from their patients on behalf of third-party payors may, ethically and in their own best judgment, make a determination as to whether a reasonable charge for their time and expertise in providing such telephone case review discussions should be made, and that third-party payers that demand such case reviews by telephone be encouraged to consider payment to physicians for their reasonable charges, if any, for these medical services. (2) The AMA objects to any utilization review performed solely upon the basis of an admitting diagnosis, without actual hospital record review, as being inadequate, incomplete, and incapable of accuracy.

Utilization review (UR) refers to the process of evaluating whether health care services are medically necessary from the payer's perspective. UR determinations finding health care services to be "medically unnecessary" when a physician believes the services to be "medically indicated" typically trigger the need for an appeal of the determination.

Health plans should have adequate appeals processes in place. The process should allow physicians to meet their ethical and legal obligations to advocate on behalf of their patients for care that is medically indicated and appropriate.

The AMA recommends that the physician document all steps in a UR appeals process.

Reference

Medicolegal Forms With Legal Analysis. Chicago, Ill: American Medical Association; 1991. 199 pp.
ISBN 0-89970-402-6   OP630290
800 621-8335

Resources

American College of Medical Quality
PO Box 34493, Bethesda, MD 20827-0493
301 365-3570   Fax 301 365-3202
E-mail: acmq@aol.com

American Health Quality Association
1140 Connecticut Ave NW, Ste 1050
Washington, DC 20036
202 331-5790 Fax 202 331-9334
E-mail: ahqa@ahqa.org

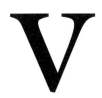

Valuation of a Medical Practice

In order to optimize the value of a practice that may be put up for sale in the managed care environment, an understanding of the implications of managed care to each of the provider groups is required to address the question of valuation sufficiently.

Practice acquisitions—primary care practices
In managed care, primary care physicians (eg, family practice, internal medicine, pediatrics, and often obstetrics and gynecology) are case managers and, therefore, the patient's first point of access to health care services. Serving in the role of coordinators of care (or "gatekeepers"), primary care physicians are experiencing increased responsibility and significance in the industry.

Capitated plans place physicians at greater risk than traditional fee-for-service structures. Success or failure depends on the flow of patients through the system and referral decisions. Losses result from overutilization of provider services since fixed fees are not increases to cover additional services. Multispecialty groups and integrated delivery systems are increasingly dependent on primary care practitioners to efficiently direct patient flow through the system.

These factors contribute to why primary care physicians' practices are those most often acquired. Intangible assets of physicians play a pivotal role in the purchase price, particularly when considering the managed care gatekeeper function.

The influence of managed care must be considered as the primary care practice is valued by the independent appraiser. In calculating the value of the intangible assets, the valuator must weigh the following characteristics and issues, particularly postacquisition, and what contribution this practice will make to the integrated delivery system and to the managed care environment in the area.
- Operating reputation of the practice and number of years in practice in the service area.
- Local health care scenes of managed care (ie, shifts from traditional payers to managed care and HMO penetration).
- Historical growth trends of the practice, including profit margins.
- Overall economic condition of the primary service area.
- Practice's historical experience of providing service in a managed care environment.
- Presence of several significant health care providers and/or payer (eg, competing hospitals, insurance companies, and HMOs).
- General demographics of the practice (ie, heavily populated urban and suburban vs rural areas).

Primary acquisitions—specialty care practices
Primary care and the role of the primary care physician as a case manager pose specific issues for specialists. Most internal medicine specialists serve in multiple roles: personal physicians to local patients; consultants to other physicians; and comanaging patient care along with colleagues from other specialties or subspecialties. Many MCOs, however, are inclined to force internists into a more limited role. Specialists in internal medicine are often given the opportunity to function as primary care physicians and coordinators of care, and internists who have subspecialized are being limited to the role of consultant. Managed care accomplishes this through the contracting process, which may specifically limit internists to one role or the other by the way they are listed in plan booklets provided to patients and in the referral mechanisms used to limit and control referrals from primary care physicians to consulting specialists.

Historically, specialists have been less pressured to control costs. Higher fees were tolerated due to medical need and expected as compensation for extending training. Compared with other providers, specialists have commanded a disproportionately higher portion of total health care spending. As cost containment pressures have mounted, managed care has placed emphasis on the primary care physician to regulate the use of specialists. Gatekeeper primary care physicians directly coordinate and authorize specialist (consultant) referrals, diagnostic testing not provided in the primary care physician's office, and other ancillary services.

These limitations have caused controversy and difficulty for specialists. Some subspecialists in internal medicine, particularly those with subspecialties involving intense use of medical technology, are uncomfortable serving as primary care physicians and prefer to remain as consultants. However, as managed care systems limit referrals for this type of care, subspecialists may find an economic inducement to broaden their practice to include the primary care role. Other specialists in internal medicine without subspecialty training or practice may want to provide subspecialty services for which they are qualified to broaden the range of care that they can make available under a given managed care arrangement. This will increase the range of services they provide and increase earning from those services.

Because of managed care, specialists face a future of reduced fee-for-service arrangements, discounted pricing, and dependence upon primary care practitioners for referral revenues. Specialists are concerned, and understandably so, when one considers that such a significant portion of their economic livelihood is beyond their control.

Certain considerations for intangible assets must be made for valuation of both primary care and specialty practices. In addition, the following contribute significant value to the intangible assets of specialty practices:
- The reputation and prominence of the medical specialist.
- The size of the medical specialty and its correlated market share within the service area.
- The supply of medical providers in that specialty in the area vs the demands for services.

Summary
Briefly, we have explained the impact of managed care on both primary care and specialty practices and the value of the practices. The increased emphasis on primary care physicians justifies a rise in the values of these practices (under certain market conditions). The valuator of a primary care practice must consider these issues in compiling the information and calculating the value of the practice. For example, if it can be estimated that through current involvement and prospective growth in managed care its profitability will increase, a reflection of this in the valuation calculations will increase the practice's value.

Specialty practices are generally expected to experience a decline in value as managed care saturates health care. The ensuing fees and limited access to patients will drive down their margins, reducing the valuation amount.

Market dynamics in the geographic service area could justify premiums as significant intangible asset value. The relevance and appropriateness of any level of intangible asset value in a practice transfer may only be proved through extensive analysis and understanding of the operations of the practice, area market conditions, and competition.

The knowledge and experience of qualified and independent professional valuators are essential to ensure accuracy in the valuation, particularly relating to managed care and integrated delivery networks. (AVMP-1996)

Growing the value of your practice

Howard Larkin
AM News June 27, 1994 pp 29-32

As the medical market continues its unprecedented shift toward managed care and integrated delivery networks, chances are your practice situation is going to change—if it hasn't already.

It could be a purchase offer from a hospital or specialized company set up to manage practices. It could be a merger offer from an established group practice, or from several colleagues interested in starting a group.

You might want to borrow against your practice to finance a physician contracting organization. Or you might simply want to sell your practice and retire.

How you fare in any of these transactions depends in large part on the value of your practice. The more your practice is worth, the more you're likely to get—and the more leverage you will have in negotiating with financially stronger players, such as hospitals and large groups.

But what makes a practice valuable?
In abstract terms, a practice's value is largely determined by how much economic benefit it is likely to produce in the future. What that means in concrete terms varies with the circumstances.

Traditionally, a practice with an established base of mostly fee-for-service patients was considered valuable because its loyal following could be counted on to continue generating cash.

Today, however, that same practice might be considerably less valuable if it's in an area moving quickly to managed care, because it risks losing patients to practices that have already signed contracts.

Likewise, what can be done to enhance a practice's value depends on circumstances. Where the practice above in a traditional setting might benefit most from improving efficiency of office procedures, in a managed care environment the practice might gain more from signing favorable contracts and training staff to administer them.

And keep in mind that economic benefit isn't confined to practice revenue. It also includes things like referral streams, which is a big reason hospitals and multispecialty groups are buying primary care practices.

A qualified practice appraiser can help you identify exactly how to increase the value of your practice in your unique circumstances. But in general, anything that increases either the volume or the security of future revenue increases your practice's value.

Value enhancers range from something as simple as remodeling your reception area to setting up a group practice or physician contracting organization. Below are a few ideas on adding value to your practice.

Build your patient base
While managed care contracts increasingly determine where patients see physicians, a primary care doctor's patient base and a specialist's referral base are still the most valuable assets most practices have, says Robert Cimasi, president of St. Louis-based Health Capital Consultants Inc. Cimasi routinely values practices for sales, mergers, divorces and estate planning.

Enhancing your patient base can be a fairly simple task, Cimasi says. For primary care practices, he recommends programs that "enhance the patient's experience of the physician as gatekeeper to the medical system," so they will think of you first when they have a medical problem. These enhancements might include call-back programs, reminding patients they are due for a follow-up or checkup, wellness programs or patient information booklets.

Another way to build patient loyalty is to sit down with staff and identify the 10 things that irritate patients most, and five things that can alleviate those problems. You may need to help staff keep you on schedule, to add phone lines or weekend hours. "Everything you do to grow and enhance the patient base will add value," Cimasi says.

For specialists, meeting other doctors in the patient lounge or taking them out to dinner can help strengthen your referral base, Cimasi says. "But what really helps is getting a reputation for sending patients back for treatment when it's appropriate and keeping the referring doctor informed."

One thing to avoid is "anything that looks like a wind-down," Cimasi says. If you cut hours or stop seeing new patients, people will go elsewhere and the value of your practice will drop.

Get into managed care

The name of the game in practice valuation is patient flow, and managed care increasingly controls it. So playing the managed care game well can add significant value to your practice, says James Unland, president of the Chicago-based Health Capital Group.

When valuing a practice, "we look for physicians with a philosophical receptivity to managed care," says Unland, who has written two books on the subject for the AMA. He believes physicians who are "proactive" on managed care have a better chance of surviving market shakeouts than those who resist it.

Physicians with managed care contracts and those involved in contracting alliances have a value edge. Those delivering care under capitated arrangements or preparing to do so also have an edge. Practices that implement efficiency procedures, quality pathways and self-regulation through credentialing and peer review have a long-term advantage, as insurers seek to contract with groups that can handle quality matters on their own, Unland says.

But managed care is a two-edged sword, Cimasi warns. A practice that holds unprofitable contracts loses value. And a high proportion of patient volume from closed-panel HMOs can be an impediment to selling, or to bringing on a new physician who must be credentialed. Plans that never pay withholds are also problematic.

"You should only sign up for plans that provide sufficient volume and yield to make it worth your while," Cimasi says.

Join a physician organization

Unaligned physicians will have a difficult time as managed care grows, Unland believes. Therefore, those who join groups or contracting organizations add value by increasing the likelihood that their practices will continue to produce income. "We spend a lot of time getting physicians together," he says.

Modernize information systems

Capitated contracts and quality assurance associated with managed care plans require a different kind of computer system, Unland says. Where office systems traditionally focused on billing and collections, they will increasingly be used for data interchange with other providers and to track utilization and quality data.

Hire help

It can help to hire a physician assistant, nurse practitioner or even an associate physician, Cimasi says. That's because patients become loyal not only to their physician, but to whoever they receive care from.

By the same token, if you bring on the physician you are selling your practice to a year or so before you retire, your patients will have an opportunity to bond with your replacement. That adds value to your practice.

Patients also develop relationships with office staff. If your staff is stable and well trained, your patients are likely to be more loyal.

Change the practice name

Another fairly simple way to add value to your practice is to give it a name, which helps establish the practice's identity independent of your own. "If it's 'Community Primary Care' or 'Westside Family Practice' instead of 'Dr. Smith and Dr. Jones,' there is continuity when you leave," Cimasi says. This strategy works best when there is more than one physician in the practice.

Maintain and document equipment

While equipment and other hard assets generally make up only a small proportion of a practice's value, they are part of the valuation equation. If they haven't been maintained—or even if they have, but no records have been kept—they can become a significant liability.

Cimasi recommends keeping receipts for the purchase of all equipment so that the next owner can claim any depreciation still due. Maintenance records also will help establish the value of equipment, which may be assumed to be zero without records.

Clean up patient charts

Because a new physician won't know your patients, he or she will be even more dependent on your patient records than you are. Orderly and up-to-date records will be a big plus.

Maintaining patient records is also important because prospective buyers will look at them to establish how large and how loyal your patient base is. If the records aren't there, the assumption will be that the patients aren't either.

Clean up financial records

Practice-buyers are going to be looking for revenue, so they're going to be looking at your finances. Generally, a 5-year track record of profitability and low outstanding receivables are best. While it may not be feasible to establish that kind of track record now, it's better to start now than never do it at all.

Clean up the office

While it may seem like a little thing, the condition of your reception area and office furniture can make a big difference in patient loyalty. Nobody likes to sit in a dingy room on old furniture.

Simply painting, and replacing or covering old furniture, can add value by making patients feel comfortable. It also can help improve the first impression you make on a buyer.

Valuation checklist

- ☐ Copy of the physician's curriculum vitae.
- ☐ Copy of the office lease.
- ☐ Last 3 years of the practice's balance sheets and income statements.
- ☐ Federal and state income tax returns for the same period.
- ☐ Copies of insurance policies purchased through the practice and their cancellation value as of the valuation date.
- ☐ The accounts receivable in terms of age as of the valuation date.
- ☐ Retirement plan information.

- ☐ Enforceable agreements regarding assets or stock purchases.

- ☐ Copies of contractual obligations such as loan agreements, contracts with suppliers, buy-sell agreements, agreements concerning office sharing, partnership, employment, restrictive covenants.

- ☐ List of equipment and instruments, appraised by a supply house, with a letter confirming the value. If not available, list the approximate purchase price and age of equipment and/or instruments. If the practice leases any equipment, obtain a copy of the lease(s).

- ☐ Information on vehicles leased through the practice.

- ☐ Name, title, salary/wage information, and employment status/date hired on each employee working in the practice.

- ☐ A current fee schedule.

- ☐ Patient demographics schedule with patient age, payor, and zip code.

- ☐ A random sample of 50 medical records, if not computerized.

- ☐ List of payers including contracted and third-party indemnity.

- ☐ Patient charges for each year for the last 3 years (ie, 1993-94-95) and year-to-date charges for 1996.

- ☐ Adjustments to charges (contractual write-off) for the last 3 years (ie, 1993-94-95) and year-to-date charges for 1996.

- ☐ Payment (including insurance and patient payment) for the last 3 years (ie, 1993-94-95) and year-to-date charges for 1996.

- ☐ If available, the number of patient visits for the last 3 years (1993-94-95), year-to-date visits for 1995, and/or the number of new patients for these same periods. (AVMP-1996)

References

Assessing the Value of the Medical Practice: The Physician's Handbook for Measuring and Maximizing Practice Value. Chicago, Ill: American Medical Association; 1996. 100 pp.
ISBN 0-89970-787-4 OP315196

A Valuation Guide for Medical Practice: Mergers and Acquisitions. Issue 5 from *Doctors Resource Service.* Chicago, Ill: American Medical Association; 1994. 41 pp.
ISBN 0-89970-630-4 OP636194

Vascular Surgery

Society for Vascular Surgery
13 Elm St, PO Box 1565, Manchester, MA 01944-1314
508 526-8330   Fax 508 526-4018

Board Certification:
American Board of Surgery
1617 John F. Kennedy Blvd, Ste 860
Philadelphia, PA 19103
215 568-4000   Fax 215 563-5718

Veterans Benefits Administration

Veterans Benefits Administration
Department of Veterans Affairs
810 Vermont Ave NW, Washington, DC 20420
202 273-4900
Hotline for fraud, waste, and abuse:
800 488-8244

Veterinary Medicine

Veterinarian. Diagnoses and treats diseases and injuries of pets, such as dogs and cats, and farm animals, such as cattle or sheep. Examines animal to determine nature of disease or injury and treats animal surgically or medically. Tests dairy herds, horses, sheep, and other animals for diseases and inoculates animals against rabies, brucellosis, and other disorders. Advises animal owners about sanitary measures, feeding, and general care to promote health of animals. May engage in research, teaching, or production of commercial products. May specialize in prevention and control of communicable animal diseases and be designated veterinarian, public health. May specialize in diagnosis and treatment of animal diseases, using roentgen rays and radioactive substances, and be designated veterinary radiologist. (DOT-1991)

Resource

American Veterinary Medical Association
1931 N Meacham Rd, Ste 100
Schaumburg, IL 60173-4360
800 248-2862   847 925-8070   Fax 847 925-1329

Video Clinics

Network for Continuing Medical Education (NCME)
1 Harmon Plaza, 7th Fl, Secaucus, NJ 07094
800 223-0272   201 867-7600   Fax 201 867-2491

Violence

Violence

George D. Lundberg, MD, Roxanne K. Young, Annette Flanagin, RN, MA, and C. Everett Koop, MD

Murder. Arson. Drive-by-shooting. Rioting. Rape. Mugging. Stabbing. Wilding. Suicide. Assault. Incest. Spouse, partner, child, elder abuse.

A picture of American society is emerging, and it is at once both horrifying and numbing. So much so that we have been unable to stop it. We have become a society at war with itself, a nation at the mercy of a savage beast— violence.

Many of us have long recognized violence as a devastating social and public health problem. But even more of us have allowed ignorance, fear, powerlessness, and other problems that divert our attention to keep us from doing anything to resolve the problem. Certainly if violence were caused by a virus, we would have found a treatment and prevention long ago.

In an attempt to increase public and professional attention to violence, the editors of *JAMA, American Medical News,* and the American Medical Association's nine specialty journals published numerous articles on violence between January and June 1992. The best of these articles, which are collected in this compendium, include epidemiologic studies, clinical research, government reports, case descriptions, and commentaries on a wide range of violence, from firearm homicide to abuse of children and pregnant women.

For this compendium, we define violence as any human action resulting in injury or abuse, generally of the interpersonal variety, rather than that resulting from war or natural disasters. A pervasive, deceptive force, such violence destroys the basic, human foundation of our society and is best characterized with numbers:

• Homicide is the third leading cause of death among 15- to 24-year-olds and the leading cause of death among 15- to 24-year-old black males. The homicide rates for children and adolescents have more than doubled in the last 30 years.

• More than 1.5 million individuals in our country are victims of assault each year, and more than 650,000 women are victims of rape.

• 1.8 million women are beaten by their male partners each year, and 8% to 11% of pregnant women report being physically assaulted during pregnancy.

• Two to four million of our children were abused or neglected in 1991, and more than one million elderly were mistreated last year.

These statistics, although alarming, are probably underestimations. There is no denying that violence in America is a public health emergency—demanding immediate attention and corrective action.

These data paint a grotesque picture of a society steeped in violence, with such ubiquity and prevalence as to be seemingly accepted as inevitable. The authors and editors of this compendium do not accept this situation as inevitable. No civilized society should be so permeated by firearm assault, homicide, rape, and child abuse. The situation is unacceptable. Prior solutions have not succeeded. New approaches are required.

We must demand unprecedented support for additional research into the causes, prevention, and treatments, for both victims and perpetrators, of all forms of violence. We need to recognize and treat violence as more than just a social aberrancy—it is a social disease. We need to educate everyone—physicians, nurses, other health professionals, students, politicians, and the public at large—about what is now known and what can now be done to address this emergency. (VIO-1992)

JAMA Theme Issue: Violence

JAMA 1997 May 7; 277(17)

JAMA's recent issue focusing on violence in the United States (see also *JAMA* 1995 June 14; 273[22] and *JAMA* 1992 June 10; 267[22]) presents articles and editorials on screening for partner violence, clinical characteristics of women with a history of childhood abuse, and a commentary of the public health implications of a reduction in firearm advertisements.

Violence, Family

AMA Policy

Interpersonal and Family Violence: (H-515.976) CSA Rep B, A-93

Implications for the practitioner
The AMA encourages physicians to:

(1) Routinely inquire about the family violence histories of their patients, as this knowledge is essential for effective diagnosis and care; (2) Make appropriate referrals to address intervention and safety needs as a matter of course upon identifying patients currently experiencing abuse or threats from intimates; (3) Screen patients for psychiatric sequelae of violence and make appropriate referrals for these conditions upon identifying a history of family or other interpersonal violence; and (4) Become aware of local resources and referral sources that have expertise in dealing with trauma from victimization.

Violence Toward Men: Fact or Fiction? (H-515.972) CSA Rep 9 - I-94

The AMA: (1) recognizes that men also are among the victims of intimate violence, and encourages other organizations to recognize this fact. Information collected and presented on male victims of intimate violence should include data on the rate of victimization compared with women, information on the rate of injury-producing violence, the sequence of violence, and the context of the violence. This type of information should be included in AMA-sponsored publications, training programs, and curricula.

(2) will develop a protocol for physicians to use to identify men who are victimized in intimate relationships. Such a protocol should aim at distinguishing those men who are victims of physical violence and who have not physically or emotionally assaulted their partners from men who are hit and assaulted in self-defense. Moreover, the AMA believes physicians should be alert to men presenting with injuries suffered as a result of intimate violence because these men may require intervention as either victims or abusers themselves.

(3) urges hospitals, community mental health agencies, and other helping professions to develop appropriate interventions for all victims of intimate violence. Such interventions might include individual and group counseling efforts, support groups and shelters.

(4) believes it is critically important that programs be available for victims and perpetrators of intimate violence, and that these programs include training on non-violent methods to control anger and respond to threats of physical or emotional violence.

AMA Press Release

AMA report card on violence

June 1996

Family violence
Subject includes: Spousal/partner abuse; child physical/ sexual abuse; elder abuse; suicide

Grade: C

Summary of status: The grade for family violence is up from a C- last year, primarily because of a dramatic increase in public awareness and education on the issue of domestic violence over the past year. In addition, initiatives such as the Violent Crime Control and Law Enforcement Act of 1994, the largest crime bill in US history, have impacted specifically domestic violence by encouraging and funding prevention measures. This law also protects women by calling for:

- Establishment of a national, 24-hour, toll-free, bilingual hotline (800-799-SAFE) to provide immediate information and assistance to victims and care providers.
- Prohibition of firearm possession by, and sales to, persons subject to family violence restraining orders.
- Establishment of the Violence Against Women grant program to support police/prosecutor efforts, strengthen enforcement, and provide victim services. Twenty-six million dollars were made available to states in 1995, $774 million in formula grants, and over $200 million for related competitive grants for 1996–2000.
- Provision of $325 million to the Department of Health and Human Services for battered women's shelters and other prevention activities.
- Bans on juvenile possession of handguns and ammunition or transfer of arms to juveniles by adults, except under certain limited circumstances. Aimed at decreasing likelihood such guns may be used in family altercations or suicide attempts.
- Encouragement of a pro-arrest policy in domestic violence cases when police are contacted.
- Special assistance for rural efforts in domestic violence and child abuse.
- Federal prosecution of domestic violence when state lines are crossed by a perpetrator.

Corporations are also becoming more aware of family violence. More than a dozen companies, including Polaroid, Liz Claiborne, and Marshall's, have created the Workplace Resource Center to help deal with the estimated 60,000 annual incidents of on-the-job violence related to partner abuse. The center is helping companies develop and implement policies and benefits for employees who may be victims of partner violence. This includes such things as human resource employee assistance program staff training, specialized counseling and referral services, nondiscriminatory health coverage, enforcement at work of protection orders, security from stalkers, and employee relocation, in some circumstances.

However, actual incidence rates of domestic violence, child abuse, elder abuse, and suicide are not declining.

According to the National Committee to Prevent Child Abuse, more than 3.1 million cases of child maltreatment were reported in 1995. At least 1215 children died last year as a direct result of child abuse and neglect. Since 1985 the rate of child fatalities has increased by 39%. Most often these children suffer at the hands of the people who are supposed to love them the most—their protectors and families. Sadly, these young victims are more likely to be involved in violent criminal activity in the future than their nonabused peers.

Elder abuse remains deeply shrouded by the secrecy surrounding family violence. Estimates range from 1 to 2 million cases per year, but it is believed that as few as one in every 14 victimizations is reported to a public agency. Although widely acknowledged by experts as a problem, elder abuse continues to receive little attention. Reports indicate that despite the fact that 40% of reported abuse involves elders, states spend less than $3 per elder for protective services. With the elderly segment of the population rapidly increasing, it is expected that there will be a steady increase in the number of elder abuse cases.

According to 1993 (most recently released) incidence statistics from the Centers for Disease Control and Prevention (CDC), the overall suicide rate in the United States shows no appreciable change. However, there has been an increase in suicides among the elderly. The youth suicide rate is stable but remains high.

Research continues to document staggering direct and indirect costs attributable to family violence. The National Institute of Justice released a recent report measuring for the first time the actual cost of child abuse and domestic violence. The report, "Victim Costs and Consequences: A New Look," is unusually comprehensive in that it addresses not only direct costs of crime (medical, legal, lost wages, etc.) but also estimates such things as the effect on a victim's pain, suffering, and quality of life. Overall crime costs $450 billion per year, with child abuse and domestic violence accounting for one third of those total costs. The figures do not include costs of prisons, jails, parole, and probation systems, nor does it consider certain future costs as victims later become perpetrators.

Conclusion

Over the past few decades a network of support services has formed to assist victims of family violence. However, it is clear that much more needs to be done on all fronts, particularly in the area of prevention. In addition, public awareness of and response to elder abuse and suicide remains critically low.

It seems the best solutions to problems of family violence lie in community involvement. The American Medical Association and the American Bar Association have responded to this need by developing a comprehensive "Community Guide" of model grassroots antiviolence programs that exist across the country. In addition, the AMA and ABA have begun conducting a series of regional meetings to teach multidisciplinary teams from each state strategies for building coordinated community responses to problems of violence in their communities.

Efforts like these take many years to bear fruit, so it would be unfair to expect statistical changes equivalent to the changes in attitude and community activity that have begun. The "C" assigned to this category is more indicative of progress in recognition of the problem and admirable effort to rectify it (particularly domestic violence) than it is of actual progress in reducing incidence. As a country, we still have much work to do in this area. We must continue to strive for an A+.

What physicians can do: excerpts from the AMA protocols on handling family violence

AM News Jun 15, 1992 p 7

Child sexual abuse

When interviewing a child, a physician should:
- Sit near the child, not across a desk, and sit at the child's eye level.
- Conduct the interview in private, without the caretaker present.
- Find out who else has questioned the child.
- Use the child's own words and items whenever possible.

Do not
- Suggest answers.
- Leave the child unattended or with unknown persons.
- Offer rewards to the child.

When interviewing caretakers
- Reserve judgment.
- Attempt to be objective.
- Explain further actions that will be required.

Do not
- Attempt to prove abuse.
- Pry into unrelated family matters.
- Give feedback on the caretaker's explanation of how the injury occurred.

Child physical abuse

Certain types of injuries are more commonly associated with abuse; the injuries are not explained by the history, are often located on multiple body sites, and often are in various stages of healing. However, the medical recognition of abuse may be based on a single injury.

Physical findings that may be indicative of physical abuse:
- *Bruises and welts:* forming regular patterns, often resembling the shape of the article used to inflict the injury.
- *Burns:* cigar or cigarette burns, especially on the soles, palms, back, or buttocks.
- *Immersion burns.*
- *Lacerations or abrasions:* rope burns, particularly on wrist, ankles, neck, torso; to palate, mouth, gums, lips, eyes, ears; to external genitalia.

Behavioral findings of abuse include:
- Impaired interpersonal relations.
- Role reversal.
- Excessive household responsibilities, including child care.

Spouse abuse

Once abuse is recognized, a number of interventions are possible, but even if a woman is not ready to leave the relationship or take other action, the physician's recognition of her situation is important. Optimal care also depends on the physician's knowledge of community resources that can provide safety, advocacy, and support.

Thorough medical records are essential for preventing further abuse and may prove crucial in a legal case. Records should include:
- Chief complaint and description of the event, using the patient's own words.
- An opinion on whether the injuries were adequately explained.
- If the police are called, the name of the investigating officer and actions taken.

Photographs are also valuable; the physician should ask the patient for permission to take photographs.
- When possible, take photographs before the treatment is given.
- Use color film, and a color standard.
- Hold up a coin, ruler, or other object to illustrate the size of an injury.
- Include the patient's face at least once.

Diagnosing elder abuse: Guidelines for physicians

AM News Dec 14, 1992 p 2

- When examining an elderly patient, routinely ask questions directly related to abuse or neglect.
- If answers confirm abuse, follow up to learn how and when it occurs and who is responsible.
- Examine the patient thoroughly and document findings, including patient's statements, behavior, and appearance.
- Be aware that abuse may be physical, psychological, financial, or material, or any combination of these.
- When assessing mistreatment, consider the patient's safety, emotional health, and functional status, social and financial resources, and the frequency, severity, and intent of the abuse.
- Be aware that in institutions, elder abuse may be perpetrated by a staff member, another patient, an intruder, or a visitor.
- Note that many states require physicians to report suspected elder abuse and neglect to a designated state agency. Failure to do so can make doctors liable.
- Keep thorough, well-documented medical records and photographs. These provide concrete evidence and may be crucial in any legal case.
- The duty to report suspected abuse supersedes doctor-patient confidentiality issues, say most experts.

Resources

Batterers Anonymous
1850 N Riverside Ave, Ste 220, Rialto, CA 92376
909 355-1100

National Coalition Against Domestic Violence
PO Box 18749, Denver, CO 80218
303 839-1852   Fax 303 831-9251

National Council on Child Abuse and Family Violence
1155 Connecticut Ave NW, Ste 400
Washington, DC 20036
800 222-2000   818 429-6695   Fax 818 914-3636
E-mail: nccafv@compuserve.com

Violence & Traumatic Stress Research Branch
National Institute of Mental Health
Parklawn Bldg, Rm 18-105
5600 Fishers Ln, Rockville, MD 20857
301 443-3728

Contact for a listing of local safe houses and shelters:
800 333-SAFE (800 333-7233)
800 799-SAFE (800-799-7233) bilingual
(Telecommunication Device for the Hearing Impaired)
800 873-6363

Violence, Public

AMA Press Release

AMA report card on violence

June 1996

Public violence

Subject includes: Gang/juvenile violence, gun violence, civil violence, drug violence

Grade: F

Summary of status: Public violence continues to elude our control. The enormous weight of violent crime in every segment of American life has increasingly led to mounting fears and individuals "rearming" in order to protect themselves and their families by violent means. Increasing poverty, illiteracy, drug and alcohol addiction, racial unrest, disrespect for authority, and the dissolution of the American family continue to fuel a society of fear, vigilantism, paranoia, and retribution.

As outlined in our report of June 13, 1995, "daily newspaper headlines scream tragic stories of bombings in our major cities, gang violence, and homicide." We find no significant indices, trends, surveys or other authoritative evidence to suggest any meaningful and measurable improvement.

- In 1994, 39,720 Americans were killed with firearms in homicides, suicides and accidents. Averaged for the year, that is 110 Americans each day. (*Preliminary Monthly Vital Statistics Report,* 1995;43(13):10-23.
- Demographic experts predict that juvenile arrests will more than double by the year 2010, given population growth projections and trends in juvenile arrests over the past decade. (*Juvenile Offenders and Victims: 1996 Update on Violence,* U.S. Department of Justice).
- Over the past decade, arrest rates for homicides committed by 14- to 17-year-olds have more than tripled. With the number of teenagers projected to increase over the next decade, many criminologists expect a continuing surge in crime. (*States Revamping Youth Crime Laws.* May 13, 1996).
- In a nationwide profile of juvenile gun possession and use, 70% of students who said they carried a gun said they did so for protection. (McCarthy, N. *California Bar Journal,* July 1995).
- From 1990 to 1994, the number of bombings in the United States increased 52.5%. (FBI Explosives Unit-Bomb Data Center General Information Bulletin 95-2).

Conclusion

There are many positive signs and several public policy accomplishments that do offer hope for the future. The recently enacted federal antiterrorism law, the Violent Crime Control and Law Enforcement Act of 1994, the Brady Bill, the assault weapons ban, and several other federal laws each offer differing degrees of promise for more control over mounting public violence. However, the overall trends in juvenile, gun, civil, and drug violence continue to rise.

Violence rates in certain areas (homicide for example) did show stabilization and, in some cases, decline. For example, homicide rates in New York City dropped 25% from 1994 to 1995. However, these rates do not necessarily foretell a trend. In 1995, homicide rates in Minne-

apolis rose 56%. And compared to 1965, the national murder rate per capita is almost double (1965: 5.1 per 100,000; 1994: 9.0). Most troubling are the rising rates of juvenile violence and crime, which may indicate rising rates of violence in the coming years.

The country seems to rely, in large part, on an overburdened law enforcement and legal system, overcrowded prisons, and insufficient rehabilitation programs to quell crime and reduce recidivism. The core causes of violence in our streets—lack of education, opportunity, racial harmony, and adequate psychiatric resources, as well as drug abuse, and poverty—remain woefully unaddressed. Further, the total cost to society for public violence is inestimable. The cost in productivity, human suffering, and mortality is without monetary equivalent.

Again, this failing grade (F) reflects widespread societal problems currently beyond the scope of local, state, and federal officials and lack of meaningful intervention programs at all levels. Even with some hopeful signs and slight improvement in some incidence rates, the news is still not sufficient to raise our grade above an "F."

Violence, Virtual

AMA Press Release

AMA report card on violence
June 1996

Virtual violence

Subject includes: gang/juvenile violence, video games and cyberspace violence, music violence

Grade: D+

Summary of status: The grade for virtual violence is up from a D last year because of heightened public awareness and an apparent commitment on the part of government and industry to address the problem. The enactment of legislation has promised the V-Chip and a new television rating system. Rating systems are also being developed for the music and cyberspace industries. Significant new studies of violence on television have increased our understanding of the important role context plays in how violence is perceived and will provide valuable tools for those who wish to produce responsible programming in the future. A number of consumer and industry groups have put together new guidelines to help parents monitor and evaluate their children's entertainment choices.

However, scientific studies have conclusively established that exposure to violence in entertainment media increases aggressive behavior, is associated with lower levels of pro-social behavior, and contributes to Americans' sense that they live in a "mean society." There is no evidence that virtual violence is on the decline—yet. Violence is still rampant in all forms of entertainment media, and consumers are still buying it.

Television violence

When the AMA issued its *Report Card on Violence* in June of last year, it proposed several intervention strategies to help stem the tide of virtual violence, including implementation of a V-Chip to allow parents to block objectionable television programming and development of an industrywide television rating system similar to that used by the motion picture industry. Both measures are part of the new telecommunications law, enacted in February 1996.

For the first time, two important industry studies have analyzed the context in which television violence is presented. The National Television Violence Study found that context and explicitness of portrayals of violence are just as important as the quantity of violence portrayed. The study identifies and surveys such contextual factors as the nature of perpetrators and victims, what consequences are shown, the involvement of humor, and whether or not the violent act is condoned or condemned.

The study also uncovered important information about the effectiveness of rating systems and advisories that should prove helpful in devising a meaningful and effective television rating system. An earlier study by the UCLA Center for Communications Policy also evaluated televised violence in a contextual manner. That study identified continuing problems with the broadcast of films on television and with children's programming where sinister combat violence shows are increasingly dominate.

Serious concerns have also been raised about the consistency and effectiveness of the movie rating system on which the new television rating system will be based. The motion picture industry's ratings are determined by a board of concerned parents, none of whom have training in child development or the effect of mass media on children. The rating system ignores critical child development stages and focuses on how parents feel about a film rather than on how it might affect children. There are problems with consistency of ratings and no evaluation of the context in which violence occurs. Unless these problems are resolved, the television ratings system could prove as ineffective and unreliable as that of the motion picture industry.

Video game and cyberspace violence

The Internet, a global "network of networks," is not governed by any government or private entity. This vacuum leaves no checks or limits on the information maintained by and accessible to users and holds no one accountable when superhighway accidents occur.

Evidence of violence on the Internet is anecdotal, rather than statistical, in part because communication on the Internet is private. Reported cases of abuse are relatively infrequent, but as the technology continues to explode, there is potential for great harm, as well as great good.

All of the online services offer parental control devices which screen online content for certain key words, phrases, or names and then block or restrict access to the content parents identify as objectionable. Other blocking devices allow parents to block entire areas such as chat rooms and electronic bulletin boards, and to monitor their child's access. Parental control devices are also available for users who want to access the Internet directly, instead of going through an online service.

As with all parental control devices, blocking mechanisms are not effective in protecting children unless parents have the knowledge and interest to use them wisely. Unfortunately, the children most at risk on the Internet are the very children whose parents have abdicated

responsibility. No control device exists to protect those children from harm.

Internet violence may be the most troubling of all forms of virtual violence because the Internet provides a global audience. Last year, the Oklahoma bombing suspect obtained a copy of the *Turner Diaries* from the Internet. Whereas before, one would have had to know where to look and been predisposed to search for the book, the Internet made it easily accessible to a broad audience. It is that potential to exponentially increase the public's exposure to violent images and violent thoughts which causes the deepest concern and most eludes quick solutions.

The impact of violent video games upon children is not as clearly established as the impact of violent television programming. Due to their role-modeling capacity to promote real-world violence, there is concern that playing violent video games with their fully digitalized human images will cause children to become more aggressive toward other children and become more tolerant of, and more likely to engage in, real-life violence.

The video game industry recognizes that all games are not appropriate for all age groups and voluntarily rated more than 2000 videos last year. The rating system consists of both age-based classifications and an explanation of the reasons for the rating. The Video Software Dealers Association has implemented a "Pledge to Parents" program to enforce the ratings system adhered to by the Blockbuster video chain, Toys R Us, and Wal-Mart, among others.

Music violence

Public pressure continues to have an impact on the music industry. In 1985, the Parents Music Resource Center succeeded in pressuring the record industry to attach the "Parental Advisory, Explicit Lyrics" warning labels that many companies now voluntarily place on selected records. In 1995, public pressure from advocacy groups played a role in forcing Warner Music Group to sever its 50% stake in Interscope Records, home to Nine Inch Nails and controversial rap artists Snoop Doggy Dogg and Dr. Dre.

However, Time Warner's actions did not stop the flood of "gangsta" rap. Rap artists simply turned to a different distribution network, and when the CDs hit the stores, lyrics that glorified guns, rape, and murder were left intact. Efforts are once again underway to help parents evaluate the content of their children's music. Imposition of a mandatory rating system for music, however, has gained little public or legislative support.

Conclusion

Over the next year the AMA will be tracking to see if the promising new intervention programs noted in this report are successfully implemented by government and industry. New tools like music labels, the V-Chip, and voluntary rating system offer hope of reducing virtual violence. But for now, this violence is still a problem for all of us, and new tools will only be as strong and successful as the public's commitment to using them. The AMA especially encourages American parents to get involved and use these tools diligently to monitor not only their own, but also their children's exposure to virtual violence.

Vitamins

Vitamins and minerals

Vitamins are a must for good health. They help the body turn food into energy and tissues. There are 13 vitamins in all: vitamin A; the vitamin B complex, which includes thiamine, riboflavin, niacin, vitamin B_6, folic acid, vitamin B_{12}, pantothenic acid, and biotin; and vitamins C, D, E, and K.

The table lists the vitamins, what they do for the body, and some good sources.

Minerals are needed for growth and maintenance of body structures. They also help to maintain digestive juices and the fluids found in and around cells. Unlike vitamins,

Vitamins	What They Do	Good Sources
A	Important for healthy skin and development of bones	Liver; green and yellow vegetables; milk
B_1 (thiamine)	Necessary for changing starches and sugars into energy	Meat; whole-grain cereals
B_2 (riboflavin)	Helps the body use food	Milk; cheese; fish; liver; green vegetables
B_3 (niacin)	Helps the body use food to make energy	Meat; yeast; fish; liver; nuts; legumes
B_6 (pantothenic acid, biotin)	Essential for chemical reactions in the body; helps the body make protein	Meat; poultry; fish; most fruits and vegetables; dairy products
B_{12}	Helps the body make red blood cells; helps keep the nervous system healthy	Meat; dairy products; poultry
Folic acid	Helps the body make proteins; works with vitamin B_{12} to help the body make red blood cells; helps fight certain birth defects	Green leafy vegetables; organ meats; nuts
C	Helps maintain ligaments, tendons, and other supportive tissues; may help the body fight infection	Citrus fruits; green peppers; strawberries; broccoli; tomatoes
D	Necessary for the body's use of calcium	Fish-liver oil; fortified milk; eggs; formed when the skin is exposed to sunlight
E	Helps maintain cell membranes; helps protect tissues against substances thought to contribute to degenerative changes in organs	Vegetable oils; whole-grain cereals; dried beans; green leafy vegetables
K	Necessary for proper clotting of the blood	Green leafy vegetables; pork liver; cauliflower; grain products; manufactured by bacteria in the intestine

Minerals	What They Do	Good Sources
Calcium	Helps the body form and maintain bones and teeth; necessary for cardiac function	Dairy products; fish with edible bones; shellfish; green leafy vegetables
Copper	Helps with enzyme activity; helps the body use iron to build hemoglobin, which carries oxygen in the blood	Organ meats; shellfish; legumes
Fluorine	Helps strengthen teeth and bones	Seafood; fluoridated water
Iodine	Helps the body form thyroid hormones, which control the rate of energy release in the body	Seafood; iodized salt
Iron	Important part of hemoglobin; helps the body obtain energy from carbohydrates and fat	Liver; red meat; shellfish; nuts; enriched grain products
Magnesium	Helps the body make bones and teeth; needed for normal enzyme activity	Nuts; whole-grain cereals; dark green vegetables
Phosphorus	Necessary to many chemical reactions in the body	Cheese; peanuts; meat; whole-grain cereals
Potassium	Helps the body regulate its water balance; necessary to nerve and muscle function	Potatoes; bananas; legumes; dried fruits
Selenium	Helps protect against cell and tissue damage; may protect against some cancers	Seafood; meat; whole-grain cereals; dairy products
Sodium	Regulates the body's water balance; essential for nerve and muscle function	Smoked, cured, or pickled meats and fish; cheese; canned soups; table salt; bread
Zinc	Necessary for growth and helps the body make energy; helps heal wounds; maintains healthy skin and eyes	Oysters; meat; whole-grain cereals; legumes

carbohydrates, fats, and proteins, minerals are not made by plants and animals. Plants get minerals from water or soil, and animals get minerals by eating plants or plant-eating animals.

The minerals the body needs in large amounts include calcium, chlorine, magnesium, phosphorus, potassium, sodium, and sulfur. Other minerals, called trace elements, are needed in much smaller amounts. Trace elements include iron, copper, fluorine, iodine, selenium, zinc, chromium, cobalt, manganese, and molybdenum.

The table lists the more important minerals, what they do, and some good food sources.

Vitiligo

National Vitiligo Foundation
Texas American Bank Bldg, PO Box 6337
Tyler, TX 75711
903 531-0074   Fax 903 531-9767
E-mail: 73071.33@compuserve.com
WWW: http://pegasus.uthct.edu/vitiligo/index.html

Volunteerism

Volunteering across borders: healing the children

Karen Cullotta Krause
AM News Aug 12, 1996 p 10

If you have a yen for travel and a yearning to make a difference, consider a volunteer vacation. This program exports the best of US medicine to disadvantaged children in remote regions overseas.

David Hoffman, DDS, traveled to Cochabamba, Bolivia, determined to enjoy a break from the stresses of his private practice.

Dr. Hoffman, 46, led a team of 11 New York–area medical professionals on a medical mission. All were volunteers with the northeast chapter of Healing the Children, a nonprofit organization based in Spokane, Wash., that arranges specialized medical and surgical care for children whose families can't afford the treatment or whose communities don't offer it. With 14 chapters in 21 states, the group has helped tens of thousands of children worldwide since it was founded in 1979. It relies exclusively on volunteers and donations to carry out its work.

Dr. Hoffman has volunteered with Healing the Children for more than a decade. The team of professionals that accompanied him to Bolivia in April—a plastic surgeon, two anesthesiologists, a pediatric resident, three registered nurses, a dental resident, and two medical students—treated 40 children in eight days. Dr. Hoffman performed four surgeries a day.

"You have to make these trips a priority to make them happen," he said. "After more than 20 trips, I'm addicted."

Angeles Glick, executive director of HTC Northeast Inc., said the Connecticut-based chapter that organized the Cochabamba trip provided services worth more than $7.5 million to about 2,308 children in 1995.

The volunteers pay their own air fare. Housing, food, and local transportation are covered by donations or supplied by local hosts.

"Everyone appreciates what we do for these children, but it can be a delicate situation," Dr. Hoffman noted. "We don't just go and do these surgeries and leave. You have to try to be sensitive and work with the local doctors as part of your group."

Max Tardill, MD, a Cochabamba surgeon who worked alongside the team, said the children are "fine ... doing very well with no complications."

The Cochabamba trip was a project of Healing the Children's Medical Missions Abroad program. The group also offers:
• Operation Inbound, which provides specialized medical treatment and assistance to disadvantaged children in US communities.
• The Stateside Program, which enables children from 58 countries to travel to the United States for specialized care.
• The Sponsorship Program, which funds foreign children who have come to the United States for care and require further treatment.
• The Relief Program, which recruits organizations to provide supplies and refurbished equipment to Third World hospitals.

Healing the Children does not track how many physicians volunteer, a spokeswoman said. Among the specialists in demand are pediatricians, pediatric surgeons, orthopedic surgeons, plastic surgeons, neurosurgeons, otolaryngologists, cardiologists, and urologists. For information on volunteering, call 509 327-4281.

Volunteering across borders: healing Gabriela's heart

Karen Cullotta Krause
AM News Aug 19, 1996 p 12

Gabriela Mantilla was cyanotic when she arrived at Presbyterian Hospital in Albuquerque. A chest X ray, ECG, echocardiogram, and cardiac catheterization confirmed that the 2½-year-old Nicaraguan girl suffered from tetralogy of Fallot, a congenital heart defect.

Gabriela's heart was repaired by physicians who volunteer with Healing the Children, a program based in Spokane, Wash., that arranges specialized medical and surgical treatment worldwide for children whose families can't afford the care or whose communities don't offer it.

Healing the Children is one of many initiatives that enable physicians to volunteer their services to benefit disadvantaged patients around the world. Founded in 1979, the nonprofit organization operates:
• The Stateside Program, which brings children from 58 countries to the United States for treatment. About 36,000 children—including Gabriela—have been helped by volunteers in 21 states.
• Medical Missions Abroad, under which physician volunteers travel overseas to provide medical and surgical services.
• Operation Inbound, which provides medical treatment and assistance to children in US communities.
• The Sponsorship Program, which funds foreign children who have come to the United States for care and require further treatment.

• The Relief Program, which recruits organizations to provide supplies and refurbished equipment to Third World hospitals.

A network of volunteers keeps the Stateside Program afloat. Physicians enlist their hospitals to donate space, medical and support staff, and medications. Local families sign on as temporary foster parents. Airlines donate free or reduced-fare tickets. Donations defray the costs incurred.

"Gabriela had a really tough time when she arrived," said Raymond Fripp, MD, a pediatric cardiologist involved in the child's care.

"She was afraid, screaming and crying. When she was ready to go back home to Nicaragua, she had basically changed from a terrified child into a friendly, outgoing kid.

"Without the surgery, she wouldn't have survived beyond adolescence."

Dr. Fripp and his colleagues volunteer six times each year. "It's not an imposition, and there is no money lost," he said. "It's just like seeing any other patient ... we try to fit them in."

Among the specialists needed by Healing the Children, a spokeswoman said, are pediatricians, pediatric surgeons, orthopedic surgeons, plastic surgeons, neurosurgeons, otolaryngologists, cardiologists, and urologists.

For information on volunteering, call 509 327-4281.

Volunteering across borders: a "house call" in the Andes

Karen Cullotta Krause
AM News Aug 26, 1996 p 8

Flying Doctors of America offers US physicians the chance to help the poorest of the poor. This team restored sight to an elderly blind woman.

They carved out medical offices from a schoolhouse in a remote Andes mountain village. They were 18 in all, volunteers with Flying Doctors of America, a 4-year-old group dedicated to sharing the wealth of the US medical system "with those who are only hours away, but have nothing."

In June, a team of internists, pediatricians, pathologists, ophthalmologists, dentists, chiropractors, and nurses visited Huilloc, Peru.

Flying Doctors promotes its trips as adventures that call on volunteers to be "half Mother Teresa, half Indiana Jones." In Peru, the Americans set up tents in the school courtyard. At night, the temperature dipped into the 30s. Sharing their hardscrabble campsite were six Peruvian medical students who acted as translators and assistants.

The patients were indigenous Quechuan Indians, descendants of the Incas, who live in adobe homes with dirt floors and no running water or electricity. Over five days, the volunteers treated 1200 people. Shower curtains divided the departments: pediatrics and ophthalmology, triage and general medicine, dentistry and chiropractic.

Among the medical problems addressed: infections, headaches, back pain, abdominal discomfort, cataracts,

pterygium, tooth decay. Intractable living conditions included contaminated water and exposure to animal feces; poor nutrition was commonplace. The pharmacy ran out of antiparasitic medications because so many patients, young and old, needed them.

There were moving moments. On the way to Huilloc, Rene Tapia, MD, a Decatur, Ga, pathologist, encountered an 84-year-old woman who was blind. An examination revealed cataracts. Once in town, the volunteers sent a bus to fetch the woman, and Andrew Dahl, MD, an ophthalmic surgeon from Poughkeepsie, NY, was able to restore partial vision.

Flying Doctors, a division of Medical Mercy Mission Inc., based in Atlanta, Ga, is a nonprofit, nondenominational organization that sponsors 30 missions each year in the United States and abroad. The program is funded by grants and other monetary and in kind contributions. Volunteers pay a portion of their travel costs.

How to reap the benefits of volunteering

Mary Hegarty
AM News May 4, 1992 p 38

Veteran volunteers follow these guidelines to enrich the experience of working with the homeless:

• Don't be judgmental. "These are the disenfranchised," says David Freedman, MD, a Chicago family physician. "They don't have the wherewithal to go one mile to get help. They are demoralized. But everyone needs health care."

• Find a clinic that takes care of the paperwork. "They should let doctors be doctors," says Pedro Jose Greer, Jr, MD, of Miami.

• Don't burn out. Volunteer consistently, but only as often as is comfortable for you, such as once a month. "One night every month is not something people can't do," says James Wallace, MD, a Bethesda, Md, internist, who volunteers at a shelter-based clinic.

• Don't volunteer on your day off. Take time from your work day, or volunteer in the evening. "Doctors work hard," Dr. Greer says. "We deserve that day off."

JAMA Article of Note: Physician service opportunities abroad

JAMA 1993 Aug 4; 270(5): 567-571

This directory lists organizations that offer US physicians short-term and long-term service opportunities overseas. It is the fourth such directory to be published in *JAMA* since 1984. Organizations that indicated they no longer provide such opportunities have been dropped, and those heard from since 1990, when the last directory appeared, have been added. The most notable changes this time are the first inclusion of fax numbers, and the fact that a few lists of countries needing physicians include areas in Europe formerly in the Soviet sphere of influence.

Listing does not imply endorsement by the American Medical Association.

Resources

Care Medico
660 First Ave, New York, NY 10016
212 686-3110

Doctors to all people
(physicians who help civilians in war areas)
American Foundation
161 Cherry St, New Canaan, CT 06840
203 966-5195

Doctors of the World (Medicines du Monde)
(maintain database of MD volunteers—matches to missions worldwide)
65 Broadway, New York, NY 10012
212 529-1556

Health Volunteers Overseas (HVO)
PO Box 65157, Washington, DC 20035-5157
202 296-0928   Fax 202 296-8018

Medecins Sans Frontieres
(Doctors Without Borders)
8, rue St Sabin, F-75544 Paris Cedex 11, France
1 40212929   Fax 1 48066868   TX 214360F
New York Office
11 E 26th St, Ste 1904
New York, NY 10010
212 679-6800   Fax 212 679-7016

National Council for International Health
1701 K St, Ste 600, Washington, DC 20006
202 833-5900   Fax 202 833-0075
NCIH publishes a Directory of US International Health Organizations that provides information on public and private US-based organizations that are active in international health assistance. In addition, NCIH publishes *Career Network*, which provides information about domestic and overseas international health positions as well as current World Health Organization openings. (A small fee is associated with both of these publications.)

Partnerships for Health Reform
4800 Montgomery Ln, Ste 600
Bethesda, MD 20814
301 913-0500   Fax 301 652-3916
PHR is a 5-year project supported by the US Agency for International Development (USAID) that provides technical assistance, research training, and information dissemination on health sector reform issues in developing countries and transition economies around the world. The project seeks to improve people's health by enabling the health sector to provide and ensure equitable access to sustainable, quality health care services. Working in partnerships with national and local governments, communities, nongovernmental organizations, and donors, PHR technical expertise supports and promotes positive changes in health policies, regulations, financing, and the quality, organization, and management of health services from hospitals to clinics, across urban and rural areas, among public and private sector providers.

Peace Corps
Associate Volunteer Program
Washington, DC 20526
800 424-8580 ext 293

Volunteer Programs, Adolescents

Amigos de las Americas (Friends of the Americas)
(for adolescents interested in the medical field;
program visits Central and South America)
5618 Star Ln, Houston, TX 77057
800 231-7796 (in TX 800 392-4580)
713 782-5290

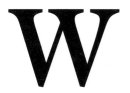

Weight Chart

Height-Weight Tables for Adults:
Metropolitan Life Insurance Co
Health and Safety Education, Dept 16W
1 Madison Ave, New York, NY 10010-3690
212 578-2211   Fax 212 578-7298

Wheelchair Exercise

National Handicapped Sports
451 Hungerford Dr, Ste 100, Rockville, MD 20850
800 966-4NHS   301 217-0960   Fax 301 217-0968

Wheelchair Sports, USA
3595 E Fountain Blvd, Ste L-1
Colorado Springs, CO 80910
719 574-1150   Fax 719 574-9840

Women in Medicine

The lady is a doctor: liberating the AMA

Dick Walt
AM News Mar 17, 1997 p 24

Women physicians' battle for acceptance in the medical profession encountered many obstacles in the AMA's early years.

In 1872, AMA President D. W. Yandall, MD, defended the right of women to practice in some specialties—though not necessarily surgery—but said public demand would be the determinant: "If those [women] now pressing forward in their studies so eagerly find their services are not wanted, they will take down their signs, get married—if they can—or turn lecturers, or to some more lucrative employment. I hope they will never embarrass us by a personal application for seats in this Association."

But despite these attitudinal barriers, Sarah Hackett Stevenson, MD, of Illinois, became the AMA's first woman member in 1876. She also was the first woman to serve on the staff of Chicago's Cook County Hospital.

World War II provided another major impetus for women to join the medical profession, and societal changes of the 1960s and 1970s added to that momentum.

Women now make up more than 20% of the nation's physicians and 40% of medical students—a trend that cuts across all specialty lines. Since 1979, the AMA has been active in efforts to foster the participation of women in all facets of organized medicine, and female membership in the AMA rose 8% from 1993 to 1995.

Today, the AMA Board of Trustees is chaired by Nancy W. Dickey, MD, whose announced candidacy for AMA president-elect would, if successful, make her the Association's first woman president. She is one of four women on the 15-member board.

A Piece of My Mind

Equal not really

Jane Marshall
JAMA 1985 Aug 16; 254(7): 953

How can it be that at the age of 35, being an accomplished, respected physician, a happily married woman for 11 years, and a mother of two beautiful children, I feel melancholy, inadequate, and guilt-ridden? Ever since I can remember, my goals have been similar to those of most men. I have enjoyed competitive, physically demanding sports and achieved multiple varsity letters in high school. Excellence in general academics, and in particular science, was more important to me than even to my brother. The resultant conflicts of being a competitive and feminine woman in our society have been numerous. Nevertheless, I have always managed. In my 20s I was able to ride the early waves of "women's liberation." But now, at 35, the waves have crashed into the shore and eroded the sand.

My 6½-year-old gentle, vulnerable, and sensitive son has developed a "mild-to-moderate stutter." Stutter, stammer, and dysfluency are all different words for basically the same problem. My husband and I were recently called into our son's private school for a conference with his first-grade teacher, speech pathologist, director of the lower school, and assistant headmaster. During our hour together, we were informed that a probable causative factor in this was my working. Not enough mother-child time was the bottom line. It was strongly recommended that I alter my schedule if I felt "it was worth it." Worth it! Of course it was worth it!

Our initial response to this conference was anger. Both my husband and I were negatively impressed with our perception of these educators' lack of sensitivity to the plight of the "working mother" and "working couple." However, after serious review of our pressured and rushed lifestyle, I arranged an extended overdue vacation that corresponded with my son's school vacation. During this more relaxed intimate time together, his speech pattern became significantly more fluent. A partial solution to my child's stutter obviously included a more permanent change in my working schedule to increase our time together.

But what about my career and all the years of social deprivation to afford me more time to study? The years of "investing for my future" would now be set aside for something certainly more "worth it"! Worst of all there was my guilt. Why was I at fault? I have spent more time with my children than many nonworking mothers. My husband and I have almost completely eliminated our social and athletic activities in order to spend our free time with our children. This obviously was not enough for our more vulnerable eldest child!

I will, of course, alter my work load. I will curtail teaching and publishing activities. I have a mind full of ideas that will not be written by me but by others.

Every time I hear my son speak, I feel his pain and frustration. I am filled with sorrow and guilt. I now know I am not equal to my male colleagues. In many ways I am better. However, I may not be allowed to show you or them because first I am a mother and wife and then I am a physician. I suppose I may continue to cry myself to sleep for many years. And when my daughter comes to me for career advice—what should I tell her?

Women in medicine in America

For the second time in the history of the United States, women are thriving in the medical profession. The first time was in the last quarter of the 19th century, soon after Elizabeth Blackwell and her sister, Emily, opened the pioneering Woman's Medical College of the New York Infirmary in 1869 because no other regular medical school in the city would accept women. More than 20 years before, in 1848, Elizabeth Blackwell had been the first American woman to receive a medical degree. Women's medical schools flourished in the latter half of the 1800s—another 16 existed—and it was not unheard of, 100 years ago, for women physicians to combine the dual demands of career and family. A year before Abraham Flexner published his watershed report on medical education in 1910, all but three of these schools had closed.

In the last quarter of this century there has been another renaissance for women entering the medical field. The number of women physicians more than quadrupled between 1970 and 1990, from 25,401 to more than 100,000. Projections suggest that 30% of physicians will be female by the year 2010.

With the publication *Women in Medicine in America,* the American Medical Association's (AMA's) Women in Medical Services is responding to a continuing desire for information about women physicians. It includes both a discussion of the issues facing women in medicine today and more than 60 statistical tables reflecting all parts of a woman's career, from medical school through practice.

In recent years, the American Medical Association has been overwhelmed with requests for the type of information found in *Women in Medicine in America.* This pursuit of information corresponds with both the growing representation of women in medicine and the questions raised when members of a formerly small minority in a profession assume a major place in its ranks.

The earlier era of prosperity for women in medicine may contain some lessons for today. Prevented from entering male medical schools, women founded their own—theirs was, of necessity, a separatist movement. The numbers were encouraging: women represented only 0.8% of the physician population in 1870, but 6% by the turn of the century. The 6% representation was a peak not attained again by women until the second half of this century.

Most female physicians were clustered in New York, Boston, and Philadelphia where the first women's medical schools and hospitals were founded. By 1900, women were more than 18% of Boston's physicians. Two surveys done on graduates of their own medical schools in the late 1800s revealed that women typically worked in private practice as general practitioners or ob/gyns, or in women's institutions. The surveys differ on marital status: One found that 47% of its graduates married, the other discovered that fewer than 20% had done so.

As the century ended, more opportunities for coeducational training unfolded, and women welcomed the attainment of their long-term goal in medical training—integration. In 1894, women made up at least 10% of the study body at 18 medical schools run by men. And when the Woman's Medical College of the New York Infirmary was absorbed by Cornell University Medical School in 1899, Emily Blackwell, one of the Infirmary's founders, said that Cornell's acceptance of women made "a separate medical school for women unnecessary." Seventy women from the women's medical school entered Cornell in 1900. But by 1903 that number had been reduced to 10.

The fall of that women's medical school and the corresponding reduction of places for women echoed elsewhere. In 1910, more than half the medical schools in America did not accept women. The lack of acceptance persisted; in 1946 the dean of a large medical school in the East admitted to limiting the enrollment of women to 6%. Even in the 1960s, women still faced small quotas when trying to enter medical schools. However, despite the quotas and the then small number of women in medicine, women were in the profession to stay. The American Medical Association opened membership to women in 1915.

Perhaps the lessons to be learned from those more difficult times are about parity and the need within the profession for a view that fully integrates, rather than excludes, those whose gender raises uncomfortable issues about training and practice. Women must be allowed to thrive in any institution and in any specialty in which they can make a contribution. Almost two thirds of women physicians are found in five specialties: pediatrics; psychiatry; family practice; internal medicine; and obstetrics/gynecology. It is not that women must become surgeons; rather, that they must be able to comfortably pursue that specialty and secure acceptance if they are to achieve parity in medicine. They must be found at all levels of administration, as heads of medical schools, clinical departments, and medical societies.

The normative patterns of training and work for physicians that now exist are often difficult for women who want to have families and have a career in medicine. Approximately 75% of female physicians are married, and 85% of those married or previously married have children. Again, the point is that all women physicians should have the option to have children and still have tenured positions, be heads of departments, and pursue specialties that require many years of training—just as do male physicians with children.

Medicine has changed women, but women are changing medicine, too. Residency programs can no longer treat a pregnant resident as an oddity; it simply happens too often. And new decisions and opportunities that reflect the needs of today's female and male physicians are being made. Maternity and paternity leave policies, expanding the time track to tenure, reducing the hours that residents are allowed to work, shared positions, child care programs in hospitals—the fact that these exist and are increasing is evidence that women are being better served as physicians. As Nancy Dickey, MD, a member if the Board of Trustees at the AMA, says, "There are still barriers, but there are very few hurdles that can't be leaped by women who are energetic and dedicated." If the extraordinary strides women in medicine have made thus far are indicative of future successes, Dr Dickey will be proven correct. (WIM-1991)

JAMA Article of Note: Promotion of women physicians in academic medicine: glass ceiling or sticky floor?

JAMA 1995 Apr 5; 273(13): 1002-1005

Resources
Advisory Panel on Women Physicians' Issues:
American Medical Association
515 N State St, Chicago, IL 60610-0174
312 464-4392

American Medical Women's Association
801 N Fairfax, Ste 400, Alexandria, VA 22314
703 838-0500   Fax 703 549-3864

Women's Health

Women's health, public welfare

Bernadine Healy, MD
JAMA 1991 Jul 24/31; 266(4): 566-568

While leafing through a pile of the press clippings that regularly cross my desk at the National Institutes of Health (NIH), I was struck particularly by two headlines in the *Philadelphia Inquirer* (May 31, 1991; sec A:1) that said, "Menopause Becoming 'Au Courant' as It Hits Women of Baby Boom" and, on another page, "Menopause Comes of Age as Medical and Social Issue." Indeed, women's health, in general—in terms of research, services, and access to care—has come of age and become a priority medically, socially, and politically.

The article "Gender Disparities in Clinical Decision Making,"[1] the report of the Council on Ethical and Judicial Affairs of the American Medical Association, is to be applauded for its important contribution to answering the question of why women's health research and care demand such particular attention and vigor. The report documents the disparity between genders in regard to access to certain critical diagnostic and therapeutic interventions—specifically, kidney dialysis and transplantation, diagnosis of lung cancer, and catheterization for coronary bypass surgery. And it asks each of us to acknowledge and consider the fact that clinical decision making is based not only on scientific indications, but also on "myriad social, economic, and cultural factors" that may result in gender disparities in the provision of health care. One sentence in the report is the anthem of its message:

"The medical community cannot tolerate any discrepancy in the provision of care that is not based on appropriate biological or medical indications."

This credo has two implications: first, that we possess the knowledge that allows us to undertake scientific evaluation; and second, that we are able to dismiss and invalidate other subtle factors that allow discrimination.

Research alone cannot correct the disparities, inequities, or insensitivities of the health care system, but it makes a critical contribution. Because much of our current knowledge is based, as the report indicates, on research in which the study populations were predominantly men, our responsibility now is to establish the science base that will permit reliable diagnoses, as well as effective treatment and prevention strategies, to provide care to women, based on "appropriate biological or medical indications." The NIH is committed to meeting this challenge directly and to addressing the important recommendations of this report. Indeed, in the NIH's mission to use the methods of science toward the interests of public health and welfare, women's health research must figure prominently.

In September 1990, the NIH established the Office of Research on Women's Health, a major step forward for women's health concerns. Charged with ensuring that research conducted and supported by the NIH appropriately addresses issues regarding women's health, it sees that women participate fully and appropriately in clinical research, including clinical trials.

The new office vigorously responded to the concerns and recommendations of the General Accounting Office report and implemented a strengthened and revitalized NIH policy on the inclusion of women in study populations (published in the *NIH Guide to Grants and Contracts,* August 24, 1990, and February 2, 1991). The seriousness of purpose with which the NIH has addressed this policy is already evident. All NIH staff responsible for review and scientific management of research grants and contracts attended training sessions; NIH peer review groups and all of the institute and center advisory councils received formal briefings on these policies; and the NIH has revised its grant application forms to require information about the composition of study populations in proposed clinical research. The NIH has taken the position that no applications will be funded in which women and minorities are not adequately represented in planned clinical research populations, as appropriate, unless compelling scientific justification is provided.

Although the major portion of research conducted or supported by the NIH benefits both men and women, there are areas of special need for new knowledge that are unique to women. Accordingly, another of the report's recommendation has already been embraced by the NIH: "More medical research on women's health and women's health problems should be pursued." The NIH has embarked on two major efforts that will dramatically affect research regarding women's health.

First, through a series of activities in 1991—including an invited scientific conference and a public hearing to gather the viewpoints of women's health advocates—the NIH Task Force on Opportunities for Research on Women's Health will assess the current status of such research, identify research opportunities and gaps in knowledge, and recommend a comprehensive NIH plan for future directions for research on women's health during the next 10 to 20 years. Experts in the fields of basic and clinical sciences, practitioners interested in women's health, and women's health advocates are being asked to recommend a research agenda focusing on diseases, disorders, and conditions unique to women, more serious in women, or having different risk factors or interventions in women. This agenda will recommend research priorities across each stage of life and will help guide such research into the next century.

Second, we have recently launched a new initiative that will be the most definitive, far-reaching study of women's health ever undertaken. The Women's Health Initiative will examine heart disease and stroke, cancer, and osteoporosis—the major causes of death, disability, and frailty in women of all races and socioeconomic strata. Comprising three components—a large prospective surveillance study, a nationally based community intervention and prevention study, and randomized clinical trials—the study will examine the effects of menopause on disease in older women, as well as diet modification, smoking cessation, use of hormones, and physical exercise. Seven NIH institutes will be involved, and coordination by the Office of Research on Women's Health will ensure that the institutes contribute their knowledge, expertise, and wisdom to an integrated, productive research program.

The Office of Research on Women's Health is also undertaking an evaluation of the medical, social, and legal barriers to inclusion of women of childbearing potential in clinical research, a project that will benefit all researchers in designing and implementing research protocols. Broader policy questions pertaining to women's health are also being investigated: Should guidelines be developed to indicate when a study should be designed specifically to evaluate gender differences? Is it feasible to develop guidelines to evaluate an intervention over the course of the menstrual cycle? Can issues such as potential fetal damage, the liability for fetal damage, and possible adverse effects on fertility be overcome in designing studies to include women? The answers to these questions are critical to progress in research on women's health.

An additional goal of the NIH and its Office of Research on Women's Health is to set an agenda for nurturing women in leadership roles in biomedical research. We applaud the recommendation in the report that "awareness of and responsiveness to sociocultural factors that could lead to gender disparities may be enhanced by increasing the number of female physicians in leadership roles and other positions of authority in teaching, research, and the practice of medicine."[1] It is our plan in 1992 to host a conference that will address on a national scale how we can better encourage, recruit, maintain, and promote women in scientific and medical careers.

Over the past years, the number of women entering medical schools has increased steadily, and the federal government now has women in two of the highest jobs in the Department of Health and Human Services—as Surgeon General and as director of the NIH. However, I would suggest that there may be one omission from the report's discussion. Progress in addressing the gender discrepancies that have been documented cannot depend alone on swelling the ranks of female researchers and physicians or on physicians who "examine their practices and attitudes for influence of social or cultural biases."[1]

Here, more may be needed. Namely, we must train all medical students, male and female, to understand the biological differences between the sexes, to take the time to listen to their patients, to respect their patients' concerns and anxieties, and, most of all—as so many women have consistently written to me—to take them seriously.

Just as the NIH had been forced to rethink and revamp its research agenda and policies regarding women, so too must other institutions reconsider their processes, philosophies, and training curricula that have contributed to gender disparities in health care. The NIH plans to work with institutional review boards and other administrators to assist in this process.

JAMA has tackled some thorny and difficult issues in the past several issues, including its recent discussions of the future of the American health care system. Access to care, access to appropriate interventions and diagnosis, and access to participation in clinical trials are all important concerns for women.

The report adopted by the House of Delegates of the American Medical Association, while providing important recommendations for change, documents a situation that cannot persist. The NIH is committed to conducting and supporting the research that will provide the important foundation on which clinical decision making depends. But solutions to the subtle factors that have allowed discrepancies in the provision of care that is not based on appropriate biological or medical indications lie not only in research, training, and education, but also within each of us.

Reference

1. Council on Ethical and Judicial Affairs, American Medical Association. Gender disparities in clinical decision making. *JAMA.* 1991;266:559-562.

Resource

Center for Research on Women and Gender
University of Illinois College of Medicine
1640 W Roosevelt Rd, Chicago, IL 60612
312 413-7752

Workers' Compensation

Workers' compensation is governed almost entirely by state rather than federal law. The purpose of the workers' compensation system is to provide a uniform method of compensating employees for on-the-job injuries at a cost that is evenly distributed through insurance or other assessments against employers. Points to remember are:
- Request all information provided by your state's Workers' Compensation Board.
- Post the required information as directed.
- Update and keep records of claims.

Employer obligations

Most states require employers to comply with the workers' compensation law in one of two ways:
- Purchasing workers' compensation insurance through a qualified carrier or a state insurance fund.

• Becoming self-insured by a process prescribed under state law.

The majority of employers are insured for workers' compensation through private carriers. Carriers base their particularly on a classification system that assigns different levels of risk to various business activities. Higher rates are generally assessed for employers whose employees are exposed to a greater degree of harm. Other rating factors are based on the likelihood of many claims being brought against a particular type of employer. In addition, rates are based on the employer's "experience rating."

Employers that fail to purchase insurance or obtain self-insurance approval lose the immunity normally afforded employers under the workers' compensation law. The system is based on the concept that once an employer complies and pays the required premiums, the employer has no further liability for workplace injuries to an employee. The employee will be compensated for injuries by the insurer without regard to fault. The employer will not be subject to lawsuits based on negligence or other fault in causing an employee's injuries.

However, employers may be subject to exposure if injuries occur under the following theories:
• *Intentional acts.* An employer may be directly liable for injuries if the employee can show that the employer specifically intended to injure the employee or that the employer knew that the injury was certain to happen. Liability also exists if the employer knowingly and intentionally exposed employees to danger without informing them of the risk.
• *Dual capacity doctrine.* This doctrine is sometimes used against medical employers that treat their own employees. If an employee is injured by an employer acting in the role of a third-party provider of medical services, the employer may be liable for injuries that result from the medical treatment.
• *Third-party liability.* In some situations an injured employee may sue a third party for work-related injuries, and the third party will turn to the employer for indemnification. This scenario usually arises from a work site where more than one employer has control over workplace safety.
• *Retaliatory action.* Most states prohibit an employer from taking an adverse employment action against an employee for exercising rights under the workers' compensation system.

Covered injuries
To be compensable under state workers' compensation laws, an injury must "arise out of and in the course of employment." Generally, an injury is considered work related if it meets two or more of the following requirements:
• Occurred during working hours.
• Occurred within the physical boundaries of the work site or where work is ordinarily done (usually includes parking lots).
• Occurred while the employee was pursuing the employer's business interest, whether directly or indirectly, or a part of the inherent conditions of employment.

Occupational diseases
Most states also cover occupational diseases under the workers' compensation system. An occupational disease is one that results from exposure to harmful conditions of employment. States that cover occupational diseases generally require that the harmful work conditions must present a greater risk to the employee than to the public at large.

Types of benefits
Most states provide that an employee can recover the following types of benefits for work-related injuries:
• *Medical benefits.* Full medical and hospitalization benefits are generally provided for a limited period, which can be extended if necessary. An employer may generally challenge excessive expenses or unnecessary treatment for an injured employee. In most states, an employer may also have an employee examined by a doctor chosen by the employer. Treatment varies by state.
• *Lost wages or lost earning capacity (also called temporary total disability).* This is usually calculated as a percentage of the employee's average weekly wage, subject to minimum and maximum benefit levels adjusted annually.
• *Temporary partial disability.* These benefits are provided when there is an actual wage loss to an employee who can return to some type of work short of full normal duties.
• *Permanent partial disability (also called specific injury benefits).* These benefits are provided when an employee suffers a permanent injury that is not totally disabling. Most state laws provide for a specific number of weeks of benefits to be paid for a specific injury (eg, 40 weeks of benefits for loss of one finger).
• *Permanent total disability.* These benefits are provided when the employee is completely incapacitated from working at any occupation or when the services the employee can do are so limited in quality, dependability, or quantity that no reasonable market exists for such skills.
• *Rehabilitation costs.* Most states provide that employers are responsible for vocational training or other reemployment costs that are necessary because of the employee's injury.
• *Death benefits.* A predetermined amount is payable to the surviving spouse and dependent children of a deceased worker. A burial allowance is usually provided.

What to do before an accident
Education makes the workplace safer and holds down costs. By making a safer workplace, managers can prevent injuries from occurring and lessen the severity of injuries that do occur, which holds down the medical expense portion of workers' compensation costs. By knowing how to act when an injury does occur, managers and supervisors can help injured workers get the benefits they are entitled to, avoid paying out unwarranted benefits, get the injured employee back to work more quickly, and avoid litigation.

By following the four principles outlined below, managers can go a long way in developing an effective "loss prevention" program.
• Involve management in any loss prevention program.
• Use the hiring process to avoid workers' compensation losses.

- Establish a safety policy.
- Train employees to eliminate accidents.

What to do after an accident

Taking good care of an injured worker pays off. During the first few days of an injury, the worker may have fears and anxieties about the effect the injury has on his/her employment. Having a good system to follow provides an effective answer to the concerns and may prevent the injured worker from going to an attorney. When the worker understands the "no-fault, no-litigation" system, the "us vs them" position is eliminated.

The first 24-hour period can be the most strategic in handling a workers' compensation claim. Every employer should have steps to follow. This can mean the difference between limiting potential costs and carrying an injured worker on the books for years.

At every opportunity, reinforce the fact that the practice has a compassionate program for taking care of its employees and that the employee will receive the best possible care. Start by telling employees how the workers' compensation system works so that they know how to report injuries. Treat every injury as legitimate and respond in the following way:

- Respond to the injured employee.
- Give first aid or make sure the employee receives medical attention.
- Document the accident.
- Explain the workers' compensation procedures.
- Be involved in the medical care given.
- Know the medical provider.
- File an accident report.
- Investigate the accident.
- Consider every injury legitimate until it is proven otherwise.
- Encourage a speedy return to work.
- Maintain contact with the injured employee.

Rehabilitation and return to work

It is crucial to return injured workers to the job quickly. Perhaps the most important and effective action an employer can take to reduce costs is to develop an aggressive return-to-work program, including making light-duty work available. Statistically, the longer a worker is out, the less likely is any return to the workplace. In most states the job taken on returning to work need not be the same job the employee had at the time of injury, but must be within the employee's vocational and physical abilities. Any payment the worker receives from the new job will reduce wage-loss benefits accordingly, since those benefits are based on the difference between the employee's before- and after-injury wages. If the new job pays about the same as the employee's before- and after-injury wages, then no wage-loss benefits need to be paid since there has been no reduction in the employee's wages. (PMMP-1996)

Resource

Federal:
230 S Dearborn, Chicago, IL 60604
312 353-5656

Workers' Compensation Statewide

Alabama Workers' Compensation Division
Department of Industrial Relations
602 Madison Ave, Montgomery, AL 36130
205 242-2868

Alaska Division of Workers' Compensation
Department of Labor
PO Box 25512, Juneau, AK 99802
907 465-2790

Arizona State Compensation Fund
3031 N Second St, Phoenix, AZ 85012
602 631-2000

Arkansas Workers' Compensation Commission
Justice Bldg, 2nd Fl, Little Rock, AR 72201
501 682-3930

California Department of Industrial Relations
Wing A, 5th Fl, 45 Fremont St
San Francisco, CA 94105
415 975-0730

Colorado Department of Labor and Employment
1515 Arapahoe, Tower 2, Ste 406
Denver, CO 80202-2117
303 575-8700

Connecticut Workers' Compensation Commission
1890 Dixwell Ave, Hamden, CT 06514
203 789-7783

Delaware Division of Industrial Affairs
Department of Labor
820 N French St, Wilmington, DE 19801
302 571-2877

District of Columbia Office of Workers' Compensation
Department of Employment
1200 Upshur St NW, 3rd Fl, Washington, DC 20011
202 576-6265

Florida Division of Workers' Compensation
Labor and Employment Security Department
Forrest Bldg, 2728 Centerview Dr
Tallahassee, FL 32399-0564
904 488-7700

Georgia State Board of Workers' Compensation
1 CNN Center, Ste 1000, Atlanta, GA 30303
404 656-2034

Hawaii Disability Compensation Division
Labor and Industrial Relations Department
830 Punchbowl St, Honolulu, HI 96813
808 548-5414

Idaho State Insurance Fund
1215 W State St, Boise, ID 83720
208 334-2370

Illinois Industrial Commission
100 W Randolph St, Ste 8-272, Chicago, IL 60601
312 814-6555

Indiana Worker's Compensation Board
402 W Washington St, W196, Indianapolis, IN 46204
317 232-7103

Iowa Division of Industrial Services
Department of Employment Services
1000 E Grand, Des Moines, IA 50319
515 281-5934

Kansas Division of Workers' Compensation
Department of Human Resources
600 Merchants Bank Tower, Topeka, KS 66612
913 296-3441

Kentucky Department of Workers Claims
Perimeter Park West, Bldg C
1270 Louisville Rd, Frankfort, KY 40601
502 564-5550

Louisiana Office of Workers' Compensation
PO Box 94094, Baton Rouge, LA 70804-9040
504 342-7555

Maine Workers' Compensation Commission
State House Station #27, Augusta, ME 04333
207 289-3751

Maryland Workers' Compensation Commission
6 N Liberty St, Rm 940, Baltimore, MD 21201
410 333-4775

Massachusetts Industrial Accident Board
600 Washington St, 7th Fl, Boston, MA 02111
617 727-4300

Michigan Bureau of Workers' Compensation
Department of Labor
PO Box 30016, Lansing, MI 48909
517 373-3480

Minnesota Workers' Compensation Division
Department of Labor and Industry
443 Lafayette Rd, North St Paul, MN 55155
612 296-2432

Mississippi Workers' Compensation Commission
1428 Lakeland Dr, Jackson, MS 39216
601 987-4200

Missouri Division of Workers' Compensation
Labor and Industrial Relations Department
722 Jefferson St, PO Box 58
Jefferson City, MO 65102
314 751-4231

Montana State Compensation and
Mutual Fund Insurance
Department of Administration
5 S Last Chance Gulch, Helena, MT 59601
406 444-6518

Nebraska Workmen's Compensation Court
State Capitol, 13th Fl
PO Box 94967, Lincoln, NE 68509
402 471-2568

Nevada State Industrial Insurance System
515 E Musser St, Carson City, NV 89714
702 687-5220

New Hampshire Workmen's Compensation Division
Department of Labor
19 Pillsbury St, Concord, NH 03301
603 271-3174

New Jersey Division of Workers' Compensation
Department of Labor
John Fitch Plaza, CN 381, Trenton, NJ 08625
609 292-2414

New Mexico Workmen's Compensation Administration
Labor and Industrial Commission
180 Randolph SE, Albuquerque, NM 87106
505 841-6000

New York State Workers' Compensation Board
180 Livingston St, Brooklyn, NY 11248
718 802-6964

North Carolina Industrial Commission
Department of Economic and Community Development
430 N Salisbury St, 6th Fl, Raleigh, NC 27611
919 733-4820

North Dakota Workers' Compensation Bureau
4007 N State St, Bismarck, ND 58501
701 224-3800

Ohio Workers' Compensation Bureau
246 N High St, Columbus, OH 43266
614 466-1935

Oklahoma Workers' Compensation Committee
1915 N Stiles, Oklahoma City, OK 73105
405 557-7600

Oregon Workers' Compensation Division
Department of Insurance and Finance
350 Winter St NE, Rm 21, Salem, OR 97310
503 945-7881

Pennsylvania Bureau of Workers' Compensation
Department of Labor and Industry
3607 Derry St, 4th Fl, Harrisburg, PA 17120
717 783-5421

Rhode Island Workers' Compensation Commission
1 Dorrance Plaza, Providence, RI 02903
401 272-0700

South Carolina Workers' Compensation Commission
PO Box 1715, Columbia, SC 29202
803 734-5744

South Dakota Division of Labor and Management
Department of Labor
Kneip Bldg, Pierre, SD 57501
605 773-3681

Tennessee Workers' Compensation
Department of Labor
501 Union Bldg, Nashville, TN 37243
615 741-2395

Texas Workers' Compensation Commission
Southfield Bldg, 400 Interstate Hwy 35 South
Austin, TX 78704
512 446-7900

Utah Industrial Commission
PO Box 146610, 160 E 300 S
Salt Lake City, UT 84114-6610
801 530-6844

Vermont Department of Labor and Industry
7 Court St, Montpelier, VT 05602
802 828-2286

Virginia Workers' Compensation Commission
PO Box 1794, Richmond, VA 23214
804 367-8666

Washington Department of Labor and Industries
Claims Section, PO Box 44291
Olympia, WA 98504-4291
800-547-8367

West Virginia Division of Workers' Compensation
PO Box 3051, Charleston, WV 25332
304 344-2580

Wisconsin Division of Workers' Compensation
Department of Workforce Development
201 E Washington, PO Box 746, Madison, WI 53707
608 267-9407

Wyoming Workers' Compensation Division
Department of Employment
122 W 25th St, Cheyenne, WY 82002
307 777-7441

American Samoa Workmen's
Compensation Commission
Legal Affairs, Pago Pago, AS 96799
684 633-5520

Guam Department of Labor
PO Box 9970, Tamuning, GU 96911
671 646-9241

Northern Mariana Islands Civil Service Commission
Personnel Management Office
Office of the Governor, Saipan, MP 96950
670 234-6925

Puerto Rico State Insurance Fund
PO Box 365028, San Juan, PR 00936
809 781-0122

US Virgin Islands Department of Labor
PO Box 890, Christiansted, St Croix, VI 00820
809 773-1994

World Health Organization

The World Health Organization (WHO) was established in 1948 as an agency of the United Nations with responsibilities for international health matters and public health. Its headquarters is in Geneva, Switzerland; there are also regional offices for Europe, Africa, North America, South America, Southeast Asia, the Eastern Mediterranean, and the Western Pacific (including Australia).

The WHO has campaigned effectively against certain infectious diseases, notably smallpox (which was officially declared eradicated throughout the world in 1980), tuberculosis, and malaria. Its other functions include sponsoring medical research programs, organizing a network of collaborating national laboratories, and providing expert advice to its 160 member states on matters such as health service organizations, family health, the use of medicinal drugs, the abuse of drugs, and mental health. The organization's current strategy is described in its campaign "Health for all by the year 2000." The plan gives specific targets for basic public health measures, such as the provision of piped water supplies and other basic sanitation, the universal provision of immunization of children against infectious diseases, and reductions in the use of tobacco and alcohol. (ENC-1989)

Headquarters:
World Health Organization
CH-1211, Geneva 27, Switzerland
22 79 12 111   Fax 22 79 10746   TX 415416
UNISANTE-GENE
Web address: http://www.who.com

Regional Office for the Americas:
525 23rd St NW, Washington, DC 20037
202 861-3200

WHO Publications Center
49 Sheridan Ave, Albany, NY 12221
518 436-9686

World Medical Association
(Association Medicale Mondiale-AMM)
28, Avenue des Alpes, F-01210
Ferney-Voltaire, France
50 40 7575   Fax 50 40 5937

World Medical Journal
Editorial information available through:
World Medical Association
Executive Editor, Dr C. A. S. Wink
100 Wigmore St, London W1H 9DR, England
Co-editor, Walter Burkhart
Hädenkampstr 5, 5000 Köln 41, Germany

World Wide Web

Web technology: coming soon to a hospital near you

Greg Borzo
AM News Nov 18, 1996 pp 5-6

The leaders of the medical informatics community, a largely academic group of physicians and scientists who develop computer and information systems for medicine, are not known to be taken in by hype.

But never have these research-oriented experts been so captivated by a concept as they are by World Wide Web technologies. In fact, many view the Web as the best way to weave together vast, disparate clinical information systems, including medical records.

"The Web is our salvation," said Clement J. McDonald, MD, last month at the American Medical Informatics Association's annual meeting. Dr McDonald is codirector of the Regenstrief Institute in Indianapolis. "Finally, we have a way to unify our incompatible, diverse, and geographically far-flung clinical information systems," he said.

"There's a revolution in the making," said V. J. Jagannathan, PhD, research associate at West Virginia University's Concurrent Engineering Research Center.

Although the Web hit the big time only a couple years ago, it already figures to play a central role in health care informatics, said J. Robert Beck, MD, vice president of information technology at the Baylor College of Medicine in Houston. "It would be hard to overexaggerate the Web's importance. Nothing has ever caught on so quickly."

Much of what these investigators are working on today is destined to become the clinical information and record system of tomorrow. Scores of them are testing prototype Web-enabled applications, and a few leading academic centers already use such new tools in caring for patients.

A study of Web-based systems at nine leading institutions concluded that Web tools can accomplish everything that could be expected of a clinical information system, although much work is still needed to make the Web-based interface ready for "mission-critical" applications.

The study was conducted in March, the Web's "Dark Ages," according to Dean F. Sittig, PhD, one of the authors and corporate manager of clinical systems research and development at Partners Health Care System, which is affiliated with Harvard Medical School. Now Dr Sittig says, "Most systems and applications will be Web based within 2 or 3 years."

A new 'front door'

The average hospital has 20 to 40 sources or repositories of computerized clinical information: medical records, lab, billing, pathology, radiology, pharmacy, intensive care monitoring, ECGs, transcribing, admitting, and so on. Typically, each one runs on a different computer system, platform, or vendor-specific program.

This diversity requires physicians caring for inpatients to track down the information they need from a confusing variety of sources. And the process starts all over again at the next hospital. As a result, doctors typically don't have all the information they need to care for patients, and much of the information they do have is inaccurate or out of date, studies indicate.

Enter the Web, which started as a giant document retrieval and text processing system but is rapidly developing into a more dynamic, multimedia, interactive platform.

Web technologies—browsers, servers, protocols, and standards—can be used to provide a common, platform-independent "front end" to virtually all health care information systems. This allows physicians to access most computerized information using a streamlined, uniform interface.

"We're developing a single front door to health care information," Dr Beck said. Furthermore, centralizing the data and melding it with other data enrich its usefulness: Physician orders are automatically sent to those who need to carry them out. Dictated notes are quickly available to other caregivers. Demographic information is used to automatically calculate drug doses. And new lab results instantaneously prompt suggested interventions.

"We're in this for the decision support benefits, not just because someone likes the idea of computerizing records," said William Stead, MD, director of informatics at Vanderbilt University Medical Center in Nashville, Tenn.

Many Web features are obtained at relatively little cost, and they do not require institutions to dump current information systems. In addition, Web-based systems are relatively easy to prototype, refine, and maintain, which helps win user support.

"Someone drops by with a suggestion, and we practically have it up before they leave the room," said James J. Cimino, MD, at Columbia University's department of medical informatics.

Meanwhile, links to the Internet allow physicians to access data from anywhere at anytime. On the other hand, those uncomfortable with sharing patient records or professional communications on the Internet can run their system on intranets, closed, secure Web-based communication networks operated on or off the Internet.

So far, the Web has proved to be an excellent way for physicians to access information. And getting physicians to the computer creates an opportunity for hospitals, managed care companies, and integrated delivery systems to introduce other potentially powerful computer-based tools, such as clinical guidelines, decision support, and quality measurement.

Down the road, newly emerging tools such as Java and JavaScript programming languages may improve interactively and facilitate data entry. This could greatly increase the number of physicians entering data at the point of care.

Leading systems

Many hospitals and integrated delivery systems are using Web technologies for clinical records and a variety of other purposes, including physician referral, research, referencing the literature, and scheduling. Here are two of the most advanced applications:

Last year, Harvard researchers implemented an on-line patient monitoring system in the 18-bed intensive care unit at Children's Hospital. Besides offering live, off-site monitoring, the system allows information from ICU monitoring systems—which is typically vendor specific—to be integrated with other information systems.

"Our work demonstrates that Web technologies can be used in a data-intensive environment—even for real-time monitoring that requires a continuous flow of data," said Kang Wang, PhD, a research associate at Children's Hospital and an instructor at Harvard Medical School.

Physicians at the Regenstrief Medical Center in Indianapolis can access most patient information on or off campus via a Web-enabled record system that gives them lab results, medications, problem lists, clinical summaries, problem-specific summaries, radiology studies, discharge summaries, high-quality ECG tracings, and other information from a database of 1.4 million patients. E-mail, weather reports, and cartoons are also available.

The system offers a common interface for the information from Indiana University Hospital, Wishard Memorial Hospital, numerous clinics, mental health centers, HMO sites, homeless centers, and other sites.

All the information from every site is not yet available, but increasing amounts are. Most of the information is automatically captured in digital form from devices and information systems; the rest has to be entered manually.

Regenstrief is not paperless, however. Most of the time, physicians still rely on the traditional chart, although an increasing number of them are using the Web-based information retrieval system.

In a couple years, when the current DOS-based physician order entry system is expected to be converted to the Web, physicians will be obliged to use the Web-based system for order entry, said J. Marc Overhage, MD, PhD, an assistant professor at the Indiana University School of Medicine and an investigator at Regenstrief. This may induce them to use the Web-based information retrieval system for most of their other information and communication needs, as well.

Meanwhile, the universality of the Web-based system allows Regenstrief to provide patient-specific information to emergency departments at nonaffiliated and even competing hospitals. "We may have the makings of a community-based medical record here," Dr McDonald said.

If physicians were to use Web-enabled systems in their practices, information sharing across the continuum of care would be facilitated.

Medical literature made easy: querying databases on the Internet

Robert Sikorski, MD, PhD; Richard Peters, MD, PhD
JAMA 1997 Mar 26; 277(12): 959

Nine tenths of wisdom consists of being wise in time.

—Theodore Roosevelt

In the new patient clinic, an oncology fellow sees a 60-year-old man who was diagnosed with gastric cancer 1 year earlier. The patient underwent surgical resection and reports that all of his tumor was removed. He has had no medical care in the interim. Since the fellow does not see many patients with gastric cancer in the clinic, he is unsure of the current treatment recommendations. Does the patient need follow-up computed tomographic (CT) scans? If so, how often? Would adjuvant chemotherapy be beneficial for this type of cancer? After seeing the patient, the physician decides to use the Internet to perform a literature search on the topic.

Reviewing the published medical literature is perhaps the primary way that practicing physicians remain aware of the latest clinical developments. Whether clarifying treatment options in a dynamic field, finding related case reports to gain perspective on a rare condition, learning about research studies that might pertain to a patient, or simply obtaining a review article to increase general knowledge on a topic, a literature consult is often the best medicine.

Traditionally, literature searches were considered a major chore. Clinicians generally had to thumb through stacks of journals at their desks or go to the library to find an appropriate abstract or article. Then came the explosive use of the personal computer and, with it, the ability to perform online literature database searches or consult CD-ROM references. This streamlined the process considerably, allowing clinicians to query the world's medical literature from the comfort of their own offices or homes. However, several factors kept these resources from being widely used. It can be cumbersome to regularly upgrade the evolving computer software needed for online searching and to constantly update CD-ROM databases. In addition, outside academia, online literature searches have been perceived as too costly and perhaps too difficult for physicians who seldom perform them.

But like everything else in medicine today, the literature search is being reinvented. The driving force is the Internet and especially the World Wide Web (WWW or Web). Now, universally available software programs (Web browsers) can serve as the gateway to instantly accessing huge, up-to-date literature databases. This article will provide some background on the origin of the best known of these literature databases—those maintained by the US government—and offer some tips as to how to best use their Internet versions.

The source

The National Institutes of Health's National Library of Medicine (NLM), located in Bethesda, Md, is the world's largest research library in a single scientific and professional field. In addition to its role as a repository of printed biomedical material for use by National Institutes of Health scientists, the NLM also provides global access to some of the best online resources in the form of searchable databases.

The outside user will usually access the main NLM databases through a software system called MEDLARS (MEDical Literature Analysis and Retrieval System). MEDLARS provides online access, for a fee, to more than 40 different information databases containing about 18 million references.[1] The databases linked through MEDLARS are diverse, ranging from disease-specific information (AIDSLINE, CANCERLIT, Physician Data Query), to the history of medicine (HISTLINE), to toxicology (TOXLINE, TOXNET), to general literature in medicine and science (MEDLINE). A complete list of MEDLARS databases can be found on the Web.[1]

To search a MEDLARS database, a user must first complete a registration form and receive a password. This account can be set up over the Internet; the NLM accepts credit cards for payment.[2] The most common software package employed on the user's computer to interface with MEDLARS is Grateful Med. It is available for both Windows and Macintosh systems, either on diskette or by downloading through the NLM's World Wide Web site. Usage fees are based on the amount of information retrieved and the time the software spends searching the MEDLARS files (with the exception of the AIDS databases, which can be searched free of charge). The complete cost for a typical search query averages about $2 to $4 (Sheldon Kotzin, National Library of Medicine, oral communication, February 14, 1997). Users are only billed during the brief time that a chosen query is sent, unlike an online service where users can be billed continuously.

When Grateful Med was first created, users could access its databases only by "dialing up" the system via a modem. Last year, however, the NLM launched an Internet version of Grateful Med as a way of providing a more global window into MEDLARS data, as well as to other biomedical information collections. Starting with MEDLINE, Internet Grateful Med now offers AIDSLINE, PREMEDLINE (unedited new references), and HealthSTAR (health care management issues). Plans are under way to make additional MEDLARS databases available through the Internet Grateful Med Web site. Costs are similar to the standard dial-up version of Grateful Med.[3]

Although the NLM serves as the focal entry point to these unique and exceptionally useful collections, MEDLARS databases also are licensed by other organizations (such as SilverPlatter or Ovid) and repackaged and sold on the WWW or on CD-ROM. In addition, portions of the PDQ database, which contains a wealth of practical information on many aspects of cancer diagnosis and treatment, can be viewed free of charge through the National Cancer Institute's CancerNet Web site. The National Cancer Institute site has chosen to display some of the most clinically useful aspects of PDQ, such as detailed staging information. Another National Cancer Institute site contains free excerpts from the CancerLit database, which includes literature references pertaining to 14 different types of cancer.

Data central

MEDLINE (MEDlars onLINE) is the most widely used scientific literature database in the world. It was established in 1971 and has searchable records dating back to 1966. MEDLINE contains citations and abstracts (though not full text articles) from more than 3800 biomedical journals and contains more than 8.5 million records.[4] About 31,000 new records are added each month alone. Chances are that every physician's major specialty journal is indexed in MEDLINE.

MEDLINE's utility comes from the fact that each article to be abstracted on MEDLINE is read by a trained NLM indexer and assigned keywords. These keywords, chosen from a special NLM dictionary called Medical Subject Headings (MeSH), are what make sophisticated searching techniques possible. MEDLINE records are generally updated at the NLM each week. An article in a popular medical journal (such as *JAMA* or the *New England Journal of Medicine*) will be indexed and available on the Net through Internet Grateful Med within about 1 month after publication. However, some articles appearing in less frequently read journals or those published in more specialized journals published outside the United States might take up to 6 months to be indexed.[4]

MEDLINE mania

In addition to Internet Grateful Med, a number of vendors license MEDLINE data and offer searchable interfaces to this resource via their WWW sites, meaning anyone with an Internet connection can use their service. These vendors include commercial ventures such as Healthgate, Avicenna, and Medscape. Other proprietary online services, such as Physicians' Online, also offer MEDLINE, but not through the Web.

Access restrictions for these commercial MEDLINE sites vary considerably. Some require no registration and charge no fees, whereas others provide free, unlimited usage but require the user to log in one time to obtain a password. Some of these free sites are supported by advertisers or underwriters and display an advertising banner above the query form and results each time a search is performed. With certain databases, users who pay a fee can obtain full text of articles, while others offer no such option. Finally, some sites may both require a password and charge a fee for all services. These sites may adjust their access or fee policies over time.

All that glitters is not gold

We wondered whether all of the Web sites that offer MEDLINE access are equivalent. To answer this question, we asked two medical librarians at the National Institutes of Health to compare several search sites. They queried each site on the same topic (macular degeneration) and looked at the quantity of results obtained, the overall quality of the user interface, and the speed of data retrieval at each site.

Their work yielded some surprising results. First, the number of relevant citations varied from site to site (ranging from 3 to 20), even though a similar query approach was used.[5] This range may be due to the specific search software used at each site or the frequency

with which the MEDLINE data is updated. MEDLINE tapes licensed for Web use are updated at the discretion of the vendor—and may occur as often as once a week or as infrequently as once every 6 months to 1 year. Second, the overall ease of use of the search results they obtained varied substantially. Finally, the interface through which the user is prompted to perform searches differs from site to site, with each having its own look and feel and offering different levels of detail.

The lesson seems to be that, depending on the type of data a user is seeking (a case report, review article, or survey of a topic), one should be aware of the strengths and limitations of a particular search site. Also, a site's offerings may change behind the scenes in the future, either for better or worse.

These variables aside, and even taking into account other problems inherent in using a still nascent medium, the Web affords easy and even free access to collections of the world's medical and scientific knowledge. Additional databases are being made available on the Web regularly, as the marketplace discovers the utility of linking repositories of quality clinical data to the populations that most need to use them.

A detailed version of our Internet MEDLINE comparison and a section on frequently asked questions about MEDLINE searching can be found in the NetSight add-on column established on our Web site (http://www.MedsiteNavigator.com/) as an adjunct to the NetSight column available on the *JAMA* Web site (http://www.ama-assn.org/jama/).

Sites to see: a Net resource guide

The National Library of Medicine (NLM)
http://www.nlm.nih.gov/
NLM home page

NLM Online Databases and Databanks
http://www.nlm.nih.gov/pubs/factsheets/online_databases.html
A listing and description of the more than 40 databases available through NLM

Frequently Asked Questions About Searching MEDLARS Databases
http://www.nlm.nih.gov/databases/medlars_faq.html
The details about registration, costs, and use of NLM databases

Internet Grateful Med
http://igm.nlm.nih.gov/
Internet Grateful Med home page

PDQ Detection and Prevention
http://wwwicic.nci.nih.gov/clinpdq/screening.html
A subset of PDQ dealing with cancer detection and prevention

PDQ Treatment for Patients
gopher://gopher.nih.gov:70/11/clin/cancernet/pdqinfo/pif/
A subset of PDQ dealing with treatment targeted to patients

PDQ Treatment for Physicians
gopher://gopher.nih.gov:70/11/clin/cancernet/pdqinfo/soa/
A subset of PDQ dealing with treatment targeted to physicians

National Cancer Institute (NCI) CancerNet Cancer Information for Patients and the Public
http://wwwicic.nci.nih.gov/patient.htm
Sections of PDQ along with NCI cancer facts

CANCERLIT Topics
gopher://gopher.nih.gov:70/11/clin/cancernet/cancerlit/topics/
CANCERLIT entries on 14 different tumor types, including breast and leukemia

MEDLINE Search Tools
http://www.MedsiteNavigator.com/medline/medline.html
A metasite with links to free and charging MEDLINE search engines

Mention of a Web site, company, or product in this article or the accompanying list does not imply endorsement by the authors, editors, *JAMA*, or the American Medical Association.

Corresponding author: Robert Sikorski, MD, PhD, Bldg 49, Room 4B56, National Cancer Institute, Bethesda, MD 20892.

References

1. National Library of Medicine WWW site (http://www.nlm.nih.gov/publications/factsheets/onlinedatabases.html). Accessed February 14, 1997.

2. National Library of Medicine WWW site (http://access.nlm.nih.gov:443/index.html). Accessed February 14, 1997.

3. National Library of Medicine WWW site (http://www.nlm.nih.gov/databases/medline.html). Accessed February 14, 1997.

4. National Library of Medicine WWW site (http://igm.nlm.nih.gov:80/Html/documents/splash/igm20/charges.html). Accessed February 14, 1997.

5. Medsite Navigator WWW site (http://www.medsitenavigator.com/medline/medlinereview.html). Accessed February 14, 1997.

Writers

Good scientific writing

Charles G. Roland, MD

"If you know, you can utter it in English."

—Martin H. Fischer

In this essay I shall try to answer three questions. One is the query my readers will expect to have answered: "What is good scientific writing?" The second, both more difficult and more important, can be posed thus: "Does the goodness of scientific writing, or its badness, really matter?" Finally, and logically, the question arises, "How does one learn to write well?" Any of my editor-writer colleagues who have wrestled with these problems will perhaps sympathize with my diffidence when I admit that I cannot answer my own questions. But then, many important questions are not truly answerable. The thought which invests a seriously proposed answer justifies the attempt.

Before proceeding I must make one comment. Any definition of good scientific writing must, for reasons which will become evident, be subjective. Readers will find areas of disagreement. I hope these areas will be small, but their existence is inevitable and should not invalidate the general concepts.

What is good scientific writing?

Scientific writing is a phenomenon. It is not itself science. Rather, it is art applied to the task of describing science. The appropriateness of a heavy emphasis on medical writing lies in the fact that medicine is a classic example of the interdependence of art and science. And this relation leads me to suggest a close analogy between scientific writing and laboratory practice, for I have no doubt that much art is required to experiment productively, but my background in the laboratory is too slight to leave me comfortable in pursuing the analogy in detail.

Medical practice demands both art and science. Whether the physician practices well or practices badly depends, of course, upon both his acquisition of the art and his mastery of the science. But in this discussion, both of medical practice and of scientific writing, I propose that we consider the science invariable; the hypothetical physicians of my essay shall all know the same "amount" of science, and the writing will all be equally "true" or "valid" scientifically. The variables then are artistic, in the broadest sense.

Now I have established the rules. By doing so I have simplified the analogy to the point where it is elemental. When Dr Smith, a "good" physician, practices he melds his scientific knowledge with the art of medicine. If Dr Smith is a good writer also—by no means an inevitable combination—then he presents his scientifically valid information (or hypothesis) melded with literary artistry.

Because I have use the words *art, artistic,* and *artistry,* perhaps I should make clear an important differentiation. Literary ability, in my discussion of scientific writing, does not mean literary genius. What it does mean is the ability to write clearly, unequivocally, concisely, and pleasingly. Most of us who write are merely adequate practitioners. Literary genius I know nothing about. If a physician who had literary genius came to me asking for instruction in writing, I hope I would have the good sense to leave him alone.

Genius finds, or makes, its own ways.

Good writing is not necessarily the absence of error; strictly correct writing can be dreadfully dull and, therefore, bad. Nevertheless science would be vastly improved if two categories of faults—errors and infelicities—could be eliminated. The first, and the most obvious, is the true error: the nonsentence, the incorrect subject reference, the use of the passive voice, boring repetitiveness of sentence structure. These last infelicities cause more difficulty, simply because they are relative rather than absolute faults.

By the time a medical article is published, most of the true errors will have been eliminated by the journal's editorial staff, if it has one; so the major difficulty with the published literature is infelicitous presentation. Nevertheless, every effort to improve scientific writing must direct itself to both kinds of error.

All writing is literary activity. But science has become dissociated from the humanities, and physicians seem to think that scientific writing is not a literary form; the very word "literary" frightens many, who believe that science is objective while literature is subjective. They pursue this belief to its questionably logical conclusion by supposing that science is only objective, and that therefore it must be antiliterary. And from this belief, rarely expressed but common, comes a contempt for good writing—not for writing, but for doing it well.

Does good writing matter?

The attitude I have just described does exist. How common it may be, I do not know. But to anyone who has this attitude of contempt, the answer to the question "Does good writing matter?" is "No." Nevertheless they are wrong, on several counts.

It does matter to write well. Good writing has been described as good manners. Those who cannot or will not write well epitomize bad manners. Moreover, they forget that writing unread, or read but not understood, is irrelevant trivia, totally worthless. So both good manners and good sense should lead the physician to want to write better.

The aim of science is not just to discover new facts and create new hypotheses: the aim is to discover fact, make hypotheses, and disseminate these to the rest of the scientific world for study, evaluation, acceptance, and incorporation into Science. Good scientific writing is clear and unequivocal, and thus good writing will be more easily read, understood, and evaluated than will bad writing. Indeed, this fact occasionally makes the reader suspicious that a badly written article may have been so prepared deliberately, to disguise the scientific deficiencies of the work. Richard Asher, writing in the *Lancet* (August 27, 1949), remarked that "obscurity is bad, not only because it is difficult to understand but also because it is confused with profundity, just as a shallow muddy pool may look deep."

There is another reason to write well, a completely practical one. In these days when we are being overwhelmed by the burgeoning mass of the literature, attention to its dimensions has largely been limited to considering the number of journals, and the number of articles each contains. Not usually considered is the number of words in an article. But consider this passage, published in a major scientific periodical in this country.

> The thesis herein offered is that woman (like man) is a biologic, social, and cultural creature, and as such is dependent for health on the acceptance, approval, support, and encouragement of significant individual members of the social group to which she belongs. In other words, her self-evaluation is determined, in the last analysis, on how she perceives and symbolizes this attitude, behavior, expectations, etc., of the group of which she is a member. Intimate human relations and interactions are so essential to health that one's sanity and potential for self-fulfillment are jeopardized for the most part by the perceived threat of disapproval, rejection, devaluation, or loss of security.

Just to read the passage, without spending any additional time trying to understand it, takes me 36 seconds. I am a reasonably rapid reader, but by no means a speed reader. Let me assume that the time I take to read this passage is the average time for physicians. Let me further suppose that this passage would be read by 50,000 readers. (Considering the journal in which this passage was published, that is a highly conservative estimate.) I can edit the passage in many ways, one of which I show here.

> Woman is a biologic, social, and cultural creature, dependent for health on the acceptance and encouragement of members of her social group. Her self-evaluation is determined by her perceptions and symbolizations of the attitudes of her group. Interactions are so essential to health that one's sanity and potential for self-fulfillment are jeopardized by perceived threats of disapproval, rejection, devaluation, or loss of security.

Without question this version is shorter. I hope you will agree that it is easier to read and understand than was the original. I would further propose that it says the same thing that the original says (which incidentally turns out to be not very much, when some of the sanctifying jargon is removed). I can read this passage in 22 seconds. And if I subtract the time is takes to read the edited version from the time to read the original, and multiply the answer by our hypothetical 50,000 readers, it appears that the author has wasted 8 days of time of his combined readership. And this calculation is based on only one paragraph, not the entire lengthy paper.

Authors complain especially bitterly about delays between acceptance and publications by journals. Yet in many published articles the author could have removed redundancies and compressed language to shorten the material by 25% to 50%. Taking the lower figure, 25%, and applying that to a monthly that published 1200 pages a year, it would require 300 fewer pages to publish the same number of articles; that is, the editor could publish 30 more 10-page papers per year than he can now. Just think what this mean to the backlog of material that seems to hang like a millstone around the neck of many an editor. The possibilities are intoxicating. Furthermore, at a time when so many scientific periodicals are instituting or have already instituted page charges, and when the complaints about payment of such page charges are increasing rapidly, editing such as I have suggested provides a way for the journal to decrease the amount of charge to an individual author while maintaining the same level of income for the journal.

Finally, a quite different reason why good writing does matter: the pursuit of excellence. This pursuit has been a sorry casualty of our age. Although many individuals feel the urge to excel intellectually, the desire is far from universal. Yet I am sufficiently old-fashioned to believe that every person has a responsibility to do everything he does as well as he possibly can. And for the physician and the scientist this means that each has a responsibility to report his scientific observations as well as he possibility can.

How to learn to write well

After the acceptance of this responsibility—one I would boldly call a moral responsibility—you naturally ask next, how can the conscientious author learn to write more skillfully? There is no simple response, no easy way. But I shall attempt to provide a few brief directions.

First, you learn to write by writing. Or perhaps I should say, you cannot learn to write if you do not do it. So the author or potential author must devote much time to this chore. Writing is not easy. It is hard work. The urge to avoid the effort is great. The man who says he is too busy to write often means that he contrives to be too busy to write. As every sensible person knows, he can find time for anything that is important to him. Finding time for writing means finding a distraction-free locale, and keeping it free of distractions. Most of these come from within—the urge to do something else, write a letter, read a journal, clean shoes, take out the garbage, knit, anything but write—that is the urge to battle against. When I suggest that you must write, I do not mean that you must publish. Writers need to practice their art, and at least occasionally they should do so as an exercise in itself.

Whether or not the work is destined to appear in print, you should try to have it criticized by someone whose judgment you respect. Ideally this critic should have exemplary patience and unlimited time, as well as some expertise in your area of knowledge and considerable literary good sense. Seek his candid comments—but skip the whole exercise if you find that you cannot react calmly and productively to candid comments.

In addition to your self-preceptorship, which is the most important part of any writer's training, you may supplement your education by attending courses on medical writing and by reading books on the subject. "Courses" that are merely series of lectures do little for the student. Workshops, on the other hand, can be most useful, and these I recommend highly. As for books about writing, they can be useful but only to supplement the hard work of writing itself.

However, one kind of reading can help the writer immeasurably. This is the reading of well written books and articles, both in your field (if you can find them) and in general literature. A process analogous to osmosis seems operative, so that some of the techniques of skillful writers insensibly become part of the reader's writing skills—but only if he reads deeply and carefully and often.

I have listed a few books in the Appendix that I have found useful, books by Hemingway and Orwell, for example. But every reader must find his own exemplars; I am sufficiently prejudiced to suggest that there is little likelihood of finding, in the current best-seller lists for fiction, an author whose style one would wish to use as a guide.

As far as reading well written prose in your field is concerned, that is what the rest of this book is about. I began to collect the examples because participants in writing workshops asked me to direct them to well written scientific articles and books. From this request came the series on "Good Scientific Writing," which has appeared in *Archives of Internal Medicine*. Each part of the series appeared under a motto by Lord Chesterfield that epitomizes the rationale for the project and for this book: "We are more than half what we are by imitation. The great point is to choose good models and to study them with care." (WRT-1983)

Resource

American Medical Writers Association
9650 Rockville Pike, Bethesda, MD 20814-3998
301 493-0003   Fax 301 493-6384
E-mail: amwa@amwa.org
Web address: gopher://cais.com:70/11/.amwa

since the time of John Morgan had never laid far below the surface. In the turmoil of the late 1840s, this trend showed itself more and more and became a dominant factor later in the century.

All the problems varied in intensity among the several states, and each state, taking account of its own environmental and social circumstances, attempted its own remedies. But the powers of the states were too localized, and the problems too complex. The inability of any single state society to deal competently with them soon became apparent to the more farsighted physicians. Over a period of 20 years, from about 1826, there were many efforts to form some sort of national medical society, excellently summarized by Stookey,[5] all proved abortive. There is no need to repeat here the story of these numerous frustrated attempts.

Cooperation had never been a prominent American trait, for "rugged individualism" more nearly expressed the American character. The earlier attempts at a national organization, in Vermont, New York, Georgia, Ohio, and New Hampshire, all came to naught. The historian naturally asks the question, Why did the earlier attempts to achieve some sort of joint cooperation all fail, until the final success of 1845-1846? The answer, I suggest, lay in an overall worsening of the situation that by 1844 had come to a climax. In that year, as we have seen, any special legal privileges enjoyed by the medical profession were generally withdrawn, and the era of "free trade" in medicine had begun.

For some authors, the founding of the AMA represents primarily a reform movement in medical education. This view stems largely from the aggressive rhetoric of Nathan Smith Davis, the "father of the AMA," whose narrative account is important source material for the period. Davis himself was especially interested in education, and he strongly emphasized the need for improved standards. The question of educational reform, however, must be placed in a broader perspective that will take account of the complexities of the situations.

The AMA came into existence under the impetus provided by the New York State Medical Society, which had been severely shaken by the legislative events of 1844. The legislature, influenced by the Thomsonians and by a populist tide, had revoked the special privileges of the regular medical profession. Although the medical license remained available, it lost all force and meaning. Anyone could practice, even without a license, and could collect any debts stemming from such practice. Free trade in medicine became a fact of life in New York (and, actually, in the rest of the country as well). The immediate reaction of the regular physicians in New York gives us a rare insight into the "embryology" of the AMA and the way that physicians perceived the changing functions of a medical society.

The new legislation was passed in May 1844. In June 1844, the Albany County Medical Society, in a special meeting, heard a report that analyzed the situation and recommended the course the society should take. The report[6] first gave a version of the way the societies came into existence. Originally, the county society provided a means whereby the members "may readily be recognized by each other and by the public, may exercise a general supervision over each other, and cooperated to promote

the common welfare." A student, after being taught "the science and art of Medicine" and passing the examination, is "admitted into the profession as one worthy of its honors and fitted to assume its duties." The society was a body of physicians "presenting certain guarantees of capacity and character...so that its members may be readily recognized by the public."

The law had thus recognized "educated physicians" and gave the public "the means of recognizing them." Supposedly, it was the height of absurdity for anyone to consult "an ignorant person when it is possible to procure the services of an educated physician." Nevertheless, some persons did commit this absurdity, and to protect the public from such "folly," the law prohibited irregular practice, under penalties. It has seemed proper to protect "a few silly persons" from "their own bad judgment."

But, the report continued, "a large portion of the public thinks that education and science are not necessary to qualify men for medical practice." Numerous sects sprang up that attracted a substantial public following. The authors modestly admitted that "we have not...the right to impose on them [the public] our ideas of wisdom"—if anyone who knows the facts is foolish enough to consult with quacks, he must suffer the consequences. Furthermore, the authors admitted, restrictive legislation was hard to enforce. It created a "cry of persecution," and might seem to place the medical profession in a false position, as if selfishly fighting for its own privileges rather than "defending the public against their own rashness and folly." The authors did not want to engage in controversy with special sects, "with ignoble adversaries."

Regarding the laws of 1844, the proper response of the medical society was not to seek restoration of privileges, but rather to put its house in order. "We ought to endeavor to infuse more spirit into our County societies, to have more frequent meetings, and to promote cordiality of feeling among the members. The rules of medical ethics should be scrupulously observed." Now that the law was changed, "it will be practicable to raise the standard of admission into the County Societies...into which those who find the requirements too high need not enter...The dignity and respectability of our profession is to be promoted not by asking for legal privileges, but by an increase of individual zeal and a more cordial cooperation." The barrier that separates the physician from the quacks is formed, not by legislation, but "by the high attainments and honorable deportment" of the physicians, and it is this barrier that "depends on us to make higher and stronger."

The report ended with a resolution, that "it would not be conducive to the interest or respectability of the medical profession" to seek any remedial legislation on "any medical subject whatsoever." The report and the resolution were unanimously adopted. The society seemed willing to stand by itself, without legislative help.

The whole report shows a remarkable mixture of resignation to the course of events, bitterness over what has transpired, and continued arrogance. Equally important, it showed a sensible recognition that the future can be salvaged through revitalizing the medical societies, and raising their standards and their level of discipline. Yet, at

AMA

that time, the members of the society did not look further than their own local society.

I suggest that after the initial shock had passed, men of greater vision looked to a broader scene. They could perceive an overall solution through a national rather than a local society.

In 1839, the New York State Medical Society had passed a resolution recommending a meeting of nationwide delegates, three from each state medical society and one from each regularly constituted medical school. Although invitations had been sent out, no one responded and no meeting took place. In 1844, at the state society meeting, the topic again came up for discussion, especially in reference to raising the standards of medical education. Dr. Davis, a newly appointed delegate, only 27 years old, had been deeply concerned with this aspect. The debate continued into the meeting of 1845. At that time a resolution was passed, urging the convocation of delegates from "medical societies and colleges in the whole Union,"[7] to meet in Philadelphia, in 1846, to consider the problem of elevating the standards of medical education. A committee was appointed to implement the resolution, with Dr. Davis as chairman. A forceful and indefatigable correspondent, he, more than any other single person, deserves the credit for bringing the convention into existence.

Davis's own account of the convention emphasized quite exclusively the educational aspects and ignored other important facets. The indispensable document for studying the founding of the AMA is the official *Proceedings* of the conventions of 1846 and 1847, containing the minutes and the committee reports. When we study these we gain a somewhat different perspective.

At the initial meeting on May 5, 1846, there was some difficulty in determining the status of the various persons who attended and just what they represented, but these problems were not of serious import. After the election of officers, a maverick resolution to adjourn the convention sine die was decisively rejected, and the delegates settled down to the main business. A committee, of which Davis had been the chairman, brought in six resolutions that were "adapted to fulfill the immediate objects contemplated by the Convention."[8]

The first resolution indicated the purpose of the Association, already quoted. The second proposed a committee to plan the organization of the next meeting, and the third proposed an invitation to all "regularly organized Medical Societies, and chartered Medical Schools" to attend the next meeting in Philadelphia, in 1847. The remaining resolutions have to do directly with the goals of the Association and their implementation, and form the essence of the proceedings. Thus, the fourth resolution recommended a "uniform and elevated standard" for the MD degree; the fifth, "a suitable preliminary education" for all who would study medicine; and the sixth a uniform code of medical ethics for the entire medical profession in the United States.

A further resolution, from the floor rather than the steering committee, recommended the separation of the teaching of medicine from the licensing to practice. This really meant that a diploma should not be an automatic license. Instead of multiple licensing bodies—local societies and medical facilities—there should be only a single

licensing board for each state. This resolution engendered much debate but was finally referred to a committee. Other resolutions passed at the convention are not relevant for our purpose.

The president of the convention appointed committees to consider these various resolutions and to report at the next meeting in 1847. Dr. Davis was appointed only to the committee on organization, and the final framework of the Association owes much to him and to his remarkable energy. However, he did not serve on any of the other committees that hammered out the doctrinal points. These committee reports, presented at the 1847 meeting, embody the representative thinking of the convention.

To appreciate the problems of the convention, we must recognize the essential guild structure, comparable to the British guilds such as the Royal College of Physicians or the Society of Apothecaries. Obviously, the overall environment in the United States in the 1840s differed markedly from that of Great Britain a century earlier. The goals, however, have much in common and include some basic components of all guild structures.

At the same time there was an important difference. Traditionally, a guild, in promoting the interest of its members, tries to establish a monopoly through appropriate legislative action. In the United States of the 1840s, the social and political climates effectively prevented any hope that legislation would approve monopolistic privileges. However, there remained scope for a voluntary organization that could promote the interests of its members through other than special legal privileges. For effectiveness, such an organization would depend on many factors, but the two most important elements come directly from essential and traditional guild practice: first, the control over apprentices (ie, over those would want to enter the guild); and second, a disciplinary control over those who were already in.

The concept of apprenticeship, for a long time traditional in American medicine, had by the mid-19th century been largely superseded by newer modes of medical education. A medical guild had to maintain standards, and this it could do, over the long run, only by controlling the entrance into the profession. If a centralized voluntary association wanted to control new admissions into the cadre of practicing physicians, there would need to be an agreement between medical societies and medical faculties. As we have already seen, there was considerable tension between these groups.

A guild would also need to exert control over those members who had finished their training and were actually engaged in their profession. In classical guild terminology, this would include all who had finished their apprenticeship to become journeymen or masters. The code of professional ethics was an instrument of control—transgression of the code would permit expulsion of the erring member from the guild.

The code, a weapon for keeping members in line and maintaining discipline, gave rise to a vast array of problems that will be treated later. We have a voluntary organization designed to further the interests of the medical profession (with subsidiary benefits overflowing to the general public); a firm organization was needed to pursue its goals; such a pursuit required a control over admission to the profession and control over the members already in practice—this would be accomplished by regulating medical education and establishing a code of ethics; and, furthermore, a voluntary organization must rely on itself and on public opinion, and not on specific legislative support. This interpretation is, of course, ex post facto, derived entirely by inference from the documents of the period and the whole course of events. The course of events proceeded as if these views were implicit at the time of the first convention, though they were not explicitly spelled out.

The convention of 1846 tried to face, squarely and honestly, the problems that affected the whole medical profession in the mid-1840s. The key to these problems (and the proposed solutions) lies in the committee reports, presented and discussed at the 1847 meeting and adopted as the framework for the AMA. I need not enter into the parliamentary aspects of the convention, nor the change in title from National to American Medical Association, that took place at the end of the 1847 meetings. I will restrict my analysis in my book to three topics—the impact of the code of medical ethics, the problems of medical education, and the concept of elitism. We will see how these topics affected the course of the AMA throughout the entire 19th century.

Bibliographic note

The most readily available account of the founding of the AMA is Morris Fishbein's *History of the American Medical Association, 1847-1947* (Philadelphia, WB Saunders Co, 1947). For more detailed discussion of special aspects, with abundant references, two helpful texts are Martin Kaufman's Homeopathy in America (Baltimore, The Johns Hopkins University Press, 1968) and William G. Rothstein's American Physicians in the Nineteenth Century (Baltimore, The Johns Hopkins University Press, 1972). An essential primary source is *The Proceedings of the National Medical Conventions* held in New York, May 1846, and in Philadelphia, May 1847, Philadelphia. Also of value is N.S. Davis's *History of the American Medical Association From Its Organization up to January, 1855* (Philadelphia, Lippincott Grambo & Co, 1855).

References

1. Proceedings of the National Medical Convention, p 17.

2. Transactions of the American Medical Association 1849;2:299.

3. Davis NS. *History of Medical Education and Institutions in the United States,* Chicago, Ill: SC Griggs & Co; 1851:116-117.

4. Coventry CB. Remarks on some of the proceedings of the New York State Medical Society. *NY J Med.* 1846;7:192-199.

5. Stookey B. Origins of the first National Medical Convention, 1826-1846. *JAMA.* 1961;177:133-140.

6. *NY J Med* 1844;3:281-286.

7. Davis, *History of the AMA,* p 23.

8. The remaining quotations come from the Proceedings, pp 16-22.

(AGE-1984)

The American Medical Association: A Chronology 1847-1997

AMA

1847

Founding of AMA at Academy of Natural Sciences in Philadelphia (Founder Nathan Davis)

AMA Committee on Medical Education appointed

AMA Code of Medical Ethics written and published

AMA sets first minimal standards for medical education

1848

AMA notes the dangers of universal traffic in secret remedies and patent medicine

1849

AMA establishes a board to analyze quack remedies and nostrums and to enlighten the public in regard to the nature and dangerous tendencies of such remedies

1858

AMA establishes Committee on Ethics

1868

AMA Committee on Ethics strongly advocates recognition of regularly educated and qualified female physicians

1869

Archives of Ophthalmology founded under title *Archives of Ophthalmology and Otology*

1870

AMA recommends that Congress pass a national system of quarantine regulations

1873

AMA Judicial Council founded to deal with ethical and constitutional controversies

1876

Sarah Hackett Stephenson becomes first woman member of AMA

AMA adopts a resolution promoting sanitary municipal water supplies and sewer systems

1882

Archives of Dermatology founded under title *Journal of Cutaneous Diseases*

1883

Journal of the American Medical Association founded; Nathan Davis is first editor

1884

AMA supports experimentation on animals as the most useful source of knowledge in medical practice

1897

AMA incorporated

AMA

1898

AMA Committee on Scientific Research is established to provide grants for fostering medical research

1899

AMA creates Committee on National Legislation to represent the Association's interest in Washington

AMA establishes Council on Exhibits to promote public health education

Dr George H. Simmons begins a 25-year appointment as editor of *JAMA* and develops the journal into an internationally recognized publication

AMA appoints a committee to report on the nature of tuberculosis, means of control, public education, and advisability of establishing national and state sanatoriums

AMA urges that local boards of health adopt laws requiring compulsory smallpox vaccination

1901

AMA reorganizes, creating the House of Delegates

1902

AMA acquires its first permanent headquarters in Chicago

1904

AMA establishes the Council on Medical Education to accelerate campaign to raise educational requirements for physicians

1905

AMA establishes Council on Pharmacy and Chemistry to set standards for drug manufacturing and advertising and fight the war on quack patent medicines and nostrum trade

AMA Council on Medical Education develops and publishes in *JAMA* minimum and ideal curriculum standards for medical schools

1906–1907

AMA Council on Medical Education inspects 160 medical schools and classifies them into three groups: A = acceptable; B = doubtful; and C = unacceptable

1906

AMA Council on Medical Education publishes directory of medical schools in the United States, detailing entrance requirements

AMA Chemical Laboratory is established to analyze nostrums and drugs submitted for AMA review (in the 1930s, leading to the AMA Seal of Acceptance)

AMA publishes first American Medical Directory listing over 128,000 licensed physicians in US and Canada

AMA membership exceeds 50,000

1908

Archives of Internal Medicine founded

1910

The Flexner Report, *Medical Education in the United States and Canada*, funded by the Carnegie Foundation and supported by the AMA, is published and facilitates new standards for medical schools. The report cites many diploma mills

AMA Council on Medical Education publishes the first edition of *Essentials of an Acceptable Medical College*, revised eight times in the next 41 years, to be superseded by the *Functions and Structure of a Modern Medical School*

1911

Archives of Pediatrics and Adolescent Medicine founded under title *American Journal of Diseases of Children*

1912

The Federation of State Medical Boards is established accepting AMA's rating of medical schools as authoritative

AMA approves a report of the standard methods for prevention and control of tuberculosis

1913

AMA establishes a "Propaganda Department" to gather and disseminate information concerning health fraud and quackery

1914

AMA Council on Medical Education sets standards for hospital internship programs and publishes first list of approved hospitals offering such programs

AMA adopts a resolution approving establishment of uniform milk standards and classification of milk

1915

AMA publishes favorable report on government-supported health care through sickness and accident insurance for employed individuals

1919

Archives of Neurology and Psychiatry founded

1920

AMA acquires *Journal of Cutaneous Diseases* and changes title to *Archives of Dermatology and Syphilology*

Archives of Surgery founded

AMA opposes compulsory health insurance through an August 1920 resolution by the House of Delegates

Council on Medical Education becomes Council on Medical Education and Hospitals

1922

Woman's Auxiliary to the AMA is organized to assist the AMA in its program for the advancement of medicine and public health

1923

Hygeia, the AMA's family health magazine, is founded

AMA adopts standards for medical specialty training

1924

Morris Fishbein begins 25-year tenure as editor of *JAMA* and *Hygeia*

The AMA begins radio broadcasts that bring health messages to the general public

1925

Archives of Otolaryngology—Head and Neck Surgery founded under title *Archives of Otolaryngology*

AMA Propaganda Department becomes Bureau of Investigation

1926

Archives of Pathology and Laboratory Medicine founded under title *Archives of Pathology*

1927

AMA Council on Medical Education and Hospitals publishes first list of hospitals approved for residency training

1929

AMA acquires *Archives of Ophthalmology*

AMA Council on Foods established as a subgroup of Council on Pharmacy and Chemistry

1930

AMA requests evaluative psychiatric services be made available to every criminal and juvenile court, and to correctional institutions

1931

AMA's Bureau of Medical Economics is established to study all economic matters affecting the medical profession

1934

Official recognition of specialty boards in medicine begins through collaborative efforts of the AMA Council on Medical Education and the Advisory Board for Medical Specialties (and later by its successor, the American Board of Medical Specialties)

1935

Social Security Act is approved. It does not include compulsory health insurance because of AMA influence

1936

AMA Council on Foods becomes Council on Foods & Nutrition; council offers AMA Seal of Acceptance to food manufacturers who pass advertising and content tests and who conform with Food and Drug Act; council encourages enriching milk with vitamin D to prevent rickets, and salt with iodine to prevent goiter

AMA membership exceeds 100,000

1937

AMA asks county medical societies to share the burden of caring for poor patients

1938

AMA Council on Foods and Nutrition publishes *The Normal Diet*, containing the first authoritative dietary recommendations for Americans

1940

Council on Pharmacy and Chemistry discontinues analysis of drugs and directs efforts to providing physicians with information on efficacy of dosage administration; encourages the advancement of new drugs by issuing development grants

1942

The AMA Council on Medical Education and the Association of American Medical Colleges establish the Liaison Committee on Medical Education to accredit programs leading to the MD degree

1943

AMA opens office in Washington, DC

AMA Council on Medical Service and Public Relations is established

1944

AMA receives a commendation from the Surgeon General for the radio series "Doctors at War," as an excellent service to the Medical Department of the US Army

1945

AMA recommends borderline limits to determine alcohol influence in the suspected drunken driver

1946

AMA begins television broadcasts that bring health messages to the general public

1947

AMA celebrates centennial of its founding

1948

AMA launches a campaign against President Truman's plan for national health insurance

1950

Hygeia becomes *Today's Health*

AMA Council on Medical Education, along with the Association of American Medical Colleges, develops and publishes a list of foreign medical schools with educational programs that meet AMA standards

1951

Joint Commission on Accreditation of Hospitals is formed by the American College of Surgeons, American College of Physicians, American Hospital Association, AMA, and the Canadian Medical Association

AMA endorses the principle of fluoridation of community water supplies

AMA Education and Research Foundation established to help medical schools meet expenses and to help medical students

AMA

1953

National Internship Matching Program is formally established

1954

AMA Council on Medical Education establishes the Internship Review Committee

First list of continuing education courses is published by AMA Council on Medical Education

AMA recommends equipping all automobiles with safety belts

AMA establishes Committee on Geriatrics to outline basic problems of aging and how to deal with them

1954–1955

Council on Foods & Nutrition discontinues Seal of Acceptance program and focuses efforts on providing nutritional information to the profession and the public

1955

Archives of Dermatology and Syphilology becomes *Archives of Dermatology*

AMA supports a 5-year program for states to improve mental health care

AMA approves extension of Water Pollution Act and programs to eliminate air pollution

1956

AMA declares alcoholism an illness

AMA Council on Pharmacy and Chemistry becomes Council on Drugs

1957

The AMA Council on Medical Education convenes discussions that lead to the formation of the Educational Council (now the Commission) for Foreign Medical Graduates

1958

American Medical Association News begins publication

1959

Archives of Neurology and Psychiatry splits to become two separate journals: *Archives of Neurology* and *Archives of General Psychiatry*

1960

AMA recommends a nationwide vaccination program against polio using the Sabin oral vaccine

AMA states that a blood alcohol level of 0.1% should be accepted as prima facie evidence of alcohol intoxication

AMA develops national policy on health care for older patients

AMA Archives is established to preserve AMA historical documents and serve as a resource center

1961

The American Medical Political Action Committee

(AMPAC) is formed to represent physicians' and patients' interests in health care legislation

AMA takes responsibility for updating *Standard Classification of the Nomenclature of Disease*

AMA establishes Continuing Education Advisory Committee to develop standards and mechanisms for the evaluation and accreditation of all programs of continuing medical education

1962

Dr Edward Annis gives speech in Madison Square Garden, in response to President John F. Kennedy's speech on Medicare delivered in the same location

AMA publishes the first edition of the *Style Book;* this becomes *the American Medical Association Manual of Style* in 1989

AMA holds the first National Congress on Mental Health

AMA establishes Committee on Medicine and Religion to encourage communication between physicians and clergy on the most effective care of patients

1963

AMA publishes first edition of *Current Medical Terminology,* a system of preferred and supplementary terms and descriptors for diseases

AMA Council on Medical Education and Hospitals becomes Council on Medical Education

AMA establishes the Committee on Environmental Health

1964

AMA adopts a report on the hazards of cigarette smoking

1965

AMA scientific meeting has largest attendance and is referred to by the *New York Daily News* as the "Biggest Doc Bash Ever"

AMA adopts a statement recognizing the dangers of air pollution and provides a medical basis for governmental action

AMA holds the first of seven Western Hemisphere Nutrition Congresses

AMA News becomes weekly publication

AMA membership exceeds 200,000

1966

AMA publishes first edition of *Current Procedural Terminology (CPT),* a system of standardized terms for medical procedures used to facilitate documentation

AMA encourages physicians to promote exercise as a means to better health

1966–1975

AMA organizes and administers Vietnam Medical School Project

1967–1973

AMA coordinates Volunteer Physicians for Vietnam program

The United States Adopted Names Council is established to determine nonproprietary designations for chemical compounds

1968

AMA Physician's Recognition Award program is established, providing certificates to physicians who qualify by completing required amounts of continuing education

AMA adopts a statement on infant mortality with 14 recommendations for reducing the infant mortality rate in the United States

1969

American Medical Association News becomes *AMNews*

1970

AMA urges the FAA to require all airlines to separate nonsmokers from smokers

AMA Center for Health Services Research and Development is established

AMA opens membership to osteopaths

1971

AMA creates Department of Field Service with 12 regional offices to provide on-site assistance to state and county offices

AMA publishes the first *Guides to the Evaluation of Permanent Impairment*

First edition of *AMA Drug Evaluations* published, a source of comparative evaluative information on drug therapy

AMA adopts report to Board of Trustees reviewing changes needed to increase the number of women physicians

1972

AMA opens membership to students and residents

AMA launches war on smoking, urging the government to reduce and control the use of tobacco products and supporting legislation prohibiting the disbursement of samples of tobacco

Liaison Committee on Graduate Medical Education established to accredit residency programs

1973

AMA urges physicians to cooperate in a national program to combat hypertension

1975

AMA establishes a National Commission on the cost of medical care

Woman's Auxiliary to the AMA becomes the AMA Auxiliary

AMA adopts resolution opposing sex discrimination in medical institutions

1976

AMA Section on Medical Schools established

AMA encourages handicapped access to public facilities

AMA endorses and encourages establishment of a permanent Office of Surgeon General of the US Public Health Service

1977

Liaison Committee on Continuing Medical Education established to accredit continuing medical education courses

AMA sponsors first meeting of the Resident Physicians Section

1978

AMA supports state legislation mandating the use of seat belts and other protective restraints for infants and children

AMA reorganizes House of Delegates to include representatives of national medical specialty societies

AMA develops national policy endorsing hospice care to enable the terminally ill to die in a more homelike environment

1980

AMA establishes the Medical Student Section

AMA launches the French edition of *JAMA*, the first of 28 international editions of the *Journal* established between 1980 and 1996

AMA holds first Health Reporting Conference

AMA Council on Medical Service issues a report on the impact of health maintenance organizations on quality, access, and costs of care

1981

AMA holds first annual Science Reporters Conference

Accreditation Council for Graduate Medical Education replaces Liaison Committee on Graduate Medical Education

AMA recommends that current studies on the effects of "Agent Orange" and dioxin be expanded and that all physicians be alerted to symptoms of exposure

Accreditation Committee for Continuing Medical Education replaces Liaison Committee on Continuing Medical Education

1982

George Lundberg begins serving as editor-in-chief of *JAMA* and Scientific Publications

AMA encourages each state medical society to seek and support legislation to raise the legal drinking age to 21

AMA Consumer Publishing program begins with the first edition of *AMA Family Medical Guide*, published by Random House

AMA initiates the Health Policy Agenda for the American People, with a 28-member steering committee

AMA

representing various health, business, and consumer organizations (which led up to Health Access America)

AMA adopts resolution calling for increased representation among women and minority physicians

American Medical Radio News begins

1983

AMA organizes Hospital Medical Staff Section, later renamed Organized Medical Staff Section

AMA urges a smoke-free society by the year 2000

AMA membership exceeds 250,000

AMA and the Health Care Financing Administration (HCFA) sign an agreement requiring the use of CPT in federal programs for the reporting of physicians' services, as part of the administration's common procedural coding system (HCPCS). Subsequently, HCFA in 1986 extends the requirement to state medical agencies using the Medicaid Management Information System

1984

AMA provides diagnostic and treatment guidelines for cases involving child abuse and neglect

1985

Judicial Council becomes Council on Ethical and Judicial Affairs

AMA encourages continuing research and studies concerning AIDS

AMA requests adequate government funding for research on AIDS

AMA calls for ban on all tobacco advertising and supports passage of legislation prohibiting smoking on public transportation

1986

AMA passes resolution opposing acts of discrimination against AIDS patients and any legislation that would lead to such categorical discrimination or that would involve patient-physician confidentiality

AMA Board of Trustees establishes the Medical School Visitation Program

AMA establishes the Young Physicians Section

AMA establishes an initiative to improve adolescent health

AMA publicizes and recommends the incorporation of CPR classes in secondary schools

AMA provides professional guidelines relating to a physician's personal, clinical, and public conduct relating to AIDS

AMA adopts policy prohibiting investment of AMA funds in tobacco stocks and urging medical schools and parent universities to eliminate investments in corporations that produce or promote use of tobacco

1987

AMA outlines a comprehensive approach for the prevention and control of AIDS and adopts an AIDS public awareness and information program

AMA establishes Department of Adolescent Health

AMA helps initiate the Surgeon General's workshop on Self-care and Public Health

AMA urges physicians to refer women for mammograms

In *School Board of Nassau County v Gene H. Arline*, US Supreme Court rules that individuals with infectious diseases are considered "handicapped" under antidiscrimination laws, protecting their employment under certain circumstances, as outlined in a friend-of-the-court brief provided by the AMA

AMA urges residency programs to revise requirements to reduce stress and fatigue caused by long hours and to increase supervision of residents

The Joint Commission on the Accreditation of Hospitals becomes the Joint Commission on the Accreditation of Healthcare Organizations

1988

AMA launches the Chinese edition of *Archives of Ophthalmology*, the first of 19 international editions of AMA specialty journals established between 1988 and 1996

AMA publishes and disseminates 420,000 copies *of HIV Blood Test Counseling: AMA Physician Guidelines*

AMA establishes Office of HIV/AIDS

AMA establishes Department of Geriatric Health

AMA works with the Educational Commission for Foreign Medical Graduates to establish the International Medical Scholars Program, to assist foreign physicians to gain access to educational opportunities in the United States

1989

AMA develops National HIV Policy reiterating physicians' ethical responsibility to treat HIV patients whose condition is within the physicians' realm of competence

AMA recommends confidential HIV testing be readily available to all who wish to be tested

AMA establishes the *JAMA* Journal Club, as a means of earning credit toward the Physician's Recognition Award for continuing education completed

AMA files brief on behalf of Cruzan family in US Supreme Court case *Cruzan v Missouri Department of Health;* AMA holds that the guardian has a right to refuse medical treatment for a patient in a persistent vegetative state. Court later rules that states have the right to regulate food withdrawal

AMA Encyclopedia of Medicine is published by Random House

1990

AMA moves into new building at 515 N State St, Chicago, Ill

AMA publishes *America's Adolescents: How Healthy Are They?*

AMA publishes *HIV Early Care: AMA Physician Guidelines* and disseminates to 350,000 physicians

AMA launches corporate identity program

AMA adopts guidelines governing gifts to physicians from industry

AMA Fellowship Residency Electronic Interactive Data Access System (FREIDA) describing residency programs in the United States is available in electronic form

1991

AMA proposes reform of the US health care system (Health Access America) to include expansion of health insurance coverage

AMA launches campaign against family violence

1992

Archives of Family Medicine founded

AMA calls on tobacco companies to refrain from engaging in advertising practices that target children

AMA adopts a recommendation from the Council on Medical Education that continued federal funding should be available for graduate medical education

AMA Council on Medical Education and Council on Medical Service submit a joint report to House of Delegates identifying major barriers to adequate health care for the inner-city poor and present recommendations for addressing the problems

1993

AMA Auxiliary becomes Alliance

AMA passes resolution declaring physician-assisted suicide is fundamentally inconsistent with the physician's professional role

AMA Council on Medical Education recommends multifaceted approach to encourage student and physician interest in primary care

1994

American Journal of Diseases of Children becomes *Archives of Pediatrics and Adolescent Medicine*

AMA drafts the Patient Protection Act, elements of which were included in every health system reform bill reported out of committee in both the House and Senate

AMA Physician's Recognition Award for completing continuing education is extended to appropriately licensed physicians in Mexico

Commission on Accreditation of Allied Health Education Programs succeeds AMA Committee on Allied Health Education and Accreditation

AMA Council on Medical Education and Council on Long Range Planning and Development submit report analyzing physician work-force planning strategies in light of the impact of health system reform on medical education and academic medical centers

1995

AMA launches grassroots campaign for professional liability reform

AMA drafts the Patient Protection Act II bill with two goals: protection for patients through increased disclosure requirement and managed care fairness; and physicians' need to have defined rights and protections from arbitrary separation from managed care plans

AMA launches its Website on the Internet, featuring highlights of *JAMA*, the specialty journals, *American Medical News*, and other AMA news of interest

JAMA publishes historic issue with six articles examining tobacco industry through corporate documents of Brown and Williamson Tobacco Company

1996

AMA Fellowship Residency Electronic Interactive Data Access System (FREIDA) describing residency programs in the United States goes online

Online CME Locator is launched by the AMA, featuring more than 2000 Category 1 activities sponsored by accredited providers

AMA, with the American College of Physicians and American College of Surgeons, begins campaign to promote organ and tissue donation for transplantation

AMA House of Delegates gives a voting seat to three organizations with long-time observer status in the House: National Medical Association, American Medical Women's Association, and the American Osteopathic Association

AMA establishes a section for International Medical Graduates with a voting seat in the House

1997

AMA celebrates the sesquicentennial of its founding

AMA launches the American Medical Accreditation Program to reassert the AMA's historic role as the rightful arbiter of physician quality

AMA offers Congress a reform plan to save Medicare for today's seniors and tomorrow's children

AMA establishes the National Patient Safety Foundation to fund research into ways to reduce medical errors and make health care delivery safer

To expand and enhance its role as the voice of professionalism and ethics for the nation's physicians, AMA establishes the Ethics Institute

(CARE-1997)

AMA American Medical Association Presidents 1847-1998

1847

47-48 Nathaniel Chapman—University of Edinburgh (Great Britain)

48-49 Alexander H. Stevens—University of Pennsylvania

49-50 John C. Warren—Harvard University

50-51 Reuben D. Mussey—Medical Institute of Dartmouth College

51-52 James Moultrie—University of Pennsylvania

52-53 Beverly R. Wellford—University of Maryland

53-54 Jonathan Knight—Yale College

54-55 Charles A. Pope—University of Pennsylvania

55-56 George B. Wood—University of Pennsylvania

56-57 Zina Pitcher—Middlebury College, Vermont

57-58 Paul F. Eve—University of Pennsylvania

58-59 Harvey Lindsly—Columbian Medical College

59-60 Henry Miller—Transylvania University

60-61 Eli Ives—Yale College

61-62 No Session Held

62-63 No Session Held

63-64 Alden March—Brown University, Providence, Rhode Island

64-65 Nathan Smith Davis—College of Physicians and Surgeons of Western New York at Fairfield

65-66 Nathan Smith Davis—College of Physicians and Surgeons of Western New York at Fairfield

66-67 D. Humphreys Storer—Harvard College

67-68 Henry F. Askew—University of Pennsylvania

68-69 Samuel D. Gross—Jefferson Medical College

69-70 William O. Baldwin—Transylvania University

70-71 George Mendenhall—University of Pennsylvania

71-72 Alfred Stille—University of Pennsylvania

72-73 David Wendell Yandell—University of Louisville

73-74 Thomas Muldrop Logan—Medical College of South Carolina

74-75 Joseph Meredith Toner—Vermont Medical College

75-76 William K. Bowling—Ohio Medical College

76-77 James Marion Sims—Jefferson Medical College

77-78 Henry I. Bowditch—Harvard Medical College

78-79 Tobias G. Richardson—University of Louisville

79-80 Theophilus Parvin—University of Pennsylvania

80-81 Lewis Albert Sayre—College of Physicians and Surgeons, Columbia University

81-82 John Thompson Hodgen—University of Missouri at St Louis

82-83 Joseph J. Woodward—University of Pennsylvania

83-84 John Light Atlee—University of Pennsylvania

84-85 Austin Flint—Harvard Medical College

85-86 Henry Frazer Campbell—Medical College of Georgia

86-87 William Brodie—College of Physicians and Surgeons, Columbia University

87-88 Elisha Hall Gregory—St Louis University

88-89 Alexander Y. P. Garnett—University of Pennsylvania

89-90 William Wirt Dawson—Medical College of Ohio

90-91 Edward Mott Moore—University of Pennsylvania

91-92 William T. Briggs—Transylvania University

92-93 Henry Orlando March—Harvard Medical College

93-94 Hunter Holmes McGuire—Winchester Medical College

94-95 James Farquhar Hibberd—College of Physicians and Surgeons, Columbia University

95-96 Donald MacLean—University of Edinburgh

96-97 Richard Beverly Cole—Jefferson Medical College

97-98 Nicholas Senn—Chicago Medical College (Northwestern University Medical School)

98-99 George M. Sternberg—College of Physicians and Surgeons, Columbia University

99-00 Joseph M. Mathews—University of Louisville

1900

00-01 William Wilson Keen—Jefferson Medical College

01-02 Charles Alfred L. Reed—Cincinnati College of Medicine

02-03 John Allen Wyeth—University of Louisville Medical School

03-04 Frank Billings—Chicago Medical School (Northwestern University Medical School)

04-05 John Herr Musser—University of Pennsylvania

05-06 Lewis Samuel McMurtry—Tulane University

06-07 William James Mayo—Indiana Medical College of LaPorte/University of Missouri

07-08 Joseph Decatur Bryant—Bellevue Hospital Medical College

08-09 Herbert Leslie Burrell—Harvard Medical School

09-10 William C. Gorgas—Bellevue Medical College

10-11   William Henry Welch—College of Physicians and Surgeons in New York

11-12   John Benjamin Murphy—Rush Medical College (Chicago)

12-13   Abraham Jacobi—University of Bonn (Germany)

13-14   John A. Witherspoon—University of Pennsylvania

14-15   Victor C. Vaughan—University of Michigan

15-16   William Lewis Rodman—Kentucky Military Institute

16-   Albert Vander Veer—Columbian Medical College (George Washington University)

16-17   Rupert Blue—University of Maryland

17-18   Charles Horace Mayo—Chicago Medical College (Northwestern University)

18-19   Arthur Dean Bevan—Rush Medical College (Chicago)

19-20   Alexander Lambert—College of Physicians and Surgeons, Columbia University

20-21   William C. Braisted—College of Physicians and Surgeons, Columbia University

21-22   Hubert Work—University of Pennsylvania

22-23   Geo. E. De Schweinitz—University of Pennsylvania

23-24   Ray Lyman Wilbur—Cooper Medical College of San Francisco

24-25   William Allen Pusey—Medical College of New York University

25-26   William D. Haggard—University of Tennessee Medical Department

26-27   Wendell C. Phillips—University Medical College of New York

27-28   Jabez North Jackson—University Medical College of Kansas City

28-29   William Sydney Thayer—Harvard Medical School

29-30   Malcom LaSalle Harris—Rush Medical College (Chicago)

30-31   William Gerry Morgan—University of Pennsylvania

31-32   Edward Starr Judd—University of Minnesota School of Medicine

32-33   Edward Henry Cary—Bellevue Hospital Medical College

33-34   Dean DeWitt Lewis—Rush Medical College (Chicago)

34-35   Walter L. Bierring—University of Iowa at Iowa City

35-36   James S. McLester—University of Virginia

36-   James Tate Mason—University of Virginia Medical School

36-   Charles Gordon Heyd—University of Buffalo

37-38   John H. J. Upham—University of Pennsylvania

38-39   Irvin Abell—Louisville Medical College

39-40   Rock Sleyster—University of Illinois School of Medicine

40-41   Nathan B. Van Etten—Bellevue Hospital Medical School

41-42   Frank H. Lahey—Harvard University Medical School

42-43   Fred Wharton Rankin—University of Maryland Medical School

43-44   James Edgar Paullin—Johns Hopkins University School of Medicine

44-45   Herman L. Kretschmer—Northwestern University/Marquette University

45-46   Roger Irving Lee—Harvard Medical School

46-47   Harrison H. Shoulders—Nashville Medical College

47-48   Edward L. Bortz—Harvard Medical School

48-49   R. L. Sensenich—Rush Medical School

49-50   Ernest E. Irons—Rush Medical School

50-51   Elmer L. Henderson—University of Louisville Medical School

51-52   John W. Cline—Harvard Medical School

52-53   Louis H. Bauer—Harvard Medical School

53-54   Edward J. McCormick—St Louis University

54-55   Walter B. Martin—Johns Hopkins University School of Medicine

55-56   Elmer Hess—University of Pennsylvania

56-57   Dwight H. Murray—Indiana University School of Medicine

57-58   David B. Allman—Jefferson Medical College of Philadelphia

58-59   Gunnar Gundersen—Columbia University

59-60   Louis M. Orr—Emory University Medical School

60-61   E. Vincent Askey—University of Pennsylvania

61-62   Leonard W. Larson—University of Minnesota School of Medicine

62-63   George M. Fister—Rush Medical School

63-64   Edward R. Annis—Marquette University School of Medicine

64-65   Norman A. Welch—Tufts College Medical School

       Donovan F. Ward—University of Iowa College of Medicine

65-66   James Z. Appel—University of Pennsylvania

66-67   Charles L. Hudson—University of Michigan

67-68   Milford O. Rouse—Baylor University Medical School

AMA

AMA

68-69	Dwight L. Wilbur—University of Pennsylvania
69-70	Gerald D. Dorman—Columbia University
70-71	Walter C. Bornemeier—Northwestern University
71-72	Wesley W. Hall—Tulane University
72-73	C. A. Hoffman—University of Cincinnati
73-74	Russell B. Roth—Johns Hopkins University School of Medicine
74-75	Malcolm C. Todd—Northwestern University
75-76	Max H. Parrott—University of Oregon
76-77	Richard E. Palmer—George Washington University
77-78	John H. Budd—Dalhousie University of Halifax, Nova Scotia
78-79	Tom E. Nesbitt—University of Texas, Southwestern—Dallas
79-80	Hoyt Gardner—University of Louisville
80-81	Robert B. Hunter—University of Pennsylvania
81-82	Daniel T. Cloud—University of Illinois
82-83	William Y. Rial—University of Pittsburgh
83-84	Frank J. Jirka, Jr—University of Illinois
84-85	Joseph F. Boyle—Temple University
85-86	Harrison L. Rogers—Emory University
86-87	John J. Coury—Case Western Reserve University
87-88	William S. Hotchkiss—University of Texas—Galveston
88-89	James E. Davis—University of Pennsylvania
89-90	Alan R. Nelson—Northwestern University
90-91	C. John Tupper—University of Nebraska
91-92	John J. Ring—Georgetown University
92-93	John L. Clowe—Albany Medical College
93-94	Joseph T. Painter—University of Texas—Galveston
94-95	Robert E. McAffee—Tufts University School of Medicine
95-96	Lonnie R. Bristow—New York University College of Medicine
96-97	Daniel H. Johnson, Jr—University of Texas—Galveston
97-98	Percy Wootton—Medical College of Virginia

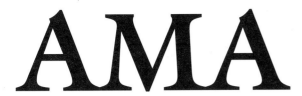

Business and Management Support Services

Publishing and Multimedia
- *JAMA*
- *American Medical News*

Multimedia Development

Business Services

Database Products and Licensing

Management Support Services
- Information Technology Steering Committee
- Information Resources (CIO)
- Corporate Services
- AMA Archives
- Marketing
- Financial Services

AMA Affiliates

The Business and Management Support Services oversee the AMA's activities in its four major revenue business areas, Publishing and Multimedia, Database Products and Licensing, Books and Products, and Investment and Real Estate. The consolidation of these activities in the Group allows for business expertise to be applied to all revenue-generating and support activities of the Association. All management support areas—including Corporate Services, Financial Services, Marketing, and Information Resources—are a part of this area. Also included in the broader definition of the AMA's businesses are its for-profit subsidiaries, AMA Solutions, Inc, and the AMA Insurance Agency, Inc, which administratively fall here as well.

Publishing and Multimedia

Publishing

The Publishing Group provides for the production, distribution, and financial support of three core businesses: *JAMA*, the Archives specialty journals, and *American Medical News* (*AMNews*). *JAMA* and *AMNews* are provided to members as a benefit of membership, generate nondues revenues, and provide the AMA with a global opportunity to promote the art and science of medicine.

Contact for author or multiple copies of reprints (ie, copies of articles from AMA periodicals on high-quality stock): 312 464-2123.

AMA Office of Permissions
Permission to use materials published in AMA journals in secondary materials is required. Permissions are not granted over the phone. Written requests to use AMA journal material should be sent to:

AMA Office of Permissions, 515 N State St, Chicago, IL 60610; Fax 312 464-5832

JAMA and Scientific Publications
With a worldwide audience of more than 2 million recipients in 146 countries and in 12 languages, the journals of the American Medical Association—the weekly *JAMA* and nine monthly specialty journals—seek to fulfill their goals of publishing peer-reviewed clinical and investigative articles in major medical disciplines, providing continuing education for physicians, offering a forum for debate on controversial issues that affect medicine, as well as informing readers about nonclinical aspects of medicine.

AMA

JAMA Instructions for Authors

Manuscript Criteria and Information

JAMA 1997 Jan 1; 277(1): 74-75

JAMA is an international, peer-reviewed, general medical journal, with simultaneous printing in the United States and United Kingdom, distribution to readers in more than 148 countries, and 22 separate international editions published in 11 languages.

Manuscript submission

All manuscripts should be sent to the Editor, George D. Lundberg, MD, *JAMA*, 515 N State St, Chicago, IL 60610, USA; telephone: 312 464-2402; fax: 312 464-5824; e-mail: JAMAms@ama-assn.org.

Manuscripts are considered with the understanding that they have not been published previously in print or electronic format and are not under consideration by another publication or electronic medium. A complete report following presentation or publication of preliminary findings elsewhere (eg, in an abstract) can be considered. Include copies of possibly duplicative material that has been previously published or is currently being considered elsewhere.[1] Authors submitting manuscripts or letters to the editor regarding adverse drug or medical device reactions, reportable diseases, and the like should also report such to the relevant government agency.

Electronic submission

Short manuscripts that do not contain tables or figures and letters to the editor may be submitted via e-mail. Send letters to JAMA-letters@ama-assn.org (see instructions below). Send short manuscripts to JAMAms@ama-assn.org. All manuscripts sent via e-mail must be copied and embedded in the actual e-mail message. Do not send attachments.

Categories of articles

JAMA publishes original contributions, review articles, brief reports, special communications, commentaries, letters to the editor, and many other categories of articles. Topics of interest include all subjects that relate to the practice of medicine and the betterment of public health worldwide. The most frequent categories of articles are described below.

Original Contributions—Randomized controlled trials (see specific instructions), intervention studies, studies of screening and diagnostic tests, outcome studies, cost-effectiveness analyses, case-control series, and surveys with high response rates. Each manuscript should clearly state an objective or hypothesis; the design and methodology (including the study's setting and time period, patients or participants with inclusion and exclusion criteria, or data sources and how these were selected for the study); the essential features of any interventions; the main outcome measures; the main results of the study; a discussion placing the results in the context of published literature; and the conclusions. For more information, see Instructions for Preparing Structured Abstracts. Typical length: 8 to 20 double-spaced manuscript pages (not including tables, figures, and references).

Reviews—Systematic critical assessments of literature and data sources pertaining to clinical topics, emphasizing factors such as cause, diagnosis, prognosis, therapy, or prevention. All articles and data sources reviewed should include information about the specific type of study or analysis, population, intervention, exposure, and tests or outcomes. All articles or data sources should be selected systematically for inclusion in the review and critically evaluated, and the selection process should be described in the paper. Meta-analyses also will be considered as reviews. Review papers that do not meet these criteria will not be accepted. For more information, see Instructions for Preparing Structured Abstracts. Typical length: 15 to 20 double-spaced manuscript pages (not including tables, figures, and references).

Brief Reports—Short reports of original studies or evaluations. We will also consider clinical cases (individual or a series), but they must be unique, first-time reports. Individual case reports are rarely accepted for publication. Typical length: 3 to 9 double-spaced manuscript pages (not including tables, figures, and references).

Letters to the Editor—Letters discussing a recent *JAMA* article are welcome. They should be received within 4 weeks of the article's publication and can be faxed to the editorial office in Chicago at 312 464-5824 or sent via e-mail to JAMA-letters@ama-assn.org. Please also send a hard copy by surface mail. Free-standing original letters that do not refer to a *JAMA* article also are welcome. All letters should be typewritten, double-spaced, and should not exceed 500 words of text and 5 references.

Criteria for manuscript acceptance

Manuscripts submitted to *The Journal* should meet the following criteria: the material is original; the writing is clear; the study methods are appropriate; the data are valid; the conclusions are reasonable and supported by the data; the information is important; and the topic has general medical interest. From these basic criteria, we assess a paper's eligibility for publication. We receive approximately 4000 papers each year, but publish only about 11% of unsolicited manuscripts. Because of this competition for space in *The Journal*, we advise authors to follow these instructions and to keep papers as brief as possible while still meeting the quality criteria described above.

Authorship information

Designate one author as correspondent and provide a complete address, telephone number, and fax number. Manuscripts should have no more than six authors; a greater number requires justification. Authors may add a publishable footnote explaining order of authorship.[2,3]

Group Authorship. If authorship is attributed to a group (either solely or in addition to one or more individual authors), all members of the group must meet the full criteria and requirements for authorship described in the following paragraphs. One or more authors may take responsibility "for" a group, in which case the other group members are not authors, but may be listed in an acknowledgment.[3]

Authorship Requirements. With the cover letter include (1) statement on authorship criteria and responsibility and (2) statement on financial disclosure and (3) one of the two statements on copyright or federal employment. Each of these three statements must be read and signed by all authors.[4] (See form that follows.)

1. *Authorship criteria and responsibility*. All persons who meet the *JAMA* criteria for authorship are listed as authors, and all authors certify that they meet the following criteria: "I have participated sufficiently in the conception and design of this work or the analysis and interpretation of the data (when applicable), as well as the writing of the manuscript, to take public responsibility for it. I believe the manuscript represents valid work. I have reviewed the final version of the submitted manuscript and approve it for publication. Neither this manuscript nor one with substantially similar content under my authorship has been published or is being considered for publication elsewhere, except as described in an attachment. If requested, I shall produce the data upon which the manuscript is based for examination by the editors or their assignees."

2. *Financial disclosure*. "I certify that any affiliations with or involvement in any organization or entity with a direct financial interest in the subject matter or materials discussed in the manuscript (eg, employment, consultancies, stock ownership, honoraria, expert testimony) are disclosed below." Research or project support should be listed in an acknowledgment.

3. *Copyright transfer*. "In consideration of the action of the American Medical Association (AMA) in reviewing and editing this submission, the author(s) undersigned hereby transfer(s), assign(s), or otherwise convey(s) all copyright ownership to the AMA in the event that such work is published by the AMA."

Federal employment
"I was an employee of the US federal government when this work was investigated and prepared for publication; therefore, it is not protected by the Copyright Act and there is no copyright of which the ownership can be transferred."

4. *Acknowledgment statement*. The corresponding author must include the following statement in the cover letter: "All persons who have made substantial contributions to the work reported in the manuscript (including writing and editing assistance), but are not authors, are named in the Acknowledgment and have given me their written permission to be named. If I do not include an Acknowledgment, that means I have not received substantial contributions from nonauthors." (See following authorship form.) Authors should obtain written permission from all individuals named in an acknowledgment, since readers may infer their endorsement of data and conclusions.[3]

Editorial review and processing
Peer Review. All submitted manuscripts are reviewed initially by a *JAMA* editor. Those manuscripts with insufficient priority for publication are returned promptly. Other manuscripts are sent to expert consultants for peer review. Peer reviewer identities are kept confidential. Author identities are not kept confidential.

The existence of a manuscript under review is not revealed to anyone other than peer reviewers and editorial staff. Information from submitted manuscripts may be systematically collected and analyzed as part of research to improve the quality of the editorial or peer review process. Identifying information remains confidential.

Rejected Manuscripts. Rejected manuscripts will not be returned to authors unless specifically requested in the cover letter. Original illustrations, photographs, and slides will be returned.[3]

Editing. Accepted manuscripts are copy edited according to AMA style[5] and returned to the author for approval. Authors are responsible for all statements made in their work, including changes made by the copy editor and authorized by the corresponding author.

Reprints. Reprint order forms are included with the edited typescript sent for approval to authors. Reprints are shipped 6 to 8 weeks after publication.

All published manuscripts become the permanent property of the AMA and may not be published elsewhere without written permission from the AMA.

Manuscript preparation
- Manuscripts should be prepared in accordance with the American Medical Association Manual of Style[5] and/or the "Uniform Requirements for Manuscripts Submitted to Biomedical Journals."[6]
- Submit the original manuscript and three photocopies; use one side of standard-sized white bond paper and 1-inch margins.
- Double-space throughout, including title page, abstract, text, acknowledgments, references, legends for illustrations, and tables. Start each of these sections on a new page, numbered consecutively, beginning with the title page.
- On the title page, include a word count for text only, exclusive of title, abstract, references, tables, and figure legends.
- Provide copy that can be scanned by an optical character reader: no smudges or pencil or pen marks. Use only standard 10- or 12-point font size. Do not use proportional spacing; use unjustified (ragged) right margins and letter-quality printing.
- On the title page type the full names, highest academic degrees, and affiliations of all authors. If an author's affiliation has changed since the work was done, list the new affiliation as well.
- Use Système International (SI) measurements only, except when "Dual report" is indicated in the SI unit conversion table in this issue.[7]
- Use generic names of drugs, unless the specific trade name of a drug used is directly relevant to the discussion.
- Do not use abbreviations in the title or abstract and limit their use in the text.

Abstract. Include a structured abstract of no more than 250 words for reports of original data, reviews (including meta-analyses), and consensus statements. (See "Instructions for Preparing Structured Abstracts" below.) For other major manuscripts, include a conventional, unstructured abstract of no more than 150 words. Abstracts are not required for Editorials, Commentaries, and special features of *The Journal*.

Informed Consent. For experimental investigations of human or animal subjects, state in the "Methods" section of the manuscript that an appropriate institutional review board approved the project. For those investigators who do not have formal ethics review committees (institutional or regional), the principles outlined in the

AMA

Declaration of Helsinki should be followed.[8] For investigations of human subjects, state in the "Methods" section the manner in which informed consent was obtained from the subjects.

Patient descriptions, photographs and pedigrees. Include a signed statement of informed consent to publish patient descriptions, photographs, and pedigrees from all persons (parents or legal guardians for minors) who can be identified in such written descriptions, photographs, and pedigrees. Such persons should be shown the manuscript before submission.

Personal Communications. Include a signed statement of permission from each individual identified as a source of information in a personal communication, either written or oral communication.

References. Number references in the order they are mentioned in the text; do not alphabetize. In text, tables, and legends, identify references with superscript arabic numerals. When listing references, follow AMA style,[5] abbreviating names of journals according to Index Medicus. Note: List all authors and/or editors up to six; if more than six, list the first three and "et al."

Examples of reference style:

1. Lyketsos CG, Hoover DR, Guccione M, et al, for the Multicenter AIDS Cohort Study. Depressive symptoms as predictors of medical outcomes in HIV infection. *JAMA.* 1993;270:2563-2567.

2. Marcus R, Couston AM. Water-soluble vitamins: the vitamin B complex and ascorbic acid. In: Gilman AG, Rall TW, Nies AS, Taylor P, eds. *Goodman and Gilman's The Pharmacological Basis of Therapeutics.* 8th ed. New York, NY: Pergamon Press; 1990:1530-1552.

Authors are responsible for the accuracy and completeness of their references and for correct text citation.

Tables. Title all tables and number them in order of their citation in the text. Double-space each table on separate sheets of standard-sized white bond paper. If a table must be continued, repeat the title on a second sheet, followed by "(con't)."

Illustrations. Submit four sets of all illustrations: (1) 5x7-inch matte-finish (or glossy) photographs for all graphs and black-and-white photographs (computer-generated graphs produced by high-quality laser printers also are acceptable); (2) high-contrast prints for X-ray films; (3) color slides (and corresponding color prints) for color illustrations. Number illustrations according to their order in the text. Affix a label with figure number, name of first author, short form of the manuscript title, and an arrow indicating "top" to the back of the print. Never mark on the print or the transparency itself. Original illustrations, photographs, and slides from rejected manuscripts will be returned to authors.

- *Legends.* Double-space legends (maximum length, 40 words) on separate pages. Indicate magnification and stain used for photomicrographs.
- *Adapting or reprinting tables and illustrations.* Acknowledge all illustrations and tables adapted or reprinted from other publications and submit written permission to reprint from the original publishers.

References

1. Lundberg GD. Statement by the International Committee of Medical Journal Editors on duplicate or redundant publication. *JAMA.* 1993;270:2495.

2. International Committee of Medical Journal Editors. Statements from the International Committee of Medical Journal Editors. *JAMA.* 1991;265:2697-2698.

3. Glass RM. New information for authors and readers: group authorship, acknowledgments, and rejected manuscripts. *JAMA.* 1992;268:99. Correction. 1993;269:48.

4. Lundberg GD, Flanagin A. New requirements for authors: signed statements of authorship responsibility and financial disclosure. *JAMA.* 1989;262:2003-2004.

5. Iverson CL, Dan BB, Glitman P, et al. *American Medical Association Manual of Style.* 8th ed. Baltimore, Md: Williams & Wilkins; 1988.

6. International Committee of Medical Journal Editors. Uniform requirements for manuscripts submitted to biomedical journals. *JAMA.* 1993;269:2282-2286.

7. Lundberg GD. SI unit implementation: the next step. *JAMA.* 1988;260:73-76.

8. 41st World Medical Assembly. Declaration of Helsinki: recommendations guiding physicians in biomedical research involving human subjects. *Bull Pan Am Health Organ.* 1990;24:606-609.

JAMA Instructions for Authors

Instructions for preparing structured abstracts

JAMA 1997 Jan 1; 277(1): 77-83

All reports of original data, reviews, including meta-analyses, and consensus statements should be submitted with structured abstracts as described below. The following is adapted from Haynes RB, Mulrow CD, Huth EJ, Altman DG, Gardner MJ. More informative abstracts revisited. *Ann Intern Med.* 1990;113:69-76.

Reports of original data

Authors submitting manuscripts reporting original data should prepare an abstract of no more than 250 words under the following headings: Objective, Design, Setting, Patients (or Other Participants), Interventions (if any), Main Outcome Measure(s), Results, and Conclusions. The content following each heading should be as follows:

1. Objective. The abstract should begin with a clear statement of the precise objective or question addressed in the report. If more than one objective is addressed, the main objective should be indicated and only key secondary objectives stated. If an a priori hypothesis was tested, it should be stated.

2. Design. The basic design of the study should be described. The duration of follow-up, if any, should be stated. As many of the following terms as apply should be used:

a. *Intervention studies:* randomized control trial (see Glossary for the definition of this and other technical terms); nonrandomized control trial; double-blind; placebo control; crossover trial; before-after trial.

b. *For studies of screening and diagnostic tests:* criterion standard (that is, a widely accepted standard with which a new or alternative test is being compared; this term is preferred to "gold standard"); blinded or masked comparison.

c. *For studies of prognosis:* inception cohort (subjects assembled at a similar and early time in the course of the disorder and followed thereafter); cohort (subjects followed forward in time, but not necessarily from a common starting point); validation cohort or validation sample if the study involves the modeling of clinical predictions.

d. *For studies of causation:* randomized control trial; cohort; case-control; survey (preferred to "cross-sectional study").

e. *For descriptions of the clinical features of medical disorders:* survey; case series.

f. *For studies that include a formal economic evaluation:* cost-effectiveness analysis; cost-utility analysis; cost-benefit analysis.

For new analyses of existing data sets, the data set should be named and the basic study design disclosed.

3. Setting. To assist readers to determine the applicability of the report to their own clinical circumstances, the study setting(s) should be described. Of particular importance is whether the setting is the general community, a primary care or referral center, private or institutional practice, ambulatory or hospitalized care.

4. Patients or Other Participants. The clinical disorders, important eligibility criteria, and key socio-demographic features of patients should be stated. The numbers of participants and how they were selected should be provided (see below), including the number of otherwise eligible subjects who were approached but refused. If matching is used for comparison groups, characteristics that are matched should be specified. In follow-up studies, the proportion of participants who completed the study must be indicated. In intervention studies, the number of patients withdrawn for adverse effects should be given.

For selection procedures, these terms should be used, if appropriate: random sample (where "random" refers to a formal, randomized selection in which all eligible subjects have a fixed and usually equal chance of selection); population-based sample; referred sample; consecutive sample; volunteer sample; convenience sample. These terms assist the reader to determine an important element of the generalizability of the study. They also supplement (rather than duplicate) the terms used by professional indexers when articles are entered into computerized databases.

5. Intervention(s). The essential features of any interventions should be described, including their method and duration of administration. The intervention should be named by its most common clinical name (for example, the generic term "chlorthalidone"). Common synonyms should be given as well to facilitate electronic textword searching. This would include the brand name of a drug if a specific product was studied.

6. Main Outcome Measure(s). The primary study outcome measurement(s) should be indicated as planned before data collection began. If the paper does not emphasize the main planned outcomes of a study, this fact should be stated and the reason indicated. If the hypoth-

esis being reported was formulated during or after data collection, this information should be clearly stated.

7. Results. The main results of the study should be given. Measurements that require explanation for the expected audience of the manuscript should be defined. Important measurements not included in the presentation of results should be declared. As relevant, it should be indicated whether observers were blinded to patient groupings, particularly for subjective measurements. Due to the current limitations of retrieval from electronic databases, results must be given in narrative or point form rather than tabular form if the abstract is to appear in computerized literature services such as MEDLINE. If possible, the results should be accompanied by confidence intervals (for example, 95%) and the exact level of statistical significance. For comparative studies, confidence intervals should relate to the differences between groups. For nonsignificant differences for the major study outcome measure(s), the clinically important difference sought should be stated and the confidence interval for the difference between the groups should be given. When risk changes or effect sizes are given, absolute values should be indicated so that the reader can determine the absolute as well as relative impact of the finding. Approaches such as "number needed to treat" to achieve a unit of benefit are encouraged when appropriate; reporting of relative differences alone is usually inappropriate. If appropriate, studies of screening and diagnostic tests should use the terms "sensitivity," "specificity," and "likelihood ratio." If predictive values or accuracy is given, prevalence or pretest likelihood should be given as well. No data should be reported in the abstract that do not appear in the rest of the manuscript.

8. Conclusions. Only those conclusions of the study that are directly supported by the evidence reported should be given, along with their clinical application (avoiding speculation and overgeneralization), and indicating whether additional study is required before the information should be used in usual clinical settings. Equal emphasis must be given to positive and negative findings of equal scientific merit.

To permit quick and selective scanning, the headings outlined above should be included in the abstract. For brevity, parts of the abstract can be written in phrases rather than complete sentences. (For example: "2. Design. Double-blind randomized trial," rather than "2. Design. The study was conducted as a double-blind, randomized trial.") This technique may make reading less smooth but facilitates selection scanning and allows more information to be conveyed per unit of space.

Review manuscripts (including meta-analyses)
Authors submitting review manuscripts and reports of the results of meta-analyses should prepare an abstract of no more than 250 words under the following headings: Objective, Data Sources, Study Selection, Data Extraction, Data Synthesis, and Conclusions. The manuscript should also include a section addressing the methods used for data sources, study selection, data extraction, and data synthesis. Each heading should be followed by a brief description:

1. Objective. The abstract should begin with a precise statement of the primary objective of the review. The focus of this statement should be guided by whether the

AMA

review emphasizes factors such as cause, diagnosis, prognosis, therapy, or prevention. It should include information about the specific population, intervention, exposure, and test or outcome that is being reviewed.

2. Data Sources. A succinct summary of data sources should be given, including any time restrictions. Potential sources include experts or research institutions active in the field, computerized databases and published indexes, registries, abstract booklets, conference proceedings, references identified from bibliographies of pertinent articles and books, and companies or manufacturers of tests or agents being reviewed. If a bibliographic database is used, the exact indexing terms used for article retrieval should be stated, including any constraints (for example, English language or human subjects).

3. Study Selection. The abstract should describe the criteria used to select studies for detailed review from among studies identified as relevant to the topic. Details of selection should include particular populations, interventions, outcomes, or methodologic designs. The method used to apply these criteria should be specified (for example, blind review, consensus, multiple reviewers). The proportion of initially identified studies that met selection criteria should be stated.

4. Data Extraction. Guidelines used for abstracting data and assessing data quality and validity (such as criteria for causal inference) should be described. The method by which the guidelines were applied should be stated (for example, independent extraction by multiple observers).

5. Data Synthesis. The main results of the review, whether qualitative or quantitative, should be stated. Methods used to obtain these results should be outlined. Meta-analyses should state the major outcomes that were pooled and include odds ratios or effect sizes and, if possible, sensitivity analyses. Numerical results should be accompanied by confidence intervals, if applicable, and exact levels of statistical significance. Evaluations of screening and diagnostic tests should address issues of sensitivity, specificity, likelihood ratios, receiver operating characteristic curves, and predictive values. Assessments of prognosis should include summarizations of survival characteristics and related variables. Major identified sources of variation between studies should be stated, including differences in treatment protocols, cointerventions, confounders, outcome measures, length of follow-up, and dropout rates.

6. Conclusions. The conclusions and their applications should be clearly stated, limiting generalization to the domain of the review. The need for new studies may be suggested.

Consensus statements

Authors submitting manuscripts reporting consensus statements should prepare an abstract of no more than 250 words under the following headings: Objective, Participants, Evidence, Consensus Process, and Conclusions. This format should also be used to report clinical practice guidelines that were developed by consensus. While the descriptions are summarized in the abstract, they should be expanded in the text. References supporting the text should be provided. The content under each heading is as follows:

1. Objective. Describe the issue, purpose, and intended audience for the consensus statement. The issue may be framed as a series of key questions; as a targeted health problem with relevant patients and providers; or as practice options with health and economic outcomes. The purpose may be to guide clinical practice; to develop public policy; to determine whether insurance will cover innovative therapy; or to set norms for evaluating clinical performance. The audience may include primary care clinicians, specialist physicians, researchers, health planners, and/or the public.

2. Participants. Explain how people became participants (eg, selection by staff members of the sponsoring agency, nomination by supporting associations, or self-designation). Explain whether meetings were open or closed. Describe the number of participants (particularly panel members or subgroups responsible for developing the statement) and their areas of expertise. Disclose the sponsor or funding source.

3. Evidence. Describe data sources, selection, abstraction, and synthesis. (See "Review Manuscripts" for more information.) If a formal literature review was prepared, describe who wrote it and whether it was reviewed. Explain the use of unpublished data and the influence of expert opinion and comments from other participants.

4. Consensus Process. Describe the basis for drawing conclusions (some techniques involve causal pathways, decision rules, or assigning values to alternative outcomes). Explain the process by which consensus was achieved, such as voting, the Delphi technique, group meetings, or the nominal group process. Explain who wrote the statement (a single person or a writing committee); whether it was drafted before it was presented to the group or after the group had expressed its opinions; and the time during which it was written. Describe who reviewed the statement and how suggestions for revision were incorporated.

5. Conclusions. Summarize the consensus statement. Conclusions may include what benefits, harms, and costs are expected if the recommendations were implemented. Include important minority views.

JAMA Instructions for Authors

Glossary of Methodologic Terms

JAMA 1995 July 5; 274(1): 93-95

Before-after trial—Investigation of therapeutic alternatives in which individuals of one period and under one treatment are compared with individuals at a subsequent time, treated in a different fashion. If the disorder is not fatal and the "before" treatment is not curative, the same individuals may be studied in the before and after periods, strengthening the design through increased group comparability for the two periods. See also **Crossover trial.**

Blind or blinded—Masked. Unaware. The term may be modified according to the purpose of the blinding. For example, clinicians or patients can be blind to the treatments that patients are receiving and observers can be blind to each other's assessments, making their observations uninfluenced by one another (see also **Double-blind**). To avoid confusion, the term Masked is preferred in studies in which vision loss is an outcome of interest.

Case-control study (Case-referent or Case-comparison study)—Study generally used to test possible causes of a disease or disorder, in which individuals who have a designated disorder are compared with individuals who do not have the disorder with respect to previous or current exposure to a putative causal factor. For example, persons with hepatic cancer (cases) are compared with persons without hepatic cancer (controls) and history of hepatitis B is determined for the two groups. A **Case-control study** is often referred to as a **Retrospective study** (even if patients are recruited prospectively) because the logic of the design leads from effect to cause.

Case series—A series of patients with a defined disorder. The term is usually used to describe a study reporting on a consecutive collection of patients treated in a similar manner, without a concurrent control group. For example, a surgeon might describe the characteristics of and outcomes for 100 consecutive patients with cerebral ischemia who received a revascularization procedure. See also **Consecutive sample**.

Cohort—A group of persons with a common characteristic or set of characteristics. Typically, the group is followed for a specified period to determine the incidence of a disorder or complications of an established disorder (that is, prognosis), as in **Cohort analytic study** (prospective study) (see also **Inception cohort**).

Cohort analytic study—Prospective investigation of the factors that might cause a disorder in which a cohort of individuals who do not have evidence of an outcome of interest but who are exposed to the putative cause are compared with a concurrent cohort who are also free of the outcome but not exposed to the putative cause. Both cohorts are then followed to compare the incidence of the outcome of interest.

Confounder, confounding variable—A factor that distorts the true relationship of the study variables of central interest by virtue of being related to the outcome of interest but extraneous to the study question and unequally distributed among the groups being compared. For example, age might confound a study of the effect of a toxin on longevity if individuals exposed to the toxin were older than those not exposed.

Consecutive sample—Sample in which the units are chosen on a strict "first come, first chosen" basis. All individuals who are eligible should be included as they are seen.

Convenience sample—Individuals or groups selected at the convenience of the investigator or primarily because they were available at a convenient time or place.

Cost-benefit analysis—A form of economic assessment, usually from society's perspective, in which the costs of medical care are compared with the economic benefits of the care, with both costs and benefits expressed in units of currency. The benefits typically include reductions in future health care costs and increased earnings due to the improved health of those receiving the care.

Cost-effectiveness analysis—An economic evaluation in which alternative programs, services, or interventions are compared in terms of the cost per unit of clinical effect (for example, cost per life saved, cost per millimeter of mercury of blood pressure lowered, or cost per quality-adjusted life-year gained). The last form of measuring outcomes (and equivalents such as "healthy days of life gained") gives rise to what is also referred to as Cost-utility analysis.

Cost-utility analysis—See **Cost-effectiveness analysis**.

Criterion standard—Preferred term to "gold standard." A method having established or widely accepted accuracy for determining a diagnosis, providing a standard to which a new screening or diagnostic test can be compared. The method need not be a single or simple procedure but could include follow-up of patients to observe the evolution of their conditions or the consensus of an expert panel of clinicians. **Criterion standard** can also be used in studies of the quality of care to indicate a level of performance, agreed to by experts or peers, to which the performance of individual practitioners or institutions can be compared.

Crossover trial—A method of comparing two or more treatments or interventions in which subjects or patients, on completion of the course of one treatment, are switched to another. Typically, allocation to the first treatment is by random process. Participants' performance in one period is used to judge their performance in others, usually reducing variability. See also **Before-after trial**.

Dataset—Raw data gathered by investigators.

Double-blind or Double-mask—(1) Neither the subject nor the study staff (those responsible for patient treatment and data collection) are aware of the group or intervention to which the subject has been assigned. (2) Any condition in which two different groups of persons are purposely denied access to information in order to keep that information from influencing some measurement, observation, or process.

Economic evaluation—Comparative analysis of alternative courses of action in terms of both their costs and consequences.

End point—See **Outcomes**.

Gold standard—See **Criterion standard**.

Inception cohort—A designated group of persons, assembled at a common time early in the development of a specific clinical disorder (for example, at the time of first exposure to the putative cause or at the time of initial diagnosis), who are followed thereafter (see also **Cohort**).

Likelihood ratio—For a screening or diagnostic test (including clinical signs or symptoms), expresses the relative odds that a given test result would be expected in a patient with (as opposed to one without) a disorder of interest.

Masked—See **Blind**.

Matching—The deliberate process of making a study group and a comparison group comparable with respect to factors that are extraneous to the purpose of the investigation but that might interfere with the interpretation of the study's findings (for example, in case-control studies, individual cases might be matched or paired with a specific control on the basis of comparable age, gender, clinical features, or a combination).

AMA

Nonrandomized control trial—Experiment in which assignment of patients to the intervention groups is at the convenience of the investigator or according to a preset plan that does not conform to the definition of **Random.** See also **Randomized control trial.**

Outcomes—All possible changes in health status that may occur in following subjects or that may stem from exposure to a causal factor or from preventive or therapeutic interventions. The narrower term **End points** refers to health events that lead to completion or termination of follow-up of an individual in a trial or cohort study, for example, death or major morbidity, particularly related to the study question.

Primary care—Medical care provided by the clinician of first contact for the patient. Typically, the primary care physician is a general practitioner, family physician, general internist, or general pediatrician. Primary care may also be administered by health professionals other than physicians, notably, specially trained nurses (nurse practitioners) and physician assistants. Primary care is typically provided in continuity. Usually, a general practitioner, family physician, nurse practitioner, or physician assistant provides only primary care services but a person with specialty qualifications may provide primary care, alone or in combination with referral services (see also **Referred care**). Thus, it is the nature of the contact (first compared with referred) that determines the care designation rather than the qualifications of the practitioner.

Primary care center, Primary care setting—Medical care facility that offers first-contact health care only. Patients requiring specialized medical care are referred elsewhere. Some primary care centers provide a mixture of primary and referred care. Thus it is the nature of the service provided (first contact) rather than the setting per se that distinguishes primary from more advanced levels of care. See also **Primary care, Referred care, Tertiary care center.**

Prospective study—See **Cohort** and **Cohort analytic study.**

Random—Governed by a formal chance process in which the occurrence of previous events is of no value in predicting future events. The probability of assignment of, for example, a given subject to a specified treatment group is fixed and constant (typically 0.50) but the subject's actual assignment cannot be known until it occurs.

Random sample—A sample derived by selecting sampling units (for example, individual patients) such that each unit has an independent and fixed (generally equal) chance of selection. Whether a given unit is selected is determined by chance (for example, by a table of randomly ordered numbers).

Randomization, random allocation—Allocation of individuals to groups by chance, usually done with the aid of a table of random numbers. Not to be confused with systematic allocation (for example, on even and odd days of the month) or allocation at the convenience or discretion of the investigator.

Randomized trial (Randomized control[led] trial, Randomized clinical trial, RCT)—Experiment in which individuals are randomly allocated to receive or not receive an experimental preventive, therapeutic, or diagnostic procedure and then followed to determine the effect of the intervention.

Referred care—Medical care provided to a patient when referred by one health professional to another with more specialized qualifications or interests. There are two levels of referred care: secondary and tertiary. Secondary care is usually provided by a broadly skilled specialist such as a general surgeon, general internist, or obstetrician. Tertiary care is provided on referral of a patient to a subspecialist, such as an orthopedic surgeon, neurologist, or neonatologist. See also **Tertiary care center.**

Retrospective study—See **Case-control study.**

Secondary care—See **Referred care.**

Sensitivity—The sensitivity of a diagnostic or screening test is the proportion of people who truly have a designated disorder who are so identified by the test. The test may consist of or include clinical observations.

Sequential sample—See **Consecutive sample.**

Specificity—The specificity of a diagnostic or screening test is the proportion of people who are truly free of a designated disorder who are so identified by the test. The test may consist of or include clinical observations.

Survey—Observational or descriptive, nonexperimental study in which individuals are systematically examined for the absence or presence (or degree of presence) of characteristics of interest.

Tertiary care—See **Referred care.**

Tertiary care center—A tertiary care center is a medical facility that receives referrals from both primary and secondary care levels and usually offers tests, treatments, and procedures that are not available elsewhere. Most tertiary care centers offer a mixture of primary, secondary, and tertiary care services so that it is the specific level of service rendered rather than the facility that determines the designation of care in a given study. See also **Referred care.**

JAMA Instructions for Authors

Manuscript Checklist

JAMA 1997 Jan 1; 277(1):74

1. Include original manuscript and three photocopies.

2. Include statements signed by each author on (*a*) authorship criteria and responsibility, (*b*) financial disclosure, and (*c*) copyright transfer or federal employment.

3. Include statement signed by corresponding author that written permission has been obtained from all persons named in the Acknowledgment.

4. Include research or project support/funding in an acknowledgment.

5. Double space manuscript (text and references) and leave right margins unjustified (ragged).

6. Check all references for accuracy and completeness. Put references in proper format in numerical order, making sure each is cited in the text.

7. Send four sets of all illustrations.

8. Provide and label an abstract.

9. Include written permission from each individual identified as a source for personal communication.

10. Include informed consent forms for identifiable patient descriptions, photographs, and pedigrees.

11. Include written permission from publishers to reproduce or adapt previously published illustrations and tables.

12. On the title page, designate a corresponding author and provide a complete address, telephone and fax numbers, e-mail address, and word count.

Regularly appearing issues of *JAMA*

JAMA has several issues that appear regularly to address predefined needs. A brief description of each type of issue follows:

Medical Education defines the state of medical education in a given year. Sections on Undergraduate and Graduate Education, and Continuing Medical Education make up the body of the issue. Many statistical tables, appendices, and articles of topical interest add to the usefulness of this annual issue.

Contempo takes the opinions of physicians in the field to describe developments in their specialties over the previous year. Each issue varies in content, but the basic premise remains the same year to year.

Pulse is prepared by the Pulse editors and *JAMA* staff and is published monthly from September through May as a special section in *JAMA*. It provides a forum for the ideas, opinions, and news that affect medical students and showcases student writing, research, and artwork.

AMA Official Call is published semiannually after the AMA Annual and Interim House of Delegates meetings. It lists the number of representatives from state associations, members of the House of Delegates, alternative delegates, with their state or organizational affiliation, current AMA officials, and members of the councils and reference committees of the AMA.

An **Index** is published in the last issue of each volume (twice a year). This source indexes materials from that current volume, and some materials that are not included in other indexing sources, such as the Book Reviews, Poetry, and the *JAMA* covers.

Reference Directories can be found regularly in *JAMA* to aid in basic references to addresses of government and specialty organizations and meetings that are helpful to the health care professional. See the table of contents in each *JAMA* to locate the latest directory in each classification.

Meetings in the United States is published in the first issue of every month. It is a list of meetings of medical interest, with notations as to language (if not English), display of exhibits, whether the meeting is scientific or administrative in nature, and the sponsoring organization of the event. It is not intended to be a complete list and tends to cover meetings held in an approximately 6-month period.

Meetings Outside the United States is published once per volume (twice a year), and contains information similar to that of US meeting listing.

State Associations and Examinations and Licensure is published once per volume (twice a year). Phone numbers of the associations are not included, but addresses, information on each state association's annual meeting, and the chief executives' names are. Medical Specialty Board examination date information is also included.

Organizations of Medical Interest is an alphabetical listing of many specialty organizations and their addresses, including voting membership number, contact phone number, president, annual meeting date, and location, and proves to be a valuable resource to clip and keep handy.

The *JAMA* Cover

Until 1964, the *JAMA* cover simply listed the contents of each issue. For a brief history on the development the covers of *JAMA*:

Breo DM. Therese Southgate, MD—The woman behind "The Cover." *JAMA*. 1990;263:2107-2112.

JAMA Cover Essay

M. Therese Southgate, MD
JAMA. 1992 Oct 14; 268(14): 1808

Her likeness is perhaps the most instantly recognizable in all of Western painting, her portrait the most famous. It has inspired poetry, reams of prose (not always so inspired), and even other paintings. The author has been analyzed by Freud, and the relationship among painter, sitter, and sitter's husband has been speculated upon. The mysterious smile has been dissected, parodied, analyzed, and satirized. Her neck and bosom have been probed with a laser beam. She has even been criticized. Yet, after nearly 500 years she has yet to reveal her secret. All that is known for sure is that her name is Lisa di Antonio Maria Gherardine. She is 24 years old and she is the wife of the prosperous Florentine citizen Francesco del Giocondo, a man who, but for his wife, would long ago have been forgotten. In her portrait, she is known familiarly as Mona Lisa, sometimes La Gioconda. The artist is the aging, bearded Leonardo, born half a century earlier in the nearby town of Vinci (1452-1519).

As the mother of mystery, the quintessential enigma, neither the Mona Lisa nor its creator has been spared the scrutiny of the centuries. The early 20th-century French painter Marcel Duchamp, for example, put a moustache on the portrait and renamed it L.H.O.O.Q. Some thought the act (and the bawdy title) sacrilegious, others that art had at last been put in its place. Andre Salmon agreed: "[Her smile] was for too long, perhaps, the Sun of Art. The adoration of her is like a decadent Christianity—peculiarly depressing, utterly demoralizing." The sculptor George Moore said he outgrew her: "her hesitating smile which held my youth in a little tether has come to seem to me but a grimace." And Renoir was simply bored.

The 19th-century Renaissance scholar Walter Pater, on the other hand, recalls how he succumbed to her spell: "She is older than the rocks among which she sits; like

AMA

the vampire, she has been dead many times, and learned the secrets of the grave." And going back to the 16th century, while the painting was still in the state Leonardo had intended, Georgio Vasari wrote that "This figure of Leonard's has such a pleasant smile that it seems rather divine than human, and was considered marvelous, an exact copy of nature." A compliment of another sort came from whoever stole the portrait from the Louvre in 1911. It was not returned until two years later. But the sincerest judgment is from Leonardo himself. He lavished 3 years on the portrait, meanwhile relieving the tedium of the sittings by engaging, as Vasari recounts, "people to play and sing, and jesters to keep her merry, and remove that melancholy which painting usually gives to portraits." When it was finished he decided not to give it up. He kept it for the remaining 16 years of his life, even taking it with him to France, where he died in 1519 at age 67.

Millions have stood before the Mona Lisa in the Louvre, millions more have stood before it when it visited New York City and Washington, DC. Every last manifestation of Leonardo's genius has been remarked upon—from the innovative pose to the perfect hands, from the hair on the shoulder whose tendrils blend with the rocky outcropping on the left to the highlighted shawl over the left shoulder that leads to the bridge on the right, from the deepening blue as the landscape recedes into the distance to the smoky "sfumato" veil Leonardo has placed between the viewer and figure. Parallels have been drawn between woman and earth, to the female figure as generative nourished by a background that is nutritive. She has been thought to be pregnant or to be recovering from a paralysis of the facial nerve. She is thought once to have been wearing a necklace, which Leonardo removed.

There are 500 years of speculation, examination, and analyses of the Mona Lisa. Yet, in spite of the fact that the paint has been subject to age and to sometimes inept cleanings, in spite of the fact that today one can view the painting only through glass or in not-so-accurate reproductions, the fact remains that the Mona Lisa is universally recognized as a masterpiece and her author as a universal genius. Yet no one has fathomed the painting's ultimate mystery: What is a masterpiece? Perhaps that is why she still smiles.

Department of Specialty Journals

This department provides a contact at AMA headquarters for the editorial staffs of the various specialty journals, who are located across the country.

Archives Journals

Archives of Dermatology

Archives of Family Medicine

Archives of General Psychiatry

Archives of Internal Medicine

Archives of Neurology

Archives of Ophthalmology

Archives of Otolaryngology—Head and Neck Surgery

Archives of Pediatrics and Adolescent Medicine

Archives of Surgery

American Medical News

American Medical News (*AMNews*) is the Association's weekly socioeconomic newspaper that covers the social and business concerns of medicine. It aims to be first and best at interpreting for physicians what is happening and what is ahead in their profession. It provides, timely, credible, and balanced reporting on issues in medicine and health care that is unavailable in a similar format. Articles appear in four sections. The news section covers issues, events, and trends in medicine; the business section offers practice management advice and business coverage geared specifically toward physicians' concerns; the feature section includes articles highlighting people, programs, and trends that explore the personal side of medicine. The commentary section includes editorials, letters to the editor, and op-ed pieces.

As Texas editor heads *American Medical News*, former chiefs recall the paper's origin, history

Phil Gunby
JAMA 1997 Apr 16; 277(15); 1184-1187

Still thirtysomething but nearing its 40th year, *American Medical News* welcomes its seventh editor this week.

She is Kathryn Trombatore, who moves to Chicago from Texas Medical Association headquarters in Austin, where she directed the Division of Communication.

As the first editor since its founder not to come out of the ranks of *American Medical News*, she assumes responsibilities previously undertaken by a succession of Kansas newspapermen followed by the paper's first woman editor (who also was the first *AMNews* editor to hold an AMA vice presidency).

Most, if not all, encountered major challenges during their editorships. Yet Trombatore's six predecessors apparently are a hardy breed, relocated from coast to coast and remaining active in a variety of pursuits.

Trombatore also will be directing a staff many of whose alumni have moved on quietly or otherwise to major editorial, public relations, law, teaching, or other positions.

September 1958 debut

The first complete issue of the tabloid newspaper that Trombatore now will edit rolled off the press in Waterloo, Wis, September 22, 1958, as *The AMA News*, a name later changed following a public relations consultant's recommendation to *American Medical News*.

Three months earlier, a sample front page of the proposed publication was circulated to physicians attending the 107th annual meeting of the American Medical Association (AMA).

That preview page included a photo of mustached Jim Reed, editor of the Topeka, Kan, Daily Capital for 8 years, whom the AMA hired in June 1958 to start its fledgling newspaper. Physicians attending the meeting were urged to look for "the man with the mustache," share their ideas for articles, or "drop him a line when you get home."

Reed, now 81, retired for 16 years, just completing his sixth book and enjoying fishing for trout or painting watercolors in Cotter, Ark, says, "I recall that most of the physicians said, Don't let any doctors write for it."

Reed organized a staff that summer of 1958 (four reporters—two from the Topeka paper plus himself and a secretary), designed a format, and helped select the firm that still prints *American Medical News*. In his first editorial, he recalls, he wrote, "It will be the goal of the editors to pack more news of interest to MDs—today this would include DOs—into each issue of The News than can be found per minute of reading in any other package." At the time, he says, "there were more than 1000 English-language medically related publications, and the idea that the AMA could steal even more of the physician's precious reading time with a new publication was beyond the comprehension of many, including some AMA staffers."

Physicians and readers from other fields including many opinion leaders promptly embraced the biweekly publication, Reed recalls, and it "quickly became the centerpiece of AMA's public relations efforts; it took off much quicker than anyone had anticipated because we were lucky enough to have selected the right format, content, and distribution for the times."

Weekly publication begun
When Reed was promoted to AMA Communications Division director in August 1961, Robert W. Riley, managing editor of *The AMA News* from its beginning and formerly news editor of the Topeka paper, became editor. "In my time," Riley recalls, "the paper was limited to 16 pages; in recent years, a single issue sometimes has exceeded 100 pages. There were no pharmaceutical ads, there was very little medical science news, and we emphasized shortness, believing the busy physician would not read long articles."

For several months, until early 1965, Riley also was editor of what now is the Medical News & Perspectives section of *The Journal*. During his editorship, also in 1965, the paper became a weekly.

Today, perhaps surprisingly, Riley suggests that "publications like *The News* may be unnecessary within 10 years. Great changes in communication already are upon us and these will be more personalized and more direct. There may still be print communication for specific audiences but I should think it would be useful largely as a guide to and perhaps review for the electronic news programs."

Riley, now retired in Scottsdale, Ariz, in turn was promoted within AMA to assistant director, Communications Division, and Marvin L. Rowlands, the paper's managing editor and still another member of the group sometimes known within AMA's halls as "the Kansas Mafia," became editor. A graduate of the University of Kansas, Rowlands was a reporter on the Cincinnati, Ohio, *Times-Star* when hired in August 1958.

Rowlands, who retired in 1990 as senior vice president, communications, McGraw-Hill Financial Services Co, New York, NY, now lives in North Chatham, Mass. He served as editor for approximately a decade, longer than anyone else to date, and is the only *AMN* editor known to have found what looked suspiciously like a bullet hole in his office window.

Rowlands recalls that "the top priority was to produce the quality journalism that would fulfill the mandate given to me by AMA's Board of Trustees and the executive vice president, to make *American Medical News* an honest, responsible newspaper. The phrase often used was to make *AMN* the *Wall Street Journal* of medicine."

He says that "the period 1965 to 1975 was a great time to be editor of a publication and it certainly was an extraordinary time to be editor of *AMNews*. Medicine was in turmoil, as was most of the nation, and to have the opportunity to report events, issues, and personalities to the AMA's members was an exciting, stimulating responsibility."

In the more than 2 decades since then, he says, "any good publication changes over time and *AMN* has done that. I think that in the period 1965 to 1975 the editorial content had more of a hard news approach, but that may not be what is needed today."

Larry D. Boston, a newsman for some years ("Dan Rather and I were cub reporters together"), who taught journalism at the University of Kansas and had worked at AMA for the Science News Department, *The Journal's* news section, and *American Medical News*, moved from AMA's Washington, DC, office to Chicago to succeed Rowlands. Now retired in San Francisco after 13 years as director of communications for the American Academy of Ophthalmology, he sought to establish *AMNews* as medicine's most comprehensive and reliable source of news; in other words, publish a good newspaper about medicine.

"That was my only priority. If that could be established, then loyal readership, increasing advertising income, and widespread recognition of AMA's policies and programs would follow naturally."

A believable newspaper
What should be kept in perspective, Boston says, "are the enormous pressures that the AMA leadership received then and continues to receive from all quarters. Sophisticated leaders and AMA senior management wisely resisted the temptation to make the newspaper a house organ, recognizing that physicians see through mere propaganda. If *AMNews* has had any success, it is as a reliable, believable newspaper for physicians."

With Boston's departure for San Francisco in March 1982, Dick Walt, yet another Kansan, who joined the staff in September 1961 and who had been managing editor and executive editor, moved into the editor's chair and served until March 1991.

Walt, who says he "pretty much failed Retirement 101" and continues to do a lot of writing (including the text for AMA's sesquicentennial book), editing, and consulting while working on his already very good golf game in Durham, NC, says his top priority overall was "to bring *AMN* into the 20th century—in 1982, we were still writing copy on electric typewriters and faxing it to the printer. . . . There was virtually no use of color and the paper had a middle-1960s look. . . . I felt we had to become more visually appealing and reader-friendly."

Like the other former editors, Walt gives major credit for achievements during his tenure to the newspaper's staff. In addition to excellent staff, he says, "particularly in the early stages of my watch, I had 100% enthusiastic backing

AMA

from my immediate supervisor and from the AMA executive vice president. This enabled us to experiment, to change, to innovate."

Among other challenges, he presided over the introduction of computerized journalism to *American Medical News* and its move from its long-time home in the 535 North Dearborn Street building to its present 515 North State Street headquarters in 1990, as well as over a growing number of *AMN* pages and staff members.

It's important, he says, that the editor be able to protect the staff from interference by the rest of the organization and be able to balance the demands of producing a quality publication ("it is a benefit of membership and one of the AMA's most visible products") with the association's other goals.

As long as association publications continue to produce high-quality editorial content, he says, "I think the future is bright. The good ones—*AMNews* included—are widely respected in the profession and by competing media. Being part of an association enables them to ride out downswings in the advertising market better than their for-profit competitors; in upswings, there is a lot of revenue to be had."

Challenge and reorganization

Barbara Bolsen, who began as a copy editor in 1973, left for a time, then later was an *AMNews* reporter in Chicago and Washington, DC, before serving as executive editor from 1982 until becoming editor in 1991 (and later an AMA vice president), continued the newspaper's award-winning efforts. Among the challenges that she recalls was "to create an organizational structure that would allow us to focus our coverage on the issues most interesting to physicians and to accompany that coverage with clear and concise informational graphics. . . . We reorganized the reporting staff into teams focused on professional issues, the changing health system, and public health."

Now completing a master of divinity degree at Chicago Theological Seminary and teaching graduate students of Northwestern University's Medill School of Journalism, Bolsen says her priorities as editor included making *AMN* timely, readable, and credible. And she adds another goal that seems to have been shared by Reed, Riley, Rowlands, Boston, and Walt: "To make the paper the most compelling source available covering news and trends affecting physicians."

Multimedia Development

Division of Publishing & Multimedia Application Development. Past, present, and future

Lisa Smialek
AMA Reporter, April 1997, p 10

In August 1995, the AMA made a decision that would affect the way physicians (members and potential members) and patients around the world would view the AMA. It was at this time that the AMA launched its Internet Web site at: http://www.ama-assn.org.

Initially, the AMA's Web site was used strictly for AMA publications, including *The Journal of the American Medical Association* (*JAMA*), *American Medical News*,

and the *Archives*, and received approximately 5000 hits—the number of times an inquiry comes into the Web site—a day. However, in November of 1995, the AMA expanded the Web site to include information from other AMA areas. And when word of this great new vehicle spread, the Web site expanded even further. "Even people who weren't exactly sure what a Web site was wanted to get on," said Doug Stone, Director of Publishing & Multimedia Application Development.

Today, the AMA's award-winning Web site receives over 60,000 hits a day, and continues to grow. A large part of the population is looking to the AMA for all sorts of medical information. One of the current focuses for the Web site is to provide more information not only to physicians, but to patients as well. "After all," says Stone, "informed patients make better patients."

The AMA Physician Select is just one example of AMA's efforts to help patients. With information on over 650,000 licensed physicians, Physician Select is a great resource for people looking to find a new physician or information on their current physician or specialist.

The Division of Publishing & Multimedia Application Development is also working with the Science and Marketing areas on a section of the AMA's home page dedicated solely to offering information on various specific conditions. The section will start by covering asthma and migraine headaches, and will expand as time goes on.

In the future, there will be a connection between the condition-specific areas and the Physician Select, allowing a patient to not only look up information on various conditions, but also to be linked to physicians specializing in that field.

Following are just a few other things to look for on the AMA home page in the future: (1) an area for publicizing meetings or conferences, giving users pertinent information about when and where the conference is, the content of the meeting, who the speakers are, what hotels, activities, and restaurants are in the area, and eventually allowing on-line registration; (2) ordering membership, subscriptions, AMA products and more, on-line with a credit card, made possible by a secured commerce software; (3) monthly surveys to find out what people like and would like to see more of, and much much more!

The AMA hopes to have 500,000 pages viewed by October 1, 1997.

Getting on the Web

The AMA's home page is open to all units who want to relay something valuable to physicians and patients. To get information on the Web site, first contact the Division of Publishing & Multimedia Application Development. Together with the Publishing and Marketing areas, they will evaluate material prior to its being placed on the Web. Once the information has been reviewed, Stone and his staff of seven will work with text, sent in electronic format—either on disk or over e-mail—graphics, and photos, to design the pages, making sure that its appearance conforms to the AMA home page style. However, before information actually appears on the Web site, it must be coded in HTML (hypertext markup language), which tells an Internet browser what format the text and graphics should appear. Units interested in utilizing the AMA home page are encouraged to start small and periodically expand and update information—keeping their section current.

The AMA home page is a great resource for patients and physicians dedicated to their patients.

Business Services

Database Products and Licensing

Department of Physician Data Services
Physician Data Services provides physician biographies for businesses, hospitals, and others with a need for them in the form of a *Physician Profile*. A *Physician Profile* is a computerized printout of biographical information on individual physicians that is used by health care organizations to verify physician credentials. A new *Electronic Profile Option*, in which requests for profiles are submitted on disk or tape in a predetermined format, is also available for those who need information on a large number of physicians. Information on recently deceased physicians is also available through Physician Data Services.

Contact Physician Data Services at 312 464-5195.

The department services the public need, however, through the mail: To receive a free biography of an MD (the requests must be in writing), an interested party should send a stamped self-addressed envelope to:

Physician Profile
Department of Physician Data Services
American Medical Association
515 N State, Chicago, IL 60610

Related publications include:

Physician Characteristics and Distribution in the United States

US Medical Licensure Statistics and Current Licensure Requirements

Database Licensing Services
The AMA Physician Masterfile is considered to be the most comprehensive source of physician-related data in the United States. It contains names and addresses, demographics, credentials, and practice characteristics of all physicians in the United States.

The AMA is a major supplier of information to firms and institutions interested in providing goods and services to physicians and group practices. To do this, Database Licensing is responsible for releasing AMA's Physician Masterfile data to database licensees to generate revenues. Availability of the Masterfile to a wide variety of publishers and commercial and educational data users enables physicians, for instance, to receive information on continuing medical education, free current awareness periodicals called "throwaway" journals that are distributed to specialists as defined in the Masterfile, and materials on pharmaceutical and other health-related items that will assist them in the daily practice of medicine.

Department of Physician Biographic Records
The database from which mailing and subscription lists are drawn is maintained here. Physicians' address changes to the system are directed to this department.

A physician should call the department at 312 464-5153 to change his/her database record.

Department of Masterfile Information Programs
This area makes AMA data available to various health-related organizations that provide data to the AMA Physician Masterfile and others. Current and historical data are made available to meet the data needs of these organizations for health manpower planning, policy development, research studies, and other purposes.

Department of Physician's Professional Activities
Records regarding the type of practice, employment, primary, secondary, and tertiary self-designation practice specialties, and hospital and group affiliation that are used in the Masterfile are kept current by this unit. Information on the number of hours worked, routinely updated by the department, is often used as the primary basis for classifying physicians.

Division of Systems Programming
The major activities of the Division of Systems Programming are designed to ensure that all administrative and business systems are available to the AMA throughout the business day and to ensure that the corporate data are integral, secure, and accurate. The division also seeks to identify emerging business technologies and leverage them against the AMA's and Federation's growing need for information. Through expanded access to information, the AMA can better serve the Association's members and target/tailor its marketing activities and products.

Department of Library Services
The activities of the AMA Library support the needs of the profession and related fields for medical and socio-economic information. The library provides document delivery on topics in medicine from its journal and microfilm collection. The library's journal and monograph collection is made available to other libraries through established library networks.

AMA Management Support Services

The AMA's management support services provide the administrative expertise necessary to ensure the success of the AMA as a professional association and as a business. In addition to providing standard corporate support services—Financial Services, Human Resources, Corporate Services, Marketing and Information Resources—the AMA's special position as the leading supplier of physician and medical information has led to the formation of a special AMA-wide committee, the Information Technology Steering Committee, to direct the development and application of the latest electronic information systems to the AMA's business and professional activities.

Information Technology Steering Committee
Its objective is to explore the application of new technologies to existing information products and services and to the development of new products and services

AMA

that build upon the AMA's preeminent position in the medical information field. The committee also aims to apply technical solutions to certain identified business needs of the AMA.

Information Resources

This unit is responsible for developing and managing the enterprise-computing environment that supports the AMA's Information Systems. This division constructs this strategic business tool, consisting of mainframe and minicomputers, operating systems, teleprocessing systems, and data communications through planning, evaluation, hardware and software implementation and support, consultation, and other data processing services in the support of the AMA's business and publishing units. The success of the AMA is directly tied to how efficiently it manages the flow of information internally and how effectively it communicates information to its members and other constituencies. IR's objectives are to maintain AMA data collection and database management systems and to align information systems with business goals and make these responsive to the needs of users.

Corporate Services

The overall objective of Corporate Services is to ensure that the AMA's physical plant and internal support services provide a productive, efficient, and cost-effective environment for staff.

Division of Corporate Facilities

The management of the AMA's corporate facilities located in Chicago, Washington, DC, and New York is key objectives consistent with general management and administration guidelines. The primary objective is to maintain these properties in the most cost-effective manner while protecting the Association's assets and provide an attractive, comfortable, and safe environment for employees.

Division of Office Services

This area, in addition to providing high-quality, cost-effective communications systems for the AMA and all its operating units, also sees as a primary objective enhancing employee productivity and esprit de corps by providing a cafeteria and an on-site catering operation that serves refreshments at a reasonable cost in a comfortable environment. The Departments of Telecommunications, Distribution and Records Management, including the Archives, and of Reprographic Services are parts of this division.

AMA Archives

The American Medical Association Archives documents the rich history of the nation's most respected and influential medical organization. Composed of more than 50 major collections, the Archives preserves documents, photographs, films, books, memorabilia, and artifacts that cover the full range of AMA initiatives and activities from medical ethics and medical education to clinical research, public health, and scores of other professional issues.

Share the history

The Archives is more than a repository of information. It is a dynamic resource for AMA members, medical societies, and health care researchers to use for their own exploration, education, and illumination. A member or researcher may:

- Read the original 1847 *AMA Code of Ethics* advising the physician "not to abandon a patient because the case is deemed incurable; for his attendance may be highly useful to the patient by alleviating pain...and by soothing mental anguish..."
- Read the letter of an AMA volunteer physician in Vietnam in 1967, reporting "the work is hard and is continuous, however...one does not have the paperwork headaches of the United States."
- Experience the "curative" lights of the Spectro-Chrome, a quack device that promised to relieve everything from indigestion to impotence.

Highlights of the collection

Historical Health Fraud and Alternative Medicine. The nation's finest collection on medical quackery is the result of nearly 70 years of activity by the AMA's Department of Investigation. The collection contains nearly 1000 boxes of advertising pamphlets, letters, product containers, and actual equipment relating to more than 3500 practitioners, products, and businesses that the AMA investigated between 1906 and 1975. Frequently used to compare present and past quackery practices, the collection has provided vital information for countless books, papers, and documentaries.

Photographs, Memorabilia, and Other Artifacts. Used for AMA Archives exhibits at the Annual, Interim, and other selected meetings, this collection contains photographs, posters, and artifacts that tell the story of the AMA and American medicine. Artifacts range from founder Nathan Davis' microscope and 19th century surgical kits to member badges worn at Annual Meetings throughout the nation from 1898 until the late 1950s.

The extensive photograph collection records medical events and AMA activities from the late 19th century until the present and is highly utilized by members and other researchers for videos, documentaries, slide presentations, publication illustrations, and exhibits.

Rare Books and Journals. This collection contains complete sets of AMA publications, such as *Hygeia*, the consumer health magazine (1923-49), *Transactions and Proceedings of AMA meetings from 1847-present*, and the *Journal of the American Medical Association* (1883-present)—one of the few bound sets in the nation containing advertising pages that document the social side of medical history. Rare books range from Nathan Davis' 1855 *History of the American Medical Association* to the landmark *Medical Education in the United States and Canada* by Abraham Flexner (1910) to sex education pamphlets published by the AMA in 1913.

Films, Videos, and Audiotapes. Many AMA-produced films have been converted to VHS format and are available for loan. Among these is the 1962 film of Dr. Edward Annis (AMA president, 1963-64) responding in an empty Madison Square Garden to President Kennedy's Medicare speech presented in the same amphitheater. Other films include *Bac Si My*, about the Volunteer Physicians for Vietnam project (1967-73) and *Quackery*, an interview with longtime AMA Bureau of Investigation director Oliver Field, among many others. Audiotapes chronicle public health issues, graduate medical education, and the lives of well-known doctors. The most recent accession to this collection is a set of tapes documenting the Conference on Ethics and American

Medicine held in March, 1997 in Philadelphia as part of the AMA sesquicentennial celebration.

Make a contribution to history

If someone should have photographs, illustrations, rare books, medical equipment, or other artifacts that reflect the history of the AMA or American medicine in general, please call the Archives at 312 464-4083 or 312 464-4179, or write to the AMA headquarters. Contributions to the collective memory of the American Medical Association are welcome.

How to use the Archives

Whether writing an article, a paper, or book; producing a documentary film or video; or preparing slide presentation or exhibition; or simply entertaining an interest in AMA history, visitors are invited to come to the Archives at the AMA headquarters in Chicago. Hours of operation are 9 am - 4 pm, Monday through Friday. For an appointment, or schedule of reproduction and use fees, call or write:

The Archives
American Medical Association
515 N State St, Chicago, IL 60610
312 464-4083   312 464-4179   Fax 312 464-4184

AMA art collection

Under the auspices of Governance comes a unique aspect of AMA headquarters itself—a substantial art collection.

Images, in the form of words or pictures, have a profound place in our world. They are a means of communicating information, sharing ideas, storing memories, delighting us. It has been said that a picture is worth a thousand words, and if that saying is true, the AMA collection is worth volumes. As a "contemporary" collection of American art this group of drawings, paintings, photographs, prints, and sculpture reflects preoccupations and concerns of artists in the late 20th century in the United States. Within this collection are not only a range of techniques, but more importantly, a range of emotions and thoughts that mirror our contemporary world, and make comment on the culture of the current moment. Since ours is a time with a mix of thought on design, there is no one answer, direction, or point of view, and no one artist has a corner on what is correct and accepted as the sole standard of excellence. There is instead throughout the current art world, and so reflected in the AMA collection, a shared ability on the part of artists to respond artistically and intellectually to a complex world.

Like the artworks, which cover a cross section of contemporary directions, the artists, both men and women, represent a geographic cross section from all over the country. Each artist represented in the collection has established a reputation and has shown his or her work at museums and serious galleries. While the majority have solid academic backgrounds, and a knowledge of art history, individuals among the group have chosen to veer from the norms of the past. What is "pictured" is less central for artists who are interested in abstract forms or abstract ideas, such as Christian Eckhart or Marcia Hafif. Also included in the collection are artists who continue to acknowledge traditional standards and who work within established conventions: for these artists who have used recognizable imagery to create cityscapes or figure studies, such as Richard Haas or Leslie Machinest, what

is pictured is still very important. Still other artists, such as the team of Helen Mayer and Newton Harrison, have mixed a concern for science into their palette, and have turned our attention to the ecology of our planet, making what is pictured a new way of addressing serious questions of the earth's survival.

The philosophic points raised visually in AMA's artworks can be gently implied—like the dark quiet of Lois Lane's paintings, or shouted with bright energy—like the works by Nancy Graves or John Torreano. There is humor, seriousness, sheer beauty, a sense of history, even a taste for technology and mysticism in our sampling.

Since nothing is off-limits, no area of study or imagination or material, anything is possible for the artist. When at his or her best, the artist becomes the conjurer who can open up our world by offering his or her vision. Such visions can be very tied to the real, like the sculptural reliefs of John Ahearn or the landscapes of Mel Pekarsky, or they can be illusions like the drawings of Alan Saret or the recording of the real world into a more perfect world system by Matt Mullican.

To anchor this abundance of differing directions in our late 20th century, and to suggest that art has always presented many possibilities, the AMA collection includes two 19th century examples of excellence in American art: the traditional nature studies of John James Audubon and the revolutionary ornamentation of the architect Louis H. Sullivan.

(AMA Art Collection Handbook-1992)

Marketing

The primary thrust of the AMA's product marketing function is to ensure that the identified needs of AMA members and others are met with products and services that are developed, priced, promoted, and distributed according to conventional marketing standards for quality, customer satisfaction, and product performance as identified by market needs analysis. This is accomplished by providing support services such as market analysis and product planning, product development, promotional execution, customer service, and telemarketing. Critical activities include creation of a true product development process and refinement of the new fulfillment/customer service program.

Division of Marketing Operations

Several initiatives make up this division. AMA Product Marketing designs the product catalog of materials the AMA distributes. AMA Customer Services is there to help callers obtain AMA materials, check on problems with orders, begin a subscription to a journal, or order a back issue of an AMA serial publication that is no older that 18 months. As an outreach to the public, this division has developed a tool for bringing AMA products into the marketplace.

Contact AMA Subscriber Services at:
800 262-2350   312 670-7827

Books and Products

The Books and Products (B & P) business is divided into three broad product lines—professional books, trade books, and consumer retail activities.

AMA

The B & P area of Marketing is organized to:

- Develop new products and services in two major lines: (1) professional products, including reimbursement, science and statistics, legal, and managed care titles; and (2) trade products, including adult reference books and children's nonfiction.
- Develop new partnerships with retailers to distribute AMA publications and products.
- Offer discounts on AMA products and publications to AMA members as a benefit of membership.
- Resell consumer health products through a consumer catalog.

AMA Book Source is a member benefit that aids members in locating and purchasing medical books. The Book Source has more than 25,000 titles in stock and has access to most titles available in print.

Contact the AMA Book Source at:
1851 Diplomat Rd, Dallas, TX 75234
800 451 2262

Financial Services

Financial Services is responsible for the accounting, budgeting, corporate taxation, and internal audit functions of the Association. The activities of these functions include the safeguarding of Association assets through the establishment of a sound system of internal controls; providing timely and accurate financial information; ensuring compliance with generally accepted accounting principles, government regulations, and sound business practices; and establishing a financial reporting framework to allow meaningful measurement of financial performance. Efforts are directed to the continued development of the financial control process to improve investment and operating returns through the careful analysis of costs and productivity.

Editorial

Tobacco-free investing

AM News April 14, 1997 p 49

Editorials represent the opinions of the authors and *AMNews* and not those of the American Medical Association.

Mutual funds offer investors convenience combined with expert management—they make all the buy/sell decisions for you. For investors who would rather not subsidize the tobacco industry, that convenience can actually be a problem.

As an analysis conducted for the AMA last year indicates, mutual fund investors have at least a fair chance of having their money go to support tobacco companies. The look at roughly 7000 mutual funds found that 1474 held investments in any of 13 publicly traded tobacco companies. (That list will be updated soon based on first-quarter 1997 reports from funds.)

The AMA now has a way for mutual fund investors to opt out of supporting tobacco companies. The AMA's Coalition for Tobacco-free Investments is made up of 53 mutual funds that don't hold stock or bonds from any of 17 US tobacco companies. We've listed the coalition funds on this page. Others may soon be added.

To qualify for the coalition, a fund must not have any current tobacco holdings and must pledge not to purchase any. That's an important condition, because mutual funds typically revise their portfolios constantly in search of optimal returns.

To give the devil its due, tobacco funds have historically been good performers. No wonder. The nicotine in tobacco is physically addictive, an unquestionable marketing edge. Nor does it seem that they are adversely affected by having so many of their customers die young. Not so long as it's easy to hook young people and the tobacco export market is going strong.

Still, tobacco's latest legal problems appear to be taking away some of its investment luster, at least in the short term. Upon news of a recent Mississippi Supreme Court ruling allowing a tobacco lawsuit to move forward, the value of stock tobacco giants Philip Morris and RJR Nabisco Holdings each fell about 8%. The day their competitor, the Liggett Group, announced its settlement of a class action suit against it by 22 state attorneys general, Morris took a 5% drop and RJR dipped 2.3%. Who knows what damage the documents Liggett has turned over will do to the other tobacco firms?

AMA investing

As far as the funds in the AMA coalition go, to our extremely untrained eyes many seem worth a second look. Translation: There was a plus sign in front of their earnings figures. But before taking our word for it and writing a check—as with any investment—carefully read the prospectus. Note that the AMA does not endorse any investment and, of course, does not guarantee any rate of return.

While we're on the subject of disclosure, since 1986 the AMA has ordered its investment managers not to buy tobacco stocks when investing the Association's reserves and pension funds. That covers most of what the AMA has under investment. The AMA does not have the same control over the institutional funds where it has a small part of its portfolio. However, when we checked, none of those funds appeared on the list of 1474 tobacco-stock holders.

That leaves 401(k) retirement accounts individually owned by employees. As of now, employees are limited to five investment options. A small percentage of tobacco holdings has been found in one stock fund and one bond fund appears on the tobacco list (fiduciary concerns warranted the choice of the mutual funds). In order to ensure a tobacco-free retirement fund option for AMA employees, the Association will soon announce the addition of a tobacco-free mutual fund.

With that change, employees will have a choice about investing even a dime with tobacco companies. If that's an option that's important to you, the funds from the AMA's coalition at least provide some places to start.

The list of funds in the AMA's Coalition for Tobacco-free Investments can be found on the Internet at http://www.ama-assn.org/ad-com/releases/1996/tobstock.htm

A complete listing of the 1474 funds holding tobacco stocks can be found at http://www.ama-assn.org/ad-com/releases/1996/tobsmoak.htm

AMA Affiliates

The AMA serves a variety of the needs of physician members and their families through arrangements with the following groups and subsidiaries.

AMA Alliance, Inc

The American Medical Association Alliance, Inc, is a nationwide volunteer organization of 60,000-plus physicians' spouses who work to improve community health and provide support to the medical profession. As the volunteer arm of the AMA, the AMA Alliance's major focuses include promoting good health, fund-raising for medical education, and advocating sound local, state, and national health legislation.

The AMA Alliance promotes health education and services to make people aware of family violence and to provide support to its victims through a variety of initiatives:

- Four hundred programs for older Americans, including day care, educational forums, equipment loans, hospice care, meals and transportation services, and medication record programs;
- One thousand programs for children and youth on birth defects, safe babysitting, immunization, general health, sex education, teen suicide, and pregnancy
- Twelve hundred community education and service programs on such topics as AIDS, CPR, drunk driving, nutrition, organ donation, parenting, and substance abuse; 200 medical family support programs, including educational seminars and discussion groups on well-being, marriage, and the effects of health system reform;
- Four hundred safety programs to promote the use of child restraints and seatbelts, as well as home, street, and water safety;
- One hundred seventy-five screening programs for cancer, hearing, hypertension, learning disabilities, scoliosis, and vision.

Alliance celebrates 75

Lisa Smialek
AMA Reporter, July 1997 p 12

The AMA is not alone in celebrating a milestone. This year, the AMA Alliance, Inc. celebrates its 75th anniversary.

The 1997 Annual Session of the AMA Alliance, June 22-24 at the Drake Hotel in Chicago, was held to highlight the accomplishments of the past year; to develop policies on issues affecting physicians' spouses, families and communities; and to commemorate the organization's past 75 years. The session included a keynote address by Daniel H. Johnson, Jr, MD, guest speakers, including Dr Timothy Johnson, a 75th gala reception, and champagne brunch to honor past AMA Alliance presidents.

The AMA Alliance, Inc is, as its tag line reads, an organization of "physician spouses dedicated to the health of America." It is a national organization of 60,000 physicians' spouses dedicated to promoting better health, ensuring sound health legislation, and fund-raising for medical education.

In 1922, the AMA House of Delegates approved the organization of a women's auxiliary to assist the AMA in the advancement of medicine and public health. Thus, the Women's Auxiliary of the AMA was formed with 24 women from 11 states who attended their first session. The next year, 60 women from 17 states attended the annual meeting, and dues were set at $5 per state.

The Auxiliary continued to grow each year, increasing membership, forming policies and procedures, establishing relationships with other organizations, initiating community and public health programs, developing member communication, and building a strong reputation for their commitment to America's health.

In 1975, the Women's Auxiliary of AMA changed its name to the AMA Auxiliary. Almost 20 years later, in 1992, the Auxiliary once again changed its name to what it is today, the AMA Alliance, Inc.

Over the years, the AMA Alliance has been a great supporter of the AMA Education and Research Foundation (AMA-ERF) and has dealt with a great number of public health issues. Following are just a few:

- Medicare
- Children's safety
- Eldercare
- Home-centered health care
- Drug and alcohol abuse
- Dangers of smoking
- Physical fitness
- Child abuse and neglect
- Drunk driving
- Pre- and post-natal care
- AIDS health education

Perhaps one of the largest initiatives of the AMA Alliance was their 1995 launch of the nationwide SAVE Program to Stop America's Violence Everywhere. In 1996, the Alliance partnered with the AMA to launch SAVE-A-Shelter on the second annual "SAVE Today." Currently, there are more than 700 community SAVE programs across the country, fighting to end violence.

As the only national physicians' spouses organization in America today, the AMA Alliance has contributed greatly to American health in the last 75 years, and looks forward to all that lies ahead.

Resource

American Medical Association Alliance
515 N State St, Chicago, IL 60610
312 464-4470 Fax 312 464-5020
E-mail: AMAA@ama-assn.org

AMA Insurance Agency

The AMA Insurance Agency provides a full range of top-quality insurance products for physicians and their families and continues to expand and improve its range of products while making them available at competitive group rates. Some of the programs offered are intended to meet professional needs, while others are designed for the personal security needs of physicians and their families.

To contact: 800 458-5736

AMA

AMA Solutions, Inc

This program brings together sources that provide products and services that address the personal and professional needs of physicians and office-based practices. Through AMA PersonalLink, home financing opportunities, home sale and buying assistance, automobile leasing, car rental savings, student loans and student loan consolidation, credit card, and personal investment services are coordinated for optimal use by physicians.

Through AMA PracticeLink, information technology services, advice from health care consultants, educational programs, credit card acceptance capabilities, medical and office equipment services, medical, pharmaceutical, and surgical supplies, and long-distance savings can be found.

The programs offered are designed to help physicians and medical societies reduce operating expenses and remain competitive in today's changing health care environment.

To contact: 800 366-6968

Doctors Advisory Network

The Network is a national group of over 300 legal and consulting experts that provide hands-on assistance to AMA members as they respond to the managed care environment. The network includes managed care attorneys and consultants, physicians who have prospered in managed care, and experts in antitrust and practice management.

To contact the Network: 800 AMA-1066

AMA

Professional Standards

Professional Standards

Ethical Standards

Office of Quality and Managed Care

American Medical Accreditation Program

Science, Technology, and Public Health Standards

Council on Scientific Affairs

DATTA program

Medical Education Standards

Undergraduate, Graduate and Continuing Medical Education

At the AMA, the Professional Standards Group, along with Communications, identifies needs among the medical and scientific communities, channeling the AMA's resources to find effective solutions to meet those needs. This is accomplished by developing and nurturing inter-organizational and interprofessional liaisons, including those with the nursing community and other related health professions, by encouraging support for AMA policies and activities among the scientific and academic elements of the profession; and by professionally directing and administering the AMA's scientific and medical education activities.

Ethics Standards

The AMA seeks to facilitate acceptance and implementation of its ethical standards into every aspect of medical endeavors. It is clear that ethics is the pedestal upon which all of the components of quality standards rest; therefore, one of the goals of the Health Care Practice Quality Standards area is to support this initiative. Taking the lead in directing the specific interdepartmental approach toward this goal will ensure the cross-disciplinary handling of issues required.

The Ethics Institute

AMA Press Release

Chicago, March 14, 1997

AMA launches new institute for ethics

The AMA announced on Friday, March 14, 1997, that it will establish an "Institute for Ethics" that will serve as an ethical compass for the nation's medical profession.

The announcement was timed to coincide with the AMA's "Ethics and American Medicine" conference, held in Philadelphia March 14-15 in honor of the 150th anniversary of the AMA's Code of Ethics.

The new institute will provide a forum for the timely exploration and discussion of the ethical dilemmas facing physicians now and in the future. Working cooperatively with the AMA's Council on Ethical and Judicial Affairs (CEJA), the Institute will conduct research on ethics-related issues, establish practical outreach initiatives, and identify guidelines for ethical conduct in a variety of professional areas.

It will also host seminars and conferences across the country to foster open discussion

CEJA will continue to set official ethical policy and issue ethical opinions on myriad topics through the AMA's Code of Medical Ethics.

AMA To be headquartered at the AMA's Chicago office, the Institute will focus on, but not be limited to, ethical and practical issues in four major areas: end-of-life care, genetics, managed care, and professionalism. Each area will be staffed by ethics scholars and visiting fellows, each well versed in their respective area of expertise.

For more information about the Institute for Ethics, please call 312 464-4075.

The AMA gets a new code of ethics

In the celebrations that marked the centennial year 1876, medicine shared in the general self-congratulation; yet despite the rhetoric, a note of caution made itself heard. The president of the American Medical Association commented, in 1876, on the code of ethics. This he called "the best ever given for the government of medical men," and he observed that most of the members might think it "as perfect as the Decalogue, and as incapable of improvement." Nevertheless, it did not seem to work very well. Even eminent physicians, sticklers for the "inviolability of the Code," tried to find the "easiest way of getting round its provisions without a flagrant violation of them." Such physicians "feel that they are hampered by the rules that are unjust and oppressive." The code of ethics was violated every day, "not only by the rank and file, but by men high in the profession." He pointed out that sooner or later modification would be necessary to keep up with the changing times.[1]

The AMA delegates disregarded the cautionary note of their president, but some New York physicians, in their State Society meeting, took direct and forceful action that produced a major schism. The root of the problem was the consultation clause. The president of the State Society indicated, in 1881, the need for change and appointed a special committee to present suggestions at the next annual meeting.

When the committee reported in 1882, it recommended a completely new and much abbreviated code. In reference to the consultation clause, it declared, quite simply, that members of the Medical Society of the State of New York "may meet in consultation legally qualified practitioners of medicine."[2] Gone were the stipulations regarding a "regular medical education" or the disability incurred by an "exclusive doctrine." In effect, regular physicians would be able to consult freely with homeopaths. This accorded with the laws of New York, which recognized no legal distinction between homeopaths and regulars.

After the report was moved and seconded, the parliamentary maneuvers began. Dr D. B. St John Roosa (1838-1908) wanted to abolish the code entirely and substitute a simple declaration that the only ethical offenses were "those comprehended under the commission of acts unworthy of a physician and a gentleman."[3] This statement, he thought, was adequate to cover the ordinary friction of practice, for no written formula could make a man a gentleman unless he was so by nature.

The state convention thus faced three choices—the "old code," the "new code," and the "no code." Long speeches reflected the irreconcilable differences. The "no code" proposal failed to carry, so the original proposition—the adoption of a new code—was again before the meeting. After futile attempts to send the matter back to committee, or to postpone consideration, the new code was adopted, 52 to 18, more than the two-thirds majority needed.

All this took place in February 1882. Over the next several months, various medical societies and journals deplored the action.[4] When the AMA held its annual meeting in May 1882, Samuel D. Gross, unable to attend, wrote an excoriating letter. He called the action "an outrage which every member of the profession should consider as a deep personal insult, and which the Association should rebuke in a most stern and uncompromising manner."[5] Indeed, the AMA had definite retaliatory powers. It refused to seat the delegates of the State Society, so that the adoption of the new code had brought about the expulsion of the State Society from the AMA.

In the New York State Society there was now a great political activity. In the meeting of February 1883, many conservatives tried unsuccessfully to get the new code repealed, and the next year the whole situation finally boiled over. Before the state convention actually met in 1884, the supporters of the old code, who wanted to maintain affiliation with the AMA, devised a bold strategy. Since the new code had become part of the bylaws, there seemed to be little hope of mustering the two-thirds majority needed to repeal it. The supporters of the old code planned a totally new rival organization to be called the New York State Medical Association, which would reaffiliate with the AMA.

This old group code met the night before the regular State Society and unanimously passed a resolution to create this new State Association. There was a proviso that first the members should attend the Society meeting the next morning. If the Society did reenact the old code, the resolution creating the new Association would be void. The rump session was thus a threat, a saying in effect to the Society, either reenact the old code or we will form a rival association that will adhere to the old code.

The meeting the next morning was a mass of impassioned oratory, but the motion to repeal was defeated 105 to 124. As a result, the Association went ahead to complete its organization and then held its first annual meeting in November 1884.[6] For a number of years New York had two medical organizations. The "Society" was the original State organization that held to the new code and remained independent of the AMA. The "Association" was the freshly created rival that maintained the old code and affiliated with the AMA. The schism was not healed until 1903.

Of the some 5000 physicians in the state, a considerable majority probably favored the old code. The new-code adherents came mostly from New York City, while the old-code adherents were preponderantly upstate. The adoption of the new code was probably a carefully planned political group. Certainly, the total vote, 52 to 18, was extremely small considering the importance of the issue. All attempts to secure a reconsideration or to postpone definite action until the subject was referred to the grass roots were defeated. Once the code was changed it was firmly locked in. Quite probably the new-code faction had deliberately used surprise tactics to attain its objective.

A frequently voiced complaint indicted the new-code men for acting arbitrarily and not referring the matter to the AMA as a whole. The reasons for not doing so were simple. The supporters of the new code "knew the history of the American Medical Association too well to expect for a moment that it would listen to any proposition looking toward the liberalization of the profession." The "practical management and the dictation of its policy have been in the hands of one man," who used his power "as an obstacle to the scientific and political advancement of the profession."[7] The reference pointed to Nathan Smith Davis. In the meetings of the AMA he invariably opposed any liberalization and, we shall see, actual reforms took place only shortly before he died, when he was far too old to exert any further influence.

The old-code supporters charged that the drive for a new code had as its motivation the desire of urban specialists to make more money by getting referrals from homeopaths and thus tapping into their extensive practice. This charge, in any crude sense, is not tenable. Actually, the new code reflected the changing total environment. It recognized the complex interactions of emerging social, economic, and scientific factors, and of elements not operative in the 1840s, when the old code was propounded. A new era was well under way, with a broad socioeconomic base and an irresistible momentum. The proponents of the new code, aware of the coming changes, felt that the old code had outlived its usefulness, but the AMA needed 20 more years to become officially aware of the fact.

As part of their objections to the new code, the conservatives noted the sharp opposition between the homeopaths and the regulars and emphasized the total incompatibility of doctrines. "Physicians who consent to consult with persons who differ from them as light from darkness, whose views can not mingle any more than oil can mingle with water, are guilty of perpetrating fraud, and a robbery in taking a fee for it." The author later declared, "This so-called code ... encourages a spirit of lawlessness and sanctions fraud ... its adoption sent a thrill of joy through the heart of every quack in the land and gave pain to the wisest and best of our associates in the regular profession."[8]

Supporters of this attitude drew comfort from the repeated assertions that homeopaths were not "scientific," and as evidence they pointed to the extravagant claims of Hahnemann's original writings earlier in the century. Particularly objectionable was the use of incredible dilutions, often to the 20th or 30th decimal dilution. Actually, however, in the 1880s homeopathic practice was a far cry from the extravaganzas that Hahnemann had recommended 50 to 75 years earlier. A hard core of homeopaths did indeed maintain the infallibility of Hahnemann's tenets, but a strong movement of liberalization had been under way, dividing the "high-potency" faction (holding to the efficacy of fantastic dilutions) from the "low-potency" practitioners who held to modest dilutions. A physician commented in 1883 that although homeopathy still included "some so-called high dilutionists, its leaders have long since ceased to insist upon infinitesimal dosage as an essential principle of treatment."[9] The homeopaths themselves were in the throes of conflict[10] and, except for the extremists, were narrowing the differences between themselves and the regulars.

In 1878, the Homeopathic State Society indicated that their members could "make use of any established principle in medical science or any therapeutic facts founded on experiment and verified by experience."[11] The "exclusive dogma" that the AMA had condemned in 1847 was no longer exclusive. Then, too, the education of the homeopaths was approximately that of the regulars, and liberal physicians were recognizing the similarities.

For many physicians, the major objection to homeopathy was not so much the special details of its doctrines as the name, which set its practitioners apart from the regular profession. According to Austin Flint, Sr, a stalwart among conservatives, what really bothered the profession was not the special teachings of the homeopaths but their opposition to the regulars. The homeopaths were refused fellowship because of "a name and an organization distinct from and opposed to the medical profession." There would be no restriction on consultation if only the homeopaths "abandon the organization and the name."[12] Apparently, the homeopaths needed only to cease publicizing any opposition to regular medicine.

The rupture between the Society of Medicine of New York and the AMA tended to polarize the medical profession. The direct and most dramatic result of this conflict was the quarrel over the International Congress of Medicine of 1887.

An international congress, held every 3 years, had become a powerful force in promoting international communication and general good will. The eighth such congress was held in Copenhagen in the fall of 1884. A few months earlier, when the AMA met in May 1884, President Austin Flint, Sr, suggested that the ninth Congress be invited to meet in Washington, DC, in 1887. The AMA convention authorized a "committee of seven" (that actually became eight) to extend the invitation at the Copenhagen meeting. If this was accepted, the appointees would then "act as the Executive Committee, with full power to fix the time and make all necessary and suitable arrangements." The committee was empowered to add to its membership and "perfect its organization."[13] The Congress in Copenhagen accepted the invitation.

When the "original committee" (the nomenclature will prove to be important) returned to the United States in 1884, it added to itself 18 additional members; then this enlarged committee, known as the general committee, promptly set to work. It established a permanent organization, made rules for membership and selection of delegates, and set up 18 sections for the presentation of papers. Later, for each section a preliminary list of officers and council members was announced. The listings included the outstanding physicians in their respective fields, such as Francis Delafield, William Pepper, T. M. Prudden, William Welch, Christian Fenger, Reginald Fitz, George Sternberg, and James Tyson. It was truly a list to be proud of.[14]

All this vast and effective preliminary work was completed, published, and generally circulated. Then, at the annual meeting of the AMA in New Orleans (April 28-May 1, 1885), it was presented as a report. At this point

AMA

there began an episode that had a major impact on American medicine.

At the convention in New Orleans, the reactionary component of American medicine was clearly in control. When Dr John S. Billings (1838-1913), as Secretary General of the Congress, presented the report of his committee, the AMA refused to accept it. The delegates were piqued that it had already been published prior to AMA approval. Clearly, the Committee had considered itself empowered to make all arrangements, but the AMA convention thought differently. A resolution was introduced whose preamble indicated the root objections, namely, that "The committee have proceeded, *without authority from this body,* to appoint the several officers of section and committees" (emphasis added). The AMA "declined to indorse or accept these appointments."[15]

What was wrong with the appointments? In the parliamentary jockeying, before any actual resolution was passed, a substitute motion was introduced that showed the real objection. A Dr Saunders, of Ohio, proposed that the actions of the Committee, "so far as they have gone, be approved by this body, provided all new-code men be left out." This was a clear indication that the convention would not tolerate the presence, whether on the general committee or among the officers of the special section, of any physician who had rejected the AMA code and embraced the new code. This substitute motion of Dr Saunders, with its blunt statement and even more blunt implications, failed to pass, 88 to 129. There were more subtle ways of accomplishing the same end.

The AMA convention reorganized the whole mechanism for conducting the Congress. It provided for a new committee that would include one member for each state. The new general committee thus consisted of the original eight members appointed in 1884, plus 38 new men selected by the state delegations. The first general committee had become a nonentity, and the new general committee was charged to repair the work already done.[16]

Disturbed by the rapidly mounting adverse comment, the editor of *JAMA*, Nathan Smith Davis, tried to justify the actions of the convention. The original general committee, he said, had selected section officers "solely on account of their reputation at home and abroad, without regard to their membership in medical societies." As a result, the committee had included "some who have placed themselves in organizations of the profession, by openly repudiating the national Code of Ethics." The reference, of course, was to the members of the New York State Society. A second alleged error was the failure "to appreciate the importance of so distributing the officers of Sections as to represent ... the members of the profession in all the leading geographical divisions of our country."

The AMA in New Orleans had aimed "only to correct these alleged errors," and for this purpose gave the newly enlarged committee the right "to review, alter, and amend" what had already been done. This was a polite way of saying, to eliminate all heretics. The AMA had the right to alter the personnel of the committee, and the new committee, "men of sound conservative qualities ...

will be found disposed to make no unnecessary changes in the work already done."[17]

The new general committee promptly met on June 24. It did not want "to make any revolutionary or radical changes" in the appointments, and it removed "only four" of the section chairmen. Most notable was Dr Abraham Jacob of New York, the outstanding pediatrician in the United States but also a leader of the new-code adherents. The Committee also changed the rules for membership in the Congress. The American members, it decreed, "shall consist of delegates from the American Medical Association, and from Medical Societies in affiliation with the American Medical Association." As the *Medical News* commented, this reduced membership in the Congress to the constituency of the AMA.

The independent physicians began a vigorous counterattack. In Philadelphia, 29 outstanding men signed a resolution condemning the changes as "detrimental to the interests of the medical profession" and declined to hold "any office whatsoever in connection with the said Congress." The signers included such internationally recognized leaders as D. Hayes Agnew, J. M. De Costa, Louis Duhring, Samuel W. Gross, S. Weir Mitchell, William Osler, William Pepper, and Alfred Stille. In other cities, prominent physicians quickly added their remonstrances. The signatories in Boston, for example, included Henry P. Bowditch, Reginald Fitz, Francis Minot, J. Collins Warren, O. W. Holmes, David Cheever, and James C. White.[18]

JAMA reacted quite intemperately. The editor, N. S. Davis, criticized the signatories for not suggesting improvements that would have aided the committee. Had they done so, he continued, they would then have shown "more regard for the honor and interests of the profession than for their own personal prejudices and dislikes; in other words they would have acted like men, and not like half-grown school boys."[19] The implication that William Osler, O. W. Holmes, and S. Weir Mitchell were acting like half-grown school boys suggests what a raging fury must have overtaken Davis.

The New York State Medical Association—the group that adhered to the AMA code—suggested that there be two types of members: those who might take part in both the business meetings and the scientific proceedings, and those who might participate only in the scientific sessions. All voting privileges would be limited to members and affiliates of the AMA, but any physician, regardless of affiliation, could take part in the scientific sessions. *JAMA*, however, felt that all this was too cumbersome and that simpler means might guard against the admission of delegates who had "repudiated the National Code of Ethics."[20]

On September 3, 1885, the new general committee, apparently heeding the swelling protests, capitulated in regard to membership and made a simple rule: "The Congress shall consist of members of the regular profession of medicine," with no mention of adherence to the AMA or its code of ethics.[21] Then the Committee, having already driven away the leaders in American medicine, tried to woo back some of the prominent men who had previously been dismissed or who had refused to participate. The attempt to bring back the dissidents as officers of the Congress was not successful.

Nevertheless, by early 1886 the excitement was pretty well over. The Committee did put together a list of appointments. Austin Flint, who had been president of the Congress, died, and N. S. Davis was appointed in his place. The roster of officers was presented to the AMA at its annual meeting in May 1886 and duly accepted.[22] Many foreign dignitaries were included in the final list, but the Americans made a sorry aggregate when compared with the list that Billings and his committee had put together in 1885. Only rarely did a prominent name appear.

The Congress itself was held in Washington September 5-10, 1887. It was generally accounted a success. After the event, *JAMA*, in several editorials, expressed its satisfaction. The British journal, *The Lancet*, had declared the Congress "worthy of its predecessors." Davis hoped that now the medical press, "instead of nursing old prejudices ... will henceforth labor for the unity and advancement of the profession as a whole"—clear call to the medical profession to accept the AMA viewpoint.[23]

With the Congress out of the way, the road might have seemed clear to a unification of the warring factions. Certainly, each side had made a point. The AMA had succeeded in mounting a well-attended and generally satisfactory international congress, in spite of the damaging publicity and the condemnation of leading medical figures.

The image of the AMA was undoubtedly somewhat tarnished. As one result, the outstanding physicians were turning away from the AMA toward their own specialty societies, as the focus of their professional attention. Such specialty groups assumed increasing prominence in the 1880s. There were many reasons for the expansion, and dissatisfaction with the AMA was certainly one of them. There did not result an increase of scientific knowledge, but another result was the weakening of the AMA in public esteem.

Forty years had elapsed since the code was devised, and much had changed. The homeopaths, for example, had established medical schools, were studying anatomy, physiology, and chemistry, were using textbooks written by regular physicians, and were no longer practicing an "exclusive system of medicine." In the Hahnemann Medical College, at least two thirds of the textbooks were "unquestionably orthodox." The practitioners no longer taught an exclusive system, and the most prominent homeopathists "publicly deny that their practice is based exclusively upon" such a doctrine. Although the writer was kindly disposed to homeopaths, other physicians continued to excoriate them and pointed to the claims that Hahnemann made as "utterly irreconcilable with the principles and practice of medicine and with the sciences upon which medicine is founded."[24]

Neither side was taking a balanced view. Certainly, some homeopaths were still adhering to the worst possible absurdities of Hahnemann, obviously incompatible with the medical sciences. Other homeopaths were extremely well educated and well versed in the sciences. And there were all stages in between. Then, of course, among the regular practitioners some were unbelievably ignorant of the medical sciences and were incomparably worse practitioners than were homeopaths.

The real question was, should the old hostility be perpetuated, or should there be a gradual accommodation? Whatever determined the answers had little to do with the amount of scientific knowledge that the homeopath might or might not possess, but rather with the personalities of the physicians themselves. The conservatives were looking more to the past; the liberals, more to the future.

The AMA convention in 1892 took cognizance of the problem and tried to defuse the situation by "interpreting" relevant passages in the code of ethics. The real point at issue was the question of consultations. An "explanatory declaration" tried to please everyone. Mere differences in "doctrine of belief" did not exclude anyone from "professional fellowship" and nothing in the code would interfere with the "most perfect liberty of individual opinion of practice." However, anyone who adopted a name indicating some sectarian system, or who belonged to an association "antagonistic to the general medical profession," would be considered to have made "a voluntary disconnection or withdrawal from the medical profession proper." Nothing would make it proper "to enter into formal professional consultations with those who have voluntarily disconnected themselves from the regular medical profession," as defined previously.[25]

This interpretation showed the real point at issue. Any form of practice, especially in therapeutics, was acceptable if only it did not openly proclaim opposition to regular medicine. The type of treatment was secondary, but using the name of homeopath was unforgivable.

In the convention of 1892 there had been enough doubts to impel two relevant steps. Reexamination of the code seemed in order. The president appointed a committee of five to study the code and recommend any changes deemed wise. Then, in the hope of settling the New York dissension, another committee was appointed, of which Davis was chairman. This had the task of conferring with suitable committees from each of the two New York medical groups, the Society and the Association, "for the purpose of adjusting all questions of eligibility of members of said State Medical Society of New York to membership in this association."[26]

Preliminary reports were rendered at the AMA convention of 1893. The Committee to examine the Code of Ethics rendered only a partial statement and needed more time for a definite report, but meanwhile the chairman indicated in part what the majority of the committee had in mind. They advised a new interpretation of the word *consultation*. The term would properly apply only when two physicians jointly shared the management of a case. It would not apply when a practitioner transferred to a specialist the entire responsibility for the care of the patient. Such an interpretation would seem to clear the way for a specialist to accept referrals from homeopaths, who would then drop out of the picture.

The majority of the Committee also proposed some verbal changes. The importance of a "thorough medical education" was recognized. The committee suggested the statement, "No intelligent practitioner, who has a license to practice from some medical board of known and acknowledged legal authority...and who is in good moral and professional standing in the place in which he

AMA

resides, should be refused consultation, when it is requested by the patient."[27]

Only four of the five members signed this provisional statement. The fifth, Dr Didama, who had led the old-code faction in New York, filed a minority report. The existing code, he said, "is explicit, liberal, broad, humane, and founded on truth, justice, and reason," and has no "superfluous details."[28]

In 1893, Davis also reported. The New York Medical Society refused to appoint a committee to meet with him until the AMA had removed the differences that prevented "cordial relations." This meant, said Davis, "a deliberate abolition of the national code of ethics," which of course he rejected. His report, the minutes stated, "was received with great applause."[29]

The issues were clear. The New York Society would not rejoin the AMA until the code was revised. The special committee appointed to study the question, by a majority of four to one, wanted to change the code; however, Didama and Davis had strongly resisted changes.

Since the Committee had not made its definitive report until 1894, the actual vote on a new code could not take place until 1895. When the proposed changes did come up for a vote, the minutes give little information. We learn that the motion to adopt the new code of ethics, as recommended by the majority report, was "indefinitely postponed." The move to liberalize the code was dead. Didama and David had acted as principal executioners, but they had the support of the convention.[30]

Nevertheless, the separation of New York physicians into two distinct organizations had become unendurable. After the turn of the century, the *New York Medical Journal* pointed out that unification could "readily be brought about if reason should prevail." The 13,000 physicians in New York "fail to find any underlying principle of sufficient importance to justify the existing division"—an elliptic way of saying that the question of consultation with homeopaths no longer held its former significance.[31] Any unification would, of course, require a vast amount of behind-the-scenes work with the AMA. Since N. S. Davis no longer exerted any active influence, the chances for revising the code were for the first time really bright.

Negotiations between the AMA and the State Association must have begun shortly after the turn of the century. In the AMA meeting of 1902, a resolution offered a whole new code that had already been approved by the council of the New York Medical Association. The new code was referred to a special committee of the AMA, to report for the final action the following year.

Meanwhile, tortuous negotiations were going on between the two state organizations. The State Association wanted the two groups to combine as a new entity, with a new charter. The State Society flatly refused. It had a continuous existence since 1806, and under no circumstances would it accept any plan that would interrupt its legal continuity even for an instant. The State Association had to yield, and the plans called for the two to unify into the Medical Society of the State of New York. The State Medical Association was thus rejoining the State Society from which it had seceded in 1884.

However, before the union could take place the AMA had to adopt a new code of ethics. This it did at the annual meeting of 1903. The minutes declared that the resolution moving the new code "was unanimously adopted amid tumultuous applause."

Only a small part of this new code concerns us here. The articles on consultation contained no statement at all concerning who may properly consult with whom, but there was a bland statement relative to sects. The new version declared, "It is incompatible to designate their practice as based on an exclusive dogma or a sectarian system of medicine."[32] In a sense, this was inviting the homeopaths to stop calling themselves homeopaths and to throw their lot in with the regular profession.

After the AMA adopted the new code, the union of the two state organizations was a formality, but not without emotion, barely hinted at in the minutes. The motion for union was passed unanimously and was received with enthusiastic applause.

Actually, some legal technicalities caused delay, and the final judicial order consolidating the two groups was not signed until December 9, 1905. The unification then became effective. In January 1906, the *New York State Journal of Medicine*, which had been the official journal of the State Association, now carried on its masthead, "Published Monthly by the Medical Society of the State of New York." The Association, a product of secession, had ceased to exist. There was again unity among the New York physicians, and the AMA had a new Code of Ethics.

Bibliographic Note

For the detailed story behind the Code of Ethics, the primary sources must be consulted. These include the Transactions of the American Medical Association, of the Medical Society of the State of New York, and later of the New York State Medical Association. The contemporary journals, especially the *New York State Medical Journal*, the *Boston Medical and Surgical Journal of the American Medical Association*, and the *Medical Record*, are indispensable.

References

1. *Trans AMA.* 1876;27:96.

2. *Trans Med Soc State NY.* 1882:75.

3. Ibid. pp 26-50.

4. The reactions of medical societies, quotations from their resolutions, and letters from physicians are extensively presented in *Medical News* for the year 1882, vol 40, passim.

5. *Trans AMA.* 1882;33:3.

6. *Trans NY State Med Assoc.* 1884;1:505-528. See also *Trans Med Soc State NY.* 1884:36-62.

7. Piffard HG. The status of the medical profession in the State of New York, fifth article. *NY Med J.* 1883;37:589-592.

8. *Trans Med Soc State NY.* 1883:49, 91.

9. Beard RO. The schools of medicine. *Pop Sci Monthly.* 1883;22:535-539.

10. Piffard, Status, third article. *NY Med J.* 1883;37:484-487. See also Kaufman M. *Homeopathy in America.* Baltimore, Md: Johns Hopkins Press; 1971:116-124.

11. Quoted by Piffard, op cit, p 486.

12. Flint A. Medical ethics and etiquette, fourth article. *NY Med J.* 1883;37:369-376.

13. *JAMA.* 1885;4:605.

14. *JAMA.*1884;3:499, 632, and 1885;4:415-419.

15. *JAMA.*1885;4:605-607. The editorial summaries the "official" view promulgated at the AMA convention in New Orleans.

16. *JAMA.*1885;4:548-552. See also 1885;5:136-138.

17. *JAMA.*1885;4:605-607, emphasis added.

18. *Medical News.* 1885;47:26, 27, 53, 83.

19. *JAMA.*1885;5:71.

20. Ibid, p 155.

21. Ibid, p 443.

22. *JAMA.*1886;6:602-603, and 1886;7:192-194.

23. *JAMA.*1887;9:497-498.

24. Jackson E. Against sectarianism in medicine. *Medical News.* 1889;55:425-427; Solis-Cohen S. An ethical question. Ibid, 427-435.

25. *JAMA.*1892;19:611-612.

26. *JAMA.*1893;20:693. See also *JAMA.*1892;18:1803.

27. *JAMA.*1893;20:691-692; also 1894;22:508.

28. *JAMA.*1893;20:591-593, and 1894; 22:556-558.

29. *JAMA.*1893;20:693.

30. *JAMA.*1895;24:761-762.

31. *NY Med J.* 1903;77:259-264.

32. *JAMA.*1903;40:1379-1381.

Council on Ethical and Judicial Affairs

The functions of the Council on Ethical and Judicial Affairs are:

- To interpret the *Principles of Medical Ethics* of the American Medical Association.
- To interpret the Constitution, Bylaws, and rules of the Association.
- To investigate general ethical conditions and all matters pertaining to the relations of physicians to one another or to the public, and make recommendations to the House of Delegates or the constituent associations.
- To receive appeals filed by applicants who allege that they, because of color, creed, race, religion, ethnic origin, national origin, or sex, have been unfairly denied membership in a component and/or constituent association, to determine the facts in the case, and to report the findings to the House of Delegates. If the Council determines that the allegations are indeed true, it shall admonish, censure, or, in the event of repeated violations, recommend to the House of Delegates that the constituent association involved be declared to be no longer a constituent member of the American Medical Association.
- To request the president to appoint investigating juries to which it may refer complaints or evidences of unethical conduct that in its judgment are of greater than local concern. Such investigative juries, if probable cause for action be shown, shall submit formal charges to the President, who shall appoint a prosecutor to prosecute such charges against the accused before the Council on Ethical and Judicial Affairs in the name and on behalf of the American Medical Association. The Council may acquit, admonish, suspend, or expel the accused.
- To approve applications and nominate candidates for affiliate membership as otherwise provided for in B-1.141 of the AMA's bylaws. (C&B-1997)

AMA

Published Reports of the Council on Ethical and Judicial Affairs 1997-1990

1997

AMA Policy: Covenants not to compete are unethical for physicians in training. Council on Ethical and Judicial Affairs, American Medical Association. *JAMA* 1997 Aug 20: 278(7): 530an

Abstract: Physician participation in capital punishment: evaluating competence of condemned prisoners; treating condemned prisoners to restore competence. Council on Ethical and Judicial Affairs, American Medical Association. *Tex Med* 1997 Feb; 93 (2): 50-2

1996

Report 59 of the AMA Board of Trustees (A-96). Physician-assisted suicide.

Reference Committee on Amendments to Constitution and Bylaws. *J Okla State Med Assoc* 1996 Aug; 89 (8): 281-93

1995

The use of anencephalic neonates as organ donors. Council on Ethical and Judicial Affairs, American Medical Association. *JAMA* 1995 May 24-31; 273 (20): 1614-8

Financial incentives for organ procurement: Ethical aspects of future contracts for cadaveric donors. Council on Ethical and Judicial Affairs. *Arch Intern Med* 1995 Mar 27; 155(6): 581-9

Ethical issues in managed care. Council on Ethical and Judicial Affairs. *JAMA* 1995 Jan 25; 273(4): 330-5

Ethical considerations in the allocation of organs and other scarce medical resources among patients. Council on Ethical and Judicial Affairs. *Arch Intern Med* 1995 Jan 9; 155(1): 29-40

1994

Disputes between medical supervisors and trainees. Council on Ethical and Judicial Affairs. *JAMA* 1994 Dec 21; 272(23): 1861-5

Reporting Adverse Drug and Medical Device Events. Council on Ethical and Judicial Affairs. *Food Drug Law* 1994; 49: 359-65

Ethical issues in health systems reform: The provision of adequate health care. Council on Ethical and Judicial Affairs. *JAMA* 1994 Oct 5; 272(13): 1056-62

Strategies for cadaveric organ procurement: mandated choice and presumed consent. Council on Ethical and Judicial Affairs. *JAMA* 1994 Sep 14; 272(10); 809-12

Ethical issues related to prenatal genetic testing. Council on Ethical and Judicial Affairs. *Arch Fam Med* 1994;3:633-642

Report of the Council on Ethical and Judicial Affairs, American Medical Association. Physician assisted suicide. *Issues Law Med* 1994 Summer; 10(1): 91-7

AMA

Gender discrimination in the medical profession. Council on Ethical and Judicial Affairs. *Women's Health Issues* 1994 Spring; 4(1): 1-11

1993

Physician participation in capital punishment. Council on Ethical and Judicial Affairs. *JAMA* 1993 Jul 21; 270(3): 365-8

Caring for the poor. Council on Ethical and Judicial Affairs. *JAMA* 1993 May 19; 269(19): 2533-7

Mandatory parental consent to abortion. Council on Ethical and Judicial Affairs *JAMA* 1993 Jan 6; 269(1): 82-6
Abstract: This report analyzes the ethical issues raised by requirements that parents be involved when minors seek an abortion. Parents are generally supportive and understanding and can provide helpful guidance to their children. In some cases, however, parents may respond abusively to the knowledge that their minor child is pregnant or is considering an abortion. In addition, privacy in matters of health care is a profound need of minors as well as adults. Accordingly, the Council concludes that, while minors should be encouraged to discuss their pregnancy with their parents and other adults, minors should not be required to involve their parents before deciding whether to undergo an abortion.

1992

Confidentiality of HIV status on autopsy reports. Council on Ethical and Judicial Affairs. *Arch Pathol Lab Med* 1992 Nov 116(11): 1120-3
Abstract: The medical profession has long recognized the need to maintain the confidentiality of a patient's medical condition, particularly when stigmatizing conditions, like human immunodeficiency virus infections, are involved. The obligation to maintain confidentiality continues after the death of the patient. At the same time, there may be public health concerns that justify limited disclosure of a deceased person's human immunodeficiency virus status. This report provides guidelines that balance the need for confidentiality with public health concerns when a deceased person infected with the human immunodeficiency virus undergoes an autopsy.

Physicians and domestic violence: Ethical considerations. Council on Ethical and Judicial Affairs. *JAMA* 1992 Jun 17; 267(23): 3190-3

Conflicts of interest: Physician ownership of medical facilities. Council on Ethical and Judicial Affairs. *JAMA* 1992 May 6; 267(17): 2366-9
Abstract: In this report, the Council on Ethical and Judicial Affairs revisits the question of referral of patients to medical facilities in which physicians have financial interests ("self-referral"). The Council issued safeguards in 1986 to prevent abuses of self-referral and most recently updated the guidelines in 1989. Recent studies, however, have suggested that problems with self-referral persist; these problems undermine the commitment of physicians to professionalism. The Council has concluded that, in general, physicians should not refer patients to a health care facility outside their office practice at which they do not directly provide care or services when they have an investment interest in the facility. Physicians may invest in and refer to an outside facility if there is a demonstrated need in the community for the facility and alternative financing is not available.

Decisions near the end of life. Council on Ethical and Judicial Affairs. *JAMA* 1992 Apr 22/29; 267(16): 2229-33

Requirements or incentives by government for the use of long-acting contraceptives. Board of Trustees. *JAMA* 1992 Apr 1; 267(13): 1818-21

1991

Sexual misconduct in the practice of medicine. Council on Ethical and Judicial Affairs. *JAMA* 1991 Nov 20; 266(19): 2741-5
Abstract: The American Medical Association's Council on Ethical and Judicial Affairs recently reviewed the ethical implications of sexual or romantic relationships between physicians and patients. The Council has concluded that (1) sexual contact or a romantic relationship concurrent with the physician-patient relationship is unethical; (2) sexual contact or a romantic relationship with a former patient may be unethical under certain circumstances; (3) education on the ethical issues involved in sexual misconduct should be included throughout all levels of medical training; and (4) in the case of sexual misconduct, reporting offending colleagues is especially important.

Use of genetic testing by employers. council on ethical and Judicial Affairs. *JAMA* 1991 Oct 2; 266(13): 1827-30

Gender disparities in clinical decision making. Council on Ethical and Judicial Affairs *JAMA*. 1991 Jul 24-31; 266(4); 559-62

Guidelines for the appropriate use of do-not-resuscitate orders. Council on Ethical and Judicial Affairs. *JAMA* 1991 Apr 10; 265(14) 1868-71
Abstract: Cardiopulmonary resuscitation (CPR) is routinely performed on hospitalized patients who suffer cardiac or respiratory arrest. Consent to administer CPR is presumed since the patient is incapable at the moment of arrest of communicating his or her treatment preference, and failure to act immediately is certain to result in the patient's death. Two exceptions to the presumption favoring CPR have been recognized, however. First, a patient may express in advance his or her preference that CPR be withheld. If the patient is incapable of expressing a preference, the decision to forgo resuscitation may be made by the patient's family or other surrogate decision maker. Second, CPR may be withheld if, in the judgment of the treating physician, an attempt to resuscitate the patient would be futile. In December 1987, the American Medical Association's Council on Ethical and Judicial Affairs issued a series of guidelines to assist hospital medical staffs in formulating appropriate resuscitation policies. The Council's position on the appropriate use of CPR and do-not-resuscitate orders is updated in this report.

Gifts to physicians from industry. Council on Ethical and Judicial Affairs. *JAMA* 1991 Jan 23/30; 265(4): 501

1990

Conflicts of interest in medical center/industry research relationships. Council on Scientific Affairs and Council on Ethical and Judicial Affairs. *JAMA* 1990 May 23/30; 263(20): 2790-3

Frozen pre-embryos. Board of Trustees. *JAMA* 1990 May 9; 263(18): 2484-7

Black-white disparities in health care. Council on Ethical and Judicial Affairs. *JAMA* 1990 May 2; 263(17): 2344-6
Abstract: Persistent, and sometimes substantial, differences continue to exist in the quality of health among Americans. Blacks have higher infant mortality rates and shorter life expectancies than whites. Underlying the disparities in the quality of health among Americans are differences in both need and access. Moreover, recent studies have suggested that even when blacks gain access to the health care system, they are less likely than whites to receive certain surgical or other therapies. These studies have examined treatments in several areas, including cardiology and cardiac surgery, kidney transplantation, general internal medicine, and obstetrics. Whether the disparities in treatment decisions are caused by differences in income and education, sociocultural factors, or failures by the medical profession, they are unjustifiable and must be eliminated. In this report, the Council on Ethical and Judicial Affairs of the American Medical Association emphasizes the need for (1) greater access to necessary health care for black Americans, (2) greater awareness among physicians of existing and potential disparities in treatment, and (3) the continued development of practice parameters, including criteria that would preclude or diminish racial disparities in health care decisions.

Medical applications of fetal tissue transplantation. Council on Scientific Affairs and Council on Ethical and Judicial Affairs. *JAMA* 1990 Jan 26; 263(4): 565-70
Abstract: Fetal tissue transplantation has been attempted for a limited number of clinical disorders, including Parkinson disease, diabetes, immunodeficiency disorders, and several metabolic disorders. Fetal tissue has intrinsic properties—ability to differentiate into multiple cell types, growth and proliferative ability, growth factor production, and reduced antigenicity—that make it attractive for transplantation research. At this time the results from fetal tissue grafts for Parkinson disease and diabetes have not demonstrated significant long-term clinical benefit to patients with these disorders. Further research will be necessary to determine the potential value of fetal tissue transplantation. For these clinical investigations to proceed, specific ethical guidelines are needed to ensure that fetal tissue derived from elective abortions is used in a morally acceptable manner. These guidelines should separate, to the greatest extent possible, the decision by a woman to have an abortion from her consent to donate the postmortem tissue for transplantation purposes. Such ethical guidelines are offered in this report.

Persistent vegetative state and the decision to withdraw or withhold life support. Council on Scientific Affairs and Council on Ethical and Judicial Affairs. *JAMA* 1990 Jan 19; 263(3): 426-30
Abstract: Persons with overwhelming damage to the cerebral hemispheres commonly pass into a chronic state of unconsciousness (ie, loss of self-awareness) called the vegetative state. When such cognitive loss lasts for more than a few weeks, the condition has been termed a persistent vegetative state, because the body retains the functions necessary to sustain vegetative functions. Recovery from the vegetative state does occur, but many persons in persistent vegetative states live for months or years if provided with nutritional and other supportive measures.

The withdrawal of life support from these persons with loss of higher brain function is a controversial issue, as highlighted by public debates and judicial decisions. This article provides criteria for the diagnosis of permanent unconsciousness and reviews the available data that support the reliability of these criteria. Significant legal decisions have been made with regard to withdrawal of life support to patients in persistent vegetative states, and the trends in this area are discussed.

Related publications include:
Code of Medical Ethics, Current Opinions With Annotations

Advanced Medical Directives: A Guide to Living Wills and Powers of Attorney: for Patients

Advanced Medical Directives: A Guide to Living Wills and Powers of Attorney: for Physicians

Office of Quality and Managed Care

To assist physicians in their various roles as providers of patient care, the emphasis on quality standards for patient care and on the analysis of performance is a goal of this unit. A growing part of this concern is the area of setting standards for patient care and outcomes assessment.

This group focuses on issues directed toward the development and appropriate use of practice parameters, clinical indicators, utilization review, and outcomes measurement tools.

Division of Accreditation

AMA Press Release

Chicago, May 19, 1997
New physician accreditation program announces standards: requirements and supplemental points make up national standard of excellence.

The program that will—in the near future—accredit American physicians based on a single scale of excellence today announced its first standards for that accreditation.

The American Medical Accreditation Program (AMAP) will ask physicians to meet 12 core standards addressing education, licensure, ethics, and practice operations, and to score an additional minimum number of points from among 13 other requirements, which address the physician's qualifications and professional performance.

"Not every physician will meet AMAP's exacting requirements," said Randolph D. Smoak, Jr, MD, Chair of the AMAP Governing Body. "Those who do can demonstrate to patients that they have acquired and maintained the education and training, and that they meet the high ethical and performance standards that the public should expect in choosing a physician."

Required AMAP accreditation standards include:
• Satisfactory medical, postgraduate, and continuing medical education.

AMA

- Unrestricted medical licensure and controlled substances registration.
- No violation of the AMA Principles of Medical Ethics.
- No record of felony or fraud convictions.
- No state or federal disciplinary action of any kind within the past 5 years.
- A satisfactory score on a review of the medical office.

Accredited physicians must agree to abide by the American Medical Association's Principles of Medical Ethics. They must also participate in a medical organization where their performance undergoes peer review. Beginning July 1, 1998, accredited physicians must also complete one or more AMAP-approved self-assessment programs.

The AMAP office site review criteria address five areas of medical practice quality:

1. Safety of the physical environment, including infection control and hazardous materials.
2. Physical appearance and access to the office.
3. Office administrative systems, including appointments, triage procedures, and patient follow-up.
4. Staffing and staff performance.
5. Medical records.

Supplementary accreditation standards include:
- Specialty board certification and recertification.
- Above average professional liability claims experience.
- Continuing education focused in the specialty of practice.
- Current participation in data systems for evaluation of clinical performance and/or patient care results.

AMAP, created to replace the current duplicative and fragmented system of physician assessment, is being phased in on a state-by-state basis and will begin accepting applications from physicians in selected states by the fall of 1997.

Division of Clinical Performance Standards

The central focus of this office is to strengthen the AMA's position as a leader in the efforts of organized medicine to ensure and improve the quality of medical care. This is accomplished by ensuring that clinical practice guidelines are developed and implemented in consonance with the professional standards of the medical profession. The benefits of these activities include more effective clinical practice and appropriate utilization of health care resources.

Office publications include:

Directory of Clinical Practice Guidelines (formerly known as the *Directory of Practice Parameters*)

This annual publication is a bibliography of practice parameters produced by physician organizations and others. Developed in cooperation with the Practice Parameters Partnership and Practice Parameters Forum, this 158-page document is the only complete source of information on practice parameters, and is available in both printed and CD-ROM formats. By controlling the contents of the *Directory*, the AMA maintains a strategically central role in the development, dissemination, and implementation of practice parameters. The *Directory* also offers a subscription to *Practice Parameter Update*, which is available separately as well.

Outcomes Research Resource Guide: A Survey of Current Activities

The *Outcomes Research Resource Guide* provides information regarding the outcomes activities of almost 150 physician organizations and other groups.

Science, Technology, and Public Health Standards

Recognizing that the quality of care can be no better than the science on which it is based, the Council on Scientific Affairs (CSA) has called for increasing emphasis on setting standards in science and biomedical research. The Science, Technology, and Public Health Standards area is prepared to address these concerns. It also acknowledges that America is faced with a series of large public health epidemics including AIDS, violence, tuberculosis, drug abuse, and sexually transmitted diseases. Since the ultimate solution to many of these activities is linked to biomedical and behavioral science, the AMA's public health activities are therefore parallel to other initiatives within this area.

Council on Scientific Affairs

The functions of the Council on Scientific Affairs are:
- To advise on substantial and promising developments in the scientific aspects of medicine and biomedical research that warrant public attention.
- To advise on professional and public information activities that might be undertaken by the AMA in the field of scientific medicine.
- To assist in the preparation of policy positions on scientific issues raised by the public media.
- To advise on policy positions on aspects of government support, involvement in or control of biomedical research.
- To advise on opportunities to coordinate or cooperate with the scientific activities of national medical specialty societies, voluntary health agencies, other professional organizations, and governmental agencies.
- To consider and evaluate the benefits that might be derived from joint development of domestic and international programs on scientific affairs.
- To propose and evaluate activities that might be undertaken by the AMA as major scientific projects, either individually or jointly with state and local medical societies. (C&B-1997)

Reports of the Council on Scientific Affairs

Published reports by year:

1996

Health care needs of gay men and lesbians in the United States. Council on Scientific Affairs, American Medical Association. *JAMA* 1996 May 1; 275 (17): 1354-9

Alcoholism in the elderly. Council on Scientific Affairs, American Medical Association. *JAMA* 1996 Mar 13; 275 (10): 797-801

Good care of the dying patient. Council on Scientific Affairs, American Medical Association. *JAMA* 1996 Feb 14; 275 (6): 474-8

1995

Female Genital Mutilation. Council on Scientific Affairs. *JAMA* 1995 Dec 6; 274(21); 1714-6
Abstract: Female genital mutilation is the medically unnecessary modification of female genitalia. Female genital mutilation typically occurs at about 7 years of age, but mutilated women suffer severe medical complications throughout their adult lives. Female genital mutilation most frequently occurs in Africa, the Middle East, and Muslim parts of Indonesia and Malaysia, and it is generally part of a ceremonial induction into adult society. Recent political and economic problems in these regions, however, have increased the numbers of students and refugees to the United States. Consequently, US physicians are treating an increasing number of mutilated patients. The Council on Scientific Affairs recommends that US physicians join the World Health Organization, the World Medical Association, and other major health care organizations in opposing all forms of medically unnecessary surgical modification of the female genitalia.

Dehydration. Evaluation and management in older adults. Council on Scientific Affairs, American Medical Association. *JAMA* 1995 Nov 15; 274 (19): 1552-6
Abstract: The objective of this report was to review published literature regarding dehydration in older individuals and formulate a consensus on the evaluation and treatment of this unrecognized cause of hospitalizations, morbidity, and mortality. The literature concerning dehydration in the elderly population from MEDLINE was reviewed from 1976 through 1995. Search terms included dehydration, elderly, evaluation, hospitalization, and treatment. Particular emphasis was placed on articles describing original research leading to the development of new information on the evaluation and treatment of dehydration and review articles relating to the epidemiology, detection, treatment, and health outcomes of this syndrome common in the geriatric population, including frail, institutionalized individuals. Data contributing to a broad scientific understanding of dehydration were initially grouped according to topic areas of the physiology of normal aging, illness-associated clinical reports of dehydration in the elderly population, and diagnostic and therapeutic interventions. The authors developed a consensus based on the weight of evidence presented and the authors' experience in the field. The conclusions of this report were found to be that early diagnosis is sometimes difficult because the classical physical signs of dehydration may be absent or misleading in an older patient. Many different etiologies place the elderly at particular risk. In patients identified as being at risk for possible dehydration, an interdisciplinary care plan with regard to prevention of clinically significant dehydration is critical if maximum benefit is to result.

1994

Helmets and preventing motorcycle- and bicycle-related injuries. Council on Scientific Affairs, American Medical Association. *JAMA* 1994 Nov 16; 272(19): 1535-8

1993

Silicone gel breast implants. Council on Scientific Affairs, American Medical Association. *JAMA* 1993 Dec 1; 270 (21): 2602-6

Adolescents as victims of family violence. Council on Scientific Affairs, American Medical Association. *JAMA* 1993 Oct 20; 270 (15): 1850-6
Abstract: Adolescents experience maltreatment at rates equal to or exceeding those of younger children. Recent increases in reported cases of maltreatment have occurred disproportionately among older children and adolescents. However, adolescents are less likely to be reported to child protective services and are more likely to be perceived as responsible for their maltreatment. Adolescent girls are reported as victims more often than boys, especially in sexual abuse. However, boys may be less likely to be identified or reported and often are abused by non–family members. Parents of adolescent victims have higher average income and educational levels and are less likely to have a parental history of abuse than parents of younger children. A wide range of serious adolescent risk behaviors is associated with maltreatment. These include increased risk of premature sexual activity, unintended pregnancy, emotional disorders, suicide attempts, eating disorders, alcohol and other drug abuse, and delinquent behavior. Incarcerated youth, homeless or runaway youth, and youth who victimize siblings or assault parents have been shown to have high rates of prior maltreatment. Signs of maltreatment are often ambiguous for adolescents. Screening questions have been effective in prompting self-disclosure of abuse. Adolescents also experience problems in the child welfare system that offers fewer and less appropriate services for this age group. Recommendations are made regarding screening of adolescents for maltreatment, the development of better services for adolescents, research on parenting to prevent maltreatment, and training of school staff to identify and refer victims of maltreatment.

The use of pulse oximetry during conscious sedation. Council on Scientific Affairs, American Medical Association. *JAMA* 1993 Sept 22/29; 270(12): 1463-8

Users and uses of patient records. Report of the Council on Scientific Affairs. Council on Scientific Affairs, American Medical Association. *Arch Fam Med* 1993 Jun; 2(6): 678-81
Abstract: At present, there is significant momentum for developing and implementing computer-based patient records systems. It is essential that their development be guided by the functional requirements of the users and uses of patient records. Users can be grouped into seven categories: providers, patients, educators, researchers, payers, managers and reviewers, and licensing and accrediting agencies and professional associations. Uses of patient records include fostering continuity of care, supporting diagnosis and choice of therapy, assessing and managing health risks, documenting the services provided, maintaining accurate medical histories, billing and verifying payment, documenting professionals' experience, teaching students, preparing conferences and presentations, conducting research, formulating practice guidelines, and providing data to support utilization review, quality assurance, accreditation, and licensure. Patient records can be classified as primary records used by professionals while providing health care services or secondary records derived from primary records to aid nonclinical users. Protecting the confidentiality of patient information will restrict access to primary records for some users and should prevent inclusion of sensitive data in secondary records. The design features to be incorpo-

AMA

rated into computer-based record systems should expand the record's function from that of a simple device for documenting events into a powerful tool for providing and managing care.

Physicians and family caregivers. A model for partnership. Council on Scientific Affairs, American Medical Association. *JAMA* 1993 Mar 10; 269 (10): 1282-4

Abstract: Primary care physicians need a strong and effective model to guide their relationships with family caregivers, key resources for the frail elderly. Caregivers provide a significant proportion of the home care needed by the rapidly growing number of frail elderly living in the community. Caregiving exacts a physical, psychological, social, and emotional toll that no intervention strategies have proven powerful enough to offset. An effective relationship model would acknowledge the key linkage role of the primary care physician, recognize that caregivers and patients form interdependent units, and affirm a care partnership between the physician and caregiver. In this model, the physician conducts periodic assessments of the caregiver as well as the patient; uses a comprehensive home-based approach to care and services; provides training to caregivers, particularly in managing difficult behavior; validates the role of caregiver; and acts as case manager. Educational opportunities and reimbursement structures should be modified to encourage physicians to use the partnership model.

Diet and cancer. Report of the Council on Scientific Affairs: Diet and cancer: Where do matters stand? *Arch Intern Med* 1993 Jan 11; 53(1): 50-6

Abstract: During the past decade, the scientific literature base on the putative but elusive relationship between diet and cancer expanded enormously. Increased emphasis by funding agencies, fueled in turn by broadening public interest in the topic, led to this growth. The laboratory and epidemiologic research conducted in the past decade has shown that a simple solution does not exist. The key to the diet/cancer puzzle may lie in nutrient interactions and in individual response to dietary factors, determined in turn by genetic, physiologic, and lifestyle factors. Given the rapid strides being made in furthering the understanding of the biochemistry and molecular biology of cancer, it may be possible to look forward to the day when optimal dietary and lifestyle guidelines can be tailored to a specific individualized basis.

1992

Clinical ecology. Council on Scientific Affairs. *JAMA* 1992 Dec 23-30; 268(24): 3465-7

Induced termination of pregnancy before and after *Roe v Wade:* Trends in the mortality and morbidity of women. Council on Scientific Affairs, American Medical Association. *JAMA* 1992 Dec 12; 268(22): 3231-39

Abstract: The mortality and morbidity of women who terminated their pregnancy before the 1973 Supreme Court decision in *Roe v Wade* are compared with post-*Roe v Wade* mortality and morbidity. Mortality data before 1973 are from the National Center for Health Statistics; data from 1973 through 1985 are from the Centers for Disease Control and The Alan Guttmacher Institute. Trends in serious abortion-related complications between 1970 and 1990 are based on data from the Joint Program for the Study of Abortion and from the National Abortion Federation. Deaths from illegally induced abortion declined between 1940 and 1972 in part because of the introduction of antibiotics to manage sepsis and the widespread use of effective contraceptives. Deaths from legal abortion declined fivefold between 1973 and 1985 (from 3.3 deaths to 0.4 death per 100,000 procedures), reflecting increased physician education and skills, improvements in medical technology, and, notably, the earlier termination of pregnancy. The risk of death from legal abortion is higher among minority women and women over the age of 35 years, and increases with gestational age. Legal-abortion mortality between 1979 and 1985 was 0.6 death per 100,000 procedures, more than 10 times lower than the 9.1 maternal deaths per 100,000 live births, between 1979 and 1986. Serious complications from legal abortion are rare. Most women who have a single abortion with vacuum aspiration experience few if any subsequent problems getting pregnant or having healthy children. Less is known about the effects of multiple abortions on future fecundity. Adverse emotional reactions to abortion are rare; most women experience relief and reduced depression and distress.

Assault weapons as a public health hazard in the United States. Council on Scientific Affairs, American Medical Association. *JAMA* 1992 Jun 10; 267(22): 3067-70

Violence against women. Relevance for medical practitioners. Council on Scientific Affairs, American Medical Association. *JAMA* 1992 Jun 17; 267(23): 3184-9

Abstract: Evidence collected over the last 20 years indicates that physical and sexual violence against women is an enormous problem. Much of this violence is perpetrated by women's intimate partners or in relationships that would presumably carry some protective aura (eg, father-daughter, boyfriend-girlfriend). This violence carries with it both short- and long-term sequelae for women and affects both their physical and psychological well-being. The high prevalence of violence against women brings them into regular contact with physicians; at least one in five women seen in emergency departments has symptoms relating to abuse. However, physicians frequently treat the injuries only symptomatically or fail to recognize the injuries as abuse. Even when recognized, physicians are often without resources to address the needs of abused women. This report documents the extent of violence against women and suggests paths that the physician community might take to address the needs of victims.

1991

Use of animals in medical education. Council on Scientific Affairs, American Medical Association. *JAMA* 1991 Aug 14; 266(6): 836-7

Abstract: The use of animals in general medical education is essential. Although several adjuncts to the use of animals are available, none can completely replace the limited use of animals in the medical curriculum. Students should be made aware of an institution's policy on animal use in the curriculum before matriculation, and faculty should make clear to all students the learning objectives of any educational exercise that uses animals. The Council on Scientific Affairs recognizes the necessity for the responsible and humane treatment of animals and urges all medical school faculty members to discuss this moral and ethical imperative with their students.

Asbestos removal, health hazards, and the EPA. Council on Scientific Affairs, American Medical Association. *JAMA* 1991 Aug 7; 266(5): 696-7

Abstract: Resolution 193 (A-90), which was adopted by the House of Delegates of the American Medical Association, called on the Council on Scientific Affairs to study the situation regarding asbestos abatement, the risks to health, and the appropriateness of Environmental Protection Agency regulations, policies, and control measures. This report reviews the current status of asbestos abatement as applied to schools and public buildings, which currently accounts for the major expenditure of public funds.

Ultrasonic imaging of the heart. Report of the Council on Scientific Affairs: report of the Ultrasonography Task Force. *Arch Intern Med.* 1991 Jul; 151(7): 1288-94

Abstract: The use of ultrasonography in cardiology has progressed so dramatically that not only is anatomic information available but information can also be derived about cardiac hemodynamics. Applications range from intravascular ultrasonic imaging of coronary atherosclerosis to predictions of the severity of fetal valvular pulmonic stenosis detected in utero. We reviewed cardiac ultrasonography as utilized in B-mode imaging, pulsed and continuous-wave spectral Doppler, and Doppler color flow mapping. We reviewed specialized areas, including stress echo for wall motion analysis, valvular and congenital heart disease applications, and new applications in intraoperative, transesophageal, contrast echography, coronary imaging, and fetal echocardiography. Finally, future applications of quantitative flow mapping and intraluminal and interventional ultrasonography were considered along with the required technological advances.

The future of ultrasonography. Report of the Ultrasonography Task Force. Council on Scientific Affairs, American Medical Association. *JAMA* 1991 Jul 17; 266(3): 406-9

Abstract: Future advances in ultrasonography will undoubtedly occur in three major areas: diagnostic capability, instrumentation, and clinical applications. In the area of diagnostic capability, spatial and contrast resolution offer excellent opportunities for improvement. Continued research into tissue characterization is worthwhile, even though efforts to date have been more frustrating than fulfilling. Blood flow studies and new contrast agents are among the more promising areas for future development. New techniques of signal detection, analysis, and display in Doppler imaging may overcome some present limitations, including those in color flow imaging.

Gynecologic sonography. Report of the Ultrasonography Task Force. Council on Scientific Affairs, American Medical Association. *JAMA* 1991 Jun 5; 265(21): 2851-5

Abstract: Sonography, because it is nonionizing, is the preferred imaging modality for the female pelvis. Traditionally, transabdominal, transcystic studies were performed. However, development of transvaginal and transrectal transducers has led to enhanced imaging capabilities of the pelvis. These new technologies will likely improve our ability to understand gynecologic pathology. The clinical use of pelvic ultrasonography depends on a thorough understanding of normal anatomy and cyclical changes and on the relative limitations of the imaging modality in specifically characterizing pathologic processes. This article reviews the accepted role of pelvic sonography in gynecologic disease and provides a preview of some of the potential applications of recent advances in sonographic technology.

Doppler sonographic imaging of the vascular system. Report of the Ultrasonography Task Force. Council on Scientific Affairs, American Medical Association. *JAMA* 1991 May 8; 265(18): 2382-7

Abstract: Ultrasonic vascular imaging has been used for more than 20 years to define vascular anatomy, pathologic changes in vessel size, and perivascular abnormalities. In the last decade, development of duplex Doppler technology has permitted the evaluation of both anatomic vascular features and physiologic blood flow parameters in a variety of locations. Doppler "color flow" imaging promises to expand these applications. In many instances, duplex Doppler technology has replaced more invasive angiographic procedures for evaluation of suspected vascular abnormalities. Improved ultrasound duplex technology, combined with the relatively inexpensive, rapid, noninvasive aspects of ultrasonography, has made it a valuable screening examination for suspected flow abnormalities.

Health effects of radon exposure. Report of the Council on Scientific Affairs, American Medical Association. *Arch Intern Med.* 1991 Apr; 151(4): 674-7

Abstract: The consensus of scientists is that exposure to radon is hazardous, but disagreement exists about the effects of lower radon concentrations. Studies of underground miners have indicated that the risk of lung cancer increases in proportion to the intensity and duration of exposure to radon, and a recent authoritative report (BEIR IV) has concluded that estimates based on those studies are appropriate for estimating risks for occupants of homes. The BEIR IV report concluded that smoking cigarettes increases the risk of lung cancer associated with radon. Average radon levels in US homes range from 0.055 to 0.148 Bq/L (1.5 to 4 pCi/L), depending on the circumstances of measurement. Few studies have investigated health outcomes in occupants of homes with high radon levels. In advising patients about reducing the risks associated with radon, physicians should consider the costs, as well as the benefits, of remedial actions, and they should emphasize that, by far, the best way to avoid lung cancer is to stop smoking.

Ultrasonic imaging of the abdomen. Report of the Ultrasonography Task Force. Council on Scientific Affairs, American Medical Association. *JAMA* 1991 Apr 3; 265(13): 1726-31

Abstract: As new imaging modalities emerge and existing technologies improve, indications for a particular imaging method may change. This article examines current indications for abdominal and prostatic ultrasound examination and, where possible, compares ultrasound with other imaging techniques. This is not an attempt to list all possible ultrasound indications or examinations, but rather an attempt to serve as an aid to informed imaging selection based on current literature and equipment.

AMA

Biotechnology and the American agricultural industry. Council on Scientific Affairs, American Medical Association. *JAMA* 1991 Mar 20; 265(11): 1429-36
Abstract: To meet the needs of a rapidly growing population and minimize the toxic influences of traditional farming practices on the environment, the American agricultural industry has applied molecular technology to the development of food crops and livestock. By placing genes specific for highly desirable phenotypes into the DNA of plants, animals, and bacteria, farmers have increased crop and livestock survival, enhanced the nutritional quality of foods, increased industry productivity, and reduced the need for toxic pesticides and herbicides. However, introduction of genetically modified foods into the marketplace has raised a spectrum of public health issues. Physicians, as the most proximal scientific resource for most individuals, are uniquely positioned to address patient concerns regarding the safety of genetically altered foods. This report provides an overview of the inherent risks and benefits of "agrogenetics" and offers a series of recommendations designed to promote the education of the medical community and dispel public misconception regarding genetic manipulation.

Medical diagnostic ultrasound instrumentation and clinical interpretation. Report of the ultrasonography task force. Council on Scientific Affairs. *JAMA* 1991 Mar 6; 265(9): 1155-9
Abstract: Over the past 20 years, there has been a dramatic increase in the use of ultrasonography as an imaging modality. The introduction of real-time ultrasonography and Doppler units for the measurement of blood flow in the 1970s, recent advances in transducer design, signal processing, and miniaturization of electronics, along with the lack of radiation exposure, have been primarily responsible for the increased use of ultrasound. However, although ultrasonography can provide diagnostic information safely and easily, interpretation of the information requires an understanding of the physics behind ultrasound, how that physics is translated into ultrasound instrumentation, recognition of artifacts that are associated with the various types of ultrasonography, and identification of these artifacts in specific anatomic locations.

Educating physicians in home health care. Council on Scientific Affairs and Council on Medical Education [corrected] [published erratum appears in *JAMA* 1991 May 8; 265(18):2340]. *JAMA* 1991 Feb 13; 265(6): 769-71
Abstract: A growing proportion of health care, especially long-term care, should best and most appropriately be provided in the home setting. Physicians have largely remained on the periphery of this reemerging area of health care. Yet if home health care is to reach its full potential, physicians must fulfill their essential role as members of the home health team. Direct physician input and participation are needed to ensure that home health care is safe and medically appropriate. Physician involvement will enhance the supervision of medical care in the home, and physicians' expertise is also much needed for home health care quality assurance and clinical research. Role models and training experiences must be developed for new physicians so that they can integrate home health care skills and values into their future practices. Although most of the usual physician objections to home health care involvement can be addressed by education, the problem of inadequate reimbursement is substantive and must be addressed by policy change.

Hispanic health in the United States. Council on Scientific Affairs. *JAMA* 1991 Jan 9; 265(2): 248-52
Abstract: Hispanics are the fastest-growing minority in the United States. Typically, they are divided into five subgroups: Mexican American, Puerto Rican, Cuban American, Central or South American, and "other" Hispanics. Risk factors for morbidity and mortality vary among these subgroups. Use of health care services is affected by perceived health care needs, insurance status, income, culture, and language. Compared with whites, Hispanics are more likely to live in poverty, be unemployed or underemployed, and have little education and no private insurance. Hispanics are at an increased risk for certain medical conditions, including diabetes, hypertension, tuberculosis, human immunodeficiency virus infection, alcoholism, cirrhosis, specific cancers, and violent deaths. Proportionate to their representation in the population, there are few Hispanic health providers, emphasizing the need for all medical personnel to be knowledgeable about Hispanic health care needs.

1990

Medical and nonmedical uses of anabolic-androgenic steroids. Council on Scientific Affairs. *JAMA* 1990 Dec 12; 264(22): 2923-7
Abstract: Recent trends in the use, abuse, and diversion of steroids for nonmedical purposes illustrate a growing problem that not only imposes health risks but presents ethical dilemmas as well. Concern over the known adverse effects, the limited research into the long-term effects, and the ethics of engineering body size and performance through anabolic-androgenic steroid use has led to legislative, legal, and education responses. Increased penalties for distribution to minors and stricter controls in prescribing practices have been enacted through state legislation and federal initiatives. Government, some health professional organizations, and some sports groups have denounced the nonmedical use of anabolic-androgenic steroids and have developed materials to educate their members, other professionals, athletes, educators, and the public at large.

The IOM report and public health. Council on Scientific Affairs *JAMA* 1990 Jul 25; 264(4): 503-6
Abstract: A recent Institute of Medicine report defined "public health" as what society must do to keep people healthy and further defined it as involving the collection of data, assessment of problems, and assurance of health protection. Public health professionals include physicians, nurses, sanitarians, biostatisticians, engineers, and administrators, and epidemiology is public health's basic science. Past successes in the United States, such as increases in longevity and decreases in infant mortality and cardiovascular death rates, demonstrate that progress is possible; however, inequalities persist, for example, in infant mortality rates and availability of medical care to lower socioeconomic groups. The major responsibilities of public health departments include leading and coordinating public health efforts, controlling epidemics, carrying out disease and injury surveillance, collecting vital statistics, ensuring good medical and dental care for the indigent, environmental control, health education, and laboratory services.

Societal effects and other factors affecting health care for the elderly. Report of the Council on Scientific Affairs. AMA Council on Scientific Affairs. *Arch Intern Med* 1990 Jun; 150(6): 1184-9

Abstract: With advances in medical care, life expectancy of Americans has increased dramatically. The increase in the size of the elderly population has had a major impact on health care provision and will have an even greater impact on our health care system over the next several decades. Although today's medical students will spend nearly half of their collective careers caring for the elderly, insufficient numbers of students show an interest in geriatrics. American society has become in many ways less traditional, and age is no longer seen as "a pathway to wisdom." Since we are now a more mobile society, extended families tend to scatter, and the elderly are frequently alone. We examine the effects of our rapidly changing, youth-oriented society on health care for the elderly.

The worldwide smoking epidemic. Tobacco trade, use, and control. Council on Scientific Affairs. *JAMA* 1990 Jun 27; 263(24): 3312-8

A permanent US-Mexico border environmental health commission. Council on Scientific Affairs. *JAMA* 1990 Jun 27; 263(24): 3319-21

Abstract: Public health officials, physicians, and politicians have long been aware of the squalid environmental conditions existing along the US-Mexico border. Some attempts have been made to improve the environmental pollution and causes of human disease, beginning as early as the 1930s with the IBWC, established in 1889. More recent agreements and legislation have called for US and Mexican cooperation by way of each nation's corresponding environmental agency (ie, the EPA and Mexico's SEDUE) and their agencies of foreign affairs (ie, the IBWC). Nevertheless, environmental monitoring and disease incidence data continue to point out that public and environmental health along the border—the result of uncontrolled air and water pollution and lack of disease vector control—is rapidly deteriorating and seriously affecting the health and future economic vitality on both sides of the border. Many prominent public health professionals and environmental organizations are concerned that the present working relationship between the United States and Mexico is not functioning well and cannot adequately cope with existing environmental conditions; for one thing, the efforts of the EPA and SEDUE are reviewed no more frequently than once a year by a staff quartered in Washington and Mexico City. Some projects to improve these conditions have been undertaken by the EPA and SEDUE and the IBWC; at present, the prospects for success do not appear promising. Consequently, these individuals and organizations have urged creation of a US-Mexico border environmental health commission. Congress did see fit last year to give responsibility for the environment to the IBWC in the form of Public Law 100-465. This law, however, does not address the full severity of environmental and public health degradation along the border; it does not address the pollution of the New River, Agua Prieta, the San Pedro River, or the Pacific Ocean, neither does it offer remedial control of hazardous waste sites, rabies, and other disease vectors. Moreover, the IBWC is only a deliberative body, not an implementing one.

Conflicts of interest in medical center/industry research relationships. Council on Scientific Affairs and Council on Ethical and Judicial Affairs. *JAMA* 1990 May 23-30; 263(20): 2790-3

Education for health. A role for physicians and the efficacy of health education efforts. Council on Scientific Affairs. *JAMA* 1990 Apr 4; 263(13): 1816-9

Abstract: Health education efforts have grown dramatically over the past decade and seek to improve the health of individuals by providing them with information that will lead to behavioral changes and thereby result in improved health. There is now substantial evidence to support the idea that health education activities can alter health behaviors, even though the mechanisms by which health education efforts succeed are largely unknown. Physicians could add to the success of health education efforts by incorporating preventive services into their patient encounters, particularly patients in high-risk situations. There are many examples of successful physician-based interventions, and a new emphasis on preventive services in primary care is emerging.

Home care in the 1990s. Council on Scientific Affairs *JAMA* 1990 Mar 2; 263(9): 1241-4

Abstract: Home care is a rapidly growing field that is beginning to attract greater physician interest and participation. Cost-containment pressures have led to reduced institutionalization in hospitals and nursing homes and to more patients, both acutely and chronically ill, being cared for in their own homes. Undergraduate and graduate medical education programs are developing home care curricula, and academic medicine is beginning to develop a research agenda, particularly in the area of clinical outcome measurements. Medical care in the home is highly diversified and innovative. The areas of preventive, diagnostic, therapeutic, rehabilitative, and long-term maintenance care are all well represented as physicians develop new practice patterns in home care.

American Medical Association white paper on elderly health. Report of the Council on Scientific Affairs [published erratum appears in *Arch Intern Med* 1991 Feb; 151(2): 265]. *Arch Intern Med* 1990 Dec; 150:(12): 2459-72

Health status of detained and incarcerated youths. Council on Scientific Affairs. *JAMA* 1990 Feb 16; 263(7): 987-91

Abstract: Youths who are detained or incarcerated in correctional facilities represent a medically underserved population that is at high risk for a variety of medical and emotional disorders. These youths not only have a substantial number of preexisting health problems, they also develop acute problems that are associated with their arrest and with the environment of the correctional facility. Although the availability of medical services varies by the size of the institution, established standards are, in general, not being met.

Saturated fatty acids in vegetable oils. Council on Scientific Affairs. *JAMA* 1990 Feb 2; 263(5): 693-5

Abstract: Concern has been expressed about the "atherogenicity" of coconut and/or palm oil in food products. Saturated fatty acids are found primarily in animal products and in "tropical oils" (coconut, palm, and palm kernel oils). Composition of the total diet over an extended period determines nutritional status and contribution to health. Specific foods and/or food ingre-

AMA

AMA

dients need to be evaluated within the context of a person's total dietary pattern over time. Persons attempting to limit saturated fatty acid intake should be aware of the high content of saturated fatty acids in tropical oils. The American Medical Association is on record as supporting fatty acid labeling when cholesterol content is declared and cholesterol labeling when fatty acid content is declared. The American Medical Association has supported, and continues to support, voluntary efforts to increase public awareness of the composition and nutritional value of foods.

Medical applications of fetal tissue transplantation. Council on Scientific Affairs and Council on Ethical and Judicial Affairs. *JAMA* 1990 Jan 26; 263(4): 565-70
Abstract: Fetal tissue transplantation has been attempted for a limited number of clinical disorders, including Parkinson disease, diabetes, immunodeficiency disorders, and several metabolic disorders. Fetal tissue has intrinsic properties—ability to differentiate into multiple cell types, growth and proliferative ability, growth factor production, and reduced antigenicity—that make it attractive for transplantation research. At this time the results from fetal tissue grafts for Parkinson disease and diabetes have not demonstrated significant long-term clinical benefit to patients with these disorders. Further research will be necessary to determine the potential value of fetal tissue transplantation. For these clinical investigations to proceed, specific ethical guidelines are needed to ensure that fetal tissue derived from elective abortions is used in a morally acceptable manner. These guidelines should separate, to the greatest extent possible, the decision by a woman to have an abortion from her consent to donate the postmortem tissue for transplantation purposes. Such ethical guidelines are offered in this report.

Persistent vegetative state and the decision to withdraw or withhold life support. Council on Scientific Affairs and Council on Ethical and Judicial Affairs. *JAMA* 1990 Jan 19; 263(3): 426-30
Abstract: Persons with overwhelming damage to the cerebral hemispheres commonly pass into a chronic state of unconsciousness (ie, loss of self-awareness) called the vegetative state. When such cognitive loss lasts for more than a few weeks, the condition has been termed a persistent vegetative state, because the body retains the functions necessary to sustain vegetative functions. Recovery from the vegetative state does occur, but many persons in persistent vegetative states live for months or years if provided with nutritional and other supportive measures. The withdrawal of life support from these persons with loss of higher brain function is a controversial issue, as highlighted by public debates and judicial decisions. This article provides criteria for the diagnosis of permanent unconsciousness and reviews the available data that support the reliability of these criteria. Significant legal decisions have been made with regard to withdrawal of life support to patients in persistent vegetative states, and the trends in this area are discussed.

1989

Medical perspective on nuclear power. Council on Scientific Affairs. *JAMA* 1989 Nov 17; 262(19): 2724-9

Musculoskeletal applications of magnetic resonance imaging. Council on Scientific Affairs [published erratum appears in *JAMA* 1990 Jul 25; 264(4):456]. *JAMA* 1989 Nov 3; 262(17): 2420-7
Abstract: Magnetic resonance imaging provides superior contrast, resolution, and multiplanar imaging capability, allowing excellent definition of soft-tissue and bone marrow abnormalities. For these reasons, magnetic resonance imaging has become a major diagnostic imaging method for the evaluation of many musculoskeletal disorders. The applications of magnetic resonance imaging for musculoskeletal diagnosis are summarized and examples of common clinical situations are given. General guidelines are suggested for the musculoskeletal applications of magnetic resonance imaging.

Infectious medical wastes. Council on Scientific Affairs. *JAMA* 1989 Sep 22-29; 262(12): 1669-71
Abstract: A number of recent incidents involving improper handling and disposal of hospital waste have prompted the demand for more stringent legislation to cover the management of infectious hospital waste. Resolution 53 (December 1987 Interim Meeting) called for the American Medical Association to promote the passage of federal legislation for the proper disposal of infectious hospital waste. This resolution has prompted a Council on Scientific Affairs report on the current status of infectious hospital waste management and of state and federal regulations to control such waste. The Council has concluded that existing federal and state regulations for the management of hazardous waste—in conjunction with the accreditation program of the Joint Commission on Accreditation of Healthcare Organizations and the guidelines of the Environmental Protection Agency and the Centers for Disease Control, if adhered to and properly enforced—should be adequate to ensure that the public and environment are not endangered. Therefore, the Council does not favor additional federal legislation at this time and recommends that this report be accepted in lieu of Resolution 53.

Quality assurance in cervical cytology. The Papanicolaou smear. Council on Scientific Affairs. *JAMA* 1989 Sep 22-29; 262(12): 1672-9

Health care needs of homeless and runaway youths. Council on Scientific Affairs. *JAMA* 1989 Sep 8; 262(10): 1358-61
Abstract: Large numbers of homeless adolescents can be found in this country, with estimates of their numbers ranging from 500,000 to more than 2 million. Some are runaways while others are involuntarily without shelter, often having been forced out of their homes. Most receive no help from social service agencies and their lack of skills forces them into a marginal existence, leaving them vulnerable to abuse and victimization. Health problems are numerous and health care is generally inadequate for several reasons, including a lack of treatment facilities, the behavior of the adolescents themselves, the ability of providers to deal with such youths, and the questionable legal status of homeless adolescents. The Council on Scientific Affairs urges that reliable and up-to-date data on the extent of homelessness among adolescents and the nature of their needs be generated and that guidelines for the medical care of such youths be developed.

Low-level radioactive wastes. Council on Scientific Affairs. *JAMA* 1989 Aug 4; 262(5): 669-74

Abstract: Under a federal law, each state by January 1, 1993, must provide for safe disposal of its low-level radioactive wastes. Most of the wastes are from using nuclear power to produce electricity, but 25% to 30% are from medical diagnosis, therapy, and research. Exposures to radioactivity from the wastes are much smaller than those from natural sources, and federal standards limit public exposure. Currently operating disposal facilities are in Beatty, Nev, Barnwell, SC, and Richland, Wash. National policy encourages the development of regional facilities. Planning a regional facility, selecting a site, and building, monitoring, and closing the facility will be a complex project lasting decades that involves legislation, public participation, local and state governments, financing, quality control, and surveillance. The facilities will utilize geological factors, structural designs, packaging, and other approaches to isolate the wastes. Those providing medical care can reduce wastes by storing them until they are less radioactive, substituting nonradioactive compounds, reducing volumes, and incinerating. Physicians have an important role in informing and advising the public and public officials about risks involved with the wastes and about effective methods of dealing with them.

Dietary fiber and health. Council on Scientific Affairs. *JAMA* 1989 Jul 28; 262(4): 542-6

Abstract: During the last 18 years, considerable research has been conducted on the role of dietary fiber in health and disease. Interest was stimulated by epidemiologic studies that associated a low intake of dietary fiber with the incidence of colon cancer, heart disease, diabetes, and other diseases and disorders. Dietary fiber is not a single substance. There are significant differences in the physiological effects of the various components of dietary fiber. A Recommended Dietary Allowance for dietary fiber has not been established. However, an adequate amount of dietary fiber can be obtained by choosing several servings daily from a variety of fiber-rich foods such as whole-grain breads and cereals, fruits, vegetables, legumes, and nuts.

Harmful effects of ultraviolet radiation. Council on Scientific Affairs. *JAMA* 1989 Jul 21; 262(3): 380-4

Abstract: Tanning for cosmetic purposes by sunbathing or by using artificial tanning devices is widespread. The hazards associated with exposure to ultraviolet radiation are of concern to the medical profession. Depending on the amount and form of the radiation, as well as on the skin type of the individual exposed, ultraviolet radiation causes erythema, sunburn, photodamage (photoaging), photocarcinogenesis, damage to the eyes, alteration of the immune system of the skin, and chemical hypersensitivity. Skin cancers most commonly produced by ultraviolet radiation are basal and squamous cell carcinomas. There also is much circumstantial evidence that the increase in the incidence of cutaneous malignant melanoma during the past half century is related to increased sun exposure, but this has not been proved. Effective and cosmetically acceptable sunscreen preparations have been developed that can do much to prevent or reduce most harmful effects to ultraviolet radiation if they are applied properly and consistently. Other safety measures include (1) minimizing exposure to ultraviolet radiation, (2) being aware of reflective surfaces while in the sun, (3) wearing protective clothing, (4) avoiding use of artificial tanning devices, and (5) protecting infants and children.

Animals in research. Council on Scientific Affairs. *JAMA* 1989 Jun 23-30; 261(24): 3602-6

Mammographic screening in asymptomatic women aged 40 years and older. Council on Scientific Affairs. *JAMA* 1989 May 5; 261(17): 2535-42

Abstract: Currently, age-specific recommendations for screening mammograms in asymptomatic women that have been developed by professional, voluntary, and governmental organizations differ. While there is strong epidemiologic evidence that mammographic screening in asymptomatic women aged 50 years or older reduces breast cancer mortality, the evidence for mortality reduction is not as clear for women aged 40 to 49 years. However, as described in this report, findings of further mortality and survival follow-up of subjects in earlier studies, as well as observations from more recent studies, suggest reductions in mortality and better survival in younger women as well. While mammography is currently the most effective method for detecting early breast cancers, some breast cancers may develop during the intervals between screening mammograms. The costs of mammographic screening also require consideration in the process of making national screening recommendations.

Dyslexia. Council on Scientific Affairs. *JAMA* 1989 Apr 21; 261(15): 2236-9

Abstract: Experts disagree on the etiology and definition of dyslexia. Neurological research is ongoing but is not yet conclusive. Specific educational techniques for diagnosis and remediation are available. Physicians can serve on multidisciplinary diagnostic teams and can act to support and provide informational resources to affected families.

Providing medical services through school-based health programs. Council on Scientific Affairs. *JAMA* 1989 Apr 7; 261(13): 1939-42

Abstract: Resolution 162, which was adopted at the 1987 Annual Meeting by the Board of Trustees, called on the American Medical Association to study the efficacy of school-based health clinics. Recent data show that a significant number of school-aged youth are in need of an adequate source of health care. School-based health programs constitute a promising avenue for providing health services to adolescents, particularly in medically underserved areas. Although there are insufficient data to support universal establishment of school-based health programs, small-scale studies suggest that such programs are a viable means to increase access to health care for youth.

Formaldehyde. Council on Scientific Affairs. *JAMA* 1989 Feb 24; 261(8): 1183-7

Abstract: In response to Resolution 195 (A-87), the medical literature on the adverse health effects of formaldehyde was reviewed, and the potential cancer risk to anatomists and other related health professionals from exposure to the chemical is described. Though the evidence in humans is limited and controversial, both the Environmental Protection Agency and the Occupational Safety and Health Administration, in their consideration of available epidemiologic and toxicological studies, now regard formaldehyde as a possible human carcinogen and will regulate it accordingly.

AMA

Magnetic resonance imaging of the abdomen and pelvis. Council on Scientific Affairs. *JAMA* 1989 Jan 20; 261(3): 420-33

Abstract: Magnetic resonance imaging (MRI) of the abdomen presents greater inherent difficulties than other anatomic regions. However, new techniques now allow imaging comparable in quality to computed tomography (CT). Magnetic resonance imaging offers the advantages of greater tissue contrast, multiplanar imaging, and lack of ionizing radiation or risk of toxic reactions from iodinated contrast media. Its use remains limited by high cost, limited availability, lack of a bowel contrast agent, and long imaging time, which some patients cannot tolerate. In many areas of abdominal imaging, MRI is now comparable to CT, but because of the greater availability and lesser cost, CT remains the procedure of choice. Magnetic resonance imaging is more accurate for staging neoplasms of the liver, adrenal glands, kidneys, bladder, prostate, uterus, and cervix and may aid in diagnosis of hepatic, adrenal, and uterine masses. In selected patients, especially those in whom CT is inconclusive or those who cannot tolerate iodinated contrast material, MRI can provide valuable information. Development of faster scanning techniques and MRI contrast agents and wider availability will probably increase the usefulness of abdominal MRI. At this time, MRI complements other abdominal imaging procedures. In a small number of patients, however, it can provide unique information in a virtually risk-free manner.

1988

Evaluation of the health hazard of clove cigarettes. Council on Scientific Affairs. *JAMA* 1988 Dec 23-30; 260(24): 3641-4

Abstract: Resolution 43 (1987 Annual Meeting), adopted by the House of Delegates, resolved that the American Medical Association study the dangers associated with clove cigarettes, that policy recommendations regarding regulation of clove and other tobacco additives be developed, and that this information be made available to physicians and the public. Clove cigarettes are tobacco products. They therefore possess all the hazards associated with smoking all-tobacco cigarettes. In addition, inhaling clove cigarette smoke has been associated with severe lung injury in a few susceptible individuals with prodromal respiratory infection. Some individuals with normal respiratory tracts have apparently suffered aspiration pneumonitis as the result of a diminished gag reflex induced by a local anesthetic action of eugenol (the active component of cloves), which is volatilized into the smoke. The American Medical Association has an existing policy vigorously opposing the use of any tobacco product; no exemption from this policy is made for clove-containing cigarettes.

Magnetic resonance imaging of the head and neck region. Present status and future potential. Council on Scientific Affairs. Report of the Panel on Magnetic Resonance Imaging. *JAMA* 1988 Dec 9; 260(22): 3313-26

Abstract: Magnetic resonance imaging (MRI) has many bona fide applications in the head and neck region. The major strengths of its current conventional use include excellent soft-tissue contrast, multiplanar capabilities, noninvasiveness, and lack of ionizing radiation. Newer advances, including gradient-echo techniques, three-dimensional Fourier transformation, paramagnetic contrast, and more efficient receiver coils, will improve images and expand indications for MRI. The technology, however, remains relatively expensive, and the additional information compared with that of other techniques might not always justify the difference in cost. Moreover, MRI's insensitivity to calcifications, lack of depiction of fine bone detail, and, in some areas, degradation caused by motion and other artifacts make computed tomography and other noninvasive studies more appropriate as a primary imaging tool in many circumstances. Continued careful clinical research should clarify the relative role of MRI and other imaging tools during the next several years.

Positron emission tomography—a new approach to brain chemistry. Council on Scientific Affairs. Report of the Positron Emission Tomography Panel [published erratum appears in *JAMA* 1989 Jun 16;261(23):3412]. *JAMA* 1988 Nov 11; 260(18): 2704-10

Abstract: Positron emission tomography permits examination of the chemistry of the brain in living human beings. Until recently, positron emission tomography had been considered a research tool, but it is rapidly moving into clinical practice. This report describes the uses and applications of positron emission tomography in examinations of patients with strokes, epilepsy, malignancies, dementias, and schizophrenia and in basic studies of synaptic neurotransmission.

Treatment of obesity in adults. Council on Scientific Affairs. *JAMA* 1988 Nov 4; 260(17): 2547-51

Abstract: Concern with weight control should begin sufficiently early in life to reduce the risk of developing obesity. The complex etiology of obesity is, in part, responsible for the difficulty physicians encounter in treating this condition. Prevention is the "treatment" of choice. Early identification of individuals genetically at risk can be helpful in targeting those most likely to gain excess weight. Numerous dietary regimens have been devised in an attempt to achieve progressive weight loss in obese individuals. Since the ultimate goal of a weight-reduction program is to lose weight and maintain the loss, a nutritionally balanced, low-energy diet that is applicable to the patient's lifestyle is most appropriate. Increasing energy expenditure through physical activity, in addition to decreasing energy intake, generally improves results in the management of obesity. Major changes in eating and exercise behaviors are necessary to ensure long-term weight control. Diet, exercise, and behavior modification are interdependent and mutually supportive. A comprehensive weight-reduction program that incorporates all three components is more likely to lead to long-term weight control.

Cancer risk of pesticides in agricultural workers. Council on Scientific Affairs. *JAMA* 1988 Aug 19; 260(7): 959-66

Abstract: This report discusses some of the inherent limitations of cancer studies in animals and humans and presents a qualitative carcinogen risk assessment of a number of pesticides based on the judgment of national and international authorities who have reviewed the available experimental and epidemiologic evidence. A large number of pesticidal compounds have shown evidence of genotoxicity or carcinogenicity in animal and in vitro screening tests, but no pesticides—except arsenic and vinyl chloride (once used as an aerosol propellant)—

definitely have been proved to be carcinogenic in humans. Resolution 94 (1-86), which was referred to the Board of Trustees, calls for the American Medical Association, through its scientific journals and publications, to alert physicians to the potential hazards of agricultural pesticides, to provide physicians with advice on such hazards for their patients, and to urge that these substances be appropriately labeled. This report addresses the potential carcinogenicity of pesticides by review of the available literature.

Application of positron emission tomography in the heart. Council on Scientific Affairs. Report of the Positron Emission Tomography Panel. *JAMA* 1988 Apr 22-29; 259(16): 2438-45
Abstract: This report discusses experimental and clinical applications of positron emission tomography to the heart, including measurements of blood flow to the myocardium and studies of metabolism and experimental injury. Most initial clinical studies have concentrated on ischemic heart disease, but the technique also has potential for investigation of cardiomyopathies, studying the neural control of the heart, and evaluating the effects of drugs on cardiac tissues.

Positron emission tomography in oncology. Council on Scientific Affairs. *JAMA* 1988 Apr 8; 259(14): 2126-31
Abstract: This report describes the current and potential uses of positron emission tomography in clinical medicine and research related to oncology. Assessment will be possible of metabolism and physiology of tumors and their effects on adjacent tissues. Specific probes are likely to be developed for target sites on tumors, including monoclonal antibodies and specific growth factors that recognize tumors. To date, most oncological applications of positron emission tomography tracers have been qualitative; in the future, quantitative metabolic measurements should aid in the evaluation of tumor biology and response to treatment.

Cyclotrons and radiopharmaceuticals in positron emission tomography. Council on Scientific Affairs. Report of the Positron Emission Tomography Panel. *JAMA* 1988 Mar 25; 259(12): 1854-60
Abstract: Positron emission tomography (PET) can probe biochemical pathways in vivo and can provide quantitative data; for that purpose, tracers labeled with positron-emitting radioisotopes are essential. This report describes the tracers that are being used or that may have future use, their production by cyclotrons, and other needed resources for PET imaging. Current routine and automated methods for convenient production of labeled compounds, coupled with simple computer-controlled accelerators, can support the creation of clinical PET centers in any large medical institution, obviating the need for in-depth research teams. An alternate approach involves the development of regional centers that provide in-house service and that supply fluorine 18- and carbon 11-labeled compounds to nearby hospitals with PET machines.

Drug abuse in athletes. Anabolic steroids and human growth hormone. Council on Scientific Affairs. *JAMA* 1988 Mar 18; 259(11): 1703-5
Abstract: This report, the first in a three-part series on drug abuse by athletes, responds to adopted Resolution 4 (1984 Annual Meeting) and to Resolution 57 (1986 Annual Meeting), "Human Growth Hormone," which

was referred to the Board of Trustees for action. Subsequent reports will cover other classes of abused drugs (Resolution 57, A-86).

Instrumentation in positron emission tomography. Council on Scientific Affairs. Report of the Positron Emission Tomography Panel. *JAMA* 1988 Mar 11; 259(10): 1531-6
Abstract: Positron emission tomography (PET) is a three-dimensional medical imaging technique that noninvasively measures the concentration of radiopharmaceuticals in the body that are labeled with positron emitters. With the proper compounds, PET can be used to measure metabolism, blood flow, or other physiological values in vivo. The technique is based on the physics of positron annihilation and detection and the mathematical formulations developed for x-ray computed tomography. Modern PET systems can provide three-dimensional images of the brain, the heart, and other internal organs with resolutions on the order of 4 to 6 mm. With the selectivity provided by a choice of injected compounds, PET has the power to provide unique diagnostic information that is not available with any other imaging modality. This is the first of five reports on the nature and uses of PET that have been prepared for the American Medical Association's Council on Scientific Affairs by an authoritative panel.

Magnetic resonance imaging of the central nervous system. Council on Scientific Affairs. Report of the Panel on Magnetic Resonance Imaging. *JAMA* 1988 Feb 26; 259(8): 1211-22
Abstract: This report reviews the current applications of magnetic resonance imaging of the central nervous system. Since its introduction into the clinical environment in the early 1980s, this technology has had a major impact on the practice of neurology. It has proved to be superior to computed tomography for imaging many diseases of the brain and spine. In some instances it has clearly replaced computed tomography. It is likely that it will replace myelography for the assessment of cervicomedullary junction and spinal regions. The magnetic field strengths currently used appear to be entirely safe for clinical application in neurology, except in patients with cardiac pacemakers or vascular metallic clips. Some shortcomings of magnetic resonance imaging include its expense, the time required for scanning, and poor visualization of cortical bone.

Report of the organ transplant panel. Corneal transplantation. Council on Scientific Affairs. *JAMA* 1988 Feb 5; 259(5): 719-22
Abstract: Corneal transplantation is the most common form of organ transplantation practiced in the United States. Two procedures for transplantation are utilized. Penetrating keratoplasty is used in about 90% of the cases, with lamellar keratoplasty being utilized in the remaining situations. Demand for corneal transplantation exceeds the available supply of corneas. Advances in procurement and preservation must continue to meet this demand. Finally, these procedures are not without complications, and these are discussed to provide a clear risk-benefit analysis.

AMA

Magnetic resonance imaging of the cardiovascular system. Present state of the art and future potential. Council on Scientific Affairs. Report of the Magnetic Resonance Imaging Panel. *JAMA* 1988 Jan 8; 259(2): 253-9

Abstract: State-of-the-art magnetic resonance imaging (MRI) generates high-resolution images of the cardiovascular system. Conventional MRI techniques provide images in 6 to 10 minutes per tomographic slice. New strategies have substantially improved the speed of imaging. The technology is relatively expensive, and its cost-effectiveness remains to be defined in relation to other effective, less expensive, and noninvasive technologies, such as echocardiography and nuclear medicine. The ultimate role of MRI will depend on several factors, including the development of specific applications such as (1) noninvasive angiography, especially of the coronary arteries; (2) noninvasive, high-resolution assessment of regional myocardial blood flow distribution (eg, using paramagnetic contrast agents); (3) characterization of myocardial diseases using proton-relaxation property changes; and (4) evaluation of in vivo myocardial biochemistry. The three-dimensional imaging capability and the ability to image cardiovascular structures without contrast material give MRI a potential advantage over existing noninvasive diagnostic imaging techniques. This report analyzes current applications of MRI to the cardiovascular system and speculates on their future.

1987

Fundamentals of magnetic resonance imaging. Council on Scientific Affairs. *JAMA* 1987 Dec 18; 258(23): 3417-23

Magnetic resonance imaging. Prologue. Council on Scientific Affairs. *JAMA* 1987 Dec 11; 258(22): 3283-5

Aversion therapy. Council on Scientific Affairs. *JAMA* 1987 Nov 13; 258(18): 2562-6

Issues in employee drug testing. Council on Scientific Affairs. *JAMA* 1987 Oct 16; 258(15): 2089-96

In vitro testing for allergy. Report II of the Allergy Panel. Council on Scientific Affairs. *JAMA* 1987 Sep 25; 258(12): 1639-43

In vivo diagnostic testing and immunotherapy for allergy. Report I, Part II, of the Allergy Panel. Council on Scientific Affairs [published erratum appears in *JAMA* 1987 Dec 11; 258(22): 3259]. *JAMA* 1987 Sep 18; 258(11): 1505-8

In vivo diagnostic testing and immunotherapy for allergy. Report I, Part I, of the Allergy Panel. Council on Scientific Affairs. *JAMA* 1987 Sep 11; 258(10): 1363-7

Radon in homes. Council on Scientific Affairs [published erratum appears in *JAMA* 1988 Jan 1;259(1):47]. *JAMA* 1987 Aug 7; 258(5): 668-72

Autopsy. A comprehensive review of current issues. Council on Scientific Affairs. *JAMA* 1987 Jul 17; 258(3): 364-9

Scientific issues in drug testing. Council on Scientific Affairs. *JAMA* 1987 Jun 12; 257(22): 3110-4

Results and implications of the AMA-APA Physician Mortality Project. Stage II. Council on Scientific Affairs [published erratum appears in *JAMA* 1987 Aug 7;258(5):614]. *JAMA* 1987 Jun 5; 257(21): 2949-53

Vitamin preparations as dietary supplements and as therapeutic agents. Council on Scientific Affairs. *JAMA* 1987 Apr 10; 257(14): 1929-36

Introduction to the management of immunosuppression. Council on Scientific Affairs. *JAMA* 1987 Apr 3; 257(13): 1781-5

Preventing death and injury from fires with automatic sprinklers and smoke detectors. Council on Scientific Affairs. *JAMA* 1987 Mar 27; 257(12): 1618-20

Health effects of video display terminals. Council on Scientific Affairs. *JAMA* 1987 Mar 20; 257(11): 1508-12

Elder abuse and neglect. Council on Scientific Affairs. *JAMA* 1987 Feb 20; 257(7): 966-71

Radioepidemiological tables. Council on Scientific Affairs. *JAMA* 1987 Feb 13; 257(6): 806-9

1986

Autologous blood transfusions. Council on Scientific Affairs. *JAMA* 1986 Nov 7; 256(17): 2378-80

Dementia. Council on Scientific Affairs. *JAMA* 1986 Oct 24-31; 256(16): 2234-8

Polygraph. Council on Scientific Affairs. *JAMA* 1986 Sep 5; 256(9): 1172-5

Lasers in medicine and surgery. Council on Scientific Affairs. *JAMA* 1986 Aug 15; 256(7): 900-7

Health effects of smokeless tobacco. Council on Scientific Affairs. *JAMA* 1986 Feb 28; 255(8): 1038-44

Alcohol and the driver. Council on Scientific Affairs. *JAMA* 1986 Jan 24-31; 255(4): 522-7

1985

Xenografts. Review of the literature and current status. Council on Scientific Affairs. *JAMA* 1985 Dec 20; 254(23): 3353-7

Saccharin. Review of safety issues. Council on Scientific Affairs. *JAMA* 1985 Nov 8; 254(18): 2622-4

The use of cardiac pacemakers in medical practice. Excerpts from the report of the Advisory Panel. Council on Scientific Affairs. *JAMA* 1985 Oct 11; 254(14): 1952-4

Status report on the acquired immunodeficiency syndrome. Human T-cell lymphotropic virus type III testing. Council on Scientific Affairs. *JAMA* 1985 Sep 13; 254(10): 1342-5

AMA diagnostic and treatment guidelines concerning child abuse and neglect. Council on Scientific Affairs. *JAMA* 1985 Aug 9; 254(6): 796-800

Aspartame. Review of safety issues. Council on Scientific Affairs. *JAMA* 1985 Jul 19; 254(3): 400-2

Effects of toxic chemicals on the reproductive system. Council on Scientific Affairs. *JAMA* 1985 Jun 21; 253(23): 3431-7

Guidelines for reporting estimates of probability of paternity. Council on Scientific Affairs. *JAMA* 1985 Jun 14; 253(22): 3298

SI units for clinical laboratory data. Council on Scientific Affairs. *JAMA* 1985 May 3; 253(17): 2553-4

Scientific status of refreshing recollection by the use of hypnosis. Council on Scientific Affairs. *JAMA* 1985 Apr 5; 253(13): 1918-23

Current status of therapeutic plasmapheresis and related techniques. Report of the AMA panel on therapeutic plasmapheresis. Council on Scientific Affairs. *JAMA* 1985 Feb 8; 253(6): 819-25

1984

Methaqualone: Abuse limits its usefulness. Council on Scientific Affairs. *JAMA* 1983 Dec 9; 250(22): 3052

Early detection of breast cancer. Council on Scientific Affairs. *JAMA* 1984 Dec 7; 252(21): 3008-11

A physician's guide to asbestos-related diseases. Council on Scientific Affairs. *JAMA* 1984 Nov 9; 252(18): 2593-7

The acquired immunodeficiency syndrome. Commentary. Council on Scientific Affairs. *JAMA* 1984 Oct 19; 252(15): 2037-43

Caffeine labeling. Council on Scientific Affairs. American Medical Association. *JAMA* 1984 Aug 10; 252(6): 803-6 (Resolution 74, I-82)

Exercise programs for the elderly. Council on Scientific Affairs. *JAMA* 1984 Jul 27; 252(4): 544-6

Combined modality approaches to cancer therapy. Council on Scientific Affairs. *JAMA* 1984 May 11; 251(18): 2398-407

Effects of pregnancy on work performance. Council on Scientific Affairs. *JAMA* 1984 Apr 20; 251(15): 1995-7

Percutaneous transluminal angioplasty. Council on Scientific Affairs. *JAMA* 1984 Feb 10; 251(6): 764-8

Effects of physical forces on the reproductive cycle. Council on Scientific Affairs. *JAMA* 1984 Jan 13; 251(2): 247-50

1983

Calcium channel blocking agents. Council on Scientific Affairs. *JAMA* 1983 Nov 11; 250(18): 2522-4

Pharmaceutical dissolution of gallstones. *JAMA* 1983 Nov 4; 250(17): 2373-4

Dietary and pharmacologic therapy for the lipid risk factors. *JAMA* 1983 Oct 14; 250(14): 1873-9

In utero fetal surgery. Council on Scientific Affairs. *JAMA* 1983 Sep 16; 250(11): 1443-4

Cochlear implants. *JAMA* 1983 Jul 15; 250(3): 391-2

Automobile-related injuries. *JAMA* 1983 Jun 17; 249(23): 3216-22.

Fetal effects of maternal alcohol use. *JAMA* 1983 May 13; 249(18): 2517-21

Medical evaluations of healthy persons. Council on Scientific Affairs. *JAMA* 1983 Mar 25; 249(12): 1626-33

Sodium in processed foods. *JAMA* 1983 Feb 11; 249(6): 784-9

Estrogen replacement in the menopause. Council on Scientific Affairs. *JAMA* 1983 Jan 21; 249(3): 359-61

Brain injury in boxing. Council on Scientific Affairs. *JAMA* 1983 Jan 14; 249(2): 254-7

1982

Continuous ambulatory peritoneal dialysis. Council on Scientific Affairs. *JAMA* 1982 Nov 12; 248(18): 2340-1

Health effects of Agent Orange and dioxin contaminants. Council on Scientific Affairs. *JAMA* 1982 Oct 15; 248(15): 1895-7

Dimethyl sulfoxide. Controversy and current status— 1981. Council on Scientific Affairs. *JAMA* 1982 Sep 17; 248(11): 1369-71

Health care needs of a homosexual population. Council on Scientific Affairs. *JAMA* 1982 Aug 13; 248(6): 736-9

Genetic counseling and prevention of birth defects. Council on Scientific Affairs. *JAMA* 1982 Jul 9: 248 (2): 221-4

Maternal serum alpha-fetoprotein monitoring. Council on Scientific Affairs. *JAMA* 1982 Mar 12; 247(10): 1478-81

Drug abuse related to prescribing practices. Council on Scientific Affairs. *JAMA* 1982 Feb 12; 247(6): 864-6

1981

Electronic fetal monitoring. Council on Scientific Affairs. *JAMA* 1981 Nov 20; 246(20): 2370-3

Organ donor recruitment. Council on Scientific Affairs. *JAMA* 1981 Nov 13; 246(19): 2157-8

Marijuana. Its health hazards and therapeutic potentials. Council on Scientific Affairs. *JAMA* 1981 Oct 16; 246(16): 1823-7

Carcinogen regulation. Council on Scientific Affairs. *JAMA* 1981 Jul 17; 246(3): 253-6

Physician-supervised exercise programs in rehabilitation of patients with coronary heart disease. Council on Scientific Affairs. *JAMA* 1981 Apr 10; 245(14): 1463-6

Medical care for indigent and culturally displaced obstetrical patients and their newborns. Committee on Maternal, Adolescent, and Child Health. Council on Scientific Affairs. *JAMA* 1981 Mar 20; 245(11): 1159-60

Hypnotic drugs and treatment of insomnia. Council on Scientific Affairs. *JAMA* 1981 Feb 20; 245(7): 749-50.

1980

Hypoglycemic treatment. Guidelines for the non-insulin-dependent diabetic. Council on Scientific Affairs. *JAMA* 1980 May 23/30; 243(20): 2078-9

Smoking and health. *JAMA* 1980 Feb 22-29; 243(8): 779-81

1979

Indications for aortocoronary bypass graft surgery, 1979. Council on Scientific Affairs. *JAMA* 1979 Dec 14; 242(24): 2709-11

American Medical Association concepts of nutrition and health. Council on Scientific Affairs. *JAMA* 1979 Nov 23; 242(21): 2335-8

1978

Adoption of international system of units for clinical chemistry. Council on Scientific Affairs. *JAMA* 1978 Dec 8; 240(24): 2664

Health evaluation of energy-generating sources. AMA Council on Scientific Affairs. *JAMA* 1978 Nov 10; 240(20): 2193-5

Council on Scientific Affairs: Unpublished Reports

The following list contains Council on Scientific Affairs reports that have been requested by the House of Delegates in addition to the published materials above. Here they are listed in alphabetical order by the year and meeting they were first presented to the House by a representative of the Council.

1997

Annual Meeting

Alternative Medicine

Calcium Supplementation, Hormone Replacement Therapy, and Osteoporosis

"Crossover" Use of Donated Blood

Diagnosis and Treatment of Attention Deficit Disorders in School Age Children

Drivers Impaired by Alcohol

Folk Remedies Among Ethnic Subgroups

Guide to Clinical Preventive Services, 2nd Edition

Harm Reduction

Heat-Related Illness

HIV Home Collection Kits

Immunization of Health Care Workers With Varicella Vaccine

Silicone Elastomer Cerebrospinal Fluid Shunt Systems

The Advisability of Screening Younger Women for Breast Cancer

Unlabeled Indications of Food and Drug Administration Approved Drugs

Use of Restraints for Patients in Nursing Homes

1996

Annual Meeting

Fatigue, Sleep Disorders, and Motor Vehicle Crashes

Federal Block Grants and Public Health

Hyponatremic Seizures Among Infants Fed With Commercial Bottled Drinking Water

Principles of Discharge and Discharge Criteria

Thiamin Addition to Alcohol

Interim Meeting

Alternative Therapies for the Symptoms of Menopause

Conference: Clinical Research: Assessing the Future in a Changing Environment

Establishment of a National Vaccine Authority

Genetic Susceptibility Testing for Breast and Ovarian Cancer

HIV Home Test Kits Update

On-Site Physician Home Health Care

Silicone Breast Implants and Disease

Thiamin Addition to Alcohol

Annual 1996 Joint CSA/CEJA Report

Ethical Issues in Assisted Reproductive Technology

1995

Annual Meeting

Barriers to Optimal Pain Management

Guidelines for Evaluating Spinal Impairments Under the Americans With Disabilities Act

Impact of 24-Hour Postpartum Stay on Infant and Maternal Health (Res 135, A-94)

Maternal HIV Screening and Treatment to Reduce the Risk of Perinatal HIV Transmission: An Update Report

Prevention of Sexually Transmissible Diseases (Res 411, A-94)

Substance Abuse Among Physicians

Interim Meeting

Adolescent Immunization

American Hospital Association (AHA) "Management Advisory" on No-Cause Drug Testing of the Medical Staff

Emerging Laboratory Tests for the Diagnosis of *Chlamydia trachomatis* Infection

Folic Acid Relationships to Spinal Closure Birth Defects and Adult Vascular Disease

Intake of Dietary Calcium to Reduce the Incidence of Osteoporosis

1994

Annual Meeting

American Hospital Association "Management Advisory" on No-Cause Drug Testing of the Medical Staff

Environmental Tobacco Smoke: Health Effects and Prevention Policies

Lead Poisoning Among Children

Memories of Childhood Abuse

Management of Disorders of Cholesterol, Triglyceride, and Lipoprotein Metabolism

Maternal HIV Screening and Treatment to Reduce the Risk of Perinatal HIV Transmission

The Potential Impact of Health System Reform Legislative Proposals on Biomedical Research and Clinical Investigation

Science and Biomedical Research: Opportunities, Challenges, and Health System Reform

Uniform State Laws for Transient Lapse of Consciousness

Interim Meeting

American Hospital Association "Management Advisory" on No-Cause Drug Testing of the Medical Staff

Endorsement of Standards for Pediatric Immunization

Educational and Informational Strategies to Reduce Pesticide Risk

Effects of Electric and Magnetic Fields

Lead Poisoning Among Children

Methadone Maintenance in Private Practice

Violence Against Men: Fact or Fiction

1993

Annual Meeting

Alcohol, Drugs, and Family Violence

Mental Health Consequences of Interpersonal and Family Violence: Implications for the Practitioner

Thermography Update

Update on AMA Policies on Human Sexuality and Family Life Education

Interim Meeting

Irradiation of Food (Res 502, I-92)

Uniform State Laws for Transient Lapse of Consciousness (Res 519, I-92)

Interim Meeting Informational Report

Environmental Tobacco Smoke: Health Effects and Prevention Policies

1992

Annual Meeting

Benzodiazepine Education (Res 413, I-91)

Food and Drug Administration Regulations Regarding the Inclusion of Added L-Glutamic Acid Content on Food Labels (Res. 187, A-91)

Recommendations for Ensuring the Health of the Adolescent Athlete

Perinatal Addiction: Issues in Care and Prevention (Res 233, A-90)

Police Chase and Chase-Related Injuries (Res 106, A-91)

US Nuclear Regulatory Regulations Affecting Outpatient Treatment with Radiopharmaceuticals (Res 22 and 23, A-91)

Annual Meeting Informational Reports

Feasibility of Assuring Confidentiality and Security of Computer-Based Patient Records

Improving Patient Records

Modern Component Usage in Transfusion Therapy, 1992

Interim Meeting

Autologous Blood Transfusion

Clinical Preventive Services: Implications for Adolescent, Adult, and Geriatric Medicine

Confidential Health Service for Adolescents

Performance Testing

Rapid Laboratory Tests for the Identification of Mycobacterium

Interim Meeting Informational Report

Tuberculosis

Interim Meeting Joint Report of CSA/CMS

Payment for Patients Enrolled in Clinical Trials (Res 115, I-91)

1991

Annual Meeting

Adding "Tobacco Contribution" to Death Certificates

Carrier Screening for Cystic Fibrosis

Commercial Weight Loss Systems and Programs

The Impact of the Marketing-Distribution System for Clozapine on Patient Access

Physicians and Retirement

Annual Meeting Informational Reports

Comorbidity

The Recognition and Treatment of Depression in Medical Practice

Treatment of Depression by Primary Care Physicians: Pharmacological Approaches

Treatment of Depression by Primary Care Physicians: Psychotherapeutic Treatments for Depression

Interim Meeting

Biotechnologies Targeting the Diseases of the Aged

Children and Youth With Disabilities

Financial Incentives for Autopsies

Food Safety: Federal Inspection Programs

Health Claims by Manufacturers of Breakfast Cereal

Over-the-Counter Availability of Veterinary Medications

Silicone Breast Implants

US Nuclear Regulatory Regulations Affecting Outpatient Treatment With Radiopharmaceuticals

Interim Meeting Informational Reports

Carpal Tunnel Syndrome

Diagnostic Evaluation of the Differential Diagnosis of Thyroid Nodules

Systemic Therapy for Breast Cancer

Interim Meeting Joint Report of CSA/CME

Federal Research Grant Indirect Cost Policy

Interim Meeting Joint Report of CSA/CMS

Seat Lift Chairs

1990

Annual Meeting

Mandatory Random Drug Testing in Competitive Sports

Organ Transplantation

Statement of Concern Regarding Destructive Themes Contained in Rock Music

Annual Meeting Informational Reports

Alternatives to Animal Use in Biomedical Research

Alternative Psychological Methods in Patient Care

Ultrasonographic Evaluation of the Fetus

Annual Meeting Joint Report of CSA/CMS

Radiographic Contrast Media—Interim Report

Interim Meeting

Drug Testing

Economic and Public Policy Issues Involving Bovine Somatotropin

The Etiology of Depression in Adults

Genetic Testing and the Potential Basis for Job Discrimination

The Need for Increased Research and Development in Nuclear Fusion to Reduce Environmental Pollution

Physician and Medical Student Support for HIV Education Programs for Adolescents

AMA

Interim Meeting Informational Reports

Extra Low Frequency Electric and Magnetic Fields and the Question of Cancer

Home Total Parenteral Nutrition

Infant Mortality and Access to Care

Interim Meeting Joint Report of CSA/CME

Radiographic Contrast Media

Technology Assessment in Medicine

1989

Annual Meeting

Global Climate Change: The Greenhouse Effect

Mammographic Criteria for Surgical Biopsy of Nonpalpable Breast Lesions

The Viability of Cancer Clinical Research

Annual Meeting Information Reports

Health Effects of Video Display Terminals: An Update

Recognition of Childhood Sexual Abuse as a Factor in Adolescent Health Issues

Interim Meeting Policy Reports

DATTA Evaluations

Nationwide Reporting of Elevated Blood Lead Levels

Potential Health Effects of the Biological Defense Research Program of the Department of Defense

Stewardship of the Environment

Viability of Clinical Research: Coverage and Reimbursement

Interim Meeting Joint Report of CSA/CEJA

Scientific Fraud and Misrepresentation

Interim Meeting Informational Reports

Establishing Mammographic Criteria for Recommending Surgical Biopsy

HIV Infection and Disease—Monographs for Physicians and Other Health Care Workers

1988

Annual Meeting

Disseminating Scientific Health Information to the Public

Reducing Transmission of Human Immunodeficiency Virus (HIV) Among and Through Intravenous Drug Abusers

Annual Meeting Informational Report

Venomous Snakebites in the United States and Canada

Interim Meeting

Fraud and Misrepresentation in Science

Recommendations for HIV Testing

Interim Meeting Informational Reports

Effects of Pregnancy on Work Performance

The Health Hazards of Lead in Drinking Water

HTLV-I Testing of Blood Donors

Hyperthyroidism in the Elderly

1987

Annual Meeting

Issues in Employee Drug Testing

Religious Exemptions From Immunizations

Annual Meeting Informational Reports

Acid Rain Update

AIDS and the Obstetrician/Gynecologist: Commentary

Biology of HIV Infection

Blood Transfusions and AIDS

The Challenge of AIDS for Physicians Today

Classification of the Clinical Spectrum of HIV Infection in Adults

Clinical Trials of Drugs for the Treatment of AIDS

Commercial Hair Analysis

Epidemiology of Acquired Immunodeficiency Syndrome: A Brief Overview

Evaluation of Routine Infant Circumcision

Issues in Health Fraud: Colonic Irrigation

Pediatric Acquired Immunodeficiency Syndrome

Real and Perceived Risks of AIDS in the Family and Household

Real and Perceived Risks of AIDS in the Health Care and Work Environment

Serologic Tests for Human Immunodeficiency Virus (HIV)

Treatment of Infertility

Interim Meeting

Accuracy of the ELISA and the Western Blot Serologic Tests for HIV Infection

AIDS Education

Firearms as a Public Health Problem in the US: Injuries and Deaths

Smoking Cessation

Interim Meeting Informational Report

Ozone Report

1986

Annual Meeting

AIDS and School Discrimination (Res 96 and 97, I-85)

Drugs and Athletes—Progress Report

The Heimlich Maneuver—Interim Report (Res 52, I-85)

Herpes Simplex and School Children

Over-the-Counter Diet Preparations Containing Phenylpropanolamine (Res 100, I-85)

Safe Use of Radioactive Materials in Medical Practice (Res 66, A-85)

Annual Meeting Informational Reports

Glucocorticoid-Induced Osteonecrosis

Statement on Liver Transplantation

Interim Meeting

Consumption of Lean Beef (Res 145, A-86

Discrimination Against AIDS Patients (Res 97, I-85)

The Heimlich Maneuver (Res 52, I-85)

Warning Labels on Over-the-Counter Iron Preparations and Dietary Supplements

Interim Meeting Informational Reports

Cocaine: Phenomenology and Treatment of Abuse

Health Fraud Report

Medical Aspects of Preadolescent Participation in Sports

1985

Annual Meeting

Autopsies: Interim Report (Substitute Res 11, A-84)

Annual Meeting Informational Reports

Acid Rain

Formaldehyde in Manufactured Housing

Harmful Effects of UVA and UVB Light

Interim Meeting

Antiabortion Film "Silent Scream" (Res 143, A-85)

Antibiotics in Animal Feeds

Drugs and Athletes—Interim Report

Effects of Pesticide Exposure

Interim Meeting Informational Reports

Opioid Abuse and Dependence: Diagnosis, Referral, and Treatment

Toxic Shock Syndrome

1984

Annual Meeting

FDA Regulation of Drugs and Medical Devices (Res 71, I-83)

Prescription Abuse Data Synthesis (PADS) Project and the AMA

Prescription Drug Abuse Activity

Interim Meeting

Chelation Therapy

The Health Effects of "Agent Orange" and Polychlorinated Dioxin Contaminants

Nicotine Chewing Gum for Cessation of Smoking

1983

Annual Meeting

Choking: The Heimlich Maneuver (Abdominal Thrust) vs Back Blows

Current Issues in Pediatric Immunization

Update on Venereal Disease

Interim Meeting

AMA's Role in Technology Assessment (Res 131 (A-83)

Drug Substitution—Definition of Terms

A Guide to the Hospital Management of Injuries Arising From Exposure to or Involving Ionizing Radiation

Nonsmoking in Hospitals

Pharmaceutical Marketing (Substitute Res 77, A-82)

1982

Annual Meeting

Council on Scientific Affairs Responses to the National Center for Health Care Technology and Office of Health Research, Statistics, and Technology

Infant Formula Marketing (Res 155, A-81)

Interim Meeting

Addition of Thiamin to Alcoholic Beverages (Res 140, A-81)

AMA Involvement in Prevention and Treatment of Child Abuse and Neglect (Substitute Res 75, A-81)

Physician Mortality and Suicide: Results and Implications of the AMA-APA Pilot Study

Pneumococcal, Influenza, and Hepatitis-B Vaccine (Res 75 A-82)

Revision of AMA Guides to Impairment

1981

Annual Meeting

Acupuncture

Evaluation of Iridology

Risks of Nuclear Energy and Low-Level Ionizing Radiation

The 1980 Report of the Joint National Commission on Detection, Evaluation, and Treatment of High Blood Pressure

Interim Meeting

Prescription of Tranquilizers and Antidepressants for Women (Board of Trustees Report X, I-80)

1980

Annual Meeting

Biological Effects of Non-Ionizing Magnetic and Electromagnetic Radiation

Encouragement of Physician Investigator Training

Infant Nutrition (Res 111, I-78)

Progress in Adoption of SI Units

Interim Meeting

Alcoholism as a Disability

Health Care Technology Assessment—1980

Importance of Diagnostic Computerized Tomographic Scanning

Indications and Contraindications for Exercise Testing

The Nutritive Quality of Processed Foods: General Policies for Nutrient Additions

1979

Annual Meeting

Physical Fitness and Physical Education

Recommendations for AMA Involvement in Alcoholism Activities

Reliability of Laboratory Procedures

Statement on the Role of Dietary Management in Hypertensive Control

AMA

Interim Meeting

The Chronic Mental Patient: Commentary on the Final Report of the President's Commission on Mental Health

Chymopapain

Dietary Sodium and Potassium

Evaluation of Community Mental Health Centers

Food Safety and the Food, Drug, and Cosmetic Act

Saccharin Availability

Sentinel Deaths

1978

Annual Meeting

Heroin Reclassification

The Medical Implications of Motorcycle Helmet Usage

Reliability of Laboratory Procedures

Use of Barbiturates in Medical Practice

Interim Meeting

AMA Committee on Medical Aspects of Sports

Care for the Chronically Mentally Ill in the Community: Progress Report

CHILDSAFE Project

Community Mental Health Centers

Principles of Quality Mental Health Care

Present Status of the Medical Autopsy

Recommendations for AMA Involvement in Alcoholism Activities and Commentary on NIAAA's *National Plan to Combat Alcohol Abuse and Alcoholism*

Recommendations on Drug Development and Drug Regulation

Shortage of Human Growth Hormone

Staging of Cancer

Status of Multiphasic Health Evaluation—1978

Symptomatic and Supportive Care for Patients with Cancer

1977

Annual Meeting

Guidelines for Recombinant DNA Research

Use of Amphetamines in the Treatment of Obesity

Interim Meeting

Airbags, Seatbelts, and Prevention of Vehicle-Related Injuries

Patient Instructional Leaflets

Physicians and Sex Therapy Clinics

Statement on Parent and Newborn Interaction

Contact for copies of Council on Scientific Affairs reports:
Brenda Stewart
Council on Scientific Affairs
American Medical Association
515 N State St, Chicago, IL 60610
312 464-5334

Office of Biomedical and Clinical Research

This office was created in response to the CSA's concern to keep science, including basic and clinical research, at the center of American medicine during a time when tight research budgets and the reorganization of the delivery and funding of medical care has placed significant pressure on this function. The office will serve as an educational focal point for the Human Genome Project, advocate for animal research and organ transplant donation, and ensure that adequate resources for clinical research are available to those in the academic community who need them.

Division of Health Science

The AMA health science activities are designed to establish a responsible role for the AMA in mental health, geriatric health, nutrition, preventive medicine and public health, adolescent health, and HIV infection and AIDS. This includes the identification of existing and emerging issues in each of these areas and the development of appropriate AMA responses, which include publications, proposed policies, conferences, and reports.

Department of Mental Health

A National Coalition of Physicians Against Family Violence has been established through the AMA Department of Mental Health for physicians interested in learning more about the various abuses constituting family violence. A national advisory council of physicians representing more than 35 specialty and medical societies has been developed to continue to guide the development of the campaign. Diagnostic and treatment guidelines on child abuse, child sexual abuse, domestic violence and elder abuse have been developed and are disseminated by the Department of Mental Health.

HIV/AIDS Office

This is an area that receives major focus with planned activities such as a national primary care physicians' survey and additional professional education activities. The AMA Task Force on AIDS, an official task force designated as such by the House of Delegates, operates inherently with this office to ensure activities in support of the many issues raised by the AIDS epidemic are addressed by the Association.

Department of Adolescent Health

This department was created in 1988 to provide leadership of the AMA's efforts to improve the health status of youth. Current activities include development of the AMA National Coalition on Adolescent Health, which consists of 34 national organizations, foundations, and government agencies directly concerned with adolescents; *Guidelines for Adolescent Preventive Services* (GAPS) project, which represents the only set of clinical preventive services recommendations for adolescents; administration of a RWJF-funded program to fund and design initiatives that seek to reduce alcohol-related problems among adolescents; and a school and community demonstration project, in conjunction with the National Association of State Boards of Education, to implement recommendations of the 1990 report of the National Commission on the role of the school and community in improving adolescent health.

Department of Preventive Medicine and Public Health

This department pursues activities in the areas of smoking cessation, women's health, and environmental health.

Office of Alcohol and Other Drug Abuse

This office emphasizes two areas: (1) the reduction of youth alcohol consumption and high-risk drinking, and (2) the development of scientific papers and training on alcohol and other drug issues affecting clinical practice, public policy, and AMA activities.

The Office administers two National Program Offices with grant funds totaling $20 million for the Robert Wood Johnson Foundation: "A Matter of Degree: Reducing High-Risk Drinking Among College Students": Eight campus/community partnerships seek to reduce binge drinking and related social norms through campus and community policies, the mass media, and other local communications channels. The second, "Reducing Underage Drinking Through Coalitions," administers 12 grantees that have developed state coalitions to mobilize the public (particularly youth), raise public awareness of the benefits of reducing underage drinking, and develop and implement plans to solve the problems presented by underage drinking.

Area Publications include:

Guides to the Evaluation of Permanent Impairment

Department of Technology Assessment

The AMA is nationally recognized as a leader in the evaluation of the drugs, devices, procedures, and techniques used in the practice of medicine. Through its Diagnostic and Therapeutic Technology Assessment (DATTA) program, the AMA provides the most authoritative information available to enhance the appropriate utilization of health care technology and communicates and represents the physician's viewpoint to third-party payers, self-insurers, HMOs, hospitals, national associations, and the federal government.

The American Medical Association's Diagnostic and Therapeutic Technology Assessment Program

JAMA 1983 July 15: 250(3): 387-8

The Diagnostic and Therapeutic Technology Assessment (DATTA) program was inaugurated in 1982, with invitations extended to all medical specialty and state medical societies that are represented in the AMA House of Delegates. They were asked to submit the names of physicians whose judgment could be valued in the assessment of their specialty or in the analysis of related clinical problems. In addition, members of the previous expert panels that had served the AMA through the Council on Scientific Affairs were nominated to serve. After reviewing the nominees, the Council on Scientific Affairs appointed 483 physicians to the DATTA roster. A complete curriculum vitae and bibliography were solicited from each nominee so that his or her special interests and particular expertise could be made available on file.

The operation of the DATTA program by AMA staff is supervised by a subcommittee of three members of the Council on Scientific Affairs. The Council reviewed several questions that had come to the AMA from external sources. It also generated questions of its own for inclusion in the initial mailing in January of 1983 of six questions of broad interest to the medical profession.

Questions will be considered from any source as long as they are clearly stated in writing and focused so that a clear opinion can be rendered. They should be accompanied by appropriate bibliographic references or suitable documentation that will help to justify the question. The selection of questions will be determined by staff under the direction of the subcommittee of the Council on Scientific Affairs, which will reserve the right to accept or reject questions.

A panel of at least 20 specialists, selected for their knowledge and experience in the clinical area under examination, receives the question, which has been carefully worded in appropriate scientific and technical terms. Each correspondent is asked to respond as to whether the practice is (1) established (with clinical limitation, if any are needed for general use), (2) investigational (used under research protocol), (3) unacceptable, (4) indeterminate, or if there is (5) no opinion (because the respondent has no knowledge of the technology).

Comments are also invited with regard to the experimental basis for the rating, pros and cons of the technology, specific knowledge of controlled trials, and inherent risks as perceived by the respondent. The bibliographic resources of the AMA's library are available to each panel member. The AMA staff is expected concomitantly to research each question and be cognizant of existing assessments (in preparation or extant) from other organizations, including appropriate medical specialty societies.

Responses are based on a consensus of the panelists. When a consensus cannot be reached a special study, conference, or report may be called for by the Council on Scientific Affairs. Approved responses will be returned to the questioner and may be disseminated to the profession and the public through publication in *JAMA*. Each response will be accompanied by the following statement: "The above response is provided as a service of the American Medical Association. It is based on current scientific and clinical information and does not represent endorsement by the AMA of particular diagnostic and therapeutic procedures or treatment."

It is apparent from this description that these responses to questions are the general opinion held by the clinical specialists in that branch of medicine who should be most knowledgeable about the practice in that area. This opinion should not be considered a final judgment on the ultimate utility or inadequacy of a particular procedure, but rather an indication of how it is viewed at this particular time by knowledgeable practitioners. All of these opinions will, of course, be highly temporal and subject to revision on the basis of new information and experience.

It would be counterproductive if these opinions should lead to a reduction in investigative efforts to establish the sensitivity and specificity of a new method of diagnosis or treatment. All physicians can recall the initial rejection of a novel technique (such as hemodialysis for kidney disease) that later became accepted after the addition of a new element (the artificial arteriovenous shunt).

The Council on Scientific Affairs appreciates that the best way to establish the superiority of one technology over

AMA

another, for diagnosis or treatment of a particular disease process, is based on research data that are ultimately published in peer-reviewed medical journals. The *Journal of the American Medical Association*, since its inception, has served along with the other peer-reviewed medical journals as a forum for the publication of data on new and innovative medical technologies.

It is hoped that the DATTA program can facilitate the wide distribution of important information in support of new technologies when that is merited. It should encourage research work at an earlier stage, when proof of utility may not be as apparent to the objective outside observer as to the investigator who is involved in the developmental research.

In the final analysis, the real proof of the effectiveness of this program will depend on the care that is used in evaluating reports from respondents and in wording the responses to these questions. The first products of this new program are presented in this issue of *JAMA*. Because these are opinions, it is appropriate to present them in *JAMA* in close proximity to the usual "Questions and Answers" section. It should be recognized that these responses have only been somewhat more extensively peer-reviewed than the responses of the other experts whose opinions are presented in the section.

Published Diagnostic and Therapeutic Technology Assessment (DATTA) Opinions

1996

Laparoscopic herniorrhaphy. Diagnostic and therapeutic technology assessment. *JAMA* 1996 Apr 10; 275 (14): 1075-82
- *Objective*—To provide clinicians with a technology assessment of the safety and effectiveness of laparoscopic herniorrhaphy for the surgical repair of inguinal hernias.
- *Conclusions*—The DATTA panelists rated the use of laparoscopic herniorrhaphy as promising for safety and investigational for effectiveness for two indications: the repair of primary inguinal hernias and the repair of bilateral inguinal hernias. The use of laparoscopic herniorrhaphy to repair recurrent inguinal hernias was rated as investigational for both safety and effectiveness by the panel. This technique was rated as promising for safety and effectiveness as a method for decreasing postoperative tenderness and time until return to full activity.

1995

Continuous ambulatory esophageal pH monitoring in the evaluation of patients with gastroesophageal reflux. Diagnostic and Therapeutic Technology Assessment. *JAMA* 1995 Aug 23-30; 274 (8): 662-8
- Abstract: *Objective*—To provide clinicians with a technology assessment of the safety and effectiveness of continuous ambulatory esophageal pH monitoring (CAEpHM) in the diagnosis of pathologic gastro-esophageal reflux in adults.
- *Conclusions*—The safety of CAEpHM was considered to be established in adults with chronic heartburn, chronic hoarseness, persistent acid reflux refractory to therapy, laryngeal lesions, or noncardiac substernal chest pain. The safety of CAEpHM was considered to

be promising in adults with episodes of apnea. The effectiveness of CAEpHM was considered to be established in adult patients with clear primary symptoms that reflect esophageal damage, such as chronic heartburn, persistent acid reflux refractory to therapy, or noncardiac substernal pain; promising in adults with chronic hoarseness; and investigational in adults with episodes of apnea.

Diagnostic and therapeutic technology assessment. Transjugular intrahepatic portosystemic shunt (TIPS). *JAMA* 1995 Jun 21; 273 (23): 1824-30
- Abstract: *Objective*—To provide clinicians with a technology assessment of the safety and effectiveness of the use of a transjugular intrahepatic portosystemic shunt (TIPS) for reducing portal hypertension and its associated complications of esophageal varices and ascites.
- *Conclusions*—The safety of TIPS was considered to be established in the acute control of bleeding from esophageal varices in patients who had failed sclerotherapy. The safety of TIPS was considered to be promising for long-term control of bleeding from esophageal varices. In patients with end-stage liver disease and esophageal varices who are liver transplant candidates, the use of TIPS was considered to be an established therapy. The effectiveness of TIPS was considered to be (1) established in the acute control of bleeding in patients who failed sclerotherapy; (2) promising for long-term control of bleeding from esophageal varices; and (3) established in patients with end-stage liver disease and esophageal varices who are candidates for liver transplants.

1994

Diagnostic and therapeutic technology assessment. Hyperthermia as adjuvant treatment for recurrent breast cancer and primary malignant glioma. *JAMA* 1994 Mar 9; 271(10): 797-802

1993

Diagnostic and therapeutic technology assessment. Human papillomavirus DNA testing in the management of cervical neoplasia. *JAMA* 1993 Dec 22-29; 270(24): 2975-81

Diagnostic and therapeutic technology assessment. Use of Teflon preparations for urinary incontinence and vesicoureteral reflux. *JAMA* 1993 Jun 16; 269 (23): 2975-80

Diagnostic and therapeutic technology assessment. Lung transplantation. *JAMA* 1993 Feb 17; 269 (7): 931-6

1992

Diagnostic and therapeutic technology assessment. Distraction/compression osteosynthesis with the Ilizarov device. *JAMA* 1992 Nov 18; 268 (19): 2717-24
Abstract: Although the Ilizarov device (and technique) to treat problematic fractures and bone deformities has been used since the 1950s in the former Soviet Union, the technique was not introduced to the United States until 1984. Since that time, the technique has become increasingly popular because, in comparison with the alternatives, the Ilizarov technique involves only one surgical procedure and it appears to have fewer complications. In addition, the Ilizarov technique was designed to correct

multiple deformities simultaneously. The DATTA panelists thought that the technique was established in terms of safety and effectiveness as a treatment of limb length deformity, bone defects, and angular/rotational deformity of the long bones. The panelists thought that it was promising in terms of safety and effectiveness as a treatment of pseudarthrosis. However, this overall endorsement of the technique was tempered by comments that the technique was associated with a lengthy learning curve, was very labor intensive, and required a large degree of patient cooperation.

Diagnostic and therapeutic technology assessment. Radiofrequency catheter ablation of aberrant conducting pathways of the heart [published erratum appears in *JAMA* 1993 Jan 13; 269(2): 216]. *JAMA* 1992 Oct 21; 268 (15): 2091-8
Abstract: Radiofrequency catheter ablation has very quickly generated considerable enthusiasm among electrophysiologists because it offers a less invasive alternative to an open surgical procedure and potentially offers an alternative to lifelong drug therapy. Early literature on RF catheter ablation focused on the technical aspects of the procedure. In contrast, the literature of the past several years is dominated by very favorable reports of large series of patients and the experience of individual institutions. The larger series have focused on the treatment of accessory pathways as opposed to AV nodal reentry pathways. The opinions of the DATTA panelists parallel the literature. The panelists considered the technology to be established in terms of its safety and effectiveness as a curative treatment of accessory pathways, and promising in terms of its safety and between promising and established in terms of its effectiveness as a treatment of AV nodal reentrant tachycardias.

Diagnostic and therapeutic technology assessment. Surrogate markers of progressive HIV disease [published errata appear in *JAMA* 1992 Dec 2; 268(21): 3074 and 1993 Jan 13; 269(2): 216]. *JAMA* 1992 Jun 3; 267(21): 2948-52

Diagnostic and therapeutic technology assessment. Surrogate markers of progressive HIV disease. *JAMA* 1992 Jun 3; 267(21): 2948-52

Diagnostic and therapeutic technology assessment. Endoscopic balloon dilation of the prostate. *JAMA* 1992 Feb 26; 267(8): 1123-4, 1127-8

Diagnostic and therapeutic technology assessment. Measurement of bone density with dual-energy X-ray absorptiometry (DEXA). *JAMA* 1992 Jan 8; 267(2): 286-8, 290-4

1991

Diagnostic and therapeutic technology assessment. Vasoactive intracavernous pharmacotherapy for impotence: intracavernous injection of prostaglandin E1. *JAMA* 1991 Jun 26; 265(24): 3321-3
Abstract: The DATTA panelists consider PGE1 to be a useful addition to the family of vasoactive agents used to treat organic impotence. It is associated with fewer side effects than either papaverine or phentolamine. Although most patients can achieve an erection with PGE1, some will not, and the other vasoactive agents may be of benefit in these cases. Synergy has been demonstrated when papaverine and PGE1 are used together, and a combination of the two in reduced dosages may be effective in

producing an erection with a reduction in side effects. Intracavernosal therapy should be prescribed and monitored by a urologist who is experienced in the treatment of impotence and who is able to treat any of the potential side effects. Whether long-term use of local injections will produce additional complications is yet to be determined.

Diagnostic and therapeutic technology assessment. Reassessment of automated percutaneous lumbar diskectomy for herniated disks. *JAMA* 1991 Apr 24; 265(16): 2122-3, 2125
Abstract: Although the safety of the APLD procedure is clearly established both by reports in the published literature and by a consensus of the DATTA panelists, there was no consensus among the DATTA panelists on the effectiveness of the procedure. The average 75% success rate reported in the larger studies contrasts with the 95% success rate reported for laminectomy and diskectomy. For APLD, careful patient selection is essential. Candidates must have failed an adequate trial of conservative therapy (bed rest and limitation of activity) and have disk herniation documented by appropriate imaging studies. These studies are important because they can demonstrate not only the degree of herniation, but also whether it is contained within the annulus and if any free fragments are present. For herniated lumbar disks with nuclear material outside and contiguous with the annulus, a statistically significant consensus of DATTA panelists believed that APLD is an inappropriate procedure. Another study has shown that the procedure can be taught to other surgeons without compromising patient safety, and, as reported, this holds with large numbers of cases. In appropriately selected patients, the clinical trade-off of APLD appears to be between a procedure with a 75% success rate with low risk and rapid recovery vs one with a 95% success rate and a more prolonged recovery. A research question is whether APLD could be extended to patients who have undergone previous surgery whose disks reherniate after a successful laminectomy. Conversely, does an APLD procedure that fails to relieve symptoms complicate subsequent laminectomy? It is recognized that there is a need for prospective, controlled, randomized clinical trials comparing APLD with laminectomy to resolve these and other issues.

Diagnostic and therapeutic technology assessment. Pancreatic transplantations. *JAMA* 1991 Jan 23-30; 265(4): 510-4

1990

Diagnostic and therapeutic technology assessment. Allogenic bone marrow transplantation for chronic myelogenous leukemia. *JAMA* 1990 Dec 26; 264(24): 3208-11

Diagnostic and therapeutic technology assessment. Dorsal rhizotomy. *JAMA* 1990 Nov 21; 264(19): 2569-70, 2572, 2574

Diagnostic and therapeutic technology assessment. Alpha-interferon and chronic myelogenous leukemia. *JAMA* 1990 Oct 24-31; 264(16): 2137-40

Diagnostic and therapeutic technology assessment. Laminectomy and microlaminectomy for treatment of lumbar disk herniation. *JAMA* 1990 Sep 19; 264(11): 1469-72

AMA

Diagnostic and therapeutic technology assessment. Vasoactive intracavernous pharmacotherapy for impotence: papaverine and phentolamine. *JAMA* 1990 Aug 8; 264(6): 752-4

Diagnostic and therapeutic technology assessment. Rigid and flexible sigmoidoscopies. *JAMA* 1990 Jul 4; 264(1): 89-92

Diagnostic and therapeutic technology assessment. Autologous bone marrow transplantation—reassessment [published erratum appears in *JAMA* 1990 Jul 18;264(3):338]. *JAMA* 1990 Feb 9; 263(6): 881-7

Diagnostic and therapeutic technology assessment. Prophylactic treatment for opportunistic infections in HIV-positive patients: aerosolized pentamidine. *JAMA* 1990 May 9; 263(18): 2510-4

Abstract: The DATTA panelists considered aerosolized pentamidine to be both safe and effective for primary and secondary prophylaxis of PCP. T4 helper cell counts offer guidance as to the best candidates for primary prophylaxis. Patients with a T4 helper cell count of fewer than $200/mm^3$ are the most appropriate group to receive primary prophylaxis with aerosolized pentamidine. However, T4 helper cell counts are not an exclusive criterion for aerosolized pentamidine prophylaxis. Some DATTA panelists suggested that certain patients, such as those with Kaposi sarcoma and lymphomas and those with concomitant human T-cell lymphotropic virus type 1 infection, might be considered candidates for aerosolized pentamidine regardless of T4 helper cell counts. There is no current literature to support this, and this opinion is based solely on clinical experience. Perhaps the use of other markers of immune function (beta 2-microglobulin, neopterin) in conjunction with T4 helper cell counts will give a better indication of when to start primary prophylaxis. Aerosolized pentamidine is not the only potential prophylactic regimen for PCP. Other drugs, including pyrimethamine and sulfadoxine, sulfamethoxazole and trimethoprim, and dapsone, are currently being evaluated. Prior diagnosis and therapy for patients with *M tuberculosis* must occur before initiation of the use of aerosolized pentamidine. This and other appropriate environmental precautions should reduce transmission of *M tuberculosis* to health care workers and other patients. Whether any prophylactic treatment of an opportunistic infection will prolong survival in HIV-infected individuals has yet to be proved. The assumption is made, however, that a reduction in opportunistic infections should lower mortality and improve the quality of life.

Diagnostic and therapeutic technology assessment. Transrectal ultrasonography—reassessment. *JAMA* 1990 Mar 16; 263(11): 1563-8

Diagnostic and therapeutic technology assessment. Chorionic villus sampling: a reassessment. *JAMA* 1990 Jan 12; 263(2): 305-6

Abstract: The Canadian and National Institute of Child Health and Human Development trials as well as other nonrandomized studies indicate that CVS is both safe and effective. Fetal loss rates have been slightly higher with CVS (six to eight more losses per 1000 procedures), but none of these results were statistically significant. Chorionic villus sampling also probably has a slightly higher procedure failure rate than amniocentesis. The DATTA panelists are now confident that the safety of CVS approaches that of amniocentesis and that the higher procedure failure rate is offset by the opportunity of earlier diagnosis with CVS. Transcervical CVS is often preferred by women because it offers an opportunity for early prenatal diagnosis and early intervention if necessary. It is performed as an outpatient procedure and is relatively simple for the patient; however, the practitioner requires special training in CVS. Modifications of the sampling technique are also under investigation. Transabdominal CVS can also be performed early in pregnancy with a fine-bore needle under ultrasonic guidance. It may be used in cases where the placenta is inaccessible to the transcervical approach or there is vaginal infection.

1989

Diagnostic and therapeutic technology assessment. Continuous peritoneal insulin infusion and implantable insulin infusion pumps for diabetic control. *JAMA* 1989 Dec 8; 262(22): 3195-8

Diagnostic and therapeutic technology assessment. Traveler's diarrhea. *JAMA* 1989 Sep 1; 262(9): 1243

Diagnostic and therapeutic technology assessment. Continuous subcutaneous insulin infusion. *JAMA* 1989 Sep 1; 262(9): 1239-43

Diagnostic and therapeutic technology assessment. Chemonucleolysis for herniated lumbar disk [see comments]. *JAMA* 1989 Aug 18; 262(7): 953-6

Abstract: The DATTA panelists did not achieve a definitive consensus on the use of chymopapain chemonucleolysis for a protruding lumbar disk contained by the annulus. Concerns about safety, especially the risk of anaphylaxis and the risk of damage to the spinal cord, were frequent. The effectiveness of this procedure for this indication was also questioned by many of the panelists. The panel did agree that chemonucleolysis is unacceptable as either safe or effective for use in patients with a herniated lumbar disk that is extruding nucleus pulposus through the annulus. Accordingly, diagnostic imaging of any suspect disk must be performed before chemonucleolysis can be deemed appropriate for any individual patient. Current imaging techniques are not infallible and cannot confer an absolute sense of security when seeming to indicate a nonextruded protruding disk.

Diagnostic and therapeutic technology assessment. Home monitoring of uterine activity. *JAMA* 1989 May 26; 261(20): 3027-9

Diagnostic and therapeutic technology assessment. Intrauterine devices [published erratum appears in *JAMA* 1990 Jan 12;263(2):238]. *JAMA* 1989 Apr 14; 261(14): 2127-30

Abstract: The DATTA panelists emphasized the critical importance of patient selection when considering IUDs for contraception. The IUD is an acceptable method of contraception, especially for those women who are in the middle to older reproductive years, unable to take oral contraceptives, in a stable monogamous relationship, and not at risk for sexually transmitted diseases. Within these constraints, the panelists gave overwhelming support to the IUD as a safe and effective method of contraception. The minority opinion (two panelists) that these devices were not established for safety or effectiveness was based on concerns over possible infectious complications.

Diagnostic and therapeutic technology assessment. Gastric restrictive surgery [see comments]. *JAMA* 1989 Mar 10; 261(10): 1491-4

Diagnostic and therapeutic technology assessment. Noninvasive electrical stimulation for nonunited bone fracture [published erratum appears in *JAMA* 1989 Jun 9; 261(22): 3246]. *JAMA* 1989 Feb 10; 261(6): 917-9

Diagnostic and therapeutic technology assessment. Percutaneous lumbar diskectomy for herniated disks [published erratum appears in *JAMA* 1989 May 26; 261(20): 2958]. *JAMA* 1989 Jan 6; 261(1): 105-9
Abstract: Percutaneous diskectomy, particularly using the Onik nucleotome, has promise. It is too early, however, to decide if the percutaneous approach to reducing lumbar disk herniation will achieve a permanent place in the surgical armamentarium. Nevertheless, it is clear that patient selection is important. At the minimum, an adequate trial of conservative therapy must be followed by diagnostic imaging that documents a herniation that can be treated in this fashion and correlates with the patient's neurological signs and symptoms. If free fragments are found, a laminectomy of some sort will be required to remove the offending material. Patients who are at risk for general anesthesia or may be allergic to chymopapain were mentioned by the panel as special subpopulations for whom the procedure may be indicated despite the lack of wide experience with it. The rapidly rising popularity of automated percutaneous lumbar diskectomy via the nucleotome will hopefully be followed in the near future with larger studies with long-term follow-up.

1988

Diagnostic and therapeutic technology assessment. Maternal serum alpha-fetoprotein testing and Down's syndrome. *JAMA* 1988 Sep 23-30; 260(12): 1779-82

Diagnostic and therapeutic technology assessment. Penile implants for erectile impotence. *JAMA* 1988 Aug 19; 260(7): 997-1000
Abstract: Three semirigid penile prostheses (Small-Carrion, Finney Flexirod, and Jonas Silicone-Silver) and a multicomponent inflatable penile prosthesis (Scott) were considered safe and effective treatment for impotence unresponsive to medical management. Each of these prostheses has its own advantages and disadvantages. The entire semirigid prosthesis group is surgically easier to implant than the inflatable models and, except for fracturing of the silver wires in the Jonas model, has a low incidence of mechanical failure. However, the semirigid models are not as aesthetically pleasing or as sexually satisfying to both partners as are inflatable devices. Multicomponent inflatable penile prostheses have had a history of mechanical failure; however, improved design and materials have reduced this problem. Several new concepts in penile prostheses have recently been developed: the self-contained inflatable prosthesis and an articulating prosthesis made of a spring-loaded cable that runs through a series of plastic segments. The self-contained inflatable prosthesis contains a fluid reservoir within the device itself. This eliminates the need for a separate reservoir, pump, and connective tubing (AMS Hydroflex, Flexiflate). There are not yet enough long-term data available to evaluate these new single-component devices.

Diagnostic and therapeutic technology assessment. Radial keratotomy for simple myopia. *JAMA* 1988 Jul 8; 260(2): 264-7
Abstract: There was a lack of consensus among DATTA panelists about the safety and, especially, the effectiveness of radial keratotomy. For patients with a preoperative refractive error greater than −6.00 D, DATTA panelists believed that radial keratotomy has not been established as safe or effective. Concerns about effectiveness focused on the lack of predictability of the results and the continuing change in the refractive error following surgery. Daily fluctuations in visual acuity and the occurrence of anisometropia were other reported adverse events that contributed to the concern expressed by DATTA panelists. Concern over the safety and effectiveness of the procedure became greater as the magnitude of the preoperative refractive error increased. Nevertheless, there is a subpopulation of myopic patients who regard their myopia as a sufficiently severe handicap for them to undergo radial keratotomy. Such carefully chosen patients who have the procedure performed may achieve emmetropia and be free of corrective lenses.

Diagnostic and therapeutic technology assessment. Immunoaugmentative therapy. *JAMA* 1988 Jun 17; 259(23): 3477-8
Abstract: The scientific evidence to date, as well as the history of IAT, will allow no other conclusion than that IAT is unequivocally dangerous to its patients and of no proved value as a treatment for cancer. Physicians who know of patients receiving IAT must be aware of the high risk those people are incurring for life-threatening infections of several types.

Diagnostic and therapeutic technology assessment. Transrectal ultrasonography in prostatic cancer [published erratum appears in *JAMA* 1988 Aug 12; 260(6): 792]. *JAMA* 1988 May 13; 259(18): 2757-9
Abstract: The DATTA panelists believe that transrectal ultrasound is established as safe for the screening and staging of prostatic cancer. The majority did not believe, however, that the effectiveness of the procedure has been established yet for either screening or staging. The panelists and the literature indicate, however, that transrectal ultrasound may well have a significant role to play in the future treatment of prostatic cancers.

Diagnostic and therapeutic technology assessment. BCG immunotherapy in bladder cancer: a reassessment. *JAMA* 1988 Apr 8; 259(14): 2153-5
Abstract: The DATTA panelists considered BCG immunotherapy to be efficacious in reducing recurrences of transitional cell carcinoma of the bladder. It has reduced recurrences in some patients in whom chemotherapeutic agents have failed, and in recent trials it has performed better than doxorubicin in preventing recurrences and in treatment of CIS. The DATTA panelists urged close evaluation of patients undergoing BCG therapy to guarantee that the tumor does not progress during treatment. Adverse reactions to BCG were not considered serious enough to jeopardize its use.

Diagnostic and therapeutic technology assessment. Ureteral stone management: II. Ureteroscopy and ultrasonic lithotripsy. *JAMA* 1988 Mar 11; 259(10): 1557-9

Diagnostic and therapeutic technology assessment. Ureteral stone management: the use of ureteroscopy with extracorporeal shockwave lithotripsy or ultrasonic lithotripsy [published erratum appears in *JAMA* 1988 Jul 15; 260(3): 343]. *JAMA* 1988 Mar 4; 259(9): 1382-4

AMA

1987

Diagnostic and therapeutic technology assessment. Chorionic villus sampling. *JAMA* 1987 Dec 25; 258(24): 3560-3

Diagnostic and therapeutic technology assessment. Coronary rehabilitation services. *JAMA* 1987 Oct 9; 258(14): 1959-62

Diagnostic and therapeutic technology assessment. Mammographic screening for breast cancer. *JAMA* 1987 Sep 11; 258(10): 1387-9

Diagnostic and therapeutic technology assessment. Ablation of accessory pathways in the Wolff-Parkinson-White syndrome. *JAMA* 1987 Jul 24-31; 258(4): 542-4

Diagnostic and therapeutic technology assessment. Ablation of accessory pathways in the Wolff-Parkinson-White syndrome. *JAMA* 1987 Jul 17; 258(3): 384-6

Diagnostic and therapeutic technology assessment. Cardiokymography. *JAMA* 1987 Jun 5; 257(21): 2973-4

Diagnostic and therapeutic technology assessment. Bacillus Calmette-Guerin immunotherapy in bladder cancer. *JAMA* 1987 Mar 6; 257(9): 1238-40

1986

Diagnostic and therapeutic technology assessment. Garren gastric bubble. *JAMA* 1986 Dec 19; 256(23): 3282-4

Diagnostic and therapeutic technology assessment. Angelchik antireflux prosthesis. *JAMA* 1986 Sep 12; 256(10): 1358-60

Diagnostic and therapeutic technology assessment. Autologous bone marrow transplantation. *JAMA* 1986 Jul 4; 256(1): 98-101

1985

Diagnostic and therapeutic technology assessment. Enhanced computed tomography in head trauma. *JAMA* 1985 Dec 20; 254(23): 3370-1

Diagnostic and therapeutic technology assessment. Stereotactic cingulotomy. *JAMA* 1985 Nov 15; 254(19): 2817-8

Diagnostic and therapeutic technology assessment. Macular drusen. *JAMA* 1985 Oct 11; 254(14): 1994

Diagnostic and therapeutic technology assessment. Age-adjusted diagnosis of hypertension. *JAMA* 1985 Oct 11; 254(14): 1994

Diagnostic and therapeutic technology assessment. Sperm penetration assay. *JAMA* 1985 Oct 11; 254(14): 1993-4

Diagnostic and therapeutic technology assessment. Diagnostic intraoperative ultrasound. *JAMA* 1985 Jul 12; 254(2): 285-7

Diagnostic and therapeutic technology assessment. Endoscopic topical therapy of gastrointestinal tract hemorrhage. *JAMA* 1985 May 10; 253(18): 2734-5

Diagnostic and therapeutic technology assessment. Endoscopic electrocoagulation of gastrointestinal tract hemorrhage. *JAMA* 1985 May 10; 253(18): 2733-4

Diagnostic and therapeutic technology assessment. Endoscopic thermal coagulation of gastrointestinal tract hemorrhage. *JAMA* 1985 May 10; 253(18): 2733

Diagnostic and therapeutic technology assessment. Endoscopic laser photocoagulation of gastrointestinal tract hemorrhage. *JAMA* 1985 May 10; 253(18): 2732-3

Diagnostic and therapeutic technology assessment. Continuous arteriovenous hemofiltration. *JAMA* 1985 Mar 1; 253(9): 1325-6

1984

Diagnostic and therapeutic technology assessment. Endoscopic transurethral nephrolithotomy. *JAMA* 1984 Dec 21; 252(23): 3302

Diagnostic and therapeutic technology assessment. Percutaneous nephrolithotomy. *JAMA* 1984 Dec 21; 252(23): 3301-2

Diagnostic and therapeutic technology assessment. Noninvasive extracorporeal lithotripsy. *JAMA* 1984 Dec 21; 252(23): 3301

Diagnostic and therapeutic technology assessment. Gastric restrictive surgery for morbid obesity. *JAMA* 1984 Jun 8; 251(22): 3011

Diagnostic and therapeutic technology assessment. Implanted electrospinal stimulator for scoliosis. *JAMA* 1984 May 25; 251(20): 2723

Diagnostic and therapeutic technology assessment. Bone marrow transplantation in childhood leukemia. *JAMA* 1984 Apr 27; 251(16): 2155

Diagnostic and therapeutic technology assessment. Diaphanography (transillumination of the breast) for cancer screening. *JAMA* 1984 Apr 13; 251(14): 1902

Diagnostic and therapeutic technology assessment. Cranial electrostimulation. *JAMA* 1984 Feb 24; 251(8): 1094

Diagnostic and therapeutic technology assessment. Cardiokymography for noninvasive cardiological diagnosis. *JAMA* 1984 Feb 24; 251(8): 1094

Diagnostic and therapeutic technology assessment. Whole-body hyperthermia treatment of cancer. *JAMA* 1984 Jan 13; 251(2): 272

1983

Diagnostic and therapeutic technology assessment. 24-hour ambulatory EEG monitoring. *JAMA* 1983 Dec 23-30; 250(24): 3340

Diagnostic and therapeutic technology assessment. Biofeedback. *JAMA* 1983 Nov 4; 250(17): 2381

Diagnostic and therapeutic technology assessment. Implantable infusion pump. *JAMA* 1983 Oct 14; 250(14): 1906

Diagnostic and therapeutic technology assessment. Chelation therapy. *JAMA* 1983 Aug 5; 250(5): 672

Diagnostic and therapeutic technology assessment. CO_2 laser treatment of gynecologic malignant neoplasms. *JAMA* 1983 Aug 5; 250(5): 672

Diagnostic and therapeutic technology assessment. Mandatory ECG before elective surgery. *JAMA* 1983 Jul 22; 250(4): 540

Diagnostic and therapeutic technology assessment. Diathermy. *JAMA* 1983 Jul 22; 250(4): 540

Diagnostic and therapeutic technology assessment. Radial keratotomy. *JAMA* 1983 Jul 15; 250(3): 420

Diagnostic and therapeutic technology assessment. Quantitative EEG (fast Fourier transform analysis) monitoring. *JAMA* 1983 Jul 15; 250(3): 420

Technology News is developed and distributed in conjunction with DATTA evaluations and provides information and analyses of current issues involving medical technology.

Contact for single copies of DATTA evaluations:
AMA Department of Technology Assessment
800 AMA-3211 ext 4531

Medical Education Standards

The functions of the Council on Medical Education are:
- To study and evaluate all aspects of medical education, including the development of programs approved by the House of Delegates for the provision of an adequate continuing supply of well-qualified physicians to meet the medical needs of the public.
- To study and evaluate education needs in the allied health professions and services, including the development of programs approved by the House of Delegates, to ensure the provision of an adequate continuing supply of well-qualified allied health personnel.
- To review and recommend policies for medical and allied health education, whereby the AMA may provide the highest education service to both the public and the profession.
- To consider and recommend means by which the AMA may, on behalf of the public and the medical profession at large, continue to provide information, leadership, and direction to the existing inter-organizational bodies dealing with medical and allied health education.
- To consider and recommend the means and methods whereby physicians and allied health personnel may be assisted in maintaining their professional competence and the development of means and criteria for recognition of such achievement. (C&B-1997)

Liaison Committee on Medical Education
The Liaison Committee on Medical Education (LCME) is the national authority for the accreditation of medical education programs leading to the MD degree in US and Canadian medical schools. The LCME is recognized for this purpose by the US Secretary of Education, by the Council on Postsecondary Accreditation, by the US Congress in various health-related laws, and by state, provincial (Canada), and territorial medical licensure boards.

Accreditation Council for Graduate Medical Education
All of the administration and professional support services provided to the Accreditation Council for Graduate Medical Education (ACGME) and its component Residency Review Committee (RRC) for the accreditation of all residency programs in the US are included in this unit. Key activities encompass the training and effective utilization of on-site surveyors; the conduct of all surveys within the expected time frame; the provision of administrative support to the RRCs; the conduct of research; and the provision of liaison and representation with relevant agencies, offices, organizations, and individuals. The ACGME carries out its accreditation mission by serving

as the deliberative body through which standards for residency programs, as well as procedures for accreditation, are established. As part of the accreditation process, the ACGME maintains oversight of committees of volunteer physicians in each of 24 specialty areas. These committees, called Residency Review Committees, normally make the accreditation decisions within their areas of expertise. In contested accreditation decisions, the ACGME serves as the final decision-making body. Departments specific to the activities of the field staff, the RRC activities, and the research and administration involved in accrediting the programs round out the elements of this program.

Specialties accredited by the ACGME include:
- Allergy and Immunology
- Ambulatory Care/See: Internal Medicine
- Anesthesiology
- Colon and Rectal Surgery
- Critical Care
- Dermatology
- Emergency Medicine
- Family Practice
- Internal Medicine
- Neurological Surgery
- Neurology
- Nuclear Medicine
- Obstetrics/Gynecology
- Ophthalmology
- Orthopedic Surgery
- Otolaryngology
- Pathology
- Pediatrics
- Pediatric Surgery
- Physical Medicine and Rehabilitation
- Plastic Surgery
- Preventive Medicine
- Psychiatry
- Radiology
- Surgery
- Thoracic Surgery
- Transitional Year (Rotating Intern) Review Committee
- Urology
- Vascular Surgery

Resource
Accreditation Council for Graduate Medical Education
515 N State St, Chicago, IL 60610
312 464-4920

Departmental publications include:
FREIDA (Fellowship and Residency Electronic Interactive Database Access): An expanded, computerized version of the *Directory of Graduate Medical Education Programs,* FREIDA is published and updated annually. It can be accessed through the Internet off the AMA's Web page at http://www.ama-assn.org. Registered users can search through the list of 7400 ACGME-accredited programs. The area will continue to place attention on liaison activities with key leaders, researchers, and organizations in medical education. The FRIEDA Hotline (800 AMA-3211, ext 5331) should be contacted with questions regarding data contained within the service.

Directory of Graduate Medical Education Programs: Also known as "The Green Book," this directory contains the official list of ACGME accredited programs, a summary of graduate medical education statistical data, the stan-

AMA

dards for program accreditation in each specialty, requirements for board certification, and a summary of licensure regulations for each state.

Division of Undergraduate Medical Education

This division's goal is to provide educational materials and guidance to those persons interested in a career in medicine. The Department of Medical Student Services produces several aids to proceed toward that goal including their videotape called *Science and Art in the Name of Healing* that presents the rewards of a medical career, and brochures that introduce the rewards of a career in medicine to students thinking about a commitment to medicine. These include *Got That Healing Feeling, Medicine: A Chance to Make a Difference,* and *You the Doctor.*

Division of Continuing Medical Education

Fostering the AMA's commitment to excellence in the provision of continuing medical education (CME) for physicians, both nationally and internationally, is a central focus of this area. This is done by developing appropriate policies, participating in the establishment of effective accreditation standards and procedures with the Accreditation Council for Continuing Medical Education (ACCME), sponsoring high-quality CME programs, communicating timely and accurate information on CME, and supporting and cooperating with other organizations and institutions that share the AMA's interest in meeting the needs of the profession for continuing medical education of the highest quality. Greater attention will be placed on a comprehensive registry of continuing medical education to enhance clinical competence and local, regional, and national CME activities to promote the visibility of the AMA.

Physician's Recognition Award

This award program is a part of the CME division's job. Established by the House of Delegates in 1968, the Physician's Recognition Award (PRA) provides certificates to physicians who qualify by completing required amounts of continuing education of acceptable quality.

Physician's Recognition Award (PRA) certificates up 11%: online application, reciprocity agreements pay off in 1996

Dick Walt
AMA/Electronic Network, Feb 18, 1996

The American Medical Association's (AMA) Physician's Recognition Award (PRA) is the most widely accepted standard for recognizing physician completion of continuing medical education (CME). Over 640,000 certificates have been issued since the PRA's founding in 1968, making the PRA the most frequently sought of all CME certificates. In 1996, issuance of PRA certificates increased 11% due to the availability of a new online application and reciprocal arrangements with state and specialty medical societies—making the application process quicker and easier.

The AMA is using the power and popularity of its World Wide Web home page to promote the PRA. An electronic PRA application is now available (select http://www.ama-assn.org and proceed to the "Medical Science and Education" section). In addition, the new online Physician Select database, which lists all US physicians,

now includes text noting whether a physician holds the PRA certificate.

"The double-digit increase in PRA certificates is ample evidence of the reborn interest in and appreciation of the PRA among physicians," said Michael J. Scotti, Jr, MD, vice president, Medical Education. "Today's increased emphasis on accountability in health care delivery has increased the value of holding the certificate."

The AMA will continue to build on the 1996 growth by developing an online copy of the PRA handbook and using the PRA as a credential indicating CME participation in the AMA's newly launched American Medical Accreditation Program. Known as AMAP, this ambitious project seeks to provide the first comprehensive accreditation process for physicians.

To receive more information or a PRA application, call 312 464-4665. A fax application is available by calling 800 621-8335 and pressing 2.

Twenty-five years in continuing medical education: The silver anniversary of the AMA/PRA

Arthur M. Osteen, PhD
JAMA 1993 Sept 1; 270(9): 1092

The American Medical Association Physician's Recognition Award (AMA/PRA) was established by the AMA House of Delegates in December 1968. As the time approaches to celebrate the PRA's 25th anniversary, we take stock of the award, how it has changed, and how it has not. It is also an opportunity to look briefly at other ways in which the AMA has been involved in continuing medical education (CME). These other involvements have perhaps been more important to CME than the PRA award itself.

The resolution establishing the award set out the following rationale and goals:
- To provide recognition for the many thousands of physicians who regularly participate in CME.
- To encourage all physicians to keep up-to-date and to improve their knowledge and judgment by CME.
- To provide reassurance to the public that America's physicians are maintaining their competence by regular participation in CME.
- To emphasize the AMA's position as a leader in CME.
- To emphasize the importance of developing more meaningful continuing education opportunities for physicians.
- To strengthen the physician's position as the leader of the health service team by focusing attention on his or her interest in maintaining professional competence.

These remain the objectives of the PRA in 1993.

The AMA was not the first organization to develop rules for CME. The program of the American Academy of Family Physicians dates from 1947 when its predecessor, the American Academy of General Practice, set up CME requirements for membership. It was the AMA, however, that began accrediting organizations that provide CME, depending on accredited organizations to assure that CME activities were of good quality and met the needs of physicians. Organizations that succeeded in being accredited were subsequently able to designate programs for AMA/PRA category 1 credit.

In time, the standards for AMA/PRA category 1 programs came to include undertaking a needs assessment for the educational activity to be offered, preparing written educational objectives, describing the means to achieve these objectives, and devising means for evaluating whether the objectives were met. Programs were required to indicate in their announcements the intended audience, the credit awarded, and the expected educational outcomes.

The AMA also made major contributions to the quality of CME through the educational programs it sponsored in the 1960s. The two annual scientific meetings were major undertakings, with attention given to the assessment of needs for education, format for programs, preparation of syllabi, and ongoing evaluation directed toward improving the quality of offerings for the next annual or interim meeting. At the time, these procedures set the standard; they were quickly picked up by other organizations involved in CME. In retrospect, the AMA was the center of early continuing education innovation.

More recently, the AMA has contributed to CME by leading in the development of ethical principles for relations between the pharmaceutical industry and physicians and relations between industry and CME providers.

One of the most frequently used terms in CME is "AMA PRA category 1," which includes activities designated AMA PRA category 1 by an accredited sponsor and international conferences approved by the AMA for category 1 credit. Category 1 activities can take the form of lectures, seminars, use of self-study materials, self-assessment programs, miniresidencies, and use of audiovisual or computer-based materials. The term means for many physicians that the educational activity is worthwhile. When the requirements established for accreditation of an organization and for designation of an activity are observed, the CME activity should be of high quality. The AMA and the accrediting bodies—the Accreditation Council for Continuing Medical Education (ACCME) and recognized state medical societies—make every effort to assure that such will be the case. In line with this objective, the AMA recently announced that in the future it will withdraw the right to designate AMA PRA credit from organizations that have designated activities that, in the words of the 1993 PRA Information Booklet, "do not meet the definition of CME, are not in accord with the AMA's Ethical Opinion on Gifts to Physicians, and the ACCME's Standards for Commercial Support of CME, solely advocate modalities for diagnosis or treatment which are not subjects for instruction in most US medical schools, [or] promote CME activities primarily for noneducational purposes."

The AMA recognizes, however, that many educational activities of great benefit to physicians, including reading and patient consultations, cannot meet the requirements for designation as AMA PRA category 1. For that reason, the AMA recently has begun to call attention to the value of these category 2 educational activities. A new PRA certificate, the Certificate With Special Commendation for Self-Directed Learning, requires category 2 educational activities.

On June 10 of 1993, the AMA Board of Trustees approved the establishment of an AMA Institute for Continuing Physician Education. The Institute has not yet begun operation, but its objectives are to continue AMA contributions to the field of CME.

Accreditation Council for Continuing Medical Education

The Accreditation Council for Continuing Medical Education (ACCME) was organized to promote and develop principles, policies, and standards for continuing medical education (CME), and to apply them to the accreditation of institutions and organizations offering CME. The ACCME accredits institutions and organizations offering CME and develops standards by which state medical societies accredit local institutions and organizations.

Online CME Locator

AMA's CME Locator can be found on the AMA Web page. It provides a quick and convenient way to access information on continuing medical education activities. AMA CME Locator is a database of over 2000 AMA PRA Category 1 activities sponsored by CME providers accredited by the Accreditation Council for Continuing Medical Education (ACCME) or approved by the American Medical Association. Information in this database was collected by an ongoing survey of all ACCME-accredited providers.

If an ACCME-accredited CME provider or a State Medical Society wants courses, seminars, conferences, or enduring CME programs included in this database, they should contact the AMA Division of Continuing Medical Education at 312 464-4671, by fax at 312 464-5830, or by e-mail to CME@ama-assn.org.

Division publications include:

- *Continuing Medical Education Directory:* A unique, biennial resource for continuing medical education (CME) planners, the *Directory* consolidates a variety of information needed for planning, accrediting, and delivering CME opportunities for physicians into one volume. The *Directory* lists accredited state and national CME sponsors and provides a detailed Federation meeting calendar. It includes information on accreditation policies and guidelines, credentialing requirements, research, and special activities. The *Directory* provides information on AMA's long-standing involvement in continuing medical education and positions the Association as a key national leader on CME issues.

- *The Physician as Learner: Linking Research to Practice:* This book compiles the research literature on CME and relates it to the practice of medicine. The book explores three major questions related to CME: What are the characteristics of the successful physician learner? How do we measure physician competence and performance and how is this useful in developing physician learning strategies? What are the most effective methods and organizational structures for delivering CME? Richly annotated and referenced, the book is derived from extensive research literature on adult education and social and educational psychology as applied to the medical setting.

AMA Allied Health Education and Accreditation

Related publication:

The Allied Health and Rehabilitation Professions Education Directory: This source provides information on approximately 5000 educational programs accredited by the CAHEA and contains information on 2200 sponsoring institutions. The *Directory* also includes national statistics on programs, institutions, enrollments, attributions, and graduates. It also provides data reflecting program director perspectives on health personnel supply and demand.

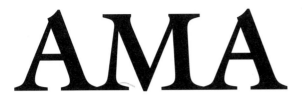 **Advocacy**

Health Policy Advocacy

Health Service Policy

Government and Political Affairs

Office of the General Counsel

Communications

The purpose of the Health Policy Advocacy Group is to promote the standards and policies that are needed for physicians to deliver good health care.

Advocacy and representation are two of the principal expectations physicians have of the AMA. They want a strong voice for the profession, manifested as legislative clout, which will make their professional lives better. They also want the organization to advocate for their responsibilities to their patients. This translates into nourishing the patient/physician relationship through advocating quality care, access, choice, and ethics.

Health Service Policy

The Association's health policy program is designed to provide the factual research information and policy alternatives needed for effective representation of physicians. Key activities include health policy research and development, the monitoring and development of the structure of medical practice financing, and payment programs such as those for coding and resource-based relative value scales.

Policy Development

The AMA's policy is developed through the input of the Association's many reporting bodies and councils that comprise the Federation of Medicine. Policy development activities provide the overall coordination and development of AMA policy on socioeconomic issues, including policy related to health system reform. A central focus in these efforts is the Council on Medical Service, which develops proactive policy recommendations and programs related to the organization, delivery, financing, and evaluation of health care services. Emphasis in 1995 will be given to the development of policy and program proposals for incremental reforms in the health system, including health care financing changes and insurance reform, patient empowerment through medical savings accounts, mergers and vertical integration, access to managed care plans, physician credentialing, care for the underserved, and electronic data interchange. Increased attention also will be placed on serving as the policy development link to the AMA's Public and Private Sector Advocacy efforts.

Council on Medical Service

The functions of the Council on Medical Service are:
- To study and evaluate the social and economic aspects of medical care; and, on behalf of the public and the profession, to suggest means for the timely development of services in a changing socioeconomic environment.
- To investigate social and economic factors influencing the practice of medicine.

AMA

- To confer with state associations, component societies and National Medical Specialty Societies regarding changing conditions and anticipated proposals that would affect medical care.
- To assist medical service committees established by state associations, component societies of the American Medical Association, and the National Medical Specialty Societies. (C&B-1997)

Reports of the AMA Council on Medical Service

1996

Annual Meeting

Electronic Data Interchange Status Report (Resolution 106, A-95)

Mental Health "Carve-Outs" (Res 121, A-95)

Definition of "Principal Care" (Res 312, A-95)

Physician and Health Plan Provision of Uncompensated Care (Res 703, A-95)

Monitoring Medicaid Managed Care

Managed Care Organizations; Use of Physicians to Provide Second Opinions to Emergency Departments

Defining Health Care Expenses

Effects of Changing Practice Organization on Physician Work Effort and Output

Enhancing Rural Physician Practices

Policy Consolidation on Physician-Specific Health Care Data

Peer Review Organization Program Status

The Financial Performance of Managed Care Plans

URAC National Network Accreditation Standards

1996

Interim Meeting

Managed Care Organizations' Use of Physicians to Provide Second Opinions to Emergency Physicians

Reexamination of Employment-Based Health Insurance

Financial Incentives Utilized in the Management of Medical Care

Definition of "Managed Care"

Physician Decision-Making in the Health Care Systems

AMA Policy on ERISA

Peer Review Organization Program Status

Policy Consolidation on Practice Parameters

Trends in Physician Practice Consolidation

Feasibility of Studying the Effects of Capitation on Physician Workforce Requirements

Status Report on the National Uniform Claim Committee and Electronic Data Interchange

1995

Annual Meeting

Trends in the Organization of Health Care Delivery Systems and the Influence on Physicians' Practices (Res 813, I-93)

Reimbursement by Medicare for Psychotherapy Provided by Residents (Res 130, A-94)

Establishing Capitation Rates (Res 113, I-94)

Informing Patients About Health Plan Participation (Res 116, I-94)

Health Benefits Plans and "Point of Service" Coverage (Res 202, 211, 224 and 240, I-94)

Cost of AMA Benefits in Different Delivery Models

Health Plan Restrictions on Mental Health Services

Improvement in Reimbursement for Primary Care Services in Rural Areas

Patient Cost Sharing

Patient Referral Guidelines

Peer Review Organization Program Status

Policy Consolidation on Health Care Costs

Producer Price Index for Physician Services

1995

Interim Meeting

Health Care Coverage of Young Adults Under Their Parents' Family Policies

Development of Health Care Priorities

Advance Directives and Utilization Review

Insurance Companies and Corporations Running Medical Clinics (Res 107, A-95)

Mandatory Point-of-Service Feature (Res 711, 713 and 715, A-95)

Access to Emergency Services

Capitation Update

Electronic Data Interchange and Telemedicine: Update

Peer Review Organization Program Status

Health Plan "Report Cards"

Policy Consolidation on Long-Term Care

1994

Annual Meeting

Access to Specialty Care

Redesigning the Traditional Hospital Structure and Orientation (Res 809, A-93)

Long-Term Care (Res 101, A-93, Res 207, A-92, and Res 133, I-92)

Health Savings Accounts: One Approach to Implementation

Electronic Data Interchange Status Report

Corporate Status of Managed Care Health Plans

Designation of Health Professional Shortage Areas

Use of Service Component of CPI in Health System Reform (Res 102, I-93)

AMA Standard Benefits Package

Peer Review Organization Program Status

AMA Opposition to Requiring Physician Participation in Health Maintenance Organizations in Order to Join a Preferred Provider Organization Panel (Res 109, I-93, First Resolve)

Medicaid Payment for Over-the-Counter Drugs When They Are the Drug of Choice

Compensation for Physicians Who Accompany Seriously Ill or Injured Patients to Hospitals (Res 102, A-93)

Evaluation of Practice Parameters (Res 717, A-93)

1994

Interim Meeting

Risk Adjustment for Community Rating

Definition of Managed Competition

Criteria for and Coverage of Specific Services

Medical Trust (Res 101, A-94)

New Durable Medical Equipment Requirements (Res 205, A-94, Second Resolve)

Access to Primary Care Services (Res 106, I-93)

Criteria for Designation of Health Professional Shortage Areas

Basic or Minimum Benefits Packages

Peer Review Organization Program Status

Electronic Data Interchange and Telemedicine Status Report

Employer Control of Health Insurance Choices

Terminology for Tax-Preferred Health or Medical Accounts

Compensation for Treatment of Victims of Family Violence (Res 805, I-92)

Behavior That Increases the Risk of Illness or Injury (Res 139, I-39)

Guidelines for Physician/Nurse Practitioner Integrated Practice

Payment for Ethics Consultations (Res 115, I-93)

1993

Annual Meeting

AMA Required Benefits Package (Res 120, I-92)

Qualifications and Credentialing of Physicians Involved in Managed Care (Res 714, I-92)

Employer-Based Health Insurance (Res 119, I-92)

Principles for the Implement of Practice Parameters at the Local/State/Regional Level

AMA Policy on Disclosure of Provider Fees and Charges (Res 113, I-92)

Payment for Concurrent Care

Financing of Care for HIV/AIDS Patients in the United States

Rural Health

Peer Review Organization Program Status

Physician Profiling

Federal Indicators of the Price of Physician Services

1993

Interim Meeting

Submission of Electronic Claims Through Electronic Data Interchange

Primary Care Physicians in the Inner City

AMA Required Standard Benefit Package (Res 128 and 140, A-93)

Telemedicine

Patient Access to Specialty Care in Managed Care Systems (Res 715, A-93)

Guidelines for Qualifications of Managed Care Medical Directors

Implementing Practice Parameters on the Local/State/Regional Level

Peer Review Organization Program Status

Emerging Trends in Utilization Management

Risk Rating and Insurance Premiums (Res 112, A-93)

Vertical Divestiture in the Health Care System

Assistance to Reservist Physicians Before, During and After Activation (Res 271, A-92)

Permanent Health Insurance (Res 106, I-92)

Expansion of Medicare Coverage for Physician Assistants' Services in Non-Health Professional Shortage Areas (Res 119, A-93)

Designation of Health Professional Shortage Areas

1992

Annual Meeting

Peer Review Organization Program Status

Rural Health

Managed Care

Health Care in the Inner City

Medicare Beneficiary Survey

Utilization Review Accreditation Commission

Regionalization of Medicare Carriers

Principles of Medical Record Documentation

Disclosure of Medical Review Criteria and Eligibility Guidelines

Cost-Effectiveness of Home Intravenous Therapy

"Tail Coverage" for Health Insurance for Existing or Chronic Illness (Resolution 89, A-91)

Extension of Practice

Defining Hospital Inpatient and Outpatient Stays (Resolution 11, I-90, and Resolution 32, A-91)

Medicare Reimbursement of Telephone Consultations (Substitute Resolution 175, A-91)

United States Health Care Spending

1992

Interim Meeting

Managed Care

Medicare Payment Schedule Conversion Factor (Res 105, I-91)

Guidelines for Disclosure of Medical Record Information to Payors

Health Insurance for Adopted Children

Medical Insurance Overhead Costs (Res 807, I-91)

Patient Responsibility of On-Call Physicians (Res 214, I-91)

Definitions of "Referral" and "Consultation" (Res 818 and 819, I-91)

Peer Review Organization Program Status

AMA Minimum Benefits Package

AMA

1991

Annual Meeting

Rural Health

Definition of Hospital Day (Res 11, I-90)

Financial Arrangements Between Hospitals and Physicians

Pro Savings vs HCFA Expenses

Definition of Quality

Practice Parameters: Their Relevance to Physician Credentialing

Economic Credentialing

Peer Review Organization Program Status

Technology Assessment in Medicine

1991

Interim Meeting

Variation in Medicare Carrier Interpretations: Interim Report

Economic Credentialing

Definition of a Hospital Day (Res 11, I-90, and Res 32, A-91)

Precertification Denials (Res 116, A-91)

Medicare Clinic Progress Notes (Res 153, A-91)

Rural Health

PRO Program Status

1990

Annual Meeting

Administrative Cost of Health Care

Closure of Rural Hospitals and Medicare's Prospective Pricing System

Preadmission Review Practices

High Cost Health Benefits Management

Medicare Social Admissions

Quality Assessment Systems

Peer Review Organization Program Status

The Quality Intervention Plan (Substitute Res 163, A-89, and Res 68, I-89)

Medical Practice in Massachusetts

Hospital Cost-Shifting

Rural Health

Disability Insurance for Medical Students and Residents

Institute of Medicine Report on Medicare Review

Purchased Diagnostic Tests (Res 115, A-89)

Preventive Medicine Services (Res 260, A-89)

1990

Interim Meeting

Case Management System for Outpatient Clinics (Res 89, A-90)

Preventive Medicine Services (Res 260, A-89)

HCFA Reimbursement in Locum Tenens Arrangements (Resolution 127, I-89)

Use of HIV Screening by Insurers (Resolution 280, A-90)

Managed Care Services (Res 173, A-90)

Pro Sanctions (Res 61, A-90)

Geographic Maldistribution of Physicians

Operation Focus (Res 187, A-90)

Prevalence of Managed Care Requirements

Disability Insurance for Medical Students and Residents —Interim Report

Medicare Policy on Inpatient Rehabilitation (Res 113, A-90)

Blue Cross/Blue Shield of Minnesota Medical Review System

Peer Review Organization Program Status

Notification of Quality Problems (Res 38, A-90)

Rural Health

Center for Health Policy Research

The AMA's health policy research program is designed to provide the factual research information and policy alternatives needed for effective representation of physicians. This area responds to the growing technical complexity of national health policy issues by providing increased support to the AMA in the form of internal consulting, providing information on physician leaders, and assisting in policy development. The research program continues to provide an authoritative source of information on medical practice in the United States through a data collection program and subsequent publication series.

Center for Health Policy Research Library

The Research Library in the Center is designed to provide resources and information services to support the Health Policy Advocacy Group in achieving its goals and mission. The Center is a full-service, socioeconomic library. The collection consists of more than 2800 books and 4500 reports, articles, monographs, and working papers (both current and historic) covering 153 topics. The Center subscribes to more than 140 journals, periodicals, newsletters, and magazines and provides online search services and Internet access.

Socioeconomic Monitoring System Core Survey

The Socioeconomic Monitoring System, which is a series of telephone surveys of physicians, was developed in 1981 to respond to an AMA need for current, credible, and unbiased data on the practice of medicine in order to represent physicians effectively. The annual core survey is conducted in the spring with approximately 4000 physicians in a 25-minute interview. Data on income and expenses, hours and weeks worked, patient visits, fees, practice arrangements, and employment status are collected. Survey results are communicated through the AMA's Center for Health Policy Research publications, special computer runs, and reports for the Office of the General Counsel, the Washington Office, and the Health Policy Group; and tabulations of special topics results for the units that requested their inclusion in the survey.

Related publications include:

Physician Marketplace Statistics
An annual reference volume presenting Socioeconomic Monitoring System data on physician income, professional expenses, fees, and selected practice characteristics, this publication was developed in response to requests from users of Socioeconomic Characteristics of Medical

Practice who wanted more detailed specialty and geographic breakdowns of information.

Socioeconomic Characteristics of Medical Practice
This annual reference volume contains SMS data on physician income, professional expenses, and selected practice characteristics.

Government and Political Affairs

Council on Legislation
The functions of the Council on Legislation are:

- To review proposed federal legislation and recommend appropriate action in accordance with AMA policy.
- To recommend changes in existing AMA policy when necessary to accomplish effective legislative goals.
- To serve as a reference council through which all legislative issues of the Association are channeled prior to final consideration by the Board of Trustees.
- To maintain constant surveillance over the legislation scene and to anticipate future legislative needs.
- To recommend to the Board of Trustees new federal legislation and legislation to modify existing laws of interest to the Association.
- To monitor the development and issuance of federal regulations and to make recommendations to the Board of Trustees concerning action on such regulations.
- To develop and recommend to the Board of Trustees models for state legislation. (C&B-1997)

Legislative Affairs Team
To establish the Association's legislative credibility and presence at both the federal and state levels, the Legislative Affairs Team monitors and analyzes federal and state legislation and regulations, develops policy positions on legislative proposals through the involvement of the Council on Legislation and others, and advocates such positions to appropriate governmental bodies. The current focus of the team is on the Association's major objectives, including health system reform and access to health care for all Americans, promotion of public health and decreased use of tobacco, continued implementation of physician payment reform, clinical laboratory reform, and reduced administrative hassles under Medicare. This is achieved through public sector advocacy, including testimony, congressional appearances, regulatory comments, and meetings with government officials and their staffs.

Advocacy Resource Center
The Center is a 1997 initiative. Its primary focus is to serve a broad set of advocacy needs of the Federation of Medicine. It will work with the Federation community to identify its advocacy needs and develop responsive products in areas such as communications, public health, state and federal legislation, legal, and managed care.

To contact the ARC:
312 464-4976   Fax 312 464 4961

Government Affairs
Providing effective advocacy of the Association's policies and positions before Congress and the Executive Branch is the primary purpose of the activities of this area. These actions are undertaken to ensure the continued availability of high-quality medical care, to represent and protect the interest of the profession and the public, and to minimize regulatory constraints on the practice of medicine.

Political Affairs
The primary objectives in this area are to provide innovative political action techniques, including direct contributions, in-kind services, independent expenditure support to congressional candidates, and state-of-the-art political education programs to stimulate legislative and political grassroots involvement by physicians.

AMA Washington Office
AMA's Washington, DC, office interacts with Congress, and works with state and specialty societies and group practices on legislation affecting physicians' practices and patients. It represents the profession before the executive branch of the federal government and various regulatory agencies.

AMA Washington Office
1101 Vermont Ave NW, Washington, DC 20005
202 789-7400   Fax 202 789-7485

American Medical Political Action Committee
The American Medical Political Action Committee (AMPAC) is a bipartisan political action committee established by the AMA over 30 years ago. AMPAC members participate in political fund-raising, campaign management, and various grassroots activities. Their goal is to persuade legislators to pass, defeat, or amend legislation of interest to physicians and, at the same time, for the well-being of their patients. AMPAC's 67,000 members receive a quarterly magazine, *Political Stethoscope*, to educate physicians and others who are running for office or working on election campaigns and promote medical community involvement through grassroots educational programs and activities.

To contact AMPAC:
1101 Vermont Ave NW, Washington, DC 20005
202 789-7462   Fax 202 789-7469

P.O.W.E.R. Network:
The American Medical Association's legislative and political grassroots network, P.O.W.E.R., provides physicians wishing to be active in the political process for the benefit of medicine the tools to do so effectively.

Office of the General Counsel

The AMA is the law firm of the profession. The AMA's legal activities are conducted to ensure that the AMA complies with applicable laws, court decisions, and other medicolegal developments that affect the practice of medicine; and that the interests of the Association and the medical profession are represented in the courts through the initiation of health policy litigation or intervention in litigation that concerns important health policy issues.

AMA for you: AMA takes assisted suicide to U.S. Supreme Court

AM News Feb 3, 1997 p 4

The AMA, in a "friend of the court" brief, is telling the U.S. Supreme Court that physician-assisted suicide violates medicine's central mission of healing and is a power

AMA

that most physicians do not want nor could control. "This brief represents a united front of the health care professionals primarily involved with patients facing death," said AMA Board Chair Nancy W. Dickey, MD. The amicus curiae brief, combined with an intensive media blitz to the American public, succeeded in raising enormous doubts about the viability of physician-assisted suicide in the United States. During court arguments on physician-assisted suicide Jan 8, several justices raised strong reservations about getting involved in the issue. At the same time, new support for our position appeared in the press across the nation. "The AMA brief had impact," said Carl Coleman, executive director of the New York State Task Force on Life and the Law. "The justices clearly were affected by the degree of consideration that the medical community had given to the issue." Here's a summary of what we did on behalf of America's physicians:

Amicus curiae brief: AMA legal staff took the lead role in filing the amicus curiae brief. Our opinion against physician-assisted suicide was supported by nearly 50 other major health organizations, including the American Nurses Association and the American Psychiatric Association.

Media blitz: Dr. Dickey represented the AMA as an observer to the oral arguments at the Supreme Court on Jan 8, and was the first person after the oral arguments to offer comments at a press conference on the Supreme Court steps. Her comments were heard and read across the country, and led the coverage by major evening newscasts. Most notable press coverage: The "Lehrer News Hour," "ABC World News Tonight," "CBS Evening News," CNN, NBC's "Today Show," CSPAN, and NPR's "All Things Considered" and "Morning Edition."

Other AMA trustees also commented during the day, including Thomas Reardon, MD, and Yank Coble, MD. The AMA viewpoint was also aired on BBC, Fox, and MSNBC and in all of the nation's major newspapers. Other steps to watch for as we continue our effort:

End-of-life-care coalition: The coalition, which promotes better end-of-life care, is planning a media training session April 17 in New York City, designed to educate reporters about issues in end-of-life care.

Health Law

The Division of Health Law helps physicians compete and prosper in their medical practices by providing the most comprehensive clearinghouse of information on medicolegal developments in the area of health care economics and regulation available to physicians. Key ongoing and planned activities of the Division focus on medical liability, litigation support, and legal issues in medicine.

The Council on Constitution and Bylaws

The functions of the Council on Constitution and Bylaws are to serve as a fact-finding and advisory committee on matters pertaining to the *Constitution and Bylaws*. The Council will recommend such changes in the *Constitution and Bylaws* as it deems appropriate for action by the House of Delegates. (C&B-1997)

Private Sector Law
The Private Sector Advocacy and Support Team (PSAT) is an interdisciplinary and interdepartmental effort created to make the American Medical Association's presence more significant as it assists physicians in the private sector. It will coordinate any managed care policy development throughout the AMA, develop private sector advocacy publications and campaign materials, and provide legal and technical assistance to members on issues ranging from development of networks to contracting and patient quality care advocacy.

Division of Representation
The AMA Division of Representation is designed to aggressively represent physicians by providing advocacy, legal, and negotiations consulting services and skills through county and state medical societies. The Division will provide advocacy materials and support, including on-site visits, as needed, to assist medical societies in various negotiations with health plans, within the limitations of antitrust laws. These representation services may include helping to organize local physicians as a more powerful negotiations force, particularly in issues related to clinical decision making and patient care, to enhance the clout of organized medicine in negotiating clinical issues of regional or national importance, such as the use of practice guidelines, to provide additional support through legislative, litigation, and media strategies, and, in some cases, upon request, to help employed physicians form collective bargaining units.

COSMO
The Center for Society Sponsored Managed Care Organizations (COSMO) was founded in 1996 to provide information, expertise, and leadership to medical societies that are interested in forming, or have formed, organizations to assist physicians such as independent practice organizations (IPAs), preferred provider organizations (PPOs), health maintenance organizations (HMOs), and management services organizations (MSOs). COSMO is targeted at medical societies and physician leaders working to provide options to physicians in a changing marketplace.

Project publications include:

Essential Characteristics of a Quality Health Plan

To contact COSMO: 312 464-5548

Other Health Law initiatives include:

The Health Care Liability Alliance is a federal coalition of physician groups, hospitals, medical product distributors, and individual physicians whose goals include ensuring that liability reform remains a component of health system reform.

The AMA/Specialty Society Medical Liability Project is a leadership effort involving 30 national medical specialty societies that has produced a number of patient safety/risk management products.

The Practice Assessment Quality Improvement program (PA/QI) is a prototype physician office risk management program that compiles information on risk management behaviors to help physicians continually improve nonclinical aspects of care and to facilitate longitudinal assessment of the effectiveness of the PA/QI program in improving care and reducing liability claims.

Traditional Health Law and Litigation Center

The Litigation Center is a medical-legal coalition of the AMA and state medical societies. The center's goal is to represent the interests of the medical profession in the courts by bringing cases of broad impact to the court system, to serve as an information and advocacy clearinghouse for medical societies and related groups by sharing amicus briefs and other legal work it generates, and to build coalitions to maximize the effect of its efforts.

The Medicine in Transition effort is designed to provide practical assistance to members' needs for information and guidance about managed care, independent fee-for-service practice in a world dominated by managed care, and other dimensions of market aggression and health system reform. A major component of this effort is the Doctors Advisory Network. The Network is a national group of over 300 legal and consulting experts who provide hands-on assistance to AMA members as they respond to the managed care environment. The network includes managed care attorneys and consultants, physicians who have prospered in managed care, and experts in antitrust and practice management.

Guidebook on Medical Society Grievance Committees
The purpose of this guidebook is to provide comprehensive direction to county and state medical grievance committees for the enforcement of professional medical ethics. This guidebook demonstrates how the disciplinary bodies of the state and county medical societies can properly and effectively enforce ethical standards of conduct. It also clarifies the legal rules implicated by ethical guidelines and ethics enforcement, so that state and county medical societies can proceed with their ethics enforcement programs without fear of legal liability.

Other division publications include:

Medicolegal Forms With Legal Analysis

Practice Parameters: A Physician's Guide to Their Legal Implications

AMA Constitution

Article I—Title and Definition
The name of this organization is the American Medical Association. It is a federacy of its state associations.

Article II—Objects
The objects of the Association are to promote the science and art of medicine and the betterment of public health.

Article III—State Associations
Constituent or state associations are those recognized medical associations of states, commonwealths, territories or insular possessions which are, or which may hereafter be, federated to form the American Medical Association.

Article IV—Component Societies
Component societies are those county or district medical societies contained within the territory of and chartered by the respective state associations.

Article V—Members
The American Medical Association is composed of individual members of state associations and others as shall be provided in the Bylaws.

Article VI—House of Delegates
The legislative and policy-making body of the Association is the House of Delegates composed of elected representatives and others as provided in the Bylaws. The House of Delegates shall transact all business of the Association not otherwise specifically provided for in this Constitution and Bylaws and shall elect the general officers except as otherwise provided in the Bylaws.

Article VII—General Officers
The general officers of the Association shall be a President, President-Elect, Immediate Past President, Secretary-Treasurer, Speaker of the House of Delegates, Vice Speaker of the House of Delegates, and 15 Trustees, including a young physician member, a resident physician member, and a medical student member. Their qualifications and terms of office shall be provided in the Bylaws.

Article VIII—Trustees
The Board of Trustees is composed of 18 members, 15 Trustees elected by the House of Delegates, including a young physician member and a resident physician member, a medical student trustee elected by the Medical Student Section Assembly, and the President, President-Elect, and Immediate Past President of the Association. It shall have charge of the property and financial affairs of the Association and shall perform such duties as are prescribed by law governing directors of corporations or as may be prescribed in the Bylaws.

Article IX—Scientific Assembly
The Scientific Assembly of the American Medical Association is the convocation of its members for the presentation and discussion of subjects pertaining to the science and art of medicine.

Article X—Conventions
The House of Delegates shall meet annually and at such other times as deemed necessary or as provided in the Bylaws, in cities or places selected by the Board of Trustees. The Scientific Assembly shall meet at such times as the Board of Trustees deems necessary, or as provided in the Bylaws, in cities or places selected by the Board of Trustees.

Article XI—Funds, Dues, and Assessments
Funds may be raised by annual dues or by assessment of the Active Members on recommendation by the Board of Trustees and after approval by the House of Delegates, or in any other manner approved by the Board of Trustees as provided in the Bylaws.

Article XII—Amendments
The House of Delegates may amend this constitution at any convention provided the proposed amendment shall have been introduced at the preceding convention and provided two thirds of the voting members of the House of Delegates registered at the convention at which action is taken vote in favor of such amendment.

Corporate Law

The Division of Corporate Law serves the interests of the AMA by providing quality and timely legal advice, counsel, and assistance to all levels of management and employees and the Board of Trustees, AMPAC, AMA-ERF, and the AMA subsidiaries in issues such as copyright

AMA

violation, employment grievances, contract disputes, and tax matters. The division also represents the AMA internationally as the AMA's delegate to the World Medical Association.

Communications

Being a strong, powerful, unified voice for the profession is the primary goal of the Communications effort.

The association-wide adoption of a communications plan enables the AMA to focus its attention on major public health issues (violence, AIDS, substance abuse, and biomedical research), public advocacy, and professionalism.

Communications Coordination Team

The establishment of a team to bring consistency and clarity to the AMA's message will bring together those with communications responsibilities from various areas together. Special projects include the inventory and assessment of the effect of the flow of AMA communications to members and nonmembers, to reduce the flow of information while improving its impact; the development of a plan to distribute communications responsibilities to various leaders in the AMA, such as the Board of Trustees and the Councils; and to enhance the ability of *AMNews* to deliver special member informational supplements and advocate for physicians.

Public Relations

Strengthening the AMA's communications outreach is the focus of the public relations program. As the public's interest in health and medical information continues to expand, media relations activities, speech writing, and science news dissemination will also increase out of Public Relations.

In 1996, a successful campaign to help raise awareness of the danger of smoking to young children was added to other initiatives to affect public health issues: the Extinguisher!

AMA Press Release

AMA's superhero joins battle against tobacco: nation's doctors will help kids smoke out the tobacco menagerie

Chicago, Nov 18, 1996—"Look out camels, cowboys, and penguins. Your days of enticing kids to take up tobacco are coming to an end," said Randolph D. Smoak, Jr, MD, member of the American Medical Association Board of Trustees. That certainly is the plan of the American Medical Association as it launches today its new cartoon superhero, "The Extinguisher," and his mentor and creator, "Doctor Nola Know," two new champions for America's kids in the fight against tobacco. Their mission is to educate and protect children from the dangers of smoking.

Together, they will help kids wage their own "kid crusades" to "smoke out" and "extinguish" the cigarette industry's advertising and marketing campaigns targeted toward America's youth.

The super duo will be featured in a new AMA nationwide public health campaign aimed at teaching elementary school–age children about the dangers of smoking and nicotine addiction. Over the next year, the AMA's Extinguisher and Dr Know will appear at antismoking events sponsored by kids, schools, and antitobacco organizations. They will even make surprise visits to Discovery Zone outlets. Discovery Zone is joining with the AMA to help keep America's schoolchildren safe from tobacco's unhealthy temptations.

The AMA will also be working with *Scholastic News* to create antismoking educational materials featuring the Extinguisher and Dr Know for use in classrooms across the country. *Scholastic News* is a current events magazine for elementary school students distributed to approximately 4 million children in 150,000 American classrooms. Kicking off the educational partnership between the AMA and *Scholastic News* will be a "Tobacco-Free Pledge Contest," in which kids will write and sign a "tobacco-free pledge," explaining how they plan to help in the fight against smoking and keep their friends, schools, and communities tobacco-free. The contest will commence in the November 15, 1996, issue of *Scholastic News*.

According to the cartoon narrative, the Extinguisher wasn't always a superhero. A short time ago, he was a young man on the brink of death. His diseased lungs had 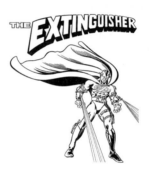 been so weakened by tobacco that desperate measures were needed to save him. A smart, savvy physician, Dr Know, not only brought him back to life, but turned him into a scientific wonder with artificial lungs and "super powers," including increased brain power and special heat-seeking devices able to detect cigarettes from miles away. "I wanted to make sure the Extinguisher was able to kick butts wherever he finds them," Dr Know said, explaining her creation.

A study published in the *Journal of the American Medical Association* in 1991 showed that children as young as 6 years old were as familiar with 'Old Joe Camel' as they were with Mickey Mouse, and that such familiarity is a known risk factor for smoking and tobacco addiction. "We know that every day in the United States 3000 young people begin to smoke—that's more than a million new smokers each year," said Dr Smoak. "Each day our children are replacing the smokers who die prematurely from tobacco-related diseases, the number one preventable cause of death in the United States. This is a terrible travesty that must end," vowed Dr Smoak.

"Smoking is not 'comic' or 'cool.' With its new cartoon characters the Extinguisher and Dr Know as its secret weapons, the AMA will take on anyone (or any animal) that threatens the health of our nation's kids."

In addition, the New York office gives the AMA daily visibility among the major print and broadcast media in the New York City area. Continued emphasis in this area is placed on scheduling AMA Officers and Trustees in key regional cities for media visits during each year. The goal of better communication with Federation public relations staffs will enhance a united front with the various audiences the AMA serves. The Division of Public Information, with its conferences for science writers and health reporters, aids in assuring quality of medical news reporting.

New York Office
600 3rd Ave, New York, NY 10016
212 867-6640   Fax 212 953-2497

American Medical Association Radio News

This activity provides radio stations, not the public or physicians, with a daily 60-second news report and a monthly feature report on a medical or health-related topic. Nearly 1000 radio stations receive the reports via telephone or satellite hook-up, one third of which use the reports three or more times per week. The Radio News Network averages 300–500 phone calls to this service per day.

Physicians who wish to rent an FM receiver should contact the Physicians' Radio Network at 203 324-1700.

Contact for general information: 800 448-9384

International film competition: medical films win 'Freddies' in international contest

AM News Dec 9, 1996 p 15

San Francisco—Forty-five producers of medical films, videos, and Web sites received medical film's highest honors last month at the 20th annual International Health and Medical Film Competition.

The mission of the film competition, presented for the first time this year by the American Medical Association, is to "promote better health through visual communication and to support the quality of health information provided to medical professionals and consumers."

Among the films honored at the event were *AIDS in India: The New Untouchables,* which won the prestigious Michael E. DeBakey, MD, Award for excellence in educational filmmaking and the award for best film in the category of community health. The video was produced by ASAP TV Film of New York City and directed by Christophe de Neuville.

The Burning Season was awarded the Robert E. Wise Cinematography Award and best film in the docudrama category. The film, produced by Home Box Office (HBO), chronicles the nonviolent fight of Chico Mendes to save the Brazilian rain forest.

The C. Everett Koop, MD, Award for best film for health professionals went to *Sub-Tenon's Anesthesia* produced by Connecticut Eye Research Foundation Inc. Author Mark Silverstein, MD, also received an award in the best surgery film category for *Sub-Tenon.*

The Helen Hayes Award for best health consumer film went to *Monitoring the Mysteries of the Fetus,* produced by the National Aeronautics and Space Administration at Ames and Michael Danty Productions of Santa Rosa, Calif. The film, also judged best in the science and technology category, details how space technology results in practical medical uses such as intrauterine fetal monitoring.

Five producers got special awards for best medical and health series programming: Mosby Productions of Chicago for *Clinical Decision and Competency Evaluation for Respiratory Care;* Toby Levine Productions of Bethesda, Md, for *Everybody Wins! Quality Care Without Restraints;* Educational Productions of Portland, Ore, for *Step 1: Beginning Language Connections;* Time/Life Medical of New York City for *At the Time of Diagnosis;* and Kaiser Permanente A-V of Oakland, Calif., for *Partners in Health.*

Bob Saget of "America's Funniest Home Videos" hosted the awards ceremony and presented a special award to the Scleroderma Foundation and its founder Sharon Monsky. Saget's sister, Gay, died of scleroderma in 1994. *For Hope,* a movie produced by Saget and based on his sister's struggle with the disease, aired last month on ABC.

Jamie Farr of TV's "M*A*S*H" joined G. W. Bailey of "The Jeff Foxworthy Show" to honor the historic frontlines medical care provided by the US Army Medical Dept. with a Lifetime Achievement Award. Brigadier General Jerome V. Foust, commander of 12 hospitals and 6500 medical personnel during Operation Desert Storm, was joined by five decorated soldier-medics of World War II, Korea, and Vietnam to accept the honor on behalf of all Army medical personnel.

Jerry Lewis and his Muscular Dystrophy Association also received a Lifetime Achievement Award from pioneer heart surgeon Michael DeBakey, MD.

The categories, winners, and producers of other Freddie-honored films—chosen from more than 600 entries—include:

Adolescent health: *This Is a Video About ... Herpes,* Healthlink Communications Inc.

Advertising: *Endosol Extra: The Bouncing Bottle,* Pacific Communications.

Basic/clinical science: *Advances in Genetics,* Glaxo Wellcome.

Caregiving: *Home Care for Children,* Children's Health System.

Children's health: *Our Heart's in All the Right Places,* Second Coming Productions.

Communications: *Grave Words,* Monsen Productions.

Coping: *Unlocking the Secrets of Schizophrenia,* Information Television Network.

Critical care: *Moments in Time,* Glaxo Wellcome.

Dentistry: *3D Obturation,* Dental Education Laboratories.

Diagnostics: *The Papanicolaou Technique,* NCCLS.

Environmental health: *Plague Fighters,* Associated Producers.

Family dynamics: *The Parent's Guide to Kidspeak,* Medical Broadcasting Co.

Fitness: *Catherine MacRae's Gentle Fitness,* Gentle Fitness Inc.

Geriatrics: *See for Yourself,* The Lighthouse Inc.

Health care administration: *Before the Earth Starts Shaking,* Kaiser Permanente A-VCR.

AMA

Health sensitivity: *Panic Disorder: Stories of Hope*, National Institute of Mental Health.

Human sexuality: *A Thousand Tomorrows*, Terra Nova Films.

Issues and ethics: *Death on Request*, First Run/Icarus Films.

Life and death: *A Heart for Olivia*, CBS News.

Managed care: *Hippocrates—What Did You Sign?* Schering-Plough.

Men's health: *Prostate Cancer at Time of Diagnosis*, Time/Life Medical.

Nutrition: *Success Without Suffering*, Zora S. Gill, MD, Inc.

Patient care: *Uncertain Journey*, Duke University Medical Center.

Patient education: *Total Knee Replacement*, Veritech.

Preventive medicine: *Burnout: Running on Empty*, Detroit Receiving Hospital.

Product presentation: *Wait No Longer*, Hewlett-Packard.

Public relations: *Point of Purchase*, Time/Life Medical.

Public service announcements: *Train*, National Institute of Mental Health.

Safety and first aid: *Baby Safe*, Hobbsco Ltd.

Special people: *Brandon Tells His Story*, The Century Council; *The Journey of Christopher Reeve*, ABC News.

Therapeutics: *Swallowing Center*, Legacy Portland Hospitals.

Tools and techniques: *Integrated Surgical Support Systems*, Greenberg Medical Instrument.

Web site: *Dermatology in the Cinema*, Dermatology Medical Group/ S.F.

Wellness: *Cholesterol: The Killer Within*, Medical Communications Resources.

Women's health: *The Lady Upstairs*, ABC News.

Corporate Relations

To contribute to the growth and effectiveness of the AMA, the Corporate Relations unit develops and manages programs that increase interaction with corporations and foundations, which results in outside financial support for the Association. It also works to cultivate new and enhance existing relationships with the pharmaceutical industry, other corporations, and national foundations.

AMA

Membership

Membership, Constituency, and Federation Relations

Membership and Federation Relations

Professional Relations

Membership, Constituency, and Federation Relations is the intersection at which point virtually all the Association's activities come together to touch physicians and medical societies. The overall mission of the area is to facilitate the participation of the Federation, Special Groups, and Sections on the policymaking process of the AMA; to marshal public support for the AMA as the principal representative of physicians; to maintain liaisons with county, state, and national societies and the group practice community; to respond to member needs; to promote physician and medical student involvement in organized medicine; and to promote and increase AMA membership.

Membership, Constituency, and Federation Relations

The AMA is, at its heart, a membership organization that exists to serve its members by serving the profession of medicine and the needs of individual members within the context of that mission.

The changing environment of medicine brings new challenges to physicians at all stages of their careers. Changing practice patterns due to the growth of group practices and managed care concerns have led to membership decisions by administrators rather than individual physicians. In addition, federal and state governments are focusing on reducing physician reimbursement from Medicare and Medicaid, putting additional strain on physician income.

Every area in the AMA is responsible for serving members and enhancing the value of AMA membership. The administration of AMA membership, including the development and implementation of member retention and recruitment programs and the collection of membership statistics, resides organizationally in the Membership unit, including areas of Membership Marketing, Membership Information Services, Membership and Federation Relations, and Group Practice Marketing.

Ongoing Membership Marketing activities of AMA and American Medical Political Action Committee (AMPAC) involve working with state, county, and specialty societies to improve AMA and AMPAC membership by providing tailored marketing plans and consultation, resources for retention and recruitment activities, and incentive programs. Peer-to-peer recruitment programs aimed at physicians, students, and residents will continue as will efforts to recruit and retain physicians through the direct program.

AMA

Strategic Membership Product Development

This area of Membership strives to establish firm relationships with consumers in order to gather feedback on issues of primary concern to the public; educates consumers on items of medical, scientific, and public health interest; and helps generate positive public opinion on issues of mutual concern to the public and physicians to help these groups understand and support AMA activities and the AMA's position on issues. This area administers the "Partners in Health" (PIH) program. PIH seeks to improve the patient-physician relationship through positioning AMA physicians and their patients as partners with a common goal: better health through information.

Group Practice Liaison and Outreach

Since 1989, the AMA has been active in outreach to the group practice community. Components of this effort include the Advisory Committee on Group Practice, which meets in conjunction with the House of Delegate Meetings and serves as an advisor to the Board of Trustees and to the AMA staff regarding policies and program activities that affect the group practice community; the Washington Advisory committee, which advises the AMA about legislative and regulatory issues of concern to groups; and an outreach group, which targets the group practice community through site visits and discussions within both the community and the AMA.

Membership Information Services

This area collects statistics on membership and tracks physicians' trends as consumers. The Member Service Center is the point where members have direct contact with the AMA for a variety of service and information needs.

Contact the Member Service Center at: 800 AMA-3211.

Professional Relations

The needs of individual physicians, regardless of their practice setting, are a primary focus of the AMA. Individual physicians need to express their viewpoints within the AMA and the Professional Relations Unit has a well-established process to accomplish that objective. This division maintains and supports democratic assemblies to achieve the objective of allowing physicians and medical students to introduce, debate, and adopt policies in support of the mission of the AMA.

One challenge in the repositioning of the AMA is to provide maximum opportunity for the leadership of all sections and advisory groups to feel pride and ownership in the AMA. Ongoing educational efforts have been implemented with all of the sections and advisory groups to promote understanding of the AMA mission and facilitate effective communications to their respective constituencies. The Governing Councils meet regularly to discuss issues pertinent to their constituents, therefore playing an advisory role to the Section Assemblies, which meet twice a year at the Interim and Annual meetings of the AMA.

Medical Student Services

These activities provide a direct voice for medical students in the AMA's policymaking process and serve the identified needs of this group by providing high-quality products and services. Key projects that address these needs include the provision of support for the Medical Student Section (MSS) and state and local section organizational development. Continued activities include a successful government relations internship program designed to expose medical students to legislative and political processes and AMA policy promotion grants for medical student groups working on community service and educational projects and activities that promote AMA policy. The MSS also sponsors a scholarship for international study that provides a third- or fourth-year medical student with a grant to study overseas.

Consortium of Medical Student Organizations

A grant from Upjohn provides funds to enable the AMA-MSS to serve as the administrative center for the Consortium of Medical Student Organizations (CMSO). The purpose of the CMSO is to facilitate the exchange of information and interaction among the 15 national medical student organization members. This role enables the AMA to be more responsive to the various medical student segments. The CMSO holds four meetings annually.

Resident Physician Services

Establishing direct access to the AMA's policymaking process for resident physicians, mainstreaming them into organized medicine, and providing information to this group are the central focus of these activities. Key projects include the Resident Physicians Section (RPS), which provides an orderly representative framework, organization-strengthening activities to foster grassroots support, and publications and communications to highlight AMA policies and the benefits of membership involvement. Special attention will be directed toward educating residents about graduate medical education issues and national health policies to train them as young physician leaders.

Glaxo Wellcome Resident Physicians Program

Made possible through a grant from Glaxo Wellcome, 40 residents receive stipends for travel and lodging to attend the AMA's Annual and Interim Meetings to participate in the policymaking process. The program requires an application, and resident selection is based on a demonstrated commitment (ie, volunteer work to the civic or medical community).

For information on the Glaxo Wellcome program contact: 800 621-8335

Young Physician Services

The primary way in which the identified needs of AMA members who are under age 40 or within the first 5 years of medical practice are serviced through the Young Physician Section (YPS). Initiatives include the establishment of the YPS as a national forum for policy deliberation and direct access to the AMA House of Delegates for young physicians. An example of the workings of the section was the major role it played in winning equal pay for young physicians under Medicare.

Department publications include:

Contracts: What You Need to Know
State Contracts

International Medical Graduates (IMG) Section

The AMA IMG Section, established by the House of Delegates at I-96 and provided for in AMA Bylaws at A-97, develops a new representational platform for IMGs.

Having existed for a number of years as an advisory committee to the AMA Board of Trustees, IMGs active within the AMA sought a section in order to have a policymaking structure that featured direct input to the AMA House of Delegates. In this way IMGs would have formal recognition and representation within the house of medicine.

The IMG issue agenda has traditionally focused on matters of discrimination, historically in the area of licensure but more recently in relation to managed care (eg, arbitrary deselection). Physician workforce planning has also emerged as a huge issue for the IMG population, in particular, how the ratcheting down of residency slots will affect IMGs seeking entry to US residency programs.

Finally, the IMG Section is open to any interested AMA member (IMG or not). There is also a provision for AMA nonmembers, who may join the Section for up to a year after which AMA membership becomes mandatory.

Organized Medical Staff Services

The AMA's Organized Medical Staff Section (OMSS) is dedicated to addressing the needs and concerns of organized hospital medical staffs and their physician members. The semiannual Assembly Meetings are the only national forum convened exclusively for hospital medical staffs. Through the OMSS, each hospital medical staff has an opportunity to participate in AMA's policymaking process. Through the Assembly meetings, educational programs, and publications, the OMSS keeps hospital medical staffs informed of current trends, conditions, and concerns affecting physicians and medical staffs. Major emphasis is placed on strengthening AMA communications to hospital medical staffs, increasing participation in the OMSS, and developing membership marketing strategies through the OMSS.

Departmental publications include:

Bylaws: A Guide for Hospital Medical Staffs

Delineation of Clinical Privileges: A Guide for Hospital Medical Staffs

Advisory Groups

These areas of the AMA support their constituents by representing their needs through an advisory relationship with the Board of Trustees.

Women Physician Services

The initiatives stemming from this area concentrate on issues of particular interest to the rapidly increasing ranks of women physicians, such as promoting and training women for leadership and mentor roles, dealing with family leave issues, sexual harassment, and other forms of gender bias. Activities consist of general outreach activities with women physicians/medical students, including providing information, support, and assistance to the Federation on Women in Medicine issues and programs; liaison activities with the AMA Board of Trustees, Councils, Section, and other special groups; site visits by Women in Medicine staff and Advisory Panel members; participation in related national and Federation meetings; and implementing the annual Women in Medicine Month campaign.

Minority Physician Services

Its advisory committee has three principal missions: to analyze pertinent data, trends, policy, and ongoing activities concerning the health status of medically underserved minorities; to increase membership and representation of minority physicians and medical students in the AMA; and to increase the number of minority physicians, students, and faculty in US medical schools.

International Medical Graduates Services

Focuses on state licensure, residency selection, and general discrimination against IMGs.

Senior Physician Services

Produces a quarterly newsletter not only to help its constituents enjoy their lives, but to offer them special insurance programs, financial, and legal information specific to their needs.

Membership and Federation Relations

This unit in the AMA is responsible for the maintenance of relations with county, state, and specialty societies, as well as with a wide variety of volunteer health agencies. This liaison serves not only to gather input from a wide base of interested groups but also to provide information to them as to the range of interest the AMA supports in the patient-physician relationship.

Federation Advisory Committee to the Executive Vice President

This committee is comprised of CEOs representing state, county, and national medical societies and AAMSE's Executive Committee. Their purpose is to advise the EVP and senior management on issues related to management and relations between the AMA and the Federation. They meet twice a year.

Several state and county medical societies have made a special commitment to the AMA. They require their members to belong to the AMA as well as to their county and state society. This special commitment contributes significantly to the AMA's membership strength.

The following are unified societies:

Unified States

Delaware (1986)

Illinois (1951)

Mississippi (1985)

Oklahoma (1950)

Pennsylvania (1989)

Unified Counties

Muskegon (MI)

Genesee (NY)

Chattanooga/Hamilton (TN)

Hill (TX)

Nueces (TX)

Panola (TX)

Runnels (TX)

Genesse/Niagara/Orleans (NY)

Special Society

American Association of Clinical Urologists

AMA

State and County Relations

This area emphasizes the building and maintaining of a strong relationship between the Federation and the AMA and that interacting with the Federation in order to build consensus and minimize potential conflict. The state and county relations group provides consultative resources for problem resolution, conveys policy and program initiatives, and informs the Federation of necessary action with respect to legislative, federal administrative, and socioeconomic issues.

The National Leadership Conference

This annual meeting for key Federation staff and elected officials is designed to serve as focal point for discussions of major national health policy issues. The Glaxo Achievement Awards program provides 25 medical students and 25 residents the opportunity to attend the AMA National Leadership Conference and interact with other physician leaders by providing each with a stipend to attend. Special receptions and educational sessions for the award winners give them further opportunities to network. An AMA selection committee chooses the winners of the award based on demonstrated nonclinical leadership skills and achievements.

AMA

Leadership

Governance

Board of Trustees

House of Delegates

Office of International Health

Board of Trustees

Within the policy guidelines set by the House of Delegates, the Board of Trustees maintains primary fiduciary and oversight responsibility for the affairs of the Association. Board members maintain active public speaking schedules, and make numerous official appearances to represent the AMA before other organizations, government bodies, the media, and the general public. The Board's public appearance program serves to maintain and enhance relationships within the profession, throughout the Federation, and with external groups and organizations. It advances the aims, purposes, and policies of the AMA as well as affording opportunities to gain a better understanding of the needs of the membership in order to provide appropriate resources and leadership guidance. The AMA provides resources and staff support to enable the Board to fulfill these essential functions, to provide interpretation and guidance, and to anticipate issues that wil! lead the AMA to appropriate scientific and public positions.

Two new trustees were named to the Board of Trustees by the AMA at its June 1997 House of Delegates annual meeting in Chicago. Newly elected trustees are Herman I. Abramowitz, MD, a family practitioner from Dayton, Ohio; and Andrew M. Thomas, MD, a resident physician in internal medicine from Columbus, Ohio.

Four trustees up for reelection for a 4-year term retained their seats. They were Yank D. Coble, MD, an endocrinologist and immunologist from Jacksonville, Fla; Timothy T. Flaherty, MD, a radiologist from Neenah, Wis; William H. Mahood, MD, a gastroenterologist from Meadow Brook, Pa; and John C. Nelson, MD, an obstetrition-gynecologist from Salt Lake City, Utah. Student trustee Pamela Petersen-Crair, from the University of California, San Francisco, was elected to serve a second 1-year term.

The House of Delegates elected Nancy W. Dickey, MD, a family physician from College Station, Tex, as president-elect, and Percy Wootten, MD, internist with a subspecialty in cardiology, from Richmond, Va, as president. The Board also elected the following officers: Thomas R. Reardon, MD, general practitioner from Portland, Ore, chair; Randolph D. Smoak, Jr, MD, surgeon from Orangeburg, SC, vice chair; D. Ted Lewers, MD, a nephrologist from Easton, Md, secretary-treasurer. In addition, Doctors Coble and Flaherty will serve on the Board's executive committee. Richard F. Corlin, MD, a Santa Monica, Calif, gastroenterologist, and John A. Knote, MD, a Lafayette, Ind, diagnostic radiologist, were reelected speaker and vice speaker of the House of Delegates, respectively.

AMA

Office of Officer Services
This program provides resources and staff support to enable the Board of Trustees to fulfill its essential functions. This contact can also provide biographical information on officers.

House of Delegates

Policy is made by the "elected" AMA. The principal policymaking body is the House of Delegates (HOD). The HOD currently has 430 voting delegates, each of whom is elected or appointed by a group; one delegate from each of the six special AMA sections (Medical Student Section, Resident Physician Section, Young Physician Section, Organized Medical Staff Services, Section for Medical Schools, International Medical Graduates); one delegate from each of the five federal services (Army, Navy, Air Force, Veterans Affairs, and Public Health Service); one delegate each from the 82 represented national medical specialty societies; and 338 delegates from states and territories allocated on a proportional basis (1:1000 AMA members). The HOD meets twice a year, with an annual meeting in June and a semiannual meeting in December. The 17-member Board of Trustees is elected by the HOD. The Board is responsible for interpreting and implementing policies established by the HOD. The President is elected and holds office as President-Elect, President, and Immediate Past President for 1 year in each office. Also noteworthy in the "elected" AMA are the seven Councils specified by the AMA Bylaws: the Council on Constitution and Bylaws, the Council on Ethical and Judicial Affairs, the Council on Legislation, the Council on Long-Range Planning and Development, the Council on Medical Education, the Council on Medical Service, and the Council on Scientific Affairs.

Annual Meeting
June 14–18, 1998—Chicago, Ill
June 20–24, 1999—Chicago, Ill

Interim Meetings
December 6–9, 1998—Honolulu, HI
December 5–8, 1999—San Diego, Calif

Office of International Medicine

The American Medical Association has a long tradition of involvement in international activities. In 1978, the Office of International Medicine was established as a focal point for coordinating these activities.

The AMA, through its Office of International Medicine, endeavors to improve the level and quality of health care worldwide by influencing standards utilized by other nations with regard to ethics, medical education, and commitment to the patient-physician relationship. To achieve this objective, the AMA maintains a membership and holds various leadership positions in the World Medical Association (WMA). In addition, the AMA works in cooperation with the World Health Organization, United Nations, Peace Corps, US Departments of State and Health & Human Services, US Agency for International Development, National Council for International Health, medical and public health schools, and other domestic and international private and public sector organizations.

Such cooperation has recently led to a Cooperative Agreement between the AMA and the US Agency for International Development—Moscow to provide support to the Russian Medical Association and the Association of Physicians of Russia in the areas of organizational development, medical education, certification, professional advocacy, and ethics.

Other activities include intervention in cases of human rights violations in cooperation with the WMA, the American Association for Advancement of Science, Amnesty International, and Physicians for Human Rights. The AMA also collaborates with international organizations to help with disaster relief and health assistance.

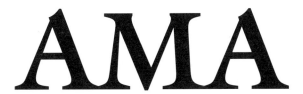

Strategic Planning

Strategic Management and Development

Strategic Planning

Strategic Market Development

Human Resources

Group on Foundation and External Relations

Each year the AMA develops a Strategic Plan that embodies the fundamental vision and objectives that the Association will pursue during its next 3 years. To enhance the process of creating and implementing this strategy a new Group on Strategic Management and Development was formed in late 1996.

Strategic Planning

Council on Long-Range Planning and Development

Strategic Planning is responsible for implementing the strategic and operational planning process at the AMA. The process involves the active participation of AMA staff, senior management, council leaders, and the Board of Trustees in the identification of critical issues for the AMA to address over the coming years. The process focuses on the needs of the medical profession, AMA members, and the public at large. Once issues are identified, strategies, activities, and products to address them are developed and are presented each year in the *AMA Strategic Plan*. Progress toward achievement of the goals stated in the plan is monitored through the AMA's strategic tracking system. The staff also provides support to the AMA and its Federation units by facilitating planning processes and providing planning-related materials.

During 1994–1995, the unit supported the "Study of the Federation," a project to identify ways to enhance working relationships among medical associations.

Strategic Advocacy Management

This area works closely with the Council on Long-Range Planning and Development to manage AMA's environmental tracking and assessment initiatives; to identify issues and strategies relating to AMA membership, organizational structure, and representation; to develop strategies to enhance the process of policy development and implementation; and to participate in the identification, analysis, and development of the long-range policy.

The communication and advocacy support activity focuses on articulating and promoting AMA policy to the various audiences, including government, business, policymakers, physicians, and the public. Emphasis is on the production of advocacy pieces on specific issues for use in addressing the various audiences. Activities and products include Advocacy Briefs, development of AMA "basic messages," and implementation of a patient-physician advocacy communications plan to assist the Federation in promoting AMA health policy.

AMA

Council on Long-Range Planning and Development

The goals of this council are:

- To study and make recommendations concerning the long-range objectives of the Association.
- To study and make recommendations concerning the projected resources, programs, and organizational structure by which the Association attempts to reach its long-range objectives in the above section.
- To serve as a focal point for the planning activities of the Association and to stimulate and evaluate planning activities throughout the organization.
- To study, or cause to be studied, anticipated changes in the environment in which medicine and the Association must function, collect relevant data, and transmit interpretations of these studies and data to the Board of Trustees for distribution to decision-making centers throughout the Association, and submit reports to the House of Delegates at appropriate times. (C&B-1997)

Area publications:

AMA Policy Compendium

This compendium is the only published source of AMA policy adopted by the House of Delegates. Arranged by policy topic and year of adoption, it provides access to more than 2000 sections of AMA policy. As of 1995, the *AMA Constitution and Bylaws* and the Council on Ethical and Judicial Affair's opinions are included in the bound volume. This material is also available, on a limited basis, electronically through a product entitled PolicyFinder.

PolicyFinder

PolicyFinder provides a MS-Windows interface to browse or search through three AMA documents: the *Policies of the AMA House of Delegates,* the *AMA Constitution and Bylaws,* and the *Current Opinions of the Council on Ethical and Judicial Affairs.* The program presents these documents in a medium called hypertext. A hypertext document allows the user to follow a series of links or jumps to quickly find a specific topic without the use of a conventional, static table of contents. PolicyFinder features full-text search capability, allowing the user to search a document for specific words or phrases, or by using multiple words or phrases in complex Boolean expressions.

Future of Medical Practice

This book was written to help physicians ready themselves for the future by presenting an analysis of the broad forces affecting the environment of medical practice. As a planning document, this book also presents a list of potential future trends that are likely to influence how medicine will be practiced in coming years.

Strategic Market Development

Division of Market Research

The Division of Market Research utilizes quantitative and qualitative research analysis methods to provide the AMA with timely and useful strategic and tactical information and intelligence to enhance AMA membership recruiting and retention; guide the AMA strategic planning, budgeting, and operations; promote existing AMA products

and activities; and identify and encourage new strategic product and program opportunities for the AMA.

Division of Payment Programs

This division has primary responsibility for physician payment issues, particularly as they relate to the Resource Based Relative Value Scale (RBRVS). Also key in the division is the ongoing development and maintenance of Current Procedural Terminology (CPT) and related coding issues. The division provides critical support to the Resource Based Relative Value Scale Update Committee (RUC), physician members and other users of CPT through the CPT-Information Service and the *CPT Assistant,* a monthly newsletter, and licenses the use of CPT through its Intellectual Property Services department.

To contact the CPT Information Service: 800 634-6922

Office of Automated Payment Systems

This office in the AMA's primary objective is related to Electronic Data Interchange (EDI) for physician practices. These activities assist in the creation of a minimum data set and of a single electronic form that is easy for physicians to use. The Association plays a role in this initiative by being active in the National Uniform Claim Committee (NUCC), which the AMA chairs and on which it performs as secretary. In addition, the Association is a liaison to the Workgroup on Electronic Data Interchange, the American National Standards Institute's Healthcare Informatics Standards Board (ANSI HISB), and other appropriate bodies.

Office of Medical Informatics

The office works to establish the AMA as an effective advocate for physicians in the development and implementation of the computer-based patient record (CPR). This project includes representation in the Computer-Based Patient Record Institute, interaction with the commercial technology and academic informatics community, and advocacy in CPR standards development groups to ensure that CPR standards reflect the needs of the practicing physician. Other activities include the development of guidelines for the evaluation of office-based clinical practice record software systems and physician education on CPRs and related practice-oriented informatics issues.

Area publications include:

Current Procedural Terminology (CPT)

Medicare Carrier Review: What Every Physician Should Know About "Medically Unnecessary Denials"

Medicare RBRVS: The Physician's Guide

New Medicare Physician Payment System: Resources for Organized Medicine

Human Resources

The objective of this program is to provide systems and services that ensure that the Association attracts, develops, and retains competent, motivated staff for its present and future needs. Major Human Resources functions include employee relations and training, compensation, placement, employee communications, planning, and corporate security. Increased attention will be placed on making the AMA more attractive to current and potential staff and increasing the motivation of staff through targeted recruiting programs, tuition reimbursement, and other compensation strategies. A recent emphasis on diversity, sexual harassment, and fitness issues for employees has kept the program current. Other directions include the implementation of programs and compensation strategies related to performance planning, benefits, cost containment, total compensation, staffing analyses, affirmative action, and community service activities.

Group on Foundation and External Relations

The Group on Foundation and External Relations develops corporate strategy for securing external funds from corporations, foundations, and government agencies. Externally funded programs must add value to the AMA and its members and meet agreed upon standards for quality, consistency, price, and AMA identification with sponsors and/or products. The group maintains a comprehensive, up-to-date, interactive clearinghouse or database of current and potential funders and funded programs. Foundation and External Relations also provides assistance on fund-raising, proposal development, and funders' priorities to other AMA units. Finally, the group manages the American Medical Association Education and Research Foundation (AMA-ERF). Founded in 1951 as an initiative to help medical schools meet expenses, the AMA-ERF makes grants to medical schools to support excellence in medical education and to help medical students. Funding for biomedical research and experimental health care projects has also been granted from this foundation. The ERF distributes over $2 million annually.

To contact the AMA-ERF: 312 464-4543

Display copies

Principles of Medical Ethics

Preamble:

The medical profession has long subscribed to a body of ethical statements developed primarily for the benefit of the patient. As a member of this profession, a physician must recognize responsibility not only to patients, but also to society, to other health professionals, and to self. The following principles adopted by the American Medical Association are not laws, but standards of conduct which define the essentials of honorable behavior for the physician.

I. A physician shall be dedicated to providing competent medical service with compassion and respect.

II. A physician shall deal honestly with patients and colleagues, and strive to expose those physicians deficient in character or competence, or who engage in fraud or deception.

III. A physician shall respect the law and also recognize a responsibility to seek changes in those requirements which are contrary to the best interests of the patients.

IV. A physician shall respect the rights of patients, of colleagues, and of other health professionals, and shall safeguard patient confidences within the constraints of the law.

V. A physician shall continue to study, apply and advance scientific knowledge, make relevant information available to patients, colleagues, and the public, obtain consultation, and use the talents of other health professionals when indicated.

VI. A physician shall, in the provision of appropriate patient care, except in emergencies, be free to choose whom to serve, with whom to associate, and the environment in which to provide medical services.

VII. A physician shall recognize a responsibility to participate in activities contributing to an improved community.

The Hippocratic Oath

I swear by Apollo the Physician, and Aesculapius, and health, and all-heal, and all the Gods and Goddesses, that, according to my ability and judgement, I will keep this oath and stipulation:

To reckon him who taught me this art equally dear to me as my parents, to share my substance with him, and relieve his necessities if required; to regard his offspring as on the same footing with my own brothers, and teach them this art, if they shall wish to learn it, without fee or stipulation; and that by precept, lecture, and every other mode of instruction, I will impart a knowledge of the art to my own sons, and those of my teachers, and to disciples bound by a stipulation and oath according to the law of medicine, but to none others.

I will follow that method of treatment which, according to my ability and judgement, I consider for the benefit of my patients, and abstain from whatever is deleterious and mischievous. I will give no deadly medicine to any one if asked, nor suggest any such counsel; further-more, I will not give to a woman an instrument to produce abortion.

With Purity and with Holiness I will pass my life and practice my art. I will not cut a person who is suffering with a stone, but will leave this to be done by men who are practitioners of this work. Into what-ever houses I enter I will go into them for the benefit of the sick and will abstain from every voluntary act of mischief and corruption; and further from the seduction of females or males, bond or free.

Whatever, in connexion with my professional practice, or not in connexion with it, I may see or hear in the lives of men which ought not to be spoken abroad I will not divulge, as reckoning that all such should be kept secret.

While I continue to keep this oath unviolated, may it be granted to me to enjoy life and the practice of the art, respected by all men at all times but should I trespass and violate this oath, may the reverse be my lot.

Hippocrates (460?–377? BC)

Patient Bill of Rights

The AMA is concerned about patients as well as physicians. The AMA feels a great responsibility to the people it serves. The AMA *Principles of Medical Ethics* for physicians is an example of this commitment. The AMA *Patient Bill of Rights* is another. Both help ensure the rights of the patient. Physicians who belong to the AMA support these six rights:

1. The patient has the right to receive information from physicians and to discuss the benefits, risks, and costs of appropriate treatment alternatives.

2. The patient has the right to make decisions regarding the health care that is recommended by his or her physician.

3. The patient has the right to courtesy, respect, dignity, responsiveness, and timely attention to his or her needs.

4. The patient has the right to confidentiality.

5. The patient has the right to continuity of health care.

6. The patient has a basic right to have available adequate health care.

Sources

ADA   *The Americans With Disabilities Act:*
A Prescription for Compliance
Chicago, American Medical Association, 1992

ADK   *America's Adolescents: How Healthy Are They?*
Janet E. Gans, PhD, et al.
Chicago, American Medical Association, 1990

AGE   *American Medicine Comes of Age 1840-1920*
Lester S. King, MD.
Chicago, American Medical Association, 1984

AHRP   *The Allied Health and Rehabilitation Profes-*
sions Education Directory, 1996-1997
Chicago, American Medical Association, 1997

ALT   *Reader's Guide to Alternative Health Methods*
Arthur W. Hafner, PhD, editor, et al.
Chicago, American Medical Association, 1993

ARTLIV   *Doctors' Rx for Health Series—Arthritis*
Chicago, American Medical Association, 1996

AVMP   *Assessing the Value of the Medical Practice:*
The Physician's Handbook for Measuring and
Maximizing Practice Value
Norcross, Ga, Coker Publishing, LLC, and
Chicago, American Medical Association, 1996

BED   *Leaving the Bedside: The Search for a*
Nonclinical Medical Career, Revised Edition
American Medical Association, Department of
Physician Licensure and Career Resources.
Chicago, American Medical Association, 1996

BIB   *Bibliography of the History of Medicine*
US Public Health Service, US Department of
Health and Human Services.
Bethesda, Md, 1992

BUS   *The Business Side of Medical Practice*
American Medical Association, Department of
Practice Service.
Chicago, American Medical Association, 1989

BUY   *Buying and Selling Medical Practices:*
A Valuation Guide
American Medical Association, Department of
Practice Development Resources.
Chicago, American Medical Association, 1990

C&B   *AMA Constitution and Bylaws*
Chicago, American Medical Association, 1997

CARE   *Caring for the Country*
Chicago, American Medical Association, 1997

CHO   *Choosing Your Physician*
Chicago, American Medical Association
(brochure)

CLO   *Closing Your Practice*
American Medical Association, Department of
Practice Development Resources.
Chicago, American Medical Association, 1988

CON   *A Physician's Guide to Selecting and Working*
With a Managed Care Attorney or Consultant
Sharyn Bills, Denise Andresen, eds.
Chicago, American Medical Association, 1993

CPT   *CPT Assistant*
American Medical Association.
Chicago, American Medical Association (serial)

CS   *Doctors' Rx for Health Series—Controlling*
Stress
Chicago, American Medical Association, 1996

DEA   *Drug Evaluations Annual 1995*
American Medical Association, Division of
Drugs and Toxicology.
Chicago, American Medical Association

DIR   *Directory of Clinical Practice Guidelines*
American Medical Association Department of
Clinical Quality Improvement.
Chicago, American Medical Association
(annual)

DOT   *Dictionary of Occupational Titles*
US Department of Labor, Employment and
Training Administration.
Washington, DC, Superintendent of Documents,
1991

DRS 1   *The Physician and Managed Care*
From *Doctors Resource Service: An Overview*
of Managed Care
Chicago, American Medical Association, 1993

DRS 9   *Techniques for Coping With Stress and Change*
From *Doctors Resource Service: Physicians*
and Change
Chicago, American Medical Association, 1994

DX-D   *Doctors' Rx for Health Series—Diabetes*
Chicago, American Medical Association, 1996

DX-FN   *Doctors' Rx for Health Series—Family*
Nutrition
Chicago, American Medical Association, 1996

DX-HBP   *Doctors Rx for Health Series—High Blood Pressure*
Chicago, American Medical Association, 1996

ENC   *American Medical Association Encyclopedia of Medicine*
Charles B. Clayman, MD, ed.
New York, Random House, and Chicago, American Medical Association, 1989

ENH   *Enhancing the Value of Your Medical Practice*
American Medical Association, Department of Practice Development Resources.
Chicago, American Medical Association, 1990

EST   *Establishing Freestanding Ambulatory Surgery Centers*
American Medical Association, Division of Professional Relations.
Chicago, American Medical Association, 1982

EVL   *Guides to the Evaluation of Permanent Impairment,* 4th edition
Chicago, American Medical Association, 1993

FAM   *The Role of the Family Physician in Occupational Health Care*
American Medical Association, Environmental and Occupational Health Program.
Chicago, American Medical Association, 1984

FIN   *Financing a Medical Practice: Start-Up, Acquisition, or Expansion*
American Medical Association Department of Practice Development Resources.
Chicago, American Medical Association, 1991

FMG   *The AMA Family Medical Guide*
Charles B. Clayman, MD, ed.
New York: Random House and Chicago, American Medical Association, 1994

GME   *Graduate Medical Education Directory, 1997-1998*
Chicago, American Medical Association (annual)

GRE   *Guidebook for Medical Society Grievance Committees and Disciplinary Committees*
American Medical Association, Office of General Counsel.
Chicago, American Medical Association, 1991

HCLA   Health Care Liability Association brochure, 1995
Web address: http://www.wp.com/HCLA/

HDS   *Physicians Resource Guide to Health Delivery Systems*
American Medical Association, Group on Health Services Policy.
Chicago, American Medical Association, 1988

HIV   *HIV Infection and Disease*
Norbert Rapoza, PhD, ed.
American Medical Association, Division of Drugs and Toxicology.

Chicago, American Medical Association, 1989

HJV   *Physician-Hospital Joint Ventures*
American Medical Association, Office of the General Counsel, Division of Medicolegal Affairs.
Chicago, American Medical Association, 1986

ICD   *The International Classification of Diseases*
Health Care Financing Administration, Department of Health and Human Services.
Washington, DC, US Government Printing Office, 1989

LIA   *Professional Liability in the '80s*
American Medical Association, Special Task Force on Professional Liability and Insurance.
Chicago, American Medical Association, 1985

LIC   *US Medical Licensure Statistics and Current Licensure Requirements*
Catherine M. Bidese, ed.
American Medical Association, Department of Credentialing Support Products.
Chicago, American Medical Association (annual)

LIFE   *The Physician's Commitment to Lifelong Learning*
American Medical Association, Division of Continuing Medical Education.
Chicago, American Medical Association, 1993

LOC   *A Guide to Locum Tenens Recruitment*
Chicago, American Medical Association, 1992 (brochure)

MAN   *American Medical Association Manual of Style,* 9th edition
Baltimore, Williams and Wilkins, 1997

MDG   *Medical Groups in the United States: A Survey of Practice Characteristics*
American Medical Association, Department of Professional Activities.
Chicago, American Medical Association, 1996

MMCMP   *Managing Managed Care in the Medical Practice: The Physician's Handbook for Success and Survival*
Norcross, Ga, Coker Publishing, LLC, and Chicago, American Medical Association, 1996

MMP   *Measuring Medical Practice*
American Medical Association, Division of Health Policy and Program Evaluation.
Chicago, American Medical Association, 1987

MPP   *Medicare RBRVS: The Physicians' Guide*
American Medical Association.
Chicago, American Medical Association, (annual)

PCD   *Physician Characteristics and Distribution in the US*
American Medical Association, Division of Survey Data Resources.
Chicago, American Medical Association (annual)

PHIV   *The Physician's Guide to HIV Prevention*
        Chicago, American Medical Association, 1996

PHM   *Physician Marketplace Statistics 1996*
        American Medical Association, Center for
        Health Policy Research.
        Chicago, American Medical Association, 1996

PHSPA   *Managing the Medical Practice: The
        Physician's Handbook for Successful Practice
        Administration*
        Norcross, Ga, Coker Publishing, LLC, and
        Chicago, American Medical Association, 1996

PMMP   *Personnel Management in the Medical Prac-
        tice: The Physician's Handbook for Successful
        Personnel Management*
        Norcross, Ga, Coker Publishing, LLC, and
        Chicago, American Medical Association, 1996

PMR   *Physicians Marketplace Report*
        American Medical Association, Center for
        Health Policy Research.
        Chicago, American Medical Association, 1994

PPP   *Principles of Practice Parameters*
        American Medical Association, Department of
        Practice Parameters.
        Chicago, American Medical Association, 1995

PREP   *Preparing a Curriculum Vitae and Other Job
        Search Tips*
        Young Physicians' Services.
        Chicago, American Medical Association, March
        1997 (brochure)

PRO   *A Physician's Guide to Professional
        Corporations*
        Alton C. Ward, et al.
        American Medical Association, Department of
        Practice Development Resources.
        Chicago, American Medical Association, 1989

SCM   *Socioeconomic Characteristics of Medical
        Practice 1997*
        American Medical Association, Center for
        Health Policy Research.
        Chicago, American Medical Association
        (annual)

SHAPE   *Shape Up for Life: Eating Disorders*
        American Medical Association Alliance.
        Chicago, American Medical Association Alli-
        ance, Inc, 1993 (brochure)

SMP   *Sexual Problems in Medical Practice*
        Harold I. Lief, MD, ed.
        Chicago, American Medical Association, 1981

SPI   *What Every Physician's Spouse Should
        Know...Impairment*
        American Medical Association Auxiliary.
        Chicago, American Medical Association
        Auxiliary, 1986 (brochure)

SPP   *What Every Physician's Spouse Should
        Know...Professional Liability*
        American Medical Association Auxiliary.
        Chicago, American Medical Association
        Auxiliary, 1986 (brochure)

TM   *Transforming Medicare: A Proposal From the
        American Medical Association*
        Chicago, American Medical Association, 1995

TMA   Texas Medical Association Web page
        http://www.texmed.org

USG   *The United States Government Manual*
        Office of the Federal Register, National
        Archives and Records Administration.
        Washington, DC, US Government Printing
        Office, 1995

VlO   *Violence: A Compendium*
        George D. Lundberg, MD, et al.
        Chicago, American Medical Association, 1992

WHG   *American Medical Association Complete Guide
        to Women's Health*
        Ramona I. Slupik, MD, ed.
        New York, Random House, and Chicago,
        American Medical Association, 1996

WIM   *Women in Medicine in America: In the
        Mainstream*
        Chicago, American Medical Association, 1991

WOR   *The Physician and Workers' Compensation*
        American Medical Association, Environmental
        and Occupational Health Program.
        Chicago, American Medical Association, 1983

WRT   *Good Scientific Writing*
        Charles G. Roland, MD.
        Chicago, American Medical Association, 1983

Index

A

Abbreviated injury scale, 1

Abbreviations, specialties, 1-2

Abdomen

    magnetic resonance imaging (AMA Council on Scientific Affairs report), 440

    ultrasonic imaging 361, 435

Abdominal surgery, 2

ABMS Compendium of Certified Medical Specialists, 330

Abnormalities

    birth defects, 36

    chorionic villus sampling (DATTA opinion), 452, 454

    cleft palate, 53//genetic counseling and birth defect prevention (AMA Council on Scientific Affairs report), 443

    kidneys, 158

    rare disorders, 288-289

Abortion, 3-4

    clinics, 4

    fetal tissue transplantation (report of AMA Council on Ethical and Judicial Affairs), 431

    film "Silent Scream" (CSA report, unpublished), 447

    mortality and morbidity trends (AMA Council on Scientific Affairs report), 434

    parental consent (report of AMA Council on Ethical and Judicial Affairs), 430

Absorptiometry, dual-energy X-ray, bone density measurement (DATTA opinion), 451

Abstracts, structured, 408-410

Academic health centers, 4, 362

Academy of Psychosomatic Medicine, 278

Academy of Rehabilitative Audiology, 27

Accent reduction, 4

Accident prevention and accidents

    abbreviated injury scale, 1

    airbags (CSA report, unpublished), 448

    alcohol and drivers (AMA Council on Scientific Affairs report), 442

    automobile-related injuries (AMA Council on Scientific Affairs report), 443

    baby sitting, 29

    drunk driving, 17, 87, 311-312

    helmets (motorcycle- and bicycle-related injuries), 311, 433, 448

    injuries, 148

    injury prevention, 311

    mountain bike injuries, 311

    muscle injuries, 217, 218

    patient safety, 312-313

    police chases (CSA report, unpublished), 445

    product safety, 269, 313

    safety, 311-313

    seat belts (CSA report, unpublished), 448

    smoke detectors and sprinklers (AMA Council on Scientific Affairs report), 442

    spinal cord injury, 335

    statistics, 340

    workers' compensation, 380-384

Accounting, 4-5

Accreditation, 5-6, see also Certification; Credentialing

    alternative nonclinical careers, 48

    ambulatory care, 18-19

    American Medical Accreditation Program, 431-432

    continuing medical education, intrastate, 65

    listing of fields, professions, 127

Accreditation Association for Ambulatory Health Care, 19

Accreditation Committee for Perfusion Education, 248, 249

Accreditation Council for Continuing Medical Education, 5, 65, 457

Accreditation Council for Graduate Medical Education, 5, 117, 356, 455

Accreditation Council for Occupational Therapy Education, 5, 127

Accreditation Manual for Hospitals, 140

Accreditation Review Committee for the Anesthesiologist's Assistant CAAHEP, 20

Accreditation Review Committee on Education for the Physician Assistant, 253

Accreditation Review Committee on Educational and Surgical Technology for the EMT-Paramedic, 93

Accrediting Commission on Education for Health Services Administration, 127

Acid rain (CSA report, unpublished), 446, 447

Acidosis, renal tubular, 158

Acne, 6

Acoustic neuroma, bibliography, 35

Acoustic Neuroma Association, 6

Acquired immunodeficiency syndrome, 13-16

    adolescent HIV education (CSA report, unpublished), 445

    aerosolized pentamidine for opportunistic infections (DATTA opinion), 452

    AMA office, 448

    autopsy confidentiality and HIV status (report of AMA Council on Ethical and Judicial Affairs), 430

    blood transfusion and (CSA report, unpublished), 446

    clinical trials (CSA report, unpublished), 446

    commentary (AMA Council on Scientific Affairs report), 443

    discrimination against patients (CSA report, unpublished), 446

    education, 13-15

    education (CSA report, unpublished), 446

    education and training centers (regional listings), 14-15

    ELISA and Western Blot tests (CSA report, unpublished), 446

    epidemiology (CSA report, unpublished), 446

    family and household risks (CSA report, unpublished), 446

    health care and work-related risks (CSA report, unpublished), 446

    HIV, AMA policies, 131-136

    HIV distinguished from, 135

    HIV infection and disease monographs (CSA report, unpublished), 446

    HIV infection biology (CSA report, unpublished), 446

    HIV prevention in primary care, 135-136

    HIV risk behavior interventions (bibliography), 31

    HIV testing recommendations (CSA report, unpublished), 446

    HIV testing, 133-134

Drunk driving, see Automobiles

Drusen, see Macular drusen

Dubost, Charles, 356

Duke University
   Medical Center, Divers Alert Network, 82
   Medical Center, Library, 162
   School of Medicine, 202

Dukes v. U.S. Healthcare, 100

Dyslexia, 87, 439

Dystrophic Epidermolysis Bullosa Research Association
      (DEBRA) of America, 74

E

Ear, see also Deafness
   AIDS hotline (hearing impaired), 15
   audiology, 26-27
   cochlear implants, 31, 443
   hearing disorder identification in children, bibliography, 34
   impairment, 128
   tinnitus, 351

Early and periodic screening, diagnosis, and treatment (managed
      care glossary), 182

East Carolina University
   Health Sciences Library, 163
   School of Medicine, 202

East Tennessee State University
   Department of Learning Resources Medical Library, 163
   James H. Quillen College of Medicine, 203

Easter Seal Society, see National Easter Seal Society

Eastern Illinois University, grammar hotline, 117

Eastern Virginia Medical School
   Medical College of Hampton Roads, 203
   Moorman Memorial Library, 163

Eating disorders, 89

Echocardiograph technicians, 89

Echocardiography, 47, 89

Ecology, 89
   clinical (AMA Council on Scientific Affairs report), 434

Economic competition, see Commerce; Cost control; Economics,
      medical

Economics, medical, see also Finances
   aging and health care spending, 10
   financing HIV care, 131
   locations for practice, 175
   physician earnings, income, 254-256
   physician fees, 256-257
   valuation of a medical practice, 363-366

ECRI, 75, 98

Ectodermal dysplasia, 74

Editorial peer review, see Journals, medical

Education, see also names of specific occupations and medical
      specialties
   AIDS, 13-15
   chiropractic schools, 53
   curriculum vitae, 67
   deaf students, 128
   dental schools, 72
   health professions, 5-6
   HIV, 132, 133

Education, medical
   adolescent health, 7
   AMA activities, 455-457

AMA foundation and, 392, 394

animal use (AMA Council on Scientific Affairs report), 434

animal use, 21

Fifth Pathway, 104

foreign medical graduates, 153-154

HIV, 132

loans, 174

medical school accreditation, 5

noncompetition covenants (report of AMA Council on Ethical
      and Judicial Affairs), 429

nutrition programs, 227

programs in US medical schools, 204

review courses, 308

Education, medical, continuing, 64-65
   accreditation, 5
   AMA activities, 456-457
   gifts to physicians, 113-116
   Physician's Recognition Award, 456-457
   video clinics, 366

Education, medical, graduate, 117, see also Residents
   accreditation, 5
   AMA activities, 455-456
   matching programs, 188
   National Residency Matching Program, 268-269
   noncompetition covenants (report of AMA Council on Ethical
      and Judicial Affairs), 429
   teaching hospitals, 345
   transitional year, 356

Educational Commission for Foreign Medical Graduates, 107,
      154, 155

Einstein, Albert, College of Medicine, see Yeshiva University

EKG, see Electrocardiography

Elder abuse, see Aging

Electric fields (CSA reports, unpublished), 444, 446

Electrocardiograph technicians, 90

Electrocardiography, 89-90
   mandatory, before elective surgery (DATTA opinion), 454

Electrocoagulation, endoscopic, of gastrointestinal tract
      hemorrhage (DATTA opinion), 454

Electrodiagnostic medicine, 90

Electroencephalography
   quantitative (Fast Fourier Transform Analysis) (DATTA
      opinion), 455
   24-hour ambulatory monitoring (DATTA opinion), 454

Electroencephalographic technicians, 90

Electromagnetic fields, bibliography, 35

Electromagnetic radiation (CSA report, unpublished), 447

Electromyographic technicians, 90

Electroneurodiagnostic technologists, 90-91

Electronic data interchange, see Computers

Electrostimulation, cranial (DATTA opinion), 454

Embolism, pulmonary, 176

Emergency medical technicians, 92-93

Emergency medicine, 93

Emergency services
   access to, 93
   ambulances, 18
   *The Guidelines for Cardiopulmonary Resuscitation and
      Emergency Cardiac Care,* 46
   Heimlich maneuver poster, 130
   identification cards, 143

Emetine, 218

Emigration and immigration, international medical graduates,
      153- 155

H

I